Asthma: A Multidisciplinary Approach

Editorial Advisor

JOEL J. HEIDELBAUGH

ELSEVIER

1600 John F. Kennedy Boulevard • Suite 1800 • Philadelphia, Pennsylvania, 19103-2899

http://www.theclinics.com

CLINICS COLLECTIONS
ISSN 2352-7986, ISBN-13: 978-0-323-35959-7

Editor: John Vassallo (j.vassallo@elsevier.com)
Developmental Editor: Patrick Manley

Clinics Collections (ISSN 2352-7986) is published by Elsevier Inc., 360 Park Avenue South, New York, NY 10010-1710. Business and editorial offices: 1600 John F. Kennedy Boulevard, Suite 1800, Philadelphia, PA 19103-2899. **POSTMASTER:** Send address changes to *Clinics Collections*, Elsevier Health Sciences Division, Subscription Customer Service, 3251 Riverport Lane, Maryland Heights, MO 63043. **Customer Service: Telephone: 1-800-654-2452** (U.S. and Canada); **1-314-447-8871** (outside U.S. and Canada). **Fax: 314-447-8029.** E-mail: **journalscustomerserviceusa@elsevier.com** (for print support); **journalsonlinesupport-usa@ elsevier.com** (for online support).

Reprints. For copies of 100 or more of articles in this publication, please contact the Commercial Reprints Department, Elsevier Inc., 360 Park Avenue South, New York, NY 10010-1710. Tel.: 212-633-3874; Fax: 212-633-3820; E-mail: reprints@elsevier.com.

Contributors

EDITORIAL ADVISOR

JOEL J. HEIDELBAUGH, MD, FAAFP, FACG
Clinical Associate Professor, Departments of Family Medicine and Urology; Clerkship Director, Department of Family Medicine, University of Michigan Medical School, Ann Arbor, Michigan; Ypsilanti Health Center, Ypsilanti, Michigan

AUTHORS

JACQUES AMEILLE, MD
Professor of Occupational Medicine, AP-HP, Unité de pathologie professionnelle, Hôpital, Raymond Poincaré, Université de Versailles, Garches, France

PETER J. BARNES, MD, PhD
Professor and Head of Respiratory Medicine, Imperial College London, Airway Disease Section, National Heart and Lung Institute, London, United Kingdom

ELLEN A. BECKER, PhD, RRT-NPS, RPFT, AE-C, FAARC
Associate Professor, Department of Respiratory Care, Rush University College of Health, Professions, Chicago, Illinois

MELISSA H. BELLIN, PhD, LCSW
Associate Professor, School of Social Work, The University of Maryland at Baltimore, Baltimore, Maryland

PIERA BOSCHETTO, MD, PhD
Associate Professor of Occupational, Medicine, Department of Clinical and Experimental Medicine, University of Ferrara, Ferrara, Italy

ARLENE M. BUTZ, ScD, MSN
Professor, Department of Pediatrics, The Johns Hopkins University School of Medicine; School of Nursing, Baltimore, Maryland

GAETANO CARAMORI, MD, PhD
Section of Respiratory Diseases, Department of Medical Sciences, Centro per lo Studio delle, Malattie Infiammatorie Croniche delle Vie, Aeree e Patologie Fumo Correlate, dell'Apparato Respiratorio (CEMICEF), University of Ferrara, Ferrara, Italy

CATHERINE D. CATRAMBONE, PhD, RN, FAAN
Associate Professor, Adult Health and Gerontological Nursing, Rush University College of Nursing, Chicago, Illinois

MARCO CONTOLI, MD, PhD
Section of Respiratory Diseases, Department of Medical Sciences, Centro per lo Studio delle Malattie Infiammatorie Croniche delle Vie Aeree e Patologie Fumo Correlate dell'Apparato Respiratorio (CEMICEF), University of Ferrara, Ferrara, Italy

JACQUES DE BLIC, MD
Professor of Pediatry, Service de pneumologie et allergologie pé diatriques,
Centre de ré férence des maladies respiratoires rares, Hôpital Necker Enfants Malades,
Assistance Publique des Hôpitaux de Paris, Université Paris Descartes, Paris, France

ANTOINE DESCHILDRE, MD
INSERM U 1019 Lung Infection and Innate Immunity, Institut Pasteur, Université de Lille 2,
Lille Cedex; Unité de pneumopé diatrie, Centre de compétence des maladies
respiratoires rares, Université Lille 2 et CHRU, Hôpital Jeanne de Flandre, Lille, France

RITA DOUMIT, PhD, RN
Instructor, University of Lebanon Byblos Campus, Byblos, Lebanon

ANNA L. EDWARDS, NP-C, MSN
Glendora, CA

SERPIL C. ERZURUM, MD
Professor and Chair, Department of Pathobiology, Lerner Research Institute, Respiratory
Institute, Cleveland, Ohio

GIACOMO FORINI, MD
Section of Respiratory Diseases, Department of Medical Sciences, Centro per lo
Studio delle Malattie Infiammatorie Croniche delle Vie Aeree e Patologie Fumo Correlate
dell'Apparato Respiratorio (CEMICEF), University of Ferrara, Ferrara, Italy

JOHN A. FORNADLEY, MD, FACS, FAAOA
Clinical Associate Professor of Surgery, Penn State University, Hershey, Pennsylvania

KEVIN D. FRICK, PhD
Professor, Department of Health Policy and Management, The Johns Hopkins University
Bloomberg School of Public Health, Baltimore, Maryland

BENJAMIN M. GASTON, MD
Professor, Department of Pediatric Pulmonary Medicine, University of Virginia School of
Medicine, Charlottesville, Virginia

MAUREEN GEORGE, PhD, RN, AE-C, FAAN
Assistant Professor, Department of Family and Community Health, University of
Pennsylvania School of Nursing; Senior Fellow, Center for Health Behavior Research,
University of Pennsylvania, Philadelphia, Pennsylvania

RACHEL GEORGOPOULOS, MD
Resident, Department of Otolaryngology, Temple University Health System, Philadelphia,
Pennsylvania

PHILIPPE GOSSET, PhD
INSERM U 1019 Lung Infection and Innate Immunity, Université de Lille 2, Institut Pasteur,
Lille Cedex, France, Paris Descartes, Paris, France

PATRICK R. HARRISON, BS, MA
Department of Psychology, Loyola University Chicago, Chicago, Illinois

CATHERINE "CASEY" S. JONES, PhD, RN, ANP-C, AE-C
Texas Pulmonary and Critical Care Consultants, PA, Texas Woman's University, Bedford,
Texas

SEBASTIAN L. JOHNSTON, MD, PhD
MRC and Asthma UK Centre in Allergic Mechanisms of Asthma, Centre for Respiratory, Infection, Imperial College London, National Heart and Lung Institute, London, United Kingdom

SARAH KLINE-KRAMMES, MD
Attending Physician, Department of Emergency Medicine, Akron Children's Hospital, Akron, Ohio

HELENE J. KROUSE, PhD, APN-BC, CORLN, FAAN
Professor of Nursing, College of Nursing, Wayne State University, Detroit, Michigan

JOHN H. KROUSE, MD, PhD
Professor and Chairman, Department of Otolaryngology - Head and Neck Surgery, Associate Dean, Graduate Medical Education, Temple University School of Medicine, Philadelphia, Pennsylvania

JOANNE KOUBA
Assistant Professor, Niehoff School of Nursing, Loyola University Chicago, Chicago, Illinois

JOAN KUB, PhD, MSN
Associate Professor, Department of Community Health, School of Nursing, Baltimore, Maryland

MANON LABRECQUE, MD, MSc
Associate Professor, Chest Department, Sacré-Coeur Hospital, Université de Montréal, Montreal, Quebec, Canada

CATHERINE LEMIERE, MD, MSc
Professor of Medicine, Chest Department, Sacré-Coeur Hospital, Université de Montréal, Montreal, Quebec, Canada

PATRICK M. LING, MD, MPH
Program Director, Division of Emergency Medicine, Royal University Hospital, University of Saskatchewan, Saskatoon, Saskatchewan, Canada

RENAUD LOUIS, MD, PhD
Professor of Respiratory Medicine, Liege University, Head of Respiratory Medicine Department, CHU Liege, Belgium

AMY MANION, PhD, RN, PNP
Pediatric Nurse Practitioner, Northwestern Children's Practice; Assistant Professor, College of Nursing, Rush University, Chicago, Illinois

BRUNILDA MARKU, MD, PhD
Section of Respiratory Diseases, Department of Medical Sciences, Centro per lo Studio delle Malattie Infiammatorie Croniche delle Vie Aeree e Patologie Fumo Correlate dell'Apparato Respiratorio (CEMICEF), University of Ferrara, Ferrara, Italy

MOLLY A. MARTIN, MD, MAPP
Assistant Professor, Department of Preventive Medicine, Rush University Medical Center, Chicago, Illinois

JONATHAN MASLAN, MD
Department of Otolaryngology, Wake Forest School of Medicine, Winston-Salem, North Carolina

ANNYCE MAYER, MD, MSPH
Division of Environmental and Occupational Health Sciences, Department of Medicine, National Jewish Health, Denver; Environmental/Occupational Health, University of Colorado Denver - Colorado School of Public Health, Aurora, Colorado

LISA K. MILITELLO, MSN, MPH, CPNP
College of Nursing, Arizona State University, Phoenix, Arizona

JAMES W. MIMS, MD
Department of Otolaryngology, Wake Forest School of Medicine, Winston-Salem, North Carolina

ARIANA MURATA, MD
Emergency Resident, Division of Emergency Medicine, Royal University Hospital, University of Saskatchewan, Saskatoon, Saskatchewan, Canada

KARIN PACHECO, MD, MSPH
Division of Environmental and Occupational Health Sciences, Department of Medicine, National Jewish Health, Denver; Environmental/Occupational Health, University of Colorado Denver - Colorado School of Public Health, Aurora, Colorado

NIKOS PAPADOPOULOS, MD, PhD
Allergy Department, 2nd Paediatric Clinic, University of Athens, Athens, Greece

ALBERTO PAPI, MD
Section of Respiratory Diseases, Department of Medical Sciences, Centro per lo Studio delle Malattie Infiammatorie Croniche delle Vie Aeree e Patologie Fumo Correlate dell'Apparato Respiratorio (CEMICEF), University of Ferrara, Ferrara, Italy

NIRALI H. PATEL, MD
Attending Physician, Department of Emergency Medicine, Akron Children's Hospital, Akron, Ohio

ALESSIA PAULETTI, MD
Section of Respiratory Diseases, Department of Medical Sciences, Centro per lo Studio delle Malattie Infiammatorie Croniche delle Vie Aeree e Patologie Fumo Correlate dell'Apparato Respiratorio (CEMICEF), University of Ferrara, Ferrara, Italy

DIRKJE S. POSTMA, MD, PhD
Department of Pulmonology, GRIAC Research Institute, University Medical Center Groningen, University of Groningen, Groningen, The Netherlands

JACQUES-ANDRÉ PRALONG, MD, MSc
Research Fellow, Research Center, Sacré- Coeur Hospital, Université de Montréal, Montreal, Quebec, Canada

HELEN K. REDDEL, MB, BS, PhD, FRACP
Research Leader, Clinical Management Group, Woolcock Institute of Medical Research, Clinical Associate Professor, University of Sydney, New South Wales, Australia

SHAWN ROBINSON, MD
Pediatric Emergency Medicine Fellow, Department of Emergency Medicine, Akron Children's Hospital, Akron, Ohio

MICHAEL P. ROSENTHAL, MD
Professor of Family and Community Medicine, Thomas Jefferson University, Chair, Department of Family and Community Medicine, Christiana Care Health System, Wilmington, Delaware

FLORENCE SCHLEICH, MD
Head of Clinic, Department of Respiratory Medicine, CHU Liege, Belgium

MINKA L. SCHOFIELD, MD
Assistant Professor, Division of Sinus and Allergy, Department of Otolaryngology - Head and Neck Surgery, The Eye and Ear Institute, Wexner Medical Center, The Ohio State University, Columbus, Ohio

ANTHONY M. SZEMA, MD
Assistant Professor of Medicine and Surgery, Chief, Allergy Section, Veterans Affairs Medical Center, Northport, New York; Department of Medicine, Stony Brook University School of Medicine, Stony Brook, New York

NICK H.T. TEN HACKEN, MD, PhD
Department of Pulmonology, Groningen Research Institute of Asthma and COPD, University Medical Center Groningen, University of Groningen, Groningen, The Netherlands

ISABELLE TILLIE-LEBLOND, MD, PhD
Professor of Pulmonology, Pulmonary Department, University Hospital, Centre de Compétence des Maladies Respiratoires Rares Medical University of Lille, Hôpital Calmette, Lille Cedex, France; INSERM U 1019 Lung Infection and Innate Immunity, Université de Lille 2, Institut Pasteur, Lille Cedex, France

MAXIM TOPAZ, RN, MA
Fulbright Fellow, University of Haifa, Israel; PhD Student, University of Pennsylvania School of Nursing, Philadelphia, Pennsylvania

ELINA TOSKALA, MD, PhD
Department of Otolaryngology, Temple University Health System, Philadelphia, Pennsylvania

THO TRUONG, MD
Assistant Professor of Medicine, Allergy and Clinical Immunology, National Jewish Health, Denver, Colorado

MAARTEN VAN DEN BERGE, MD, PhD
Department of Pulmonology, Groningen Research Institute of Asthma and COPD, University Medical Center Groningen, University of Groningen, Groningen, The Netherlands

LINDA SUE VAN ROEYEN, MS, CSN, CCRP, FNP-BC
Ann and Robert H. Lurie Children's Hospital of Chicago; Pulmonary Habilitation Program, Adjunct Faculty, DePaul University, Chicago, Illinois

BARBARA VELSOR-FRIEDRICH, PhD, RN
Professor and Faculty Scholar, Niehoff School of Nursing, Loyola University Chicago, Chicago, Illinois

Contents

Pathogenesis, Diagnosis, and Assessment of Asthma

> Asthma is an obstructive pulmonary disorder with exacerbations character-ized by symptoms of shortness of breath, cough, chest tightness, and/or wheezing. Symptoms are caused by chronic airway inflammation. There are multiple cell types and inflammatory mediators involved in its patho-physiology. The airway inflammation is frequently mediated by Th2 lympho-cytes, whose cytokine secretion leads to mast cell stimulation, eosinophilia, leukocytosis, and enhanced B-cell IgE production. Although various genes have been identified as likely contributors to asthma development, asthma is largely environmentally triggered and has a multifactorial cause. Asthma is extremely common, especially in poor, urban environments. Asthma is the third most common reason for pediatric hospitalizations.

> There are increasing data to support the "hygiene" and "microbiota" hy-potheses of a protective role of infections in modulating the risk of sub-sequent development of asthma. There is less evidence that respiratory infections can actually cause the development of asthma. There is some evidence that rhinovirus respiratory infections are associated with the development of asthma, particularly in childhood, whereas these infec-tions in later life seem to have a weaker association with the development of asthma. The role of bacterial infections in chronic asthma remains un-clear. This article reviews the available evidence indicating that asthma may be considered as a chronic infectious disease.

> Diagnosis and treatment of asthma are currently based on assessment of patient symptoms and physiologic tests of airway reactivity. Research over the past decade has identified an array of biochemical and cellular biomarkers, which reflect the heterogeneous and multiple mechanistic pathways that may lead to asthma. These mechanistic biomarkers offer hope for optimal design of therapies targeting the specific pathways that lead to inflammation. This article provides an overview of blood, urine, and airway biomarkers; summarizes the pathologic pathways that they signify; and begins to describe the utility of biomarkers in the future care of patients with asthma.

Treatment and Management of Adult Asthma

Catherine "Casey" S. Jones, Ellen A. Becker, Catherine D. Catrambone and
Molly A. Martin

The management of asthma has dramatically improved in recent years
because of a better understanding of the disease and an organized
approach to therapy. All of the various components and tools for evaluating individuals with asthma may be found in the Expert Panel Report
Guidelines by the National Heart, Lung, and Blood Institute, initially
published in 2007. These comprehensive guidelines help health care professionals care for individuals with asthma throughout their lifespan. This
article will assist the health care provider to use these evidence-based
guidelines.

Maureen George and Maxim Topaz

This article is a systematic review of complementary and alternative
medicine use for pediatric and adult asthma self-management. The aim
of the review was to summarize the existing body of research regarding
the types and patterns of, adverse events and risky behaviors associated
with, and patient-provider communication about complementary therapies in asthma. This evidence serves as the basis for a series of recommendations in support of patient-centered care, which addresses both
patient preferences for integrated treatment and patient safety.

Renaud Louis, Florence Schleich and Peter J. Barnes

Inhaled corticosteroids (ICS) have led to improved asthma control and
reduced asthma mortality in the Western world. ICS are effective in
combating T-helper type 2–driven inflammation featuring mast cell and
eosinophilic airway infiltration. Their effect on innate immunity-driven
neutrophilic inflammation is poor and their ability to prevent airway remodeling and accelerated lung decline is controversial. Although ICS remain
pivotal drugs in asthma management, research is needed to find drugs
complementary to the combination ICS/long-acting β2-agonist in refractory asthma and perhaps a new class of drugs as a first-line treatment in
mild to moderate noneosinophilic asthma.

Management of Pediatric Asthma

Michael P. Rosenthal

Childhood asthma is at historically high levels, with significant morbidity
and mortality. Despite more than two decades of improved understanding
of childhood asthma care and the evolution of beneficial medications,
widespread control remains poor, leading to suboptimal patient outcomes
and quality of life. This lack of control results in excessive emergency
department use, hospitalizations, and inappropriate and/or unnecessary

providing preventive care (family and patient attitudes and beliefs, lack of access to quality medical care, psychosocial factors, environmental factors) based on prior evidence and the authors' observation of these challenges in research with inner-city children with asthma over the past decade. Cost issues related to preventive care are addressed, and recommendations provide for pediatric nurses.

Widely researched as separate entities, our understanding of the comorbid effects of childhood obesity and asthma on quality of life is limited. This article discusses the effects of childhood obesity and asthma on self-reported quality of life in low-income African American teens with asthma. When controlling for the influence of symptom frequency, asthma classification, asthma self-efficacy, and asthma self-care levels, body mass index remains a most important factor in determining self-reported quality of life among teens with asthma. Although overweight and obesity did not change the effectiveness of the asthma intervention program, obesity did affect participants quality of life scores.

Specific Issues and Considerations in Asthma

This article discusses current best practices in asthma care and self-management. This information will support practitioners in planning intervention strategies that maximize staff resources and time, and are patient-centered.

A task force of the American Thoracic Society has defined work-exacerbated asthma (WEA) as the worsening of asthma caused by conditions at work. Occupational asthma (OA) is asthma that is initiated by occupational exposures in people without prior asthma. In contrast, WEA is asthma (*already present or coincident [new onset]*) that is worsened because of conditions at work. This difference is critical because asthma is a common disease (present in approximately 7% of working adults). Among working adults with asthma, approximately 20% may have WEA. WEA has potential implications regarding asthma morbidity, health care use, and the economy.

Control-based asthma management has been incorporated in asthma guidelines for many years. This article reviews the evidence for its utility in adults, describes its strengths and limitations in real life, and proposes areas for further research, particularly about incorporation of future risk and identification of patients for whom phenotype-guided treatment would be effective and efficient. The strengths of control-based management include its simplicity and feasibility for primary care, and its limitations include the nonspecific nature of asthma symptoms, the complex role of β2-agonist use, barriers to stepping down treatment, and the underlying assumptions about asthma pathophysiology and treatment responses.

This article summarizes the main new categories of occupational agents responsible for causing occupational asthma, with and without a latency period reported in the last 10 years. It also reports examples of occupational agents for which the fabrication processing or use have influenced the outcome of occupational asthma.

Asthma is one of the most common chronic illnesses in the world, affecting an estimated 300 million people. Globally, the prevalence of asthma has continued to spread as economic improvements in developing countries create a population trend toward urbanization and adoption of a western lifestyle. Research supports an association between obesity and asthma. Only by making weight management a priority in the treatment of asthma can the rising prevalence of both diseases be hindered and global health improved.

Consideration of the unified airway model when managing patients with rhinitis and or asthma allows a more comprehensive care plan and therefore improved patient outcomes. Asthma is linked to rhinitis both epidemiologically and biologically, and this association is even stronger in individuals with atopy. Rhinitis is not only associated with but is a risk factor for the development of asthma. Management of rhinitis improves asthma control. Early and aggressive treatment of allergic rhinitis may prevent the development of asthma. In patients with allergic rhinitis that is not sufficiently controlled by allergy medication, allergen-directed immunotherapy should be considered.

This article describes the different clinical variants of irritant-induced asthma, specifically focusing on high-dose irritant-induced asthma and irritant-induced work-exacerbated asthma, as well as reviews known causes, addresses the often adverse medical and socioeconomic outcomes of this complex condition, and considers issues of causation from an occupational and environmental medicine perspective.

Dirkje S. Postma, Helen K. Reddel, Nick H.T. ten Hacken and
Maarten van den Berge

Asthma and COPD are both heterogeneous lung diseases including many
different phenotypes. The classical asthma and COPD phenotypes are
easy to discern because they reflect extremes of a phenotypical spectrum.
Thus asthma in childhood and COPD in smokers have their own phenotypic expression with underlying pathophysiological mechanisms that
differ importantly. In older adults, asthma and COPD are more difficult to
differentiate and there exists a bronchodilator response in most but not
all patients with asthma and persistent airway obstruction in most but
not all patients with COPD where even up to 50% have been reported to
have some bronchodilator response as assessed with FEV1. Airway
obstruction is generated in the large and small airways both in asthma
and COPD, and this small airway obstruction is located more proximally
in asthma, yet is found more distally in severe and older individuals with
asthma, comparable to COPD. Though the underlying inflammation and
remodelling processes in asthma and COPD are different in their extreme
phenotypes, there are overlap phenotypes with eosinophilic inflammation
even in stable COPD and neutrophilic inflammation in longstanding and
severe asthma.

Tho Truong

Bronchiectasis should be considered as a differential diagnosis for, as well
as a comorbidity in, patients with asthma, especially severe or long-
standing asthma. Chronic airway inflammation is thought to be the primary
cause, as with chronic or recurrent pulmonary infection and autoimmune
conditions that involve the airways. Consequently, immunodeficiencies
with associated increased susceptibility to respiratory tract infections or
chronic inflammatory airways also increase the risk of developing bronchiectasis. Chronic bronchiectasis is associated with impaired mucociliary
clearance and increased bronchial secretions, leading to airway obstruction and airflow limitation, which can lead to exacerbation of underlying
asthma or increased asthma symptoms.

Preface

Each year, Elsevier's prestigious *Clinics Review Articles* series publishes more than 250 issues (3000 plus articles) encompassing nearly 60 medical and surgical disciplines. This curated collection of articles, devoted to asthma, draws from the robust *Clinics'* database to provide multidisciplinary teams with practical, clinical advice on comorbidities and complications of this highly prevalent disease. Featured articles from the *Otolaryngologic Clinics of North America*, *Clinics in Chest Medicine*, *Primary Care: Clinics in Office Practice*, *Immunology and Allergy Clinics of North America*, *Emergency Medicine Clinics of North America*, and *Nursing Clinics of North America* reflect the wide range of clinicians who manage the asthmatic patient. This multidisciplinary perspective is essential to successful team-based management.

I hope you share this volume with your colleagues and that it spurs more collaboration, deeper understanding, and safer, more effective care for your patients.

Joel J. Heidelbaugh, MD, FAAFP, FACG
Ypsilanti, MI
September 2014

Clinics Collections 2 (2014) xvii
http://dx.doi.org/10.1016/j.ccol.2014.09.001
2352-7986/14/$ – see front matter © 2014 Published by Elsevier Inc.

What is Asthma? Pathophysiology, Demographics, and Health Care Costs

Jonathan Maslan, MD, James W. Mims, MD*

KEYWORDS

- Asthma • Pathogenesis • Pathophysiology • Epidemiology • Demographics • Costs

KEY POINTS

- Cardinal asthma symptoms are shortness of breath, cough, chest tightness, and/or wheezing.
- Symptoms arise from airway inflammation, which leads to airway edema, remodeling, and hyperresponsiveness.
- The inflammation in asthma is mediated by multiple cell types including mast cells, eosinophils, lymphocytes, macrophages, neutrophils, and epithelial cells, and there is a predominantly Th2 milieu.
- The cause of asthma is a multifactorial. Active research in asthma genetics has replicated genes that likely play a role in asthma development, but phenotype expression is profoundly affected by environmental triggers.
- Roughly 8% of the US population has asthma and it is the third leading cause of hospitalization in children, accounting for roughly $56 billion per year in direct costs and lost productivity.

WHAT IS ASTHMA?

Asthma is a chronic inflammatory disorder characterized by airway obstruction and hyperresponsiveness. The medical term "asthma," which derives from the Greek for "panting," was named by Hippocrates around 400 BC. Sir William Osler described asthma in his *Principles and Practice of Medicine* in the early 20th century as "swelling of the nasal or respiratory mucous membrane, increased secretion, and…spasm of the bronchial muscles with dyspnea, chiefly expiratory." Of its treatment, he said, "Ordinary tobacco cigarettes are sometimes helpful."[1] (This position is no longer considered true.) Many decades later, it is now understood that asthma is a complex disease

This article originally appeared in Otolaryngologic Clinics of North America, Volume 47, Issue 1, February 2014.
Wake Forest School of Medicine, Medical Center Boulevard, Winston-Salem, NC 27157, USA
* Corresponding author. Department of Otolaryngology, Wake Forest School of Medicine, Medical Center Boulevard, Winston-Salem, NC 27157.
E-mail address: wmims@wakehealth.edu

Clinics Collections 2 (2014) 1–10
http://dx.doi.org/10.1016/j.ccol.2014.09.002

of airway inflammation characterized by airway edema, remodeling, and hyperresponsiveness. Asthma exacerbations are characterized by progressively worsening shortness of breath, cough, chest tightness, and/or wheezing. Under this umbrella of clinical symptoms, there is a very sophisticated interplay between underlying genotypes and environmental triggers that is only partially understood. This leads to a broad array of variable disease phenotypes and manifestations. Asthma is increasingly recognized as a syndrome, rather than an illness.[2]

Diagnosis

The diagnosis of asthma is made when episodic symptoms of airflow obstruction or airway hyperresponsiveness are present, airflow obstruction is partially reversible, and alternative diagnoses are excluded.[3] In addition to a good medical history and physical examination, spirometry is needed to demonstrate obstruction and assess reversibility.[3] Reversibility is determined by an increase in forced expiratory volume in 1 second (FEV_1) of greater than or equal to 12% from baseline or an increase greater than or equal to 10% of predicted FEV_1 after inhalation of a short-acting β_2-agonist.[3] The National Institutes of Health Guidelines for the Diagnosis and Management of Asthma recommend considering a diagnosis of asthma when certain key indicators are present (**Table 1**). The key indicators consist of specific symptoms, physical examination findings, and modifying factors and environmental exposures. There is a great deal of overlap between asthma symptoms and other disorders of the respiratory tract. The differential diagnosis for asthma symptoms includes allergic rhinitis or sinusitis, foreign body, aspiration, gastroesophageal reflux, laryngotracheomalacia, vocal cord dysfunction, bronchiolitis, chronic obstructive pulmonary disease, and cystic fibrosis, among other conditions.[3] Recurrent cough and wheezing should always alert practitioners to the possibility of asthma.

Asthma can be intermittent or persistent, and it can present with acute flares or chronic symptoms. Asthma severity is measured by objective measures of lung function (ie, spirometry or peak flow meter) and by symptoms. Measures of impairment include nighttime awakenings, need for short-acting bronchodilators, work or school

Table 1 Key indicators in asthma		
Symptoms	**Physical Examination Findings**	**Modifying Factors**
Wheezing (recurrent)	Thoracic hyperexpansion	Exercise
Cough, worse at night	Wheezing during normal breathing	Viral infection
Difficulty breathing (recurrent)	Prolonged phase of forced exhalation	Animals with fur or hair
Chest tightness (recurrent)	Rhinorrhea	Dust mites
	Nasal polyps	Mold
	Atopic dermatitis	Smoke
		Pollen
		Changes in weather
		Airborne chemicals or dusts
		Menstrual cycles

A diagnosis of asthma should be considered if any of these symptoms and physical examination findings is present, and if these findings are modified by the factors listed. The likelihood of asthma is increased if multiple key indicators are present. Spirometry is necessary for the actual diagnosis of asthma.

Adapted from National Heart, Lung, and Blood Institute. NIH expert panel report 3: guidelines for the diagnosis and management of asthma. 2007. Available at: http://www.nhlbi.nih.gov/guidelines/asthma/asthgdln.pdf. Accessed September 10, 2013.

days missed, ability to engage in normal daily activities, and quality of life assessments.[3] The frequency of exacerbations in the population with asthma varies widely. Importantly, the severity of disease (as measured by frequency of nighttime awakenings, usage of short-acting β_2-agonists, and interference with normal activity) does not correlate with the intensity of exacerbations.[3] Indeed, severe, life-threatening exacerbations can occur even in people with intermittent or mild asthma when provoked by an exposure, such as a viral illness, irritant, or allergen.[3] However, decreased FEV_1 in children demonstrates a strong association with the risk of asthma exacerbations.[4] In terms of modifying factors, viral infections are the most common cause of asthma exacerbations.[3]

There is a traditional division between allergic and nonallergic asthma. Allergic asthma is the subtype that accounts for approximately 50% to 80% of asthma cases, and is defined as asthma and positivity to skin prick test or specific IgE.[5,6] Allergic asthma is more common in younger males and associated with milder disease, whereas nonallergic asthma is more common in older females and more severe disease.[7,8] Nonallergic asthma exacerbations are more commonly triggered by infection, irritants, gastroesophageal reflux disease, stress, and exercise.[7] Despite the many overlapping phenotypes of asthma, the pattern of airway inflammation, the cellular profile, and the response of structural cells is consistent across all types of asthma.[3]

The asthma phenotype can be quite variable because of complex interactions between the environment and underlying genetic factors. Although asthma symptoms are typically episodic and reversible (either spontaneously or with treatment), there are also more long-term changes to the asthmatic airway that can occur from inflammation.[9] Multiple inflammatory cells and cytokines have been described in asthma pathogenesis, yet the mechanisms leading to the variability of disease phenotypes are still only partially understood.[3]

The Unified Airway, Asthma, and the Otolaryngologist

The unified airway model suggests that inflammatory diseases of the upper and lower airways are interconnected because of shared epithelial lining and inflammatory mediators. Pseudostratified columnar epithelium is the mucosal lining in the middle ear, nasal cavity, sinuses, and the lower airway, and the inflammatory mediators in chronic disease of the upper and lower airways, such as rhinosinusitis and asthma, are frequently the same (interleukin [IL]-4, IL-5, and IL-13).[10] Rhinitis, sinusitis, and asthma are frequently comorbid conditions. Indeed, a coincidence of upper and lower airway pathologies is suggested by self-reported symptoms in people with asthma, who list allergic rhinitis and sinusitis as their most common comorbidities.[11] A study by Corren[12] demonstrated the presence of rhinitis in 78% of people with asthma, and the presence of asthma in 38% of patients with rhinitis. Other conditions that otolaryngology patients frequently present with include vocal cord dysfunction, obstructive sleep apnea, and gastroesophageal reflux disease, all of which can masquerade as asthma, and can coexist with it. It is therefore important for otolaryngologists to be aware of the diagnosis and management of this common, complex, and treatable disease.

PATHOPHYSIOLOGY
Inflammation and Airway Remodeling

The inflammation in asthma is mediated by multiple cell types including mast cells, eosinophils, T lymphocytes, macrophages, neutrophils, and epithelial cells.[3] Asthma has allergic and nonallergic presentations, based on the presence or absence of IgE antibodies to common environmental allergens. Both variants are characterized by airway infiltration by T-helper (Th) cells, which secrete a predominantly Th2 milieu (cytokines IL-4, IL-5, and IL-13).[3,5] These cytokines stimulate mast cells, cause eosinophilia, promote leukocytosis, and enhance B-cell IgE production.

Although mild asthma symptoms are episodic and reversible, with disease progression and severity long-term and permanent airway changes can be present. Long-term changes can include airway smooth muscle hypertrophy and hyperplasia; increased mucus production (and associated risk of mucus plugs); and edema.[3] In the subepithelial layer, thickening can range from 7 to 23 μm, versus 4 to 5 μm in normal subjects, and more commonly affects the smaller airways (2–6 mm).[5,13,14] Permanent changes can include thickening of subbasement membrane, subepithelial edema and fibrosis, airway smooth muscle hypertrophy and hyperplasia, blood vessel proliferation and dilation, and mucus gland hyperplasia and hypersecretion.[3,14,15] Transforming growth factor-β, IL-11, and IL-17 are profibrotic factors that are increased in asthma and that lead to increased levels of types I and III collagen, resulting in subepithelial fibrosis.[16] Interestingly, most of the histopathologic findings noted previously are shared between asthma and chronic rhinosinusitis, and are worse when a patient has both conditions as opposed to either one.[15,17]

There is likely an occult process of bronchial inflammation that precedes clinical symptoms of asthma. Bronchial biopsies of children with early respiratory symptoms who progressed to asthma had higher concentrations of eosinophils in the bronchial mucosa and thicker subepithelial lamina reticularis than those who did not, and these findings were present before the clinical presentation of disease.[18] This suggests that an inflammatory milieu may precede clinical symptoms in people with asthma. Furthermore, in patients who had clinical symptoms of asthma that then seemed to go into remission, evidence of inflammation and remodeling persist on follow-up biopsies.[19–21] Clinical symptoms are a late manifestation of lower airway inflammation. Despite there being a robust response to anti-inflammatory medications with symptom control in many people with asthma, symptoms tend to recur when these drugs are no longer being used. Moreover, as in chronic rhinosinusitis, corticosteroids can result in symptom control, but they do not significantly impact the long-term inflammation in the disease process.[16] There are many treatments for asthma symptoms, but asthma is not a curable disease, and there is evidence that inflammation is life-long and occurs even when no symptoms are present.

Bronchoconstriction and Airway Hyperresponsiveness

The bronchoconstriction that occurs in asthma exacerbations is the main cause of obstructive symptoms. Airway hyperresponsiveness, or twitchy airways, occurs secondary to inflammation and airway remodeling. There is a distinct correlation between airway hyperresponsiveness and the degree of inflammation present. Bronchoconstriction can be induced by several pathways. Allergen-induced bronchoconstriction is caused by IgE-dependent mast cell degranulation, with resultant release of histamine, tryptase, leukotrienes, and prostaglandins.[22] Nonsteroidal anti-inflammatory disease–induced bronchoconstriction by the cyclooxygenase-2 pathway can also occur in susceptible patient populations.[23] (Approximately 10% of people with asthma are aspirin-sensitive.[24]) In addition to these mechanisms, bronchoconstriction by mast cell degranulation can also occur secondary to osmotic stimuli, which is likely the cause of exercise-induced bronchoconstriction.[3]

Genetics of Asthma

The genetics of asthma are complex and there are multiple genes that are thought to play a role, although there is not one specific gene that can explain most asthma cases. One landmark review article[25] stated that asthma susceptibility genes fall into four main groups: (1) genes associated with innate immunity and immunoregulation; (2) genes associated with Th2 cell differentiation and effector functions; (3) genes associated with epithelial biology and mucosal immunity; and (4) genes associated with lung function, airway remodeling, and disease severity. One study highlighted 43 replicated genes identified in the pathogenesis of asthma from well-conducted association studies, but how these genes interact with each other and the environment, and the role of epistasis in gene expression, requires further research.[26] An abundance of data demonstrates that the same polymorphism can lead to asthma pathology in one environment but not another.[25] Indeed, there is striking evidence among people with similar genetic backgrounds that environmental exposures can have a profound impact on asthma and wheezing incidence. For example, a comparison of people of Chinese origin showed a significantly increased prevalence of asthma in those living in Canada and Hong Kong versus mainland China.[27] A study of West Germany and East Germany shortly after reunification demonstrated an increased prevalence of asthma in the former.[28]

Risk Factors for Asthma

Numerous potential risk factors have been studied in relation to the development of asthma. Atopy is frequently identified as a strong risk factor for the development of asthma, yet there is not always a direct correlation between the two.[3,29] Some studies have demonstrated that early dust mite sensitization and maternal asthma are very significant predictors of asthma.[30,31] Parental smoking is a significant risk factor for acute lower respiratory tract infections in infants, and the development of wheezing and asthma in children.[32] However, there is also a high incidence of asthma in children not exposed to tobacco smoke. Active smoking in adults is associated with the development of asthma later in life.[33] Air pollution and viral infections are well-established triggers for asthma exacerbations,[34,35] but there is conflicting data as to whether these factors contribute to developing asthma.[28,36] Microbial exposure is inversely correlated with the development of asthma and atopy, and may account for the disparate prevalence of asthma in urban versus rural (specifically farming) environments.[2,37–39] Ultimately, it is likely that asthma develops in genetically susceptible individuals through a combination of complex environmental exposures.

DEMOGRAPHICS AND EPIDEMIOLOGY
Prevalence Internationally

There is wide variability in terms of the international prevalence of asthma, and methods by which international asthma prevalence is ascertained. Large, multinational studies that have attempted to characterize the epidemiology of asthma have determined its prevalence by such questions as: "Have you (has your child) had wheezing or whistling in the chest in the past 12 months?"[40] The European Community Respiratory Health Survey, a large, 22-country study, was based on an interviewer-led questionnaire and, when possible, objective measures, such as spirometry and skin prick testing.[41] Using these methods, there is a lower incidence of asthma in Asia and India (2%–4%) than in such countries as Canada, the United Kingdom, Australia, and New Zealand (15%–20%).[42] The European Community Respiratory Health Survey study showed a higher prevalence in Western Europe and the United States than in Eastern Europe.[41] Although asthma symptoms and prevalence increased in many countries from the 1960s through the 1990s, since that time there has been greater variability. In some countries asthma prevalence has increased significantly, whereas in others it has remained stable or even declined (**Fig. 1**).[2]

Prevalence in the United States

Within the United States, the overall prevalence of asthma has increased in recent years, although there is also wide variability geographically (**Fig. 2**). In 2011, asthma prevalence ranged from 5.5% in Tennessee to 18% in the District of Columbia.[43] In 2001, 7% of the overall US population (~20 million people) had asthma, whereas in 2009, 8% of the population (~25 million people) had asthma.[44] Women are more likely than men, and boys are more likely than girls to have asthma.[41,44] It is most common among African American children, who have an approximately one in six chance of having asthma, and as a group had the highest increase in asthma prevalence from 2001 to 2009.[44] People with asthma are more likely to be younger and unmarried, have lower educational attainment, be impoverished, and have comorbidities.[45] Asthma is the third leading cause of hospitalization among children younger than age 15.[46] In 2009, deaths caused by asthma totaled 3388, of which 157 were children.[47]

Costs

Asthma is associated with significant quality of life disruption, a decrease in work productivity, missed school, and increased health care costs. Multiple methods have been used to assess the overall costs of asthma, but one of the best studies was conducted by the Centers for Disease Control and Prevention, published in 2011, looking at direct medical costs and productivity losses caused by morbidity and mortality from asthma from 2002 to 2007.[45] The Centers for Disease Control and Prevention data came from the Medical Expenditure Panel Survey, a large, nationally representative survey that examined demographic and socioeconomic characteristics, employment, days disrupted by injury or illness, health care and medication use, medical conditions, and

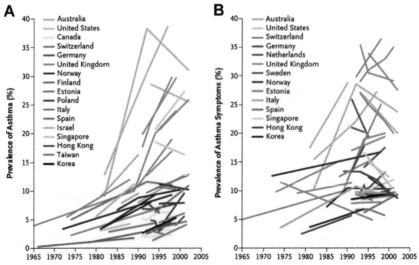

Fig. 1. Prevalence rates of asthma and asthma symptoms from around the world. Although many countries have shown increased prevalence of asthma and asthma symptoms, other countries have remained stable or even declined. (*From* Eder W, Ege MJ, von Mutius E. The asthma epidemic. N Engl J Med 2006;355:2226–35; with permission.)

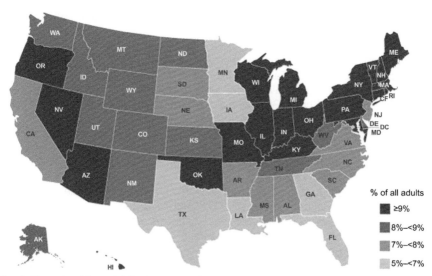

Fig. 2. There is wide variability in terms of asthma prevalence in the United States, ranging from 5.5% in Tennessee to 18% in the District of Columbia. (*From* Centers for Disease Control and Prevention. CDC vital signs. 2013. Available at: http://www.cdc.gov/VitalSigns/Asthma/index.html. Accessed September 10, 2013.)

health status. Over the 6-year period studied, costs were reported in 2009 dollars (Consumer Price Index-adjusted), as follows: the total cost per person with asthma was estimated at $3259 per year during the years 2002 to 2007. The predicted incremental cost for hospital outpatient visits was $151, for emergency department visits $110, and for inpatient visits $446.[45] On an annual basis, the cost of office-based visits for persons with asthma was estimated at $581 per year, and the additional cost of prescription medication expenditures was approximately $1680. Prescription medications accounted for the largest percentage of total medical expenditures in the adult population. This was a changing feature of asthma costs, because hospital costs accounted for most direct costs of asthma in the 1990s. Nationally, the United States population missed approximately 14.41 million work days and 3.68 million school days, with a combined estimated value of $2.03 billion per year. Overall, the study estimated that the total cost of asthma to society in 2007, including incremental direct costs and estimates of lost productivity, was approximately $56 billion.[45]

SUMMARY

Asthma is a complex disorder, affected by genetics and the environment, with a multi-factorial cause and an as yet only partially understood pathophysiology. With its unifying symptoms of shortness of breath, cough, chest tightness, and/or wheezing, and its characteristic airway edema, inflammation, remodeling, and hyperresponsiveness, it is increasingly being perceived as a syndrome rather than one specific disease entity. The societal burden of asthma is substantial, and its costs and prevalence continue to increase in the United States.

REFERENCES

1. Osler W. The principles and practice of medicine. New York, London: D. Appleton and Company; 1920.

2. Eder W, Ege MJ, von Mutius E. The asthma epidemic. N Engl J Med 2006;355: 2226–35.
3. Busse WW, et al. Expert Panel Report Three. Guidelines for the diagnosis and management of asthma. National Institutes of Health; 2007.
4. Fuhlbrigge AL, Kitch BT, Paltiel AD, et al. FEV(1) is associated with risk of asthma attacks in a pediatric population. J Allergy Clin Immunol 2001;107:61–7.
5. Cohn L, Elias JA, Chupp GL. Asthma: mechanisms of disease persistence and progression. Annu Rev Immunol 2004;22:789–815.
6. Handoyo S, Rosenwasser LJ. Asthma phenotypes. Curr Allergy Asthma Rep 2009;9:439–45.
7. Novak N, Bieber T. Allergic and nonallergic forms of atopic diseases. J Allergy Clin Immunol 2003;112:252–62.
8. Romanet-Manent S, Charpin D, Magnan A, et al. Allergic vs nonallergic asthma: what makes the difference? Allergy 2002;57:607–13.
9. Holgate ST, Polosa R. The mechanisms, diagnosis, and management of severe asthma in adults. Lancet 2006;368:780–93.
10. Bachert C, Vignola AM, Gevaert P, et al. Allergic rhinitis, rhinosinusitis, and asthma: one airway disease. Immunol Allergy Clin North Am 2004;24:19–43.
11. Dixon AE, Kaminsky DA, Holbrook JT, et al. Allergic rhinitis and sinusitis in asthma: differential effects on symptoms and pulmonary function. Chest 2006; 130:429–35.
12. Corren J. Allergic rhinitis and asthma: how important is the link? J Allergy Clin Immunol 1997;99:S781–6.
13. Roberts CR, Okazawa M, Wiggs B, et al. Airway wall thickening. In: Barnes PJ, Grunstein MM, Leff AR, et al, editors. Asthma. Philadelphia: Raven Publishers; 1997. p. 925–35.
14. Homer RJ, Elias JA. Consequences of long-term inflammation. Airway remodeling. Clin Chest Med 2000;21:331–43, ix.
15. Krouse JH, Brown RW, Fineman SM, et al. Asthma and the unified airway. Otolaryngol Head Neck Surg 2007;136:S75–106.
16. Chakir J, Shannon J, Molet S, et al. Airway remodeling-associated mediators in moderate to severe asthma: effect of steroids on TGF-beta, IL-11, IL-17, and type I and type III collagen expression. J Allergy Clin Immunol 2003;111:1293–8.
17. Dhong HJ, Kim HY, Cho DY. Histopathologic characteristics of chronic sinusitis with bronchial asthma. Acta Otolaryngol 2005;125:169–76.
18. Pohunek P, Warner JO, Turzíková J, et al. Markers of eosinophilic inflammation and tissue re-modelling in children before clinically diagnosed bronchial asthma. Pediatr Allergy Immunol 2005;16:43–51.
19. van Den Toorn LM, Prins JB, Overbeek SE, et al. Adolescents in clinical remission of atopic asthma have elevated exhaled nitric oxide levels and bronchial hyper-responsiveness. Am J Respir Crit Care Med 2000;162:953–7.
20. van den Toorn LM, Overbeek SE, de Jongste JC, et al. Airway inflammation is present during clinical remission of atopic asthma. Am J Respir Crit Care Med 2001; 164:2107–13.
21. van den Toorn LM, Overbeek SE, Prins JB, et al. Asthma remission: does it exist? Curr Opin Pulm Med 2003;9:15–20.
22. Busse WW, Lemanske RF. Asthma. N Engl J Med 2001;344:350–62.
23. Stevenson DD, Szczeklik A. Clinical and pathologic perspectives on aspirin sensitivity and asthma. J Allergy Clin Immunol 2006;118:773–86 [quiz: 787–8].
24. Vally H, Taylor ML, Thompson PJ. The prevalence of aspirin intolerant asthma (AIA) in Australian asthmatic patients. Thorax 2002;57:569–74.

25. Vercelli D. Discovering susceptibility genes for asthma and allergy. Nat Rev Immunol 2008;8:169–82.
26. Weiss ST, Raby BA, Rogers A. Asthma genetics and genomics 2009. Curr Opin Genet Dev 2009;19:279–82.
27. Wang HY, Wong GW, Chen YZ, et al. Prevalence of asthma among Chinese adolescents living in Canada and in China. CMAJ 2008;179:1133–42.
28. von Mutius E, Martinez FD, Fritzsch C, et al. Prevalence of asthma and atopy in two areas of West and East Germany. Am J Respir Crit Care Med 1994;149: 358–64.
29. Priftanji A, Strachan D, Burr M, et al. Asthma and allergy in Albania and the UK. Lancet 2001;358:1426–7.
30. Lau S, Illi S, Sommerfeld C, et al. Early exposure to house-dust mite and cat allergens and development of childhood asthma: a cohort study. Multicentre Allergy Study Group. Lancet 2000;356:1392–7.
31. Sears MR, Herbison GP, Holdaway MD, et al. The relative risks of sensitivity to grass pollen, house dust mite and cat dander in the development of childhood asthma. Clin Exp Allergy 1989;19:419–24.
32. Strachan DP, Cook DG. Health effects of passive smoking. 6. Parental smoking and childhood asthma: longitudinal and case-control studies. Thorax 1998;53: 204–12.
33. Strachan DP, Butland BK, Anderson HR. Incidence and prognosis of asthma and wheezing illness from early childhood to age 33 in a national British cohort. BMJ 1996;312:1195–9.
34. Patel MM, Miller RL. Air pollution and childhood asthma: recent advances and future directions. Curr Opin Pediatr 2009;21:235–42.
35. Corne JM, Marshall C, Smith S, et al. Frequency, severity, and duration of rhinovirus infections in asthmatic and non-asthmatic individuals: a longitudinal cohort study. Lancet 2002;359:831–4.
36. von Mutius E. Infection: friend or foe in the development of atopy and asthma? The epidemiological evidence. Eur Respir J 2001;18:872–81.
37. Braun-Fahrländer C, Lauener R. Farming and protective agents against allergy and asthma. Clin Exp Allergy 2003;33:409–11.
38. Keeley DJ, Neill P, Gallivan S. Comparison of the prevalence of reversible airways obstruction in rural and urban Zimbabwean children. Thorax 1991;46:549–53.
39. van Strien RT, Engel R, Holst O, et al. Microbial exposure of rural school children, as assessed by levels of N-acetyl-muramic acid in mattress dust, and its association with respiratory health. J Allergy Clin Immunol 2004;113:860–7.
40. Asher MI, Montefort S, Björkstén B, et al. Worldwide time trends in the prevalence of symptoms of asthma, allergic rhinoconjunctivitis, and eczema in childhood: ISAAC Phases One and Three repeat multicountry cross-sectional surveys. Lancet 2006;368:733–43.
41. Janson C, Anto J, Burney P, et al. The European Community Respiratory Health Survey: what are the main results so far? European Community Respiratory Health Survey II. Eur Respir J 2001;18:598–611.
42. Subbarao P, Mandhane PJ, Sears MR. Asthma: epidemiology, etiology and risk factors. CMAJ 2009;181:E181–90.
43. Centers for Disease Control and Prevention. Behavioral risk factor surveillance survey. Available at: http://www.lung.org/lung-disease/asthma/resources/facts-and-figures/asthma-children-fact-sheet.html. Accessed July 4, 2013.
44. Centers for Disease Control and Prevention. CDC vital signs. 2013. Available at: http://www.cdc.gov/VitalSigns/Asthma/index.html. Accessed July 4, 2013.

45. Barnett SB, Nurmagambetov TA. Costs of asthma in the United States: 2002-2007. J Allergy Clin Immunol 2011;127:145–52.
46. Centers for Disease Control and Prevention. National Center for Health Statistics, National Hospital Discharge Survey, 1995-2010. 2013. Available at: http://www.lung.org/lung-disease/asthma/resources/facts-and-figures/asthma-children-fact-sheet.html. Accessed July 4, 2013.
47. Centers for Disease Control and Prevention. Statistics. Compiled from Compressed Mortality File 1999-2009 Series 1920 No. 1920.

Asthma
A Chronic Infectious Disease?

Gaetano Caramori, MD, PhD[a], Nikos Papadopoulos, MD, PhD[b],
Marco Contoli, MD, PhD[a], Brunilda Marku, MD, PhD[a],
Giacomo Forini, MD[a], Alessia Pauletti, MD[a],
Sebastian L. Johnston, MD, PhD[c], Alberto Papi, MD[a,*]

KEYWORDS

• Asthma • Respiratory infection • Bacterial infection • Rhinovirus

KEY POINTS

• There are increasing data to support the "hygiene" and "microbiota" hypotheses of a protective role of infections in modulating the risk of subsequent development of asthma.
• There is some evidence that rhinovirus respiratory infections are associated with the development of asthma, particularly in childhood, whereas these infections in later life seem to have a weaker association with the development of asthma.
• The role of bacterial infections in chronic asthma remains unclear, but there are emerging data for a potential role of *Mycoplasma pneumoniae* and *Chlamydia pneumoniae* and gut microbiota in increasing the risk of the development of asthma and in modulating the degree of asthma control.

INTRODUCTION

The "Global Strategy for Asthma Management," prepared by a panel convened by the National Institutes of Health and the World Health Organization, defines asthma as "a chronic inflammatory disorder of the airways, in which many cells and cellular elements play a role. The chronic inflammation is associated with airway hyperresponsiveness that leads to recurrent episodes of wheezing, breathlessness, chest

This article originally appeared in Clinics in Chest Medicine, Volume 33, Issue 3, September 2012.
[a] Section of Respiratory Diseases, Department of Medical Sciences, Centro per lo Studio delle Malattie Infiammatorie Croniche delle Vie Aeree e Patologie Fumo Correlate dell'Apparato Respiratorio (CEMICEF), University of Ferrara, via Savonarola 9, 44121, Ferrara, Italy; [b] Allergy Department, 2nd Paediatric Clinic, University of Athens, 13 Levadias Street, 11527 Goudi, Athens, Greece; [c] MRC and Asthma UK Centre in Allergic Mechanisms of Asthma, Centre for Respiratory Infection, National Heart and Lung Institute, Imperial College London, Norfolk Place, London W2 1PG, UK
* Corresponding author. Sezione di Malattie dell'Apparato Respiratorio, University of Ferrara, Via Savonarola 9, 44121 Ferrara, Italy.
E-mail address: ppa@unife.it

tightness, and coughing, particularly at night or in the early morning. These episodes are usually associated with widespread, but variable, airflow limitation within the lung that is often reversible, either spontaneously or with treatment."[1]

The chronic airway inflammation seen in asthma is present even in those with very mild disease and is unique in that the airway wall is infiltrated by T lymphocytes of the T-helper (Th) type 2 phenotype, eosinophils, macrophages and monocytes, and mast cells.[1,2] In addition, an "acute-on-chronic" inflammation may be observed during exacerbations, with an increase in eosinophils and sometimes neutrophils.[1,2] Lower airway structural cells also produce inflammatory mediators. Thus, bronchial and bronchiolar epithelial cells, lung endothelial cells, lung fibroblasts, and bronchial and bronchiolar smooth muscle cells show an altered phenotype in asthma and express multiple inflammatory mediators, including cytokines, chemokines, and peptides.[2] Chronic inflammation in asthma may lead to structural changes in the lower airways, including reticular basement membrane fibrosis under the bronchial epithelium; increased thickness (mainly through hyperplasia) of lower airway smooth muscle cells; increased numbers of bronchial blood vessels (neoangiogenesis); and increased number or volume of mucus-secreting cells in the bronchial mucosa (surface epithelium and glands). These changes, often referred to as "airway remodeling," may not be fully reversible with current treatments.[3] The most objective method to confirm the diagnosis of asthma in a subject with symptoms of asthma remains the assessment of the presence of reversible airflow obstruction. The reversibility of airflow obstruction (spontaneous or induced by pharmacologic treatment) may be assessed either by measuring peak expiratory flow or FEV_1 before and after a single dose of a bronchodilator, or before and after a 3-month course of full antiasthma treatment including inhaled glucocorticoids.[4]

The cause of asthma is still unknown, and is probably multifactorial, involving complex interactions between many genetic and environmental factors. According to its presumed etiology asthma may still be defined as extrinsic (or atopic or allergic) or intrinsic. Although the term extrinsic refers to a well-recognized environmental agent, extrinsic asthma is usually defined as asthma that occurs in atopic individuals (ie, subjects with an increased amount of serum immunoglobulin E [IgE] antibodies against common environmental aeroallergens). Sometimes it is possible to identify the allergens responsible for the development and maintenance of asthma in an individual with atopy, but often it is possible to establish only the association of asthma and atopy and not the precise cause of asthma, because people with asthma and atopy can develop symptoms of asthma and airflow obstruction after exposure to a variety of provoking agents other than allergens. In addition, in some patients it is possible to identify the agents that trigger asthma exacerbations in individuals who are nonatopic. This is the case in occupational asthma induced by low-molecular-weight chemicals and in subjects with asthma induced by some drugs (eg, aspirin-induced asthma). In these cases asthma may be considered extrinsic (ie, caused by a well-defined agent), but occurring in individuals without atopy.[4]

The existence of a group of patients in whom no environmental causal agent can be identified has strongly limited the classification of asthma according to its etiology. Asthma induced by unknown causes in a subject without atopy is still defined as intrinsic. Apart from some differences in onset, severity, and natural history, and some aspects of pathology, extrinsic and intrinsic asthma are very similar, particularly from pathologic, pathophysiologic, and pharmacologic points of view.[4]

Although a genetic basis for asthma is undeniable, elucidation of polymorphisms that are "causal" is greatly hampered by variability in the clinical phenotype, which is likely caused by the multiple molecular mechanisms underlying the complex pathologic processes involved in disease development and progression.[5] However, very expensive genome-wide association studies of asthma have recently discovered many novel susceptibility genes and this may further increase the understanding of asthma.[6]

An association between respiratory infections, mainly viral, and asthma exacerbations is well documented and accepted,[7] but less conclusive, mainly epidemiologic studies also suggest a possible role of many different infections in the cause of asthma. This article reviews the available evidence indicating that asthma may be considered as a chronic infectious disease.

DUAL ROLE OF INFECTIONS IN THE ETIOLOGY OF ASTHMA

The role of infections in the cause of asthma is complex. There is mounting evidence suggesting a protective role of a greater overall exposure to infectious agents or components thereof in reducing the risk of development of asthma and less convincing data suggesting instead a role of some infections in causing the development of asthma.

INFECTIONS PROTECT FROM THE DEVELOPMENT OF ASTHMA

Many epidemiologic studies suggest that the exposure to infections in early childhood may play a protective role in the later development of asthma, the so-called "hygiene hypothesis," first proposed by Strachan[8] in 1989 demonstrating that infections and contact with older siblings or through other exposures confer protection from the development of allergy and asthma. This hypothesis has evolved in various ways exploring the role of overt viral and bacterial infections, the significance of environmental exposure to microbial compounds, and their effect on underlying responses of innate and adaptive immunity.[9]

The hygiene hypothesis proposes that a greater load of infections in early life is protective toward the eventual development of asthma.[8] These associations are supported by observations showing an inverse relationship between the age of entering day care and the incidence of asthma later in life.[10] This inverse relationship is also present between the number of siblings or family size and asthma. However, these studies have used surrogate markers for increased exposure to infections; there is a need to investigate directly the real impact of respiratory infections. Whether infections have protective effect or not may have to do also with their location, frequency, intensity, and timing.[11]

It has been proposed that the protective effect related to more frequent infections may depend on their capacity to stimulate protective Th1 immunity.[12] Indeed, neonates are born with an immune response predominantly type 2.[13] Early infections skew the immune system toward a type 1 phenotype, inducing the production of interleukin (IL)-12 by dendritic cells.[14]

Because asthma is characterized by increased Th2 immune responses, by this mechanism a reduction in childhood infectious illnesses could lead to an increase in the prevalence of asthma, especially if there is also a genetic background of impaired type 1 immunity (infants with a family history of atopic diseases).

More recent studies suggest an alternative interpretation of the evidence supporting the "hygiene hypothesis," namely the "microbiota hypothesis." Particularly, it seems that exposure to nonpathogenic microbes may be more important in directing healthy immune development and reducing the risk of asthma.

There is increasing evidence that commensal bacterial flora (human microbiome or microbiota) in various sites, including gut, skin, and lungs, is an important modulator of immune function and development and a critical contributor to the maintenance of mucosal homeostasis. However, the mechanisms by which the human microbiome influences lung immunity and inflammation and its role in the development of asthma are still not well characterized.[15]

Microbes residing in the environment might shape an exposed subject's immune responses and thereby his or her risk of asthma. There is substantial evidence that a diversity of microbial exposure can exert a protective effect, particularly in childhood, against the development of asthma.[15]

Endotoxins from gram-negative bacteria have been the first agents associated with a reduced risk for asthma. In later studies, $\beta(1 \rightarrow 3)$glucans, extracellular polysaccharides, and muramic acid from, respectively, molds and gram-positive bacteria were associated with a reduced risk of asthma separately in rural and urban populations. These results already suggested that not just one but several independent microbial signals from gram-negative and -positive bacteria, and molds, might play a role in explaining the protective effects.[16] Surprisingly, the diversity of fungal and bacterial exposure seems to have protective effects. Such a concept of diversity is challenging when aiming at refining methods of exposure assessment for future studies. In turn, it might better grasp the nature of microbial exposures, which always relate to microbial communities and the shift in such communities rather than to single microorganisms.[15]

In animal models of asthma the presence of the microbiota is essential to protect from an exaggerated Th2 response, increased airway hyperresponsiveness, and airway inflammation after sensitization and challenge with ovalbumin.[17] Furthermore, in animals, antibiotic use during infancy may indeed quantitatively or qualitatively change the intestinal microflora and thereby prevent postnatal Th1 cell maturation, thus resulting in a Th2-polarized immune deviation.[18]

Epigenetic regulation is an important mechanism by which indigenous microbiota might interact with genes involved in asthma development. For example, in pregnant maternal mice prenatal administration of the farm-derived gram-negative bacterium *Acinetobacter lwoffii* F78 prevents the development of an asthmatic phenotype in the progeny, and this effect is interferon (IFN)-γ dependent. Furthermore, the IFN-γ promoter of CD4$^+$ T cells in the offspring has a significant protection against loss of histone 4 acetylation, which is closely associated with IFN-γ expression.[19]

Although epidemiologic data support a protective effect of parasitic infection on asthma development, this may be caused by other exposures. To date, there is no conclusive evidence that parasitic infection protects against asthma development.[20]

The strongest epidemiologic evidence suggests that helminthic intestinal hookworm infections may protect subjects from developing asthma.[20] In an animal model of asthma the application of excreted and secreted products (NES) of the helminth *Nippostrongylus brasiliensis* together with ovalbumin and alum during the sensitization period totally inhibited the development of eosinophilia and goblet-cell metaplasia in the airways and also strongly reduced the development of airway hyperresponsiveness.[21] Allergen-specific IgG1 and IgE serum levels are also strongly reduced. These findings correlated with decreased levels of IL-4 and IL-5 in the airways in NES-treated animals.[21] The suppressive effects on the development of allergic responses were independent of the presence of Toll-like receptors (TLR) 2 and 4, IFN-γ, and IL-10. Paradoxically, strong helminth NES-specific Th2 responses are induced in parallel with the inhibition of asthma-like responses.[21]

Th2 responses induced by allergens or helminths share many common features. However, allergen-specific IgE can almost always be detected in patients with atopy, whereas helminth-specific IgE is often not detectable and anaphylaxis often occurs in atopy but not with helminth infections. This may be caused by T regulatory responses induced by the helminths or the lack of helminth-specific IgE. Alternatively nonspecific IgE induced by the helminths may protect from mast cell or basophil degranulation by saturating IgE binding sites. Both of these mechanisms have been implicated to be involved in helminth-induced protection from allergic responses.[22] However, a study has shown that N brasiliensis antigen (Nb-Ag1) specific IgE could only be detected for a short period of time during infection, and that these levels are sufficient to prime mast cells thereby leading to active cutaneous anaphylaxis after the application of Nb-Ag1. Taken together, at least for the model helminth N brasiliensis, the IgE blocking hypothesis can be discarded.[23] However, novel antigens binding helminth-specific IgE may be identified for other pathogenic helminths infecting humans. Identifying these antigens may aid in IgE/mast cell–dependent vaccine development for asthma.[22]

Epidemiologic studies suggest that a hookworm infection producing 50 eggs per gram of feces may protect against asthma.[24] A pilot dose-ranging study of experimental human infection with Necator americanus larvae has been performed to identify the dose of hookworm larvae necessary to achieve 50 eggs per gram of feces for therapeutic trials in asthma.[25] Experimental infection with 10 hookworm larvae in patients with asthma did not result in significant improvement in bronchial responsiveness or other measures of asthma control. However, infection was well tolerated and resulted in a nonsignificant improvement in airway responsiveness, indicating that further studies that mimic more closely natural infection are feasible and should be undertaken.[26] More controlled studies are ongoing in this area and will provide useful new data in the coming years.

RESPIRATORY INFECTIONS AND INCREASED RISK OF DEVELOPMENT OF ASTHMA

Some epidemiologic studies suggest that certain early life respiratory tract infections can favor the development of asthma later in life. However, it is unknown whether early childhood viral infections cause asthma or simply identify those who are predisposed to asthma development. Furthermore, if respiratory infections are a causal factor, it is not known which specific microorganisms are most likely to cause asthma development. Finally, the immunopathologic link between respiratory infections and asthma development is not known.

Studies that have directly analyzed infectious episodes during infancy (ie, by parental reports or doctor diagnosis) suggest that respiratory infections in early life favor the later development of asthma. Nystad and colleagues[27] have found a positive association between full-time day care and early respiratory tract infections and asthma. The association between early infections and asthma was stronger than that between day care and asthma. In this Oslo Birth Cohort, established in 1992 to 1993, early respiratory infections did not protect against the development of asthma during the first 10 years of life but increased the risk for asthma symptoms at age 10.[28] In another epidemiologic study (the Tucson study) a higher prevalence of asthma was found in children who had doctor-diagnosed pneumonia or lower respiratory tract infection, reported by parents, in early life.[29]

These studies report a positive association between asthma and infections but not the direction of this association. It is not clear whether this association is "causal" or "circumstantial." Indeed, children predisposed to asthma may simply be more likely to develop respiratory tract infections. Another hypothesis is that individuals at high risk of developing asthma are more likely to develop symptoms with respiratory tract infections, and therefore the seemingly higher incidence of infections is influenced by reporting bias. Another confounding factor to consider is the site and type of infection (ie, gastrointestinal rather than respiratory, or bacterial rather than viral) or the possibility that in the future a specific pathogenic strain associated with the subsequent onset of asthma can be identified.

RESPIRATORY VIRAL INFECTIONS AND INCREASED RISK OF DEVELOPMENT OF ASTHMA

Several epidemiologic studies suggest that infants who develop severe viral respiratory infections are more likely to have asthma later in childhood.[30] This evidence is strongest for respiratory infections caused by respiratory syncytial virus (RSV) and rhinoviruses (RVs). However, the link between respiratory viral infections and asthma development remains unclear. The four main causative mechanisms hypothesized in the association between viral respiratory infections and the subsequent development of asthma in children are (1) alterations in airway function and size; (2) dysregulation (congenital and acquired) of airway tone, (3) alterations in the immune response to infections; and (4) the genetic variants involved in immune response.[30] There is a need to better understand whether host factors, such as epithelial cell function or immune response or virulence of virus strain, are important in modulating the subsequent risk to develop asthma after a respiratory viral infection.[31]

In humans there is scarce evidence that respiratory viral infections in early life compromising the airway epithelial barrier lead to enhanced absorption of allergens across this barrier and enhance lung sensitization to aeroallergens, whereas there is more evidence that the airway epithelium of subjects with atopy and asthma is more prone to respiratory viral infections.[32–34] For example, allergens can damage antiviral responses of the airway epithelium and this can promote greater viral replication.[32]

RSV INFECTIONS AND INCREASED RISK OF DEVELOPMENT OF ASTHMA

RSV is the major cause of severe bronchiolitis in children less than 1 year of age; consequently, it is considered the most important respiratory tract pathogen of early childhood.[35] In animal studies neonatal RSV infection sensitizes the newborn to develop an asthma-like phenotype on reinfection.[30,36,37] Sigurs and colleagues[38] found that severe RSV bronchiolitis, linked to hospitalization, was associated with a significantly increased risk of asthma to 18 years of age, especially in children with a family history of atopy. These results are supported by another study conducted in Tennessee. Wu and colleagues[39] reported that children born 120 days before the peak of RSV season have the highest rate of hospitalization for wheezing illnesses and also the greatest risk of asthma between 4 and 5 years of age. Future reports from this cohort (The Tennessee Children's Respiratory Initiative) will help to clarify the complex relationship between infant respiratory viral infection severity, etiology, atopic predisposition, and the subsequent development of early childhood asthma.

However, not all the investigations have seen this positive relationship between RSV infections and a subsequent increased risk of development of asthma.[40] For example, the Tucson Children's Respiratory Study reported an association between RSV lower respiratory tract infections before 3 years of age and development of asthma in early childhood, but this association was not observed beyond age 11 years.[41] Thus, severe RSV infections did not cause asthma, but instead, interacted with other genetic, environmental, and developmental factors, changing the expression of the asthma phenotype over time. For example, in one study the infants who subsequently developed RSV bronchiolitis have lower cord blood levels of IL-12 at birth[42] suggesting that

RSV does not induce a Th2 response but that in the subjects susceptible to RSV infections there is already a preexisting impaired Th1 immunity. A possible cause of this deficiency of IL-12 is a polymorphism in the CD14 gene, with lower levels of soluble CD14 (a coreceptor along with the TLR-4 for the detection of bacterial lipolysaccharide) and consequently higher serum IgE levels and diminished Th1 function.[43] In addition, a recent study found that impaired cord-blood immune responses to RSV predict the susceptibility to acute respiratory tract illness during the first year of life.[44]

RV INFECTIONS OF THE RESPIRATORY TRACT AND INCREASED RISK OF DEVELOPMENT OF ASTHMA

RSV is not the only cause of bronchiolitis in infants; in 2% to 40% of cases the causative agent is RV infection.[45] Bronchiolitis associated with RV infections, occurring mainly during spring and fall, are associated with a 25% increased likelihood of early childhood asthma compared with those occurring during winter and associated mainly with RSV infections.[46] Furthermore, hospitalization for RV-associated wheezing illnesses during the first 2 years of life increases fourfold the risk of childhood asthma compared with hospitalization for wheezing associated with other viruses.[46]

These findings suggest that RV infection is more strongly associated with the risk of asthma development than is RSV infection. Thus, the increased risk of development of asthma associated with respiratory viral infections seems to be related not only to the type of infection but also timing of this and the recurrence or not of wheezing over time.

The COAST study has demonstrated that the age at which RV wheezing illnesses occur is very important to define subsequent asthma risk at age 6 years.[47] Particularly, children who wheezed with RV during the third year of life have about a 32-fold increase in asthma risk at age 6 years, compared with those who wheezed during the first year of life.[47]

Moreover, children who began wheezing before age 3 and continued to wheeze at school-age had impairment in lung function that persisted at least to the teenage years.[48] In summary, children with persistent rather than transient wheezing are more likely to develop asthma. Transient wheezing may depend on mechanical factors, such as small airway size, and when these children grow older and their airway caliber increases their wheezing may resolve.

There is evidence suggesting that the immune response between these groups is different. In one study the group of children with persistent wheeze has increased eosinophils and mast cell number and eosinophilic cationic protein levels in bronchoalveolar lavage.[49] Other studies have found higher levels of serum IgE and eosinophilic cationic protein during viral infections in persistent wheezers than in transient wheezers,[50,51] and eosinophil activity in early life predicts the development of childhood asthma after hospitalization for wheezing in infancy.[51,52] These findings are suggestive of an underlying Th2-predominant immune response in children with persistent wheeze. Instead, transient wheezers may have an immune response less skewed toward a Th2 differentiation and other mechanisms are important to explain their wheezing. Furthermore, in persistent wheezing, inflammatory changes and remodeling typical of asthma develop between 1 and 3 years of age and not before, emphasizing the potential importance of virus infections and probably other environmental exposures during this period.[53]

Despite RV infections being the main respiratory viral infections associated with an increased risk of subsequent development of asthma, it is likely that RV infection does not cause asthma by itself, because RV infections are very common in the general population and not all children infected by RV develop later asthma. This suggests that, in addition to early respiratory viral infections, there are other factors that contribute to asthma development, such as the viral strain that could be more "asthmagenic"; environmental factors (ie, tobacco smoke exposure and allergic sensitization during early childhood); and host factors (ie, genetic predisposition to atopy with probably impaired Th1 immunity leading to defective antiviral responses).[54,55]

For example, the barrier function of the airway epithelium is an important component of the innate immune response to respiratory viral infection. Disruption of the airway epithelium could alter host antiviral responses and increase replication of RV. This is a potential mechanism by which various environmental exposures, such as tobacco smoke and allergens, may increase viral replication and determine more severe lower respiratory illnesses.

IFN deficiencies are another potential mechanism behind the susceptibility of people with asthma to more severe RV illnesses. Bronchial epithelial cells and alveolar macrophages from subjects with atopic asthma infected in vitro with RV produce less IFN-β and IFN-λ compared with control subjects and this is associated with increased RV replication,[33,34] and peripheral blood cells from patients with atopic asthma, when exposed to respiratory viruses, produce lower levels of IFN-α.[56] Studies have linked reduced peripheral blood IFN-γ responses at first months of life to an increased risk of wheezing in school-age children.[57]

BACTERIAL INFECTIONS AND INCREASED RISK OF DEVELOPMENT OF ASTHMA

There is some evidence to support a role for chronic bacterial infection or colonization of the lower airways with an increased risk of development of asthma, but it is also possible that a subject with altered immune function, biased toward atopy, may have altered host defenses that increase susceptibility to bacterial infections and an increased risk of developing asthma.[58,59] Indeed, there is evidence of impaired IFN responses in patients with atopic asthma to bacterial polysaccharides[34] and of an approximately threefold increased risk of severe respiratory bacterial infections in people with asthma.[59]

The potential role of atypical bacterial infection in the pathogenesis of asthma is a subject of continuing debate. There is an increasing body of literature concerning the association between the atypical intracellular bacteria *Chlamydophila* (formerly *Chlamydia*) *pneumoniae* and *Mycoplasma pneumoniae* and asthma pathogenesis; however, many studies investigating such a link have been uncontrolled and have provided conflicting evidence, in part because of the difficulty in accurately diagnosing infection with these atypical pathogens.[60]

Using highly sensitive molecular techniques the genome of *M pneumoniae* and *C pneumoniae* are frequently detected in samples from the lower airways of patients with asthma, although their exact contribution to asthma development or persistence remains to be determined and a definitive diagnosis of infection is often difficult to obtain because of limitations with sampling and detection.[61] It has been previously reported that approximately 40% of adult subjects with acute asthma exacerbations had evidence of reactivation of *C pneumoniae* infection, and that those with evidence of reactivation had four times greater neutrophilic and eosinophilic airway inflammation.[62]

Small uncontrolled serologic studies suggest also that in a subgroup of adults with severe persistent asthma a chronic infection with *C pneumoniae* may amplify the inflammation that occurs in asthma and improves with antibiotic therapy effective against *C pneumonia*.[61] However, other studies have shown that seropositivity to *C pneumoniae* is common in older adults and does not correlate with asthma.[63,64]

Another study performed with methods (eg, culture, polymerase chain reaction [PCR]) that are more specific for persistent *C pneumoniae* infection than serology could not find any evidence of *C pneumoniae* infection in the airways of adults with stable persistent asthma.[65]

Numerous animal studies have outlined mechanisms by which these infections may promote allergic lung inflammation and airway remodeling.[61] *C pneumoniae* infection can induce allergic airway sensitization in animals modulating the action of T regulatory and dendritic cells.[66] There is evidence in animal models that chronic asymptomatic chlamydial infections may cause persistent airway inflammatory responses through innate and adaptive immune responses. Indeed, this chronic infection, through chronic antigenic stimulation, seems to promote continued specific IgE production, which causes bronchoconstriction, airway inflammation, and hyperreactivity.[66] Furthermore, the major *C pneumoniae* antigen, heat-shock protein 60, seems to be a powerful inducer of macrophage inflammatory response through the innate immune receptor complex TLR-4/MD-2.[67]

Case reports suggest the onset of persistent asthma after *M pneumoniae* infection[61] and a few studies suggest a chronic reduction of small airways function after childhood *M pneumoniae* infection.[61] A report has demonstrated that *M pneumoniae* is present by PCR (but not culture) in the lower airways (bronchoalveolar lavage or bronchial biopsies) of 9 of 18 adults with persistent asthma and only 1 of 11 control subjects.[65] In animals and human subjects during respiratory tract infections *M pneumoniae* is mainly localized to the cilia of bronchial epithelial cells.[61]

In animal studies *M pneumoniae* infection of the lungs is associated with an elevated IL-4/INF-*y* ratio and development of airway hyperresponsiveness.[68] Studies in mice have shown that allergic airway inflammation impairs antibacterial host defenses: it particularly reduces the expression of TLR-2 and the production of IL-6, which play an important role in *M pneumoniae* response,[39] and markedly reduces short palate, lung, and nasal epithelium clone 1 protein expression, contributing to persistent *Mycoplasma* infection in allergic airway disease.[58]

Animal studies have also suggested that mycoplasmic infections may contribute to neurogenic inflammation in the airways.[69] Neurogenic inflammation is induced in a murine model of respiratory infection with *Mycoplasma pulmonis* and sensory nerve stimulation with capsaicin. The infected rat airway demonstrates an increased neurokinin 1 expression on blood vessels and enhanced mucus production in the trachea epithelial layer.[69] Treatment with a tetracycline antibiotic in this animal model significantly reduced the airway neurogenic inflammation and the number of infecting organisms.[69] Increased expression of substance P or neurokinin 1 receptor has been shown in the lower airway tissue, especially in the bronchial epithelium, of subjects with asthma and *M pneumoniae* infection compared with normal control subjects and subjects with asthma without *M pneumoniae* infection.[69] Subjects with asthma treated with a macrolide antibiotic active against *M pneumoniae* show reduction of substance P, neurokinin 1, and mucus in the epithelium. Reduction of epithelial neurokinin 1 expression is more prominent in subjects with asthma and *M pneumoniae* than in those without *M pneumoniae* infection.[69] However, because macrolide antibiotics have been suggested to have some direct anti-inflammatory effects, it is not possible to exclude the possibility that these results may be caused by their anti-inflammatory effect. For example, clarithromycin treatment in patients with asthma could reduce the edematous area as identified by α_2-macroglobulin staining, which may lead to airway tissue shrinkage and cause an artificial increase in the number of blood vessels.[70]

It is possible that chronic airway infection by atypical bacteria promotes persistent airway inflammation that favors progression of asthma and action of viruses or allergens. The role of antimicrobials, particularly macrolide-ketolide antibiotics, directed against atypical bacteria in asthma is still under investigation.[61,71] Animal studies, case reports, and a few small, mainly uncontrolled, pilot studies suggested initially a potential benefit of these drugs in the chronic treatment of stable persistent asthma.[61,71] In a small controlled clinical trial 6 weeks of clarithromycin therapy improves lung function in adults with asthma, but only in those subjects with positive PCR findings for *M pneumoniae* or *C pneumonia*.[72]

However, more recently in a large controlled clinical trial, adding clarithromycin to fluticasone in adults with mild-to-moderate persistent asthma that was suboptimally controlled by low-dose inhaled glucocorticoids alone did not further improve asthma control. Although there is an improvement in airway hyperresponsiveness with clarithromycin, this benefit is not accompanied by improvements in other secondary outcomes.[73] In another controlled clinical trial performed in a subgroup subjects with asthma with serologic evidence of *C pneumoniae* infection, 6 weeks of treatment with roxithromycin led to an initial improvement in asthma control but this benefit is not sustained at 3 and 6 months after the end of treatment, where differences between the two groups are not significant.[74] Furthermore, in another controlled clinical trial azithromycin has not been an effective inhaled corticosteroid-sparing agent in children with moderate-to-severe persistent asthma.[75]

In analyzing the results of the controlled clinical trials using antibacterial agents for the treatment of chronic asthma it should also be noted that macrolide-ketolide antibiotics have been suggested to have in vitro and in vivo some direct anti-inflammatory, immunomodulatory, and antiviral effects independent from their antibacterial action.[76] Furthermore, telithromycin, like macrolides, is also a strong inhibitor of cytochrome P-450 (CYP) isoenzyme 3A4. Two inhaled glucocorticoids commonly used in clinical practice (budesonide and fluticasone) are metabolized to inactive catabolites predominantly by CYP3A enzymes in the liver. The CYP3A4 is also responsible for aliphatic oxidation of the long-acting inhaled β_2-agonist bronchodilator salmeterol, which is extensively metabolized by hydroxylation. Drug interactions may reduce CYP3A activity through inhibition or may increase metabolic activity through induction. Such interactions can expand the range of variability of its activity to about 400-fold.[77] Further controlled clinical trials are required to assess the role of these antimicrobals in the treatment of severe stable asthma.

A study has found that neonates colonized in the hypopharyngeal region with *Streptococcus pneumoniae*, *Haemophilus influenzae*, or *Moraxella catarrhalis*, or with a combination of these organisms, are at increased risk for recurrent wheeze and asthma early in life,[78] suggesting a potential role for neonatal extracellular bacteria colonization of the upper airways in modulating the risk of developing asthma. This interesting new area of research clearly requires more data.

Several experimental, epidemiologic, and clinical observations support the hypothesis that changes in human indigenous microbiota can be a predisposing risk factor for asthma.[79] The microbiota resides as a stable climax community. However, it is dynamic and has the ability to maintain its structure after a perturbation (resistance) and to return to its baseline structure after resistance is broken (resilience).[80] Although the adults' microbiota remains relatively stable over time, the microbiota's structure in the first months of life is strongly influenced by many environmental factors, such as antibiotic use, dietary changes, and other lifestyle differences.[81]

Chronic airway colonization by pathogenic bacteria (airway microbiota) may directly play a role in the pathogenesis of chronic asthma. Recent studies using molecular analysis of the polymorphic bacterial *16S-rRNA* gene to characterize the composition of bacterial communities from the lower airways have demonstrated that the bronchial tree is not sterile, containing a mean of 2000 bacterial genomes per square centimeter surface sampled.[82] Pathogenic Proteobacteria, particularly *Haemophilus* spp., are more frequent in bronchi of adults with asthma than control subjects and there is a significant increase in Proteobacteria in children with asthma. Conversely, Bacteroidetes, particularly *Prevotella* spp., are more frequent in control subjects than people with asthma.[82] Compared with control subjects, 16S ribosomal RNA amplicon concentrations (an index of bacterial burden) and bacterial diversity are significantly higher among patients with asthma. Furthermore, the relative abundance of particular phylotypes, including members of the Comamonadaceae, Sphingomonadaceae, Oxalobacteraceae, and other bacterial families, are highly correlated with the degree of bronchial hyperresponsiveness of the patient with asthma.[83]

The highest concentration of microbes on the mucosal surface in the human body is in the gastrointestinal tract, and this "gut microbiota" is also thought to modulate the risk of developing asthma. In epidemiologic and clinical studies there is a correlation between an alteration in the fecal microbiota and the risk of developing asthma,[79,81] and early childhood antibiotic use slightly increases the risk of later development of asthma.[84]

There is evidence for the perinatal programing of asthma by the gastrointestinal microbiome.[85] Physiologic gastrointestinal microflora dominated by lactic acid bacteria is crucial for the maturation and proper functioning of the human immune system. Gut microbiota play a central role in the maintenance of oral and airway tolerance, because they seem tightly linked.[85] The colonization of the intestine begins during the birthing process and these commensal bacteria play an important role in shaping the immune system during infancy.[85] Gut microbes induce regulatory T cells that help guide the host's Th1/Th2 balance, keeping resident dendritic cells in an immature or noninflammatory state.[85] Infants who develop asthma probably harbor a distinct gut microbiota. In particular, the pathogen *Clostridium difficile* has been associated with increased future risk of asthma.[86]

Caesarean delivery, breastfeeding, probiotics, and antibiotics are the main modifiers of infant gut microbiota in the development of asthma. The association between caesarean delivery and increased risk of developing asthma in children is controversial.[87] Caesarean delivery may prevent exposure to maternal fecal microbes, resulting in less intestinal colonization by *Bifidobacterium* and *Bacteroides* and increased colonization by *C difficile*, and this effect persist for years.[88]

Breastfeeding protects against recurrent wheeze and asthma in later childhood; however, these benefits may not apply when the nursing mother has atopy.[85] Interestingly, the milk of mothers with atopy contains significantly lower amounts of *Bifidobacterium* compared with nonallergic mothers and this may increase the risk of asthma later in childhood.[89]

Direct and indirect (infants born to mothers who received antibiotics during pregnancy or while breastfeeding) early exposure to antibiotics may suppress commensal gut bacteria and permit the emergence of asthma-associated pathogens, such as *C. difficile*,[90] and these perturbations could last for years.[91] Two recent studies have found that this association is limited to nonatopic predisposed children,[92] probably because infants of mothers with atopy inherit low levels of commensal bacteria[89] and then antibiotic exposure would be less disruptive on commensal gut bacteria. However, in childhood, the antibiotic treatment is often prescribed in response to respiratory infections,[84] suggesting that respiratory infections and not antibiotic usage may increase the risk of asthma development.

Finally, studies have shown that administration of probiotics to pregnant women, nursing mothers, or newborns can influence the composition of gut microbiota.[93] In animal studies direct and indirect supplementation of probiotics is able to attenuate allergic airway responses.[94] However, the results of the controlled clinical trials in humans have been highly variable.[95] Probiotic supplementation may have clinical benefits for school-age children with asthma. Many more good-quality studies are needed to resolve this issue.

SUMMARY

There are increasing fascinating data to support the "hygiene" and "microbiota" hypotheses of a protective role of infections (mainly viral and bacterial, but also helminthic) in modulating the risk of subsequent development of asthma. However, there is less evidence that respiratory infections can actually cause the development of asthma. There is some evidence that RV respiratory infections are associated with the development of asthma, particularly in childhood, whereas these infections in later life seem to have a weaker association with the development of asthma. The role of bacterial infections in chronic asthma remains unclear, but there are emerging data for a potential role of M pneumoniae and C pneumoniae and gut microbiota in increasing the risk of the development of asthma and in modulating the degree of asthma control.

ACKNOWLEDGMENTS

The Section of Respiratory Diseases of the University of Ferrara - Italy - received unrestricted grants for research from the Chiesi Foundation, Parma, Italy.

REFERENCES

1. Global Initiative for Asthma. Global strategy for Asthma Management and Prevention. NHLBI/WHO Workshop report 2002. NHI Publication 02-3659. Last update 2011. Available at: http://www.ginasthma.com. Accessed July 10, 2012.
2. Barnes PJ, Chung KF, Page CP. Inflammatory mediators of asthma: an update. Pharmacol Rev 1998;50:515–96.
3. Contoli M, Baraldo S, Marku B, et al. Fixed airflow obstruction due to asthma or chronic obstructive pulmonary disease: 5-year follow-up. J Allergy Clin Immunol 2010;125:830–7.
4. Maestrelli P, Caramori G, Franco F, et al. Definition, clinical features, investigations and differential diagnosis in asthma. In: Kay AB, Bousquet J, Holt P, et al, editors. Allergy and allergic disease, vol. 2, 2nd edition. London: Blackwell; 2008. p. 1597–620.
5. Barnes KC. Genetic studies of the etiology of asthma. Proc Am Thorac Soc 2011;8:143–8.
6. Torgerson DG, Ampleford EJ, Chiu GY, et al. Meta-analysis of genome-wide association studies of asthma in ethnically diverse North American populations. Nat Genet 2011;43:887–92.
7. Mallia P, Contoli M, Caramori G, et al. Exacerbations of asthma and chronic obstructive pulmonary disease (COPD): focus on virus induced exacerbations. Curr Pharm Des 2007;13:73–97.
8. Strachan DP. Family size, infection and atopy: the first decade of the "hygiene hypothesis." Thorax 2000;55(Suppl 1):S2–10.
9. von Mutius E. Allergies, infections and the hygiene hypothesis: the epidemiological evidence. Immunobiology 2007;212:433–9.

10. Ball TM, Castro-Rodriguez JA, Griffith KA, et al. Siblings, day-care attendance, and the risk of asthma and wheezing during childhood. N Engl J Med 2000;343: 538–43.

11. Oddy WH, de Klerk NH, Sly PD, et al. The effects of respiratory infections, atopy, and breastfeeding on childhood asthma. Eur Respir J 2002;19:899–905.

12. Holt PG. Postnatal maturation of immune competence during infancy and childhood. Pediatr Allergy Immunol 1995;6:59–70.

13. Prescott SL, Macaubas C, Smallacombe T, et al. Development of allergen-specific T-cell memory in atopic and normal children. Lancet 1999;353:196–200.

14. Tschernig T, Debertin AS, Paulsen F, et al. Dendritic cells in the mucosa of the human trachea are not regularly found in the first year of life. Thorax 2001;56: 427–31.

15. von Mutius E. A fascinating look at the world with a new microscope. J Allergy Clin Immunol 2012;129:1202–3.

16. Heederik D, von Mutius E. Does diversity of environmental microbial exposure matter for the occurrence of allergy and asthma? J Allergy Clin Immunol 2012;130:44–50.

17. Herbst T, Sichelstiel A, Schar C, et al. Dysregulation of allergic airway inflammation in the absence of microbial colonization. Am J Respir Crit Care Med 2011; 184:198–205.

18. Oyama N, Sudo N, Sogawa H, et al. Antibiotic use during infancy promotes a shift in the T(h)1/T(h)2 balance toward T(h)2-dominant immunity in mice. J Allergy Clin Immunol 2001;107:153–9.

19. Brand S, Teich R, Dicke T, et al. Epigenetic regulation in murine offspring as a novel mechanism for transmaternal asthma protection induced by microbes. J Allergy Clin Immunol 2011;128:618–25.

20. Cooper PJ, Barreto ML, Rodrigues LC. Human allergy and geohelminth infections: a review of the literature and a proposed conceptual model to guide the investigation of possible causal associations. Br Med Bull 2006;79–80: 203–18.

21. Trujillo-Vargas CM, Werner-Klein M, Wohlleben G, et al. Helminth-derived products inhibit the development of allergic responses in mice. Am J Respir Crit Care Med 2007;175:336–44.

22. Erb KJ. Helminths, allergic disorders and IgE-mediated immune responses: where do we stand? Eur J Immunol 2007;37:1170–3.

23. Pochanke V, Koller S, Dayer R, et al. Identification and characterization of a novel antigen from the nematode *Nippostrongylus brasiliensis* recognized by specific IgE. Eur J Immunol 2007;37:1275–84.

24. Scrivener S, Yemaneberhan H, Zebenigus M, et al. Independent effects of intestinal parasite infection and domestic allergen exposure on risk of wheeze in Ethiopia: a nested case-control study. Lancet 2001;358:1493–9.

25. Mortimer K, Brown A, Feary J, et al. Dose-ranging study for trials of therapeutic infection with *Necator americanus* in humans. Am J Trop Med Hyg 2006;75: 914–20.

26. Feary JR, Venn AJ, Mortimer K, et al. Experimental hookworm infection: a randomized placebo-controlled trial in asthma. Clin Exp Allergy 2010;40:299–306.

27. Nystad W, Skrondal A, Magnus P. Day care attendance, recurrent respiratory tract infections and asthma. Int J Epidemiol 1999;28:882–7.

28. Nafstad P, Brunekreef B, Skrondal A, et al. Early respiratory infections, asthma, and allergy: 10-year follow-up of the Oslo Birth Cohort. Pediatrics 2005;116: e255–62.

29. Castro-Rodriguez JA, Holberg CJ, Wright AL, et al. Association of radiologically ascertained pneumonia before age 3 year with asthmalike symptoms and pulmonary function during childhood: a prospective study. Am J Respir Crit Care Med 1999;159:1891–7.

30. Dakhama A, Lee YM, Gelfand EW. Virus-induced airway dysfunction: pathogenesis and biomechanisms. Pediatr Infect Dis J 2005;24:S159–69.

31. Papadopoulos NG, Gourgiotis D, Javadyan A, et al. Does respiratory syncytial virus subtype influences the severity of acute bronchiolitis in hospitalized infants? Respir Med 2004;98:879–82.

32. Rosenthal LA, Avila PC, Heymann PW, et al. Viral respiratory tract infections and asthma: the course ahead. J Allergy Clin Immunol 2010;125:1212–7.

33. Wark PA, Johnston SL, Bucchieri F, et al. Asthmatic bronchial epithelial cells have a deficient innate immune response to infection with rhinovirus. J Exp Med 2005;201:937–47.

34. Contoli M, Message SD, Laza-Stanca V, et al. Role of deficient type III interferon-lambda production in asthma exacerbations. Nat Med 2006;12:1023–6.

35. Psarras S, Papadopoulos NG, Johnston SL. Pathogenesis of respiratory syncytial virus bronchiolitis-related wheezing. Paediatr Respir Rev 2004;5(Suppl A): S179–84.

36. Dakhama A, Lee YM, Ohnishi H, et al. Virus-specific IgE enhances airway responsiveness on reinfection with respiratory syncytial virus in newborn mice. J Allergy Clin Immunol 2009;123:138–45.

37. Culley FJ, Pollott J, Openshaw PJ. Age at first viral infection determines the pattern of T cell-mediated disease during reinfection in adulthood. J Exp Med 2002;196:1381–6.

38. Sigurs N, Aljassim F, Kjellman B, et al. Asthma and allergy patterns over 18 years after severe RSV bronchiolitis in the first year of life. Thorax 2010;65: 1045–52.

39. Wu P, Dupont WD, Griffin MR, et al. Evidence of a causal role of winter virus infection during infancy in early childhood asthma. Am J Respir Crit Care Med 2008;178:1123–9.

40. Stein RT, Sherrill D, Morgan WJ, et al. Respiratory syncytial virus in early life and risk of wheeze and allergy by age 13 years. Lancet 1999;354:541–5.

41. Taussig LM, Wright AL, Holberg CJ, et al. Tucson Children's Respiratory Study: 1980 to present. J Allergy Clin Immunol 2003;111:661–75.

42. Blanco-Quiros A, Gonzalez H, Arranz E, et al. Decreased interleukin-12 levels in umbilical cord blood in children who developed acute bronchiolitis. Pediatr Pulmonol 1999;28:175–80.

43. Baldini M, Lohman IC, Halonen M, et al. A polymorphism* in the 5' flanking region of the CD14 gene is associated with circulating soluble CD14 levels and with total serum immunoglobulin E. Am J Respir Cell Mol Biol 1999;20: 976–83.

44. Sumino K, Tucker J, Shahab M, et al. Antiviral IFN-gamma responses of monocytes at birth predict respiratory tract illness in the first year of life. J Allergy Clin Immunol 2012;129:1267–73.

45. Papadopoulos NG, Moustaki M, Tsolia M, et al. Association of rhinovirus infection with increased disease severity in acute bronchiolitis. Am J Respir Crit Care Med 2002;165:1285–9.

46. Miller EK, Williams JV, Gebretsadik T, et al. Host and viral factors associated with severity of human rhinovirus-associated infant respiratory tract illness. J Allergy Clin Immunol 2011;127:883–91.

47. Jackson DJ, Gangnon RE, Evans MD, et al. Wheezing rhinovirus illnesses in early life predict asthma development in high-risk children. Am J Respir Crit Care Med 2008;178:667–72.
48. Morgan WJ, Stern DA, Sherrill DL, et al. Outcome of asthma and wheezing in the first 6 years of life: follow-up through adolescence. Am J Respir Crit Care Med 2005;172:1253–8.
49. Ennis M, Turner G, Schock BC, et al. Inflammatory mediators in bronchoalveolar lavage samples from children with and without asthma. Clin Exp Allergy 1999; 29:362–6.
50. Martinez FD, Stern DA, Wright AL, et al. Differential immune responses to acute lower respiratory illness in early life and subsequent development of persistent wheezing and asthma. J Allergy Clin Immunol 1998;102:915–20.
51. Koller DY, Wojnarowski C, Herkner KR, et al. High levels of eosinophil cationic protein in wheezing infants predict the development of asthma. J Allergy Clin Immunol 1997;99:752–6.
52. Hyvarinen MK, Kotaniemi-Syrjanen A, Reijonen TM, et al. Eosinophil activity in infants hospitalized for wheezing and risk of persistent childhood asthma. Pediatr Allergy Immunol 2010;21:96–103.
53. Saglani S, Malmstrom K, Pelkonen AS, et al. Airway remodeling and inflammation in symptomatic infants with reversible airflow obstruction. Am J Respir Crit Care Med 2005;171:722–7.
54. Miller EK, Edwards KM, Weinberg GA, et al. A novel group of rhinoviruses is associated with asthma hospitalizations. J Allergy Clin Immunol 2009;123:98–104.
55. Message SD, Laza-Stanca V, Mallia P, et al. Rhinovirus-induced lower respiratory illness is increased in asthma and related to virus load and Th1/2 cytokine and IL-10 production. Proc Natl Acad Sci U S A 2008;105:13562–7.
56. Bufe A, Gehlhar K, Grage-Griebenow E, et al. Atopic phenotype in children is associated with decreased virus-induced interferon-alpha release. Int Arch Allergy Immunol 2002;127:82–8.
57. Stern DA, Guerra S, Halonen M, et al. Low IFN-gamma production in the first year of life as a predictor of wheeze during childhood. J Allergy Clin Immunol 2007;120:835–41.
58. Chu HW, Thaikoottathil J, Rino JG, et al. Function and regulation of SPLUNC1 protein in *Mycoplasma* infection and allergic inflammation. J Immunol 2007; 179:3995–4002.
59. Talbot TR, Hartert TV, Mitchel E, et al. Asthma as a risk factor for invasive pneumococcal disease. N Engl J Med 2005;352:2082–90.
60. Johnston SL, Martin RJ. *Chlamydophila pneumoniae* and *Mycoplasma pneumoniae*: a role in asthma pathogenesis? Am J Respir Crit Care Med 2005;172: 1078–89.
61. Metz G, Kraft M. Effects of atypical infections with *Mycoplasma* and *Chlamydia* on asthma. Immunol Allergy Clin North Am 2010;30:575–85.
62. Wark PA, Johnston SL, Simpson JL, et al. *Chlamydia pneumoniae* immunoglobulin A reactivation and airway inflammation in acute asthma. Eur Respir J 2002;20: 834–40.
63. Mills GD, Lindeman JA, Fawcett JP, et al. *Chlamydia pneumoniae* serological status is not associated with asthma in children or young adults. Int J Epidemiol 2000;29:280–4.
64. Routes JM, Nelson HS, Noda JA, et al. Lack of correlation between *Chlamydia pneumoniae* antibody titers and adult-onset asthma. J Allergy Clin Immunol 2000;105:391–2.

65. Kraft M, Cassell GH, Henson JE, et al. Detection of *Mycoplasma pneumoniae* in the airways of adults with chronic asthma. Am J Respir Crit Care Med 1998;158: 998–1001.

66. Crother TR, Schroder NW, Karlin J, et al. *Chlamydia pneumoniae* infection induced allergic airway sensitization is controlled by regulatory T-cells and plasmacytoid dendritic cells. PLoS One 2011;6:e20784.

67. Bulut Y, Faure E, Thomas L, et al. Chlamydial heat shock protein 60 activates macrophages and endothelial cells through Toll-like receptor 4 and MD2 in a MyD88-dependent pathway. J Immunol 2002;168:1435–40.

68. Koh YY, Park Y, Lee HJ, et al. Levels of interleukin-2, interferon-gamma, and interleukin-4 in bronchoalveolar lavage fluid from patients with *Mycoplasma pneumoniae*: implication of tendency toward increased immunoglobulin E production. Pediatrics 2001;107:E39.

69. Chu HW, Kraft M, Krause JE, et al. Substance P and its receptor neurokinin 1 expression in asthmatic airways. J Allergy Clin Immunol 2000;106:713–22.

70. Chu HW, Kraft M, Rex MD, et al. Evaluation of blood vessels and edema in the airways of asthma patients: regulation with clarithromycin treatment. Chest 2001;120:416–22.

71. Good JT Jr, Rollins DR, Martin RJ. Macrolides in the treatment of asthma. Curr Opin Pulm Med 2012;18:76–84.

72. Kraft M, Cassell GH, Pak J, et al. *Mycoplasma pneumoniae* and *Chlamydia pneumoniae* in asthma: effect of clarithromycin. Chest 2002;121:1782–8.

73. Sutherland ER, King TS, Icitovic N, et al. A trial of clarithromycin for the treatment of suboptimally controlled asthma. J Allergy Clin Immunol 2010;126:747–53.

74. Black PN, Blasi F, Jenkins CR, et al. Trial of roxithromycin in subjects with asthma and serological evidence of infection with *Chlamydia pneumoniae*. Am J Respir Crit Care Med 2001;164:536–41.

75. Strunk RC, Bacharier LB, Phillips BR, et al. Azithromycin or montelukast as inhaled corticosteroid-sparing agents in moderate-to-severe childhood asthma study. J Allergy Clin Immunol 2008;122:1138–44.

76. Zarogoulidis P, Papanas N, Kioumis I, et al. Macrolides: from in vitro anti-inflammatory and immunomodulatory properties to clinical practice in respiratory diseases. Eur J Clin Pharmacol 2012;68:479–503.

77. Caramori G, Papi A. Telithromycin in acute exacerbations of asthma. N Engl J Med 2006;355:96.

78. Bisgaard H, Hermansen MN, Buchvald F, et al. Childhood asthma after bacterial colonization of the airway in neonates. N Engl J Med 2007;357:1487–95.

79. Noverr MC, Huffnagle GB. The 'microflora hypothesis' of allergic diseases. Clin Exp Allergy 2005;35:1511–20.

80. Allison SD, Martiny JB. Colloquium paper: resistance, resilience, and redundancy in microbial communities. Proc Natl Acad Sci U S A 2008;105(Suppl 1):11512–9.

81. Murgas Torrazza R, Neu J. The developing intestinal microbiome and its relationship to health and disease in the neonate. J Perinatol 2011;31(Suppl 1): S29–34.

82. Hilty M, Burke C, Pedro H, et al. Disordered microbial communities in asthmatic airways. PLoS One 2010;5:e8578.

83. Huang YJ, Nelson CE, Brodie EL, et al. Airway microbiota and bronchial hyper-responsiveness in patients with suboptimally controlled asthma. J Allergy Clin Immunol 2011;127:372–81.

84. Penders J, Kummeling I, Thijs C. Infant antibiotic use and wheeze and asthma risk: a systematic review and meta-analysis. Eur Respir J 2011;38:295–302.

85. Azad MB, Kozyrskyj AL. Perinatal programming of asthma: the role of gut microbiota. Clin Dev Immunol 2012;2012:932072.
86. van Nimwegen FA, Penders J, Stobberingh EE, et al. Mode and place of delivery, gastrointestinal microbiota, and their influence on asthma and atopy. J Allergy Clin Immunol 2011;128:948–55.
87. Thavagnanam S, Fleming J, Bromley A, et al. A meta-analysis of the association between caesarean section and childhood asthma. Clin Exp Allergy 2008;38:629–33.
88. Salminen S, Gibson GR, McCartney AL, et al. Influence of mode of delivery on gut microbiota composition in seven year old children. Gut 2004;53:1388–9.
89. Gronlund MM, Gueimonde M, Laitinen K, et al. Maternal breast-milk and intestinal bifidobacteria guide the compositional development of the *Bifidobacterium* microbiota in infants at risk of allergic disease. Clin Exp Allergy 2007;37:1764–72.
90. Tanaka S, Kobayashi T, Songjinda P, et al. Influence of antibiotic exposure in the early postnatal period on the development of intestinal microbiota. FEMS Immunol Med Microbiol 2009;56:80–7.
91. Jernberg C, Lofmark S, Edlund C, et al. Long-term ecological impacts of antibiotic administration on the human intestinal microbiota. ISME J 2007;1:56–66.
92. Risnes KR, Belanger K, Murk W, et al. Antibiotic exposure by 6 months and asthma and allergy at 6 years: findings in a cohort of 1,401 US children. Am J Epidemiol 2011;173:310–8.
93. Kukkonen K, Savilahti E, Haahtela T, et al. Probiotics and prebiotic galacto-oligosaccharides in the prevention of allergic diseases: a randomized, double-blind, placebo-controlled trial. J Allergy Clin Immunol 2007;119:192–8.
94. Blumer N, Sel S, Virna S, et al. Perinatal maternal application of *Lactobacillus rhamnosus* GG suppresses allergic airway inflammation in mouse offspring. Clin Exp Allergy 2007;37:348–57.
95. Forsythe P. Probiotics and lung diseases. Chest 2011;139:901–8.

Biomarkers in Asthma
A Real Hope to Better Manage Asthma

Serpil C. Erzurum, MD[a],*, Benjamin M. Gaston, MD[b]

KEYWORDS

- Asthma • Biomarkers • Asthma management

KEY POINTS

- Diagnosis and treatment of asthma are currently based on assessment of patient symptoms and physiologic tests of airway reactivity.
- This article provides an overview of blood, urine and airway biomarkers that can provide information on airway inflammation and asthma severity.
- Mechanistic biomarkers that identify pathologic pathways also provide critical insight for new therapeutic approaches for asthma.

THE CLINICAL NEED FOR BIOMARKERS TO INFORM THE CARE OF PATIENTS WITH ASTHMA

Asthma is defined as reversible airflow obstruction in the setting of airway inflammation. Asthma prevalence increased dramatically between 1970 and 2000, with more than 22 million people, of whom over 4.8 million are children, now living with asthma in the United States.[1,2] The increase of asthma has been variously ascribed to improved hygiene worldwide, acetaminophen use, increased exposure to allergens and pollution, and/or increased transmission of respiratory viruses.[3] This epidemic has occurred against a backdrop of a variety of genetic, biochemical, and immunologic host characteristics that substantially affect asthma phenotype.

This article originally appeared in Clinics in Chest Medicine, Volume 33, Issue 3, September 2012.

Funding sources: Dr Erzurum: National Heart Lung Blood Institute, American Asthma Foundation, Cardiovascular Medical Research Education Foundation, and Asthmatx Inc. Dr Gaston: National Heart Lung and Blood Institute: P01HL101871; U10HL109250; R01 HL59337.

Conflict of interests: Dr Erzurum: None. Dr Gaston: Intellectual property and minority shareholder in Respiratory Research, Inc, and In Airbase Pharmaceuticals. Intellectual property in N30 Pharma.

[a] Department of Pathobiology, Lerner Research Institute, and the Respiratory Institute, Cleveland Clinic Lerner College of Medicine-CWRU, 9500 Euclid Avenue, NC22, Cleveland, OH 44195-0001, USA; [b] Department of Pediatric Pulmonary Medicine, University of Virginia School of Medicine, Box 800386, UVA HSC, Charlottesville, VA 22908, USA

* Corresponding author.

E-mail address: erzurus@ccf.org

Currently, standard clinical practice relies on patient history of symptoms and the measure of bronchial obstruction and reactivity, which are surrogates of the inflammatory and biochemical processes that give rise to the inflammation underlying all asthma.[4] For example, the phenotype of severe asthma, which comprises up to 5% of patients with asthma, is based on a compilation of criteria, the most important of which is the documentation of the lack of clinical treatment response.[5,6] Asthma treatment is directed equally toward reversing bronchoconstriction and treating airway inflammation. Common, noninvasive measures of airflow are usually able to quantitate the efficacy of the treatment of bronchoconstriction in adults. However, commonly available methods do not precisely measure the biology of inflammation underlying the bronchoconstriction. Further, the care of children with asthma is often inadequate because of the lack of bronchial obstruction on lung function tests even when symptoms are severe, and the reluctance to prescribe corticosteroids because of actual or perceived associated morbidities in children.[7] Thus, quantifiable noninvasive biomarkers that are informative for asthma control and, optimally, for assessing the pathobiologic pathways leading to the chronic airway inflammation in a specific patient will be of clinical utility in designing successful personalized treatment plans.

Based on this rationale, the National Institutes of Health and the Agency for Health Care Quality Research have launched efforts to promote the use of biomarkers in clinical studies of new therapies of asthma and ultimately in the evaluation of routine clinical care. A recent National Heart, Lung, and Blood Institute (NHLBI) report identifies biomarkers, most of which assess atopic inflammation, such as the multiallergen screen, sputum and blood eosinophil numbers, serum IgE, exhaled nitric oxide, and urine leukotrienes.[8] Although asthma tends to be particularly problematic in patients with allergies, and more than 40% of some populations suffer from allergies, allergic diathesis genes do not seem to be uniquely associated with asthma.[2,6,9] Thus, whatever is driving the asthma epidemic, the asthma syndrome has affected a tremendous spectrum of individuals with diverse immunologic and biochemical responses.[9,10] This heterogeneity in the human population has resulted in a heterogeneity among asthma phenotypes.[10–12] Therefore, biomarker tests were recently developed and extended to identify and quantitate specific pathways of inflammation to identify specific asthma phenotypes, particularly those amenable to biologically based antiinflammatory therapy. The benefit of a noninvasive biomarker in assessing therapeutic strategies is clear; the alternative is inspection and biopsy of the airway using invasive bronchoscopy.[13]

The mechanism-based biomarker approach avoids the limitations that occur with unbiased genotyping and phenotyping approaches.[10] For example, unbiased genetic analyses did not reveal a unifying asthma gene. Rather, asthma susceptibility genes are manifest in populations depending on environmental exposures, such as secondhand cigarette smoke.[14] Similarly, unbiased asthma clinical phenotypes, although clearly revealing the heterogeneity of asthma,[15] require association with underlying pathobiologic mechanisms for clinically meaningful use. In a large asthma population of nonsevere and severe asthma, nonbiased hierarchical cluster analysis of clinical variables, such as age at asthma onset, duration of episodes, gender, race, lung functions, atopy, and questionnaire data, identified three phenotype clusters that contained patients with the most severe asthma.[15] Similar cluster analyses of children confirmed heterogeneity in childhood severe asthma.[16] This variety supports that asthma encompasses a range of underlying biochemical and immunologic disorders. Thus, an informed biochemical and pathophysiologic approach is most likely to lead directly to clinical applications. This article describes biomarkers and their potential use to stratify patients into medically meaningful unique asthma phenotypes (**Table 1**).

THE EOSINOPHILIC OR T-HELPER TYPE 2 HIGH INFLAMMATION PHENOTYPE: SPUTUM EOSINOPHILS, URINARY 3-BROMOTYROSINE, AND PERIOSTIN

Asthma phenotyping was first performed based on atopic status (ie, classification of asthma as extrinsic allergic or intrinsic nonallergic).[9] Allergic asthma is common, and documentation of this phenotype has been helpful in avoiding allergen triggers and considering immunologic-based therapies. Classification as atopic asthma, which is typified by interleukin (IL)-4, IL-5, and IL-13 cytokines, has traditionally used standard clinical tests, including circulating numbers of eosinophils and total and allergen-specific IgE. These biomarkers are used in planning immunotherapy and anti-IgE therapy. In extension of these biomarkers, several groups describe that the number of eosinophils in sputum is closely related to airway obstruction and hyperresponsiveness.[17–19] Exciting early data suggested that sputum eosinophils predict asthma control and loss of control, particularly in children who predominantly experience atopic asthma.[20,21] The presence of more than 2% eosinophils in sputum has been used to define the eosinophilic or atopic asthma phenotype, which is also usually corticosteroid-responsive.[22] A recent study of severe asthma validates that sputum eosinophils can identify individuals with poor asthma control, and greater health care use[23]; however, the test requires sputum induction, specialized processing of the sputum sample, and an experienced cytotechnologist for accurate counting, all of which have limited the use of sputum eosinophils in general clinical care. More recently, Woodruff and colleagues[24] further identified a T-helper type 2 (Th2)–high inflammation phenotype based on a combination of biomarkers, which include the presence of high serum IgE (>100 ng/mL), blood eosinophilia (>0.14 x 10^9 eosinophils/L), and high sputum eosinophils.[25] The use of microarrays has also identified a Th2-high blood biomarker, periostin, which is an IL-13–inducible protein produced by the airway epithelium. The use of periostin as a biomarker of the Th2-high phenotype to select patients who benefitted the most from treatment with an inhibitor of IL-13[25] provided a proof of concept that biomarkers may be used to stratify patients for biologic-based therapies. Conversely, the data also validate the important point that a substantial number of patients with asthma have non–Th2-predominant inflammation.

A high sputum eosinophil count correlates with a high fractional excretion of NO (FeNO) in the exhaled breath, which is often suggested as a biomarker of inflammation. However, low FeNO has been found to be a much better predictor of a noneosinophilic phenotype than a high FeNO is for an eosinophilic phenotype. Hence, FeNO should be considered as a unique metabolic biomarker of asthma, as discussed later. However, eosinophils generate high levels of reactive oxygen species,[26] and the eosinophil peroxidase is unique in its ability to convert hydrogen peroxide to hypobromous acid,[27,28] which oxidizes tyrosines to 3-bromotyrosine (BrY) (**Fig. 1**). BrY is highly stable and can be measured noninvasively in urine as a biomarker highly specific for eosinophil activation.[29,30] Because BrY is a biomarker of eosinophil activation, its levels increase dramatically after experimental or clinical asthma exacerbations,[29] and early studies show that urinary BrY in children with asthma seems highly correlated with asthma control and predicts risk of asthma exacerbations.[31] Studies are needed to evaluate the relationship of BrY and periostin in the Th2-high phenotype, but given that BrY is unrelated to IgE or blood eosinophils, these biomarkers may be nonredundant and possibly complementary in predicting asthma phenotypes for clinical treatments.

Table 1
Biomarkers of asthma

Biomarker Phenotype	Pathogenetic Pathways	Implications for Mechanistic Management
In blood		
Eosinophils[a]	Atopic; excessive Th2 pathways activation	Immunotherapy depending on clinical signs and symptoms of asthma
IgE[a]	Atopic; excessive Th2 pathways activation	Immunotherapy depending on clinical signs and symptoms of asthma
Allergen specific IgE[a]	Atopic; excessive Th2 pathways activation	Avoidance of allergens, immunotherapy, anti-IgE therapies
Periostin	IL-13–driven asthma (Th2 pathway gene)	May benefit from biologic blockade of IL-4/IL-13 receptors
Superoxide dismutase (SOD)	Oxidative and nitrative inflammation and injury leading to reducing-oxidizing (redox) imbalance and loss of SOD activity	Associated with greater airflow obstruction and bronchial hyperreactivity; evaluate environmental oxidative exposures, such as secondhand smoke and air pollutants; may benefit from redox regulation in the future
CD34+CD133+ progenitor cells	Circulating myeloid progenitors are increased in asthma, and increase further with exacerbations; differentiate into proangiogenic monocytic cells and mast cells in the airway	Promote remodeling and inflammation in the airway; anti-cKIT–directed therapies to decrease bone marrow precursors
Airway-derived		
Sputum eosinophils	Atopic asthma; excessive Th2 pathways activation	Avoidance of allergens, Immunotherapy, anti-IgE therapies
Exhaled NO (FeNO)[a]	High: excessive iNOS; when used with GSNO challenge, may indicate greater GSNO reductase or low pH	Risk for exacerbation; may need to step up antiinflammatory therapies (eg, corticosteroids decrease iNOS)
	Low or normal: limited arginine bioavailability because of consumption by arginases (activated by Th2 cytokines) or competition by methylarginines (when dimethylarginine dimethylamino hydrolase [DDAH] activity is low)	Metabolic abnormalities in arginine metabolism

Exhaled breath condensate (EBC) pH and formate	Airway acidification because of infection, low airway glutaminase, or, when formate is high, greater activity of GSNO reductase	Buffered solutions and/or glutamine inhalation
Ethyl nitrite challenge and measure of FeNO	High GSNO reductase in the airway, low levels of GSNO (loss of bronchodilator response)	Therapies to block GSNO reductase or supplement beneficial S-nitrosothiols in the airways
In urine		
Bromotyrosine (BrY)	Activation of eosinophil peroxidase for specific bromination pathways	Unstable asthma, predicts exacerbations, particularly in children; step up of antiinflammatory therapy (ie, corticosteroids)
Leukotriene E_4 (LTE_4)	Cysteinyl leukotriene pathway overactivity	Aspirin avoidance and/or desensitization; leukotriene receptor or 5-lipoxygenase inhibition
F2 isoprostanes (F2IsoP)	Nonspecific peroxidation of membrane lipids to generate F2IsoP (8-epi-$PGF_{2\alpha}$ and 2,3-dinor-8-epi-$PGF_{2\alpha}$) through excessive generation of reactive oxygen species	Nonspecific inflammation by neutrophils or eosinophils; evaluate environmental oxidative exposures, such as secondhand smoke and air pollutants; may benefit from leukotriene receptor or 5-lipoxygenase inhibition

Abbreviations: GSNO, S-nitrosoglutathione; IL, interleukin; iNOS, inducible nitric oxide synthase; NO, nitric oxide; Th2, T-helper type 2.

[a] Currently readily available to general practitioners and approved for asthma evaluation, others are not generally available or are emerging or experimental.

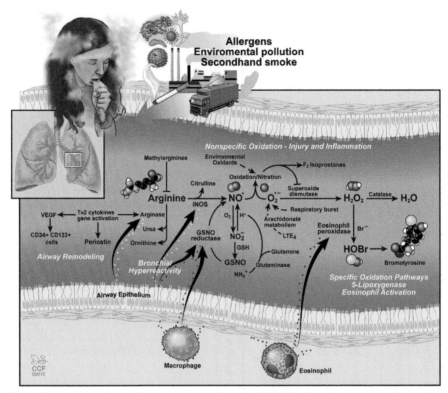

Fig. 1. Biomarkers of specific and nonspecific pathophysiologic pathways in asthma. Environmental exposures trigger and/or amplify underlying pathophysiology. *Abbreviations*: CD, cluster of differentiation; iNOS, inducible nitric oxide synthase; LTE4, leukotriene E4; TH2, T-helper 2; VEGF, vascular endothelial growth factor.

A subpopulation of patients with asthma has increased activity of the enzyme S-nitrosoglutathione (GSNO) reductase (see **Fig. 1**).[32–34] GSNO is an endogenous nitric oxide synthase (NOS) product that causes cyclic guanosine monophosphate (cGMP)–independent relaxation of human airway smooth muscle.[35,36] It can directly prevent actin-myosin interaction[37] and can S-nitrosylate G protein–coupled kinase 2 (GRK2), tachyphylaxis induced by β_2-adrenergic agonist stimulation.[38] GSNO is broken down in vivo by GSNO reductase.[32–34,39] Antigen-sensitized mice deficient in GSNO reductase are protected from methacholine-induced increased airway resistance. Further, mice deficient in GSNO reductase are prevented from having pulmonary tachyphylaxis to isoproterenol.[33] In children with asthmatic respiratory failure, GSNO reductase activity is upregulated and GSNO levels are profoundly low,[32] creating an endogenous airway smooth muscle relaxant that is deficient in the asthmatic airway. This deficiency also exacerbates refractoriness to ß2-agonist–based treatment.

Gain-of-function single nucleotide polymorphisms (SNPs) in GSNO reductase are associated with refractory asthma in certain subpopulations. Biopsies with increased GSNO reductase expression are anatomically associated with areas of poor airflow, as analyzed with hyperpolarized xenon or helium imaging. Thus, GSNO reductase is an important mechanism in the origins of a reactive asthma phenotype, but bronchoalveolar lavage studies show that GSNO reductase activity is not increased in all patients with asthma.[34] Further, essentially no differences are seen among stable, ambulatory severe, and nonsevere asthma with regard to GSNO reductase activity (Marozkina NV, unpublished observation, 2012). How can this important subpopulation with high GSNO reductase activity be identified in the clinic to target therapy with S-nitrosoglutathione replacement and/or S-nitrosoglutathione reductase inhibition? The importance of this question is highlighted by recent evidence showing that chronic excessive inhibition of S-nitrosoglutathione reductase has the potential to be associated with the development of cancer in patients exposed to chronic nitrosative stress.[40]

The authors envision the following clinical paradigm to approach this type of question. First, the clinical disease phenotype must be identified. The clinical characteristics of patients with increased airway GSNO reductase activity must be determined, which can be done through defining the phenotype of those who are identified through biochemical analysis of bronchoscopic samples. It can also be done through SNP-wide analysis of phenotype.

Next, biomarkers that validate the biochemical abnormality should be developed. In the example of GSNO reductase, there are at least two possible biomarkers. GSNO reductase also serves as an S-formylglutathione dehydrogenase.[41,42] The product of the latter enzymatic activity is formic acid, which can be measured in breath condensate. Levels are high in a subpopulation of patients with asthma, and these seem to be the same patients as those with high GSNO reductase activity. This hypothesis requires validation.

Another approach is challenge testing. In cystic fibrosis, GSNO replacement is associated with an increase of FeNO.[43] The faster the rate of GSNO breakdown, the faster the decline of FeNO after GSNO inhalation. This principle can likely also be applied to asthma. A challenge with GSNO or a GSNO precursor is associated with an increase in FeNO. The decay rate of FeNO after GSNO inhalation can be used as a surrogate for airway GSNO reductase activity. FeNO will likely be used as a readout in challenge testing for several subpopulations, including those with low pH,[36,44] high levels of eosinophils, or high levels of GSNO reductase activity. The authors believe that the challenge test may serve as a useful paradigm for identifying treatable subpopulations.

THE REDUCING-OXIDIZING IMBALANCE PHENOTYPE: LIPID OXIDATION AND LOSS OF ANTIOXIDANT SUPEROXIDE DISMUTASE

Recruitment and activation of inflammatory cells, both eosinophils and neutrophils, causes a respiratory burst in the airways that produces reactive oxygen species and reactive nitrogen species.[45–48] Certain of these species can damage proteins via specific enzyme-catalyzed oxidations or nonspecific oxidation of susceptible molecules. For example, eosinophil peroxidase and neutrophil myeloperoxidase cause halogenation, ie, bromination and chlorination respectively, of tyrosine residues; the halogenated products serve as molecular fingerprints of eosinophilic or neutrophilic inflammation. However, peroxidation of membrane lipids occurs spontaneously and results in the F_2-isoprostanes (F_2IsoPs), 8-epi-PGF$_{2\alpha}$ and its metabolite 2,3-dinor-8-epi-PGF$_{2\alpha}$. These structurally stable products are renally excreted, making them quantifiable noninvasive biomarkers of nonspecific reducing-oxidizing (redox) imbalance and inflammation.[49–51] In support of an increase of nonspecific oxidation, urine F_2IsoPs are higher in patients with asthma than healthy controls, and urine levels rise on an allergen-induced asthma exacerbation.[49,52,53] Biomarkers of enzyme-catalyzed oxidation pathways, such as urine BrY, and nonspecific oxidation pathways, such as F_2IsoPs, allow multiple opportunities to monitor asthma control and plan appropriate treatments. For example, stepping up corticosteroid therapy may be warranted in individuals with high urine BrY, but may be less helpful in those with low or normal BrY and high urine F_2IsoPs. In the latter case, neutrophilic inflammation or environmental oxidant-mediated inflammation might be suspect.

Nonspecific oxidation events also indicate a relative inadequacy of protective antioxidants. A wide array of antioxidants are present in the airways,[54] but oxidative and nitrosative stress can overwhelm these defenses, resulting in redox imbalance and oxidative injury.[10,48] The airway contains nonenzymatic antioxidants, such as glutathione, and enzymatic antioxidants, such as superoxide dismutases (SOD) and catalase (see **Fig. 1**). Asthmatic airways have increased total glutathione levels but loss of SOD and catalase enzymic activities.[48] The loss of SOD activity is found in the airways and serum of patients with asthma, allowing the serum SOD to be used as a biomarker of redox imbalance.[48,55–60] SOD activity is inversely related to airway reactivity and airflow obstruction, with higher levels of SOD related to lower airway reactivity and better airflow.[60] Murine models of asthma confirm that SOD plays a mechanistic role in airway hyperresponsiveness and inflammation (eg, SOD transgenic mice have less allergen-induced airway inflammation and reactivity than wild-type mice).[61]

In patients with asthma and in the murine model of asthma, SOD activity loss is partly related to the oxidation of the manganese SOD (MnSOD) protein and is linked to epithelial apoptosis and airway remodeling.[60,62] Low levels of serum SOD activity was an independent biomarker for airflow obstruction in patients with severe asthma nonresponsive to corticosteroids.[59] Furthermore, secondhand smoke exposure is associated with poorer lung functions and lower levels of serum SOD activity.[58] These findings suggest that strategies aimed at restoration of normal redox balance, perhaps through the use of SOD mimetics, may help patients with noneosinophilic inflammation in whom corticosteroids may have little impact on asthma control.

THE LOW PH PHENOTYPE

During acute exacerbations of asthma, breath condensate pH is decreased.[63] This reaction is associated with decreased serum and airway activity of glutaminase, activated downstream of Th1 cytokines associated with viral asthma exacerbations, preventing airway buffering.[63,64] Decreased airway pH promotes ciliary dysfunction, mucus hypersecretion, and cough.[63–65] Recent evidence suggests that this decreased airway pH might be successfully treated with inhaled buffer.[36,44] However, most patients with stable asthma seen in day-to-day practice do not have decreased pH.[66] In the NHLBI Severe Asthma Research Program (SARP) study of 572 subjects with stable asthma, only 7% had breath condensate pH less than 6.5 at baseline. This group was characterized by prominently low FeNO, low forced expiratory volume in 1 second, high body mass index, low levels of airway eosinophils, and gastric esophageal reflux symptoms, along with other features. Because most nebulized treatments are in acidic solutions, this subpopulation of outpatients with asthma with decreased airway pH might benefit from less acidic therapy, and might even experience improvement with inhaled base.

To identify these patients, initial medical suspicion should be based on the phenotype described earlier. Patients who have a characteristic phenotype can then be diagnosed through biomarker analysis. Because nitrite has a acid dissociation constant (pKa) of 3.6 and, once protonated, dissociates to form NO, increasing airway pH decreases FeNO. Therefore, inhaled buffer followed by serial FeNO measures can be used to diagnose the low pH phenotype.[36,44] Patients with a decrease in FeNO after inhaled buffer should be those whose asthma will improve with inhaled base or glutamine supplement as a targeted therapy.

AIRWAY REMODELING PHENOTYPE: AIRWAY ANGIOGENIC BIOMARKERS

Increased number of blood vessels is universally found in asthmatic airway remodeling of children and adults.[67,68] The mouse model of asthma suggests that the switch to a proangiogenic airway and neovascularization occurs early and well in advance of eosinophilic inflammation.[69] This finding suggests that angiogenesis participates in the genesis of asthma. In fact, several lines of evidence indicate that angiogenesis and chronic inflammation are mutually supportive.[70] Inflammatory cells produce many proangiogenic factors in asthmatic lungs,[71] chief among which is vascular endo-thelial growth factor (VEGF). VEGF levels are increased in asthma bronchoalveolar lavage fluid, and related to blood vessel numbers in the mucosa.[69,71] High VEGF levels in sputum are associated with airflow obstruction, and levels of VEGF increase in sputum during an asthma attack.[67] Likewise in model systems, allergen- or virus-induced inflammation increases airway VEGF levels.[72,73] In support of a mechanistic role, VEGF overexpression in airways of transgenic mice leads to an asthma-like phenotype.[74] Mast cells and eosinophils can produce high levels of proangiogenic factors, including VEGF.[75,76] Proangiogenic factors such as VEGF cause neovascula-rization largely through effects on myeloid progenitor cell proliferation and mobilization from the bone marrow. Cell surface markers CD34 and CD133 define the subset of proangiogenic myeloid progenitors,[77,78] and can thus easily be enumerated through flow cytometric analysis. Studies identify high levels of $CD34^+CD133^+$ cells in blood of patients with asthma and show that the levels correlate with airflow obstruction. Intriguingly, this same population of $CD34^+CD133^+$ cells also contains the mast cell progenitor. Further work is needed to determine if quantitation of circulating $CD34^+CD133^+$ cells can serve as a biomarker of airway remodeling and/or mast cell numbers and types in asthma.

THE ARGININE/NO PHENOTYPE: FENO, ARGINASE, METHYLARGININES

Measure of NO in the exhaled breath has been labeled as a sensitive and reliable biomarker of airway inflammation in adults and children.[79–84] Based on this finding, the U.S. Food and Drug Administration approved FeNO for evaluating antiinflamma-tory treatment responses of patients with asthma.[84] However, FeNO exhibits a broad range of values in these patients[85]; it is useful for identifying patients characterized by the greatest airflow obstruction and most frequent use of emergency care.

Inflammation, as characteristic in asthmatic airways, results in the expression of the inducible NO synthase (iNOS).[86–88] iNOS is expressed in many airway cells, but is prominent in the airway epithelial cells, where it catalyzes the conversion of L-arginine into NO and L-citrulline[86,87] (see Fig. 1). The synthesized gaseous NO may be measured noninvasively in the exhaled breath as a biomarker of chronic airway inflam-mation induction of the iNOS.[79,80,86] Eosinophils are not necessary for iNOS produc-tion of NO, and Th2 cytokines are not essential for iNOS expression. Hence, FeNO does not uniformly track with airway eosinophils, urine BrY, or periostin. Although studies suggest that monitoring antiinflammatory therapy through FeNO is useful, it does not necessarily diminish the rate of asthma exacerbations.[81,89,90] This limitation is likely because not all inflammatory processes are reflected by FeNO measure-ments.[8,91,92] This finding supports the concept that biomarkers of asthma may be more informative when used in combination with challenge testing (ie, FeNO measures with inhalation of base or in combination with other biomarkers such as urine BrY levels). In this context, although FeNO, urine BrY, and urine F_2IsoP each are useful as a biomarker of asthma, pooled together they serve as a highly sensitive and specific biomarker panel for diagnosing asthma.[93]

Although a multitude of studies focus on the meaning of high FeNO in asthma,[29,62,86,94–97] asthma patients may often have values within the normal range (<25 parts per billion). Patients with low to normal FeNO values usually do not have eosinophilic inflammation but may still have signs of inflammation and remodeling. Low FeNO is helpful in that it suggests a phenotype that is less responsive to corticosteroids, preventing excessive medication use that may cause substantial morbidity. Patients with low FeNO may have non-Th2 inflammation and/or abnormalities in arginine metabolism and/or increased oxidative consumption of NO in the airway. Additionally, FeNO may be low because of low levels of GSNO in the airways caused by catabolism by higher than normal levels of GSNO reductase. Chronic loss of airway nitrite in the context of low airway pH leads to low baseline FeNO in the low pH phenotype.

Patients with asthma often have greater metabolism of arginine via iNOS and the arginase enzymes, which identifies a subpopulation of asthma as a disease of increased arginine catabolism[98] (see **Fig. 1**). High levels of arginase activity in asthma are often associated with increased levels of methylarginines, which are endogenous NOS inhibitors. This finding suggests that methylarginines may impact arginine availability as a substrate for iNOS.[97,99,100] Serum arginase increases during acute asthma exacerbations and decreases with improved asthma control, and is inversely related to airflow.[97,98] Studies indicate that arginase expression and activity is increased by allergen-induced gene activation in asthma, and Th2 cytokines.[86,99–105] However, oxidative stress can decrease the metabolism of methylarginines through effects on dimethylarginine dimethylaminohydrolase (DDAH).[106] This diminished metabolism of methylarginines may block iNOS and contribute to low FeNO in some patients with asthma, particularly those with severe corticosteroid-resistant asthma. Serum arginase also provides insight into mechanisms of airway remodeling.[107] Arginase regulates polyamine synthesis, which is required for DNA synthesis in cell proliferation.[108,109] Arginase also regulates precursors for the synthesis of proline, required for collagen production.[110,111] Thus, serum arginase and FeNO are unique biomarkers of inflammation in severe asthma and independent of the eosinophilic phenotype. Increased arginase is associated with low FeNO in adults with severe asthma.[98] Decreased SOD activity is also associated with low FeNO in adults with severe asthma, suggesting an oxidative consumption of NO that may lead to low normal values of FeNO (see **Fig. 1**).[98]

THE LEUKOTRIENE PHENOTYPE: LEUKOTRIENE E₄, LIPOXINS AND PROTECTANTS

Endogenous lipid mediators can help maintain tissue homeostasis, yet they can also contribute to inflammation and bronchoconstriction.[112] Leukotrienes are examples of potent proinflammatory and bronchoconstricting agents. Inhibitors of the cysteinyl leukotriene receptor and the upstream cysteinyl leukotriene synthetic enzyme, 5-lipoxygenase (5-LO), are in clinical use for asthma treatment.[113] However, many patients with asthma are not effectively treated with leukotriene receptor antagonists. Further, 5-LO inhibition can cause hepatotoxicity. Therefore, identification of asthma subpopulations in whom these specific antileukotriene agents may be effective has for some time been a focus of genetic studies in asthma. Genetic testing for polymorphisms and 5-LO has also been proposed as a screening tool for identifying responsive subpopulations.[52,114] Additionally, biomarkers have been sought, including urinary leukotrienes and FeNO, to try to identify patients who would be most responsive.[115,116]

Urine leukotriene E_4 (LTE$_4$) has been validated as a biomarker of cysteinyl leukotriene overactivity. Levels of LTE$_4$ increase with acute asthma attacks and with aspirin-exacerbated respiratory disease, and decrease with cysteinyl leukotriene synthesis blockade but not with corticosteroids.[117–124] Although the use of therapies in the leukotriene pathway are valuable, lack of widespread availability of clinical testing for LTE$_4$ limit the use of this biomarker in optimizing asthma therapies. Specific lipid mediators can also prevent airway inflammation. For example, lipoxins have antiinflammatory properties affecting epithelial cells, airway leukocytes, and the pulmonary endothelium. They inhibit eosinophil and neutrophil migration into the airway and block the cytotoxicity of natural killer cells.[112,125]

The dysregulation and site of effect of lipoxins and other potentially beneficial lipid mediators (such as resolvins and protectins) in asthma is complex.[112,126] Lipoxin A4 levels are decreased in the bronchoalveolar lavage of patients with severe asthma, and lipoxin synthesis is inhibited in the circulation of many patients with severe asthma.[127,128] Decreased levels of lipoxin A4 in exhaled breath condensate have been proposed as a biomarker of lipoxin pathway abnormalities in severe asthma.

Levels of protectin D1 are similarly decreased in breath condensate during acute asthma exacerbations.[129] The identification of these biomarkers may permit targeted pharmacologic interventions for specific patients; they might ultimately be used to predict whether interventions can benefit, fail to benefit, or even harm patients based on their lipid-mediator phenotypes. It is increasingly apparent that the use of blood, sputum, and/or breath condensate biomarker analysis will be critically important in tailoring specific pharmacotherapy for specific patients with asthma.

ADDITIONAL CONSIDERATIONS FOR FUTURE STUDY

Biologic understanding is improving for several risk factors for severe asthma, including sex, race, obesity, and environmental tobacco exposure. Severe asthma is more prevalent in women after puberty.[130,131] Obesity is associated with asthma severity in adult-onset disease.[6] The greater prevalence of severe asthma among obese women may be related to menstrual cycle effects on circulating CD34$^+$CD133$^+$ cells[130] or adipose-related factors.[132,133] Additionally, circulating chitinase-like protein (YKL-40) levels are higher among patients with severe asthma in several cohorts, including SARP.[134] Asthma is characterized by air trapping.[6,15,135] Although in the early stages, CT studies may allow measurements of airways[136,137] and parenchyma,[137] which can serve as biomarkers of airway remodeling and airtrapping phenotypes. In studies of patients with severe asthma, CT determinations of air trapping were associated with disease severity.[138,139] New applications of molecular imaging promise the ability to track specific mechanistic biomarkers to specific structures using coregistered CT images, opening the door to imaging biomarkers in clinical practice. Biomarkers for severe asthma symptoms are likely to emerge from these studies.

SUMMARY

Asthma occurs in individuals with a broad range of different inflammatory and biochemical phenotypes. Most of these phenotypes have the potential to be targeted with specific treatments. Targeted treatment of the underlying disease process has the potential to be corticosteroid-sparing, particularly in patients with severe asthma. Many biomarkers are being developed to identify these specific phenotypes noninvasively. This development is grounded in a medically meaningful paradigm in which an underlying pathophysiology is suspected based on clinical presentation, a biomarker test is used to confirm the cause/diagnosis, and a targeted treatment is provided.

This article discusses several phenotypes of asthma, and more phenotypes associated with additional underlying processes almost certainly exist. The authors anticipate that each pathophysiology-based phenotype will ultimately be diagnosed by a defining biomarker, a panel of biomarkers, and/or a biomarker challenge test. Phenotypes may overlap in specific patients and may change over time. Hence, patients will likely profit from repetitive testing to define asthma pathophysiologic phenotypes and to tailor therapy. Providing targeted therapy, particularly for severe patients, based on interpretation of biomarker profiles may ultimately be the role of the asthma specialist. The authors believe that this approach will provide a clear path forward to improve treatment and minimize adverse effects.

REFERENCES

1. Yawn BP, Brenneman SK, Allen-Ramey FC, et al. Assessment of asthma severity and asthma control in children. Pediatrics 2006;118:322–9.
2. National Heart Lung and Blood Institute. Expert panel report 3: guidelines for the diagnosis and management of asthma full report. Available at: http://www.nhlbi. nih.gov/guidelines/asthma/asthgdln.pdf. Accessed July 2, 2012.
3. Wenzel S, Holgate ST. The mouse trap: it still yields few answers in asthma. Am J Respir Crit Care Med 2006;174:1173–6 [discussion: 6–8].
4. Masoli M, Fabian D, Holt S, et al. The global burden of asthma: executive summary of the GINA dissemination Committee report. Allergy 2004;59:469–78.
5. Busse WW, Banks-Schlegel S, Wenzel SE. Pathophysiology of severe asthma. J Allergy Clin Immunol 2000;106:1033–42.
6. Moore WC, Bleecker ER, Curran-Everett D, et al. Characterization of the severe asthma phenotype by the National Heart, Lung, and Blood Institute's Severe Asthma Research Program. J Allergy Clin Immunol 2007;119:405–13.
7. Paull K, Covar R, Jain N, et al. Do NHLBI lung function criteria apply to children? A cross-sectional evaluation of childhood asthma at National Jewish Medical and Research Center, 1999-2002. Pediatr Pulmonol 2005;39:311–7.
8. ATS Workshop Proceedings: exhaled nitric oxide and nitric oxide oxidative metabolism in exhaled breath condensate: executive summary. Am J Respir Crit Care Med 2006;173:811–3.
9. Wenzel SE. Asthma: defining of the persistent adult phenotypes. Lancet 2006; 368:804–13.
10. Gaston B. The biochemistry of asthma. Biochim Biophys Acta 2011;1810: 1017–24.
11. Anderson GP. Endotyping asthma: new insights into key pathogenic mechanisms in a complex, heterogeneous disease. Lancet 2008;372:1107–19.
12. Leckie MJ, ten Brinke A, Khan J, et al. Effects of an interleukin-5 blocking monoclonal antibody on eosinophils, airway hyper-responsiveness, and the late asthmatic response. Lancet 2000;356:2144–8.
13. Pavord ID, Shaw DE, Gibson PG, et al. Inflammometry to assess airway diseases. Lancet 2008;372:1017–9.
14. Meyers DA, Postma DS, Stine OC, et al. Genome screen for asthma and bronchial hyperresponsiveness: interactions with passive smoke exposure. J Allergy Clin Immunol 2005;115:1169–75.

15. Moore WC, Meyers DA, Wenzel SE, et al. Identification of asthma phenotypes using cluster analysis in the Severe Asthma Research Program. Am J Respir Crit Care Med 2010;181:315–23.
16. Fitzpatrick AM, Teague WG, Meyers DA, et al. Heterogeneity of severe asthma in childhood: confirmation by cluster analysis of children in the National Institutes of Health/National Heart, Lung, and Blood Institute Severe Asthma Research Program. J Allergy Clin Immunol 2010;127:382–9 e1–13.
17. Woodruff PG, Khashayar R, Lazarus SC, et al. Relationship between airway inflammation, hyperresponsiveness, and obstruction in asthma. J Allergy Clin Immunol 2001;108:753–8.
18. Polosa R, Renaud L, Cacciola R, et al. Sputum eosinophilia is more closely associated with airway responsiveness to bradykinin than methacholine in asthma. Eur Respir J 1998;12:551–6.
19. Louis R, Lau LC, Bron AO, et al. The relationship between airways inflammation and asthma severity. Am J Respir Crit Care Med 2000;161:9–16.
20. Covar RA, Spahn JD, Martin RJ, et al. Safety and application of induced sputum analysis in childhood asthma. J Allergy Clin Immunol 2004;114:575–82.
21. Gibson PG. Use of induced sputum to examine airway inflammation in childhood asthma. J Allergy Clin Immunol 1998;102:S100–101.
22. Berry M, Morgan A, Shaw DE, et al. Pathological features and inhaled corticosteroid response of eosinophilic and non-eosinophilic asthma. Thorax 2007;62:1043–9.
23. Hastie AT, Moore WC, Meyers DA, et al. Analyses of asthma severity phenotypes and inflammatory proteins in subjects stratified by sputum granulocytes. J Allergy Clin Immunol 2010;125:1028–36 e13.
24. Woodruff PG, Modrek B, Choy DF, et al. T-helper type 2-driven inflammation defines major subphenotypes of asthma. Am J Respir Crit Care Med 2009;180:388–95.
25. Corren J, Lemanske RF, Hanania NA, et al. Lebrikizumab treatment in adults with asthma. N Engl J Med 2011;365:1088–98.
26. MacPherson JC, Comhair SA, Erzurum SC, et al. Eosinophils are a major source of nitric oxide-derived oxidants in severe asthma: characterization of pathways available to eosinophils for generating reactive nitrogen species. J Immunol 2001;166:5763–72.
27. Aldridge RE, Chan T, van Dalen CJ, et al. Eosinophil peroxidase produces hypobromous acid in the airways of stable asthmatics. Free Radic Biol Med 2002;33:847–56.
28. Erpenbeck VJ, Hohlfeld JM, Petschallies J, et al. Local release of eosinophil peroxidase following segmental allergen provocation in asthma. Clin Exp Allergy 2003;33:331–6.
29. Wu W, Chen Y, d'Avignon A, et al. 3-Bromotyrosine and 3,5-dibromotyrosine are major products of protein oxidation by eosinophil peroxidase: potential markers for eosinophil-dependent tissue injury in vivo. Biochemistry 1999;38:3538–48.
30. Mita H, Higashi N, Taniguchi M, et al. Urinary 3-bromotyrosine and 3-chlorotyrosine concentrations in asthmatic patients: lack of increase in 3-bromotyrosine concentration in urine and plasma proteins in aspirin-induced asthma after intravenous aspirin challenge. Clin Exp Allergy 2004;34:931–8.
31. Wedes SH, Wu W, Comhair SA, et al. Urinary bromotyrosine measures asthma control and predicts asthma exacerbations in children. J Pediatr 2011;159.248–255. e1.

32. Gaston B, Sears S, Woods J, et al. Bronchodilator S-nitrosothiol deficiency in asthmatic respiratory failure. Lancet 1998;351:1317–9.
33. Que LG, Liu L, Yan Y, et al. Protection from experimental asthma by an endogenous bronchodilator. Science 2005;308:1618–21.
34. Que LG, Yang Z, Stamler JS, et al. S-nitrosoglutathione reductase: an important regulator in human asthma. Am J Respir Crit Care Med 2009;180:226–31.
35. Gaston B, Reilly J, Drazen JM, et al. Endogenous nitrogen oxides and bronchodilator S-nitrosothiols in human airways. Proc Natl Acad Sci U S A 1993;90:10957–61.
36. Gaston B, Kelly R, Urban P, et al. Buffering airway acid decreases exhaled nitric oxide in asthma. J Allergy Clin Immunol 2006;118:817–22.
37. Evangelista AM, Rao VS, Filo AR, et al. Direct regulation of striated muscle myosins by nitric oxide and endogenous nitrosothiols. PloS One 2010;5:e11209.
38. Whalen EJ, Foster MW, Matsumoto A, et al. Regulation of beta-adrenergic receptor signaling by S-nitrosylation of G-protein-coupled receptor kinase 2. Cell 2007;129:511–22.
39. Fang K, Johns R, Macdonald T, et al. S-nitrosoglutathione breakdown prevents airway smooth muscle relaxation in the guinea pig. Am J Physiol 2000;279:L716–21.
40. Marozkina NV, Wei C, Yemen S, et al. S-nitrosoglutathione reductase in human lung cancer. Am J Respir Cell Mol Biol 2011;46:63–70.
41. Jensen DE, Belka GK, Du Bois GC. S-nitrosoglutathione is a substrate for rat alcohol dehydrogenase class III isoenzyme. Biochem J 1998;331(Pt 2):659–68.
42. Greenwald R, Fitzpatrick AM, Gaston B, et al. Breath formate is a marker of airway S-nitrosothiol depletion in severe asthma. PloS One 2010;5:e11919.
43. Snyder AH, McPherson ME, Hunt JF, et al. Acute effects of aerosolized S-nitrosoglutathione in cystic fibrosis. Am J Respir Crit Care Med 2002;165:922–6.
44. Shin HW, Shelley DA, Henderson EM, et al. Airway nitric oxide release is reduced after PBS inhalation in asthma. J Appl Physiol 2007;102:1028–33.
45. Caramori G, Papi A. Oxidants and asthma. Thorax 2004;59:170–3.
46. Mak JC, Chan-Yeung MM. Reactive oxidant species in asthma. Curr Opin Pulm Med 2006;12:7–11.
47. Andreadis AA, Hazen SL, Comhair SA, et al. Oxidative and nitrosative events in asthma. Free Radic Biol Med 2003;35:213–25.
48. Comhair SA, Erzurum SC. Redox control of asthma: molecular mechanisms and therapeutic opportunities. Antioxid Redox Signal 2010;12:93–124.
49. Dworski R, Murray JJ, Roberts LJ 2nd, et al. Allergen-induced synthesis of F(2)-isoprostanes in atopic asthmatics. Evidence for oxidant stress. Am J Respir Crit Care Med 1999;160:1947–51.
50. Morrow JD, Roberts LJ. The isoprostanes: their role as an index of oxidant stress status in human pulmonary disease. Am J Respir Crit Care Med 2002;166:S25–30.
51. Wood LG, Gibson PG, Garg ML. Biomarkers of lipid peroxidation, airway inflammation and asthma. Eur Respir J 2003;21:177–86.
52. Tse SM, Tantisira K, Weiss ST. The pharmacogenetics and pharmacogenomics of asthma therapy. Pharmacogen J 2011;11:383–92.
53. Dworski R, Sheller JR. Urinary mediators and asthma. Clin Exp Allergy 1998;28:1309–12.
54. Heffner JE, Repine JE. Pulmonary strategies of antioxidant defense. Am Rev Respir Dis 1989;140:531–54.

55. De Raeve HR, Thunnissen FB, Kaneko FT, et al. Decreased Cu, Zn-SOD activity in asthmatic airway epithelium: correction by inhaled corticosteroid in vivo. Am J Physiol 1997;272:L148–54.
56. Comhair SA, Bhathena PR, Dweik RA, et al. Rapid loss of superoxide dismutase activity during antigen-induced asthmatic response. Lancet 2000;355:624.
57. Comhair SA, Erzurum SC. Antioxidant responses to oxidant-mediated lung diseases. Am J Physiol 2002;283:L246–55.
58. Comhair SA, Gaston BM, Ricci KS, et al. Detrimental effects of environmental tobacco smoke in relation to asthma severity. PloS One 2011;6:e18574.
59. Comhair SA, Ricci KS, Arroliga M, et al. Correlation of systemic superoxide dismutase deficiency to airflow obstruction in asthma. Am J Respir Crit Care Med 2005;172:306–13.
60. Comhair SA, Xu W, Ghosh S, et al. Superoxide dismutase inactivation in pathophysiology of asthmatic airway remodeling and reactivity. Am J Pathol 2005;166: 663–74.
61. Larsen GL, White CW, Takeda K, et al. Mice that overexpress Cu/Zn superoxide dismutase are resistant to allergen-induced changes in airway control. Am J Physiol 2000;279:L350–9.
62. Ghosh S, Janocha AJ, Aronica MA, et al. Nitrotyrosine proteome survey in asthma identifies oxidative mechanism of catalase inactivation. J Immunol 2006;176:5587–97.
63. Hunt JF, Erwin E, Palmer L, et al. Expression and activity of pH-regulatory glutaminase in the human airway epithelium. Am J Respir Crit Care Med 2002;165: 101–7.
64. Carraro S, Doherty J, Zaman K, et al. S-nitrosothiols regulate cell-surface pH buffering by airway epithelial cells during the human immune response to rhinovirus. Am J Physiol 2006;290:L827–32.
65. Hunt JF, Fang K, Malik R, et al. Endogenous airway acidification. Implications for asthma pathophysiology. Am J Respir Crit Care Med 2000;161:694–9.
66. Liu L, Teague WG, Erzurum S, et al. Determinants of exhaled breath condensate pH in a large population with asthma. Chest 2011;139:328–36.
67. Barbato A, Turato G, Baraldo S, et al. Epithelial damage and angiogenesis in the airways of children with asthma. Am J Respir Crit Care Med 2006;174: 975–81.
68. Hashimoto M, Tanaka H, Abe S. Quantitative analysis of bronchial wall vascularity in the medium and small airways of patients with asthma and COPD. Chest 2005;127:965–72.
69. Asosingh K, Swaidani S, Aronica M, et al. Th1- and Th2-dependent endothelial progenitor cell recruitment and angiogenic switch in asthma. J Immunol 2007; 178:6482–94.
70. Jackson JR, Seed MP, Kircher CH, et al. The codependence of angiogenesis and chronic inflammation. Faseb J 1997;11:457–65.
71. Chetta A, Zanini A, Foresi A, et al. Vascular endothelial growth factor upregulation and bronchial wall remodelling in asthma. Clin Exp Allergy 2005;35: 1437–42.
72. Psarras S, Volonaki E, Skevaki CL, et al. Vascular endothelial growth factor-mediated induction of angiogenesis by human rhinoviruses. J Allergy Clin Immunol 2006;117:291–7.
73. Avdalovic MV, Putney LF, Schelegle ES, et al. Vascular remodeling is airway generation-specific in a primate model of chronic asthma. Am J Respir Crit Care Med 2006;174:1069–76.

74. Lee CG, Link H, Baluk P, et al. Vascular endothelial growth factor (VEGF) induces remodeling and enhances TH2-mediated sensitization and inflammation in the lung. Nature Med 2004;10:1095–103.
75. Puxeddu I, Alian A, Piliponsky AM, et al. Human peripheral blood eosinophils induce angiogenesis. Int J Biochem Cell Biol 2005;37:628–36.
76. Ribatti D, Crivellato E, Roccaro AM, et al. Mast cell contribution to angiogenesis related to tumour progression. Clin Exp Allergy 2004;34:1660–4.
77. Prater DN, Case J, Ingram DA, et al. Working hypothesis to redefine endothelial progenitor cells. Leukemia 2007;21:1141–9.
78. Asahara T, Murohara T, Sullivan A, et al. Isolation of putative progenitor endothelial cells for angiogenesis. Science 1997;275:964–7.
79. Kharitonov SA, Yates D, Robbins RA, et al. Increased nitric oxide in exhaled air of asthmatic patients. Lancet 1994;343:133–5.
80. Ricciardolo FL, Gaston B, Hunt J. Acid stress in the pathology of asthma. J Allergy Clin Immunol 2004;113:610–9.
81. Smith AD, Cowan JO, Brassett KP, et al. Use of exhaled nitric oxide measurements to guide treatment in chronic asthma. N Engl J Med 2005;352:2163–73.
82. Dinakar C. Exhaled nitric oxide in pediatric asthma. Curr Allergy Asthma Rep 2009;9:30–7.
83. Nordvall SL, Janson C, Kalm-Stephens P, et al. Exhaled nitric oxide in a population-based study of asthma and allergy in schoolchildren. Allergy 2005; 60:469–75.
84. Silkoff PE, Carlson M, Bourke T, et al. The Aerocrine exhaled nitric oxide monitoring system NIOX is cleared by the US Food and Drug Administration for monitoring therapy in asthma. J Allergy Clin Immunol 2004;114:1241–56.
85. Dweik RA, Sorkness RL, Wenzel S, et al. Use of exhaled nitric oxide measurement to identify a reactive, at-risk phenotype among patients with asthma. Am J Respir Crit Care Med 2010;181:1033–41.
86. Guo FH, Comhair SA, Zheng S, et al. Molecular mechanisms of increased nitric oxide (NO) in asthma: evidence for transcriptional and post-translational regulation of NO synthesis. J Immunol 2000;164:5970–80.
87. Guo FH, Erzurum SC. Characterization of inducible nitric oxide synthase expression in human airway epithelium. Environ Health Perspect 1998;106(Suppl 5): 1119–24.
88. Guo FH, Uetani K, Haque SJ, et al. Interferon gamma and interleukin 4 stimulate prolonged expression of inducible nitric oxide synthase in human airway epithelium through synthesis of soluble mediators. J Clin Invest 1997;100: 829–38.
89. Shaw DE, Berry MA, Thomas M, et al. The use of exhaled nitric oxide to guide asthma management: a randomized controlled trial. Am J Respir Crit Care Med 2007;176:231–7.
90. Szefler SJ, Mitchell H, Sorkness CA, et al. Management of asthma based on exhaled nitric oxide in addition to guideline-based treatment for inner-city adolescents and young adults: a randomised controlled trial. Lancet 2008;372: 1065–72.
91. Khatri SB, Hammel J, Kavuru MS, et al. Temporal association of nitric oxide levels and airflow in asthma after whole lung allergen challenge. J Appl Physiol 2003;95:436–40 [discussion: 5].
92. Proceedings of the ATS workshop on refractory asthma: current understanding, recommendations, and unanswered questions. American Thoracic Society. Am J Respir Crit Care Med 2000;162:2341–51.

93. Wedes SH, Khatri SB, Zhang R, et al. Noninvasive markers of airway inflammation in asthma. Clin Transl Sci 2009;2:112–7.
94. Nelson BV, Sears S, Woods J, et al. Expired nitric oxide as a marker for childhood asthma. J Pediatr 1997;130:423–7.
95. Ceylan E, Aksoy N, Gencer M, et al. Evaluation of oxidative-antioxidative status and the L-arginine-nitric oxide pathway in asthmatic patients. Respir Med 2005; 99:871–6.
96. Li H, Romieu I, Sienra-Monge JJ, et al. Genetic polymorphisms in arginase I and II and childhood asthma and atopy. J Allergy Clin Immunol 2006;117:119–26.
97. Morris CR, Poljakovic M, Lavrisha L, et al. Decreased arginine bioavailability and increased serum arginase activity in asthma. Am J Respir Crit Care Med 2004; 170:148–53.
98. Lara A, Khatri SB, Wang Z, et al. Alterations of the arginine metabolome in asthma. Am J Respir Crit Care Med 2008;178:673–81.
99. Zimmermann N, King NE, Laporte J, et al. Dissection of experimental asthma with DNA microarray analysis identifies arginase in asthma pathogenesis. J Clin Invest 2003;111:1863–74.
100. Zimmermann N, Rothenberg ME. The arginine-arginase balance in asthma and lung inflammation. Eur J Pharmacol 2006;533:253–62.
101. Maarsingh H, Leusink J, Bos IS, et al. Arginase strongly impairs neuronal nitric oxide-mediated airway smooth muscle relaxation in allergic asthma. Respir Res 2006;7:6.
102. King NE, Rothenberg ME, Zimmermann N. Arginine in asthma and lung inflammation. J Nutr 2004;134:2830S–6S [discussion: 53S].
103. Corraliza IM, Soler G, Eichmann K, et al. Arginase induction by suppressors of nitric oxide synthesis (IL-4, IL-10 and PGE2) in murine bone-marrow-derived macrophages. Biochem Biophys Res Commun 1995;206:667–73.
104. Modolell M, Corraliza IM, Link F, et al. Reciprocal regulation of the nitric oxide synthase/arginase balance in mouse bone marrow-derived macrophages by TH1 and TH2 cytokines. Eur J Immunol 1995;25:1101–4.
105. Mistry SK, Zheng M, Rouse BT, et al. Induction of arginases I and II in cornea during herpes simplex virus infection. Virus Res 2001;73:177–82.
106. Ito A, Tsao PS, Adimoolam S, et al. Novel mechanism for endothelial dysfunction: dysregulation of dimethylarginine dimethylaminohydrolase. Circulation 1999;99:3092–5.
107. Cohen L, E X, Tarsi J, et al. Epithelial cell proliferation contributes to airway remodeling in severe asthma. Am J Respir Crit Care Med 2007;176:138–45.
108. Li H, Meininger CJ, Hawker JR Jr, et al. Regulatory role of arginase I and II in nitric oxide, polyamine, and proline syntheses in endothelial cells. Am J Physiol Endocrinol Metab 2001;280:E75–82.
109. Janne J, Alhonen L, Leinonen P. Polyamines: from molecular biology to clinical applications. Ann Med 1991;23:241–59.
110. Albina JE, Abate JA, Mastrofrancesco B. Role of ornithine as a proline precursor in healing wounds. J Surg Res 1993;55:97–102.
111. Kershenobich D, Fierro FJ, Rojkind M. The relationship between the free pool of proline and collagen content in human liver cirrhosis. J Clin Invest 1970;49: 2246–9.
112. Haworth O, Levy BD. Endogenous lipid mediators in the resolution of airway inflammation. Eur Respir J 2007;30:980–92.
113. O'Byrne PM, Israel E, Drazen JM. Antileukotrienes in the treatment of asthma. Ann Intern Med 1997;127:472–80.

114. Kalayci O, Birben E, Sackesen C, et al. ALOX5 promoter genotype, asthma severity and LTC production by eosinophils. Allergy 2006;61:97–103.
115. Montuschi P, Mondino C, Koch P, et al. Effects of montelukast treatment and withdrawal on fractional exhaled nitric oxide and lung function in children with asthma. Chest 2007;132:1876–81.
116. Rabinovitch N, Graber NJ, Chinchilli VM, et al. Urinary leukotriene E4/exhaled nitric oxide ratio and montelukast response in childhood asthma. J Allergy Clin Immunol 2010;126. 545–551. e1–4.
117. Daffern PJ, Muilenburg D, Hugli TE, et al. Association of urinary leukotriene E4 excretion during aspirin challenges with severity of respiratory responses. J Allergy Clin Immunol 1999;104:559–64.
118. O'Shaughnessy KM, Wellings R, Gillies B, et al. Differential effects of fluticasone propionate on allergen-evoked bronchoconstriction and increased urinary leukotriene E4 excretion. Am Rev Respir Dis 1993;147:1472–6.
119. O'Sullivan S, Roquet A, Dahlen B, et al. Urinary excretion of inflammatory mediators during allergen-induced early and late phase asthmatic reactions. Clin Exp Allergy 1998;28:1332–9.
120. Green SA, Malice MP, Tanaka W, et al. Increase in urinary leukotriene LTE4 levels in acute asthma: correlation with airflow limitation. Thorax 2004;59:100–4.
121. Liu MC, Dube LM, Lancaster J. Acute and chronic effects of a 5-lipoxygenase inhibitor in asthma: a 6-month randomized multicenter trial. Zileuton Study Group. J Allergy Clin Immunol 1996;98:859–71.
122. Wenzel SE, Trudeau JB, Kaminsky DA, et al. Effect of 5-lipoxygenase inhibition on bronchoconstriction and airway inflammation in nocturnal asthma. Am J Respir Crit Care Med 1995;152:897–905.
123. Pavord ID, Ward R, Woltmann G, et al. Induced sputum eicosanoid concentrations in asthma. Am J Respir Crit Care Med 1999;160:1905–9.
124. Miranda C, Busacker A, Balzar S, et al. Distinguishing severe asthma phenotypes: role of age at onset and eosinophilic inflammation. J Allergy Clin Immunol 2004;113:101–8.
125. Levy BD. Lipoxins and lipoxin analogs in asthma. Prostaglandins Leukot Essent Fatty Acids 2005;73:231–7.
126. Haworth O, Cernadas M, Yang R, et al. Resolvin E1 regulates interleukin 23, interferon-gamma and lipoxin A4 to promote the resolution of allergic airway inflammation. Nat Immunol 2008;9:873–9.
127. Planaguma A, Kazani S, Marigowda G, et al. Airway lipoxin A4 generation and lipoxin A4 receptor expression are decreased in severe asthma. Am J Respir Crit Care Med 2008;178:574–82.
128. Levy BD, Bonnans C, Silverman ES, et al. Diminished lipoxin biosynthesis in severe asthma. Am J Respir Crit Care Med 2005;172:824–30.
129. Levy BD, Kohli P, Gotlinger K, et al. Protectin D1 is generated in asthma and dampens airway inflammation and hyperresponsiveness. J Immunol 2007;178: 496–502.
130. Farha S, Asosingh K, Laskowski D, et al. Effects of the menstrual cycle on lung function variables in women with asthma. Am J Respir Crit Care Med 2009;180: 304–10.
131. Tantisira KG, Colvin R, Tonascia J, et al. Airway responsiveness in mild to moderate childhood asthma: sex influences on the natural history. Am J Respir Crit Care Med 2008;178:325–31.
132. Holguin F, Bleecker ER, Busse WW, et al. Obesity and asthma: an association modified by age of asthma onset. J Allergy Clin Immunol 2011;127:1486–93 e2.

133. Holguin F, Fitzpatrick A. Obesity, asthma, and oxidative stress. J Appl Physiol 2010;108:754–9.
134. Chupp GL, Lee CG, Jarjour N, et al. A chitinase-like protein in the lung and circulation of patients with severe asthma. N Engl J Med 2007;357:2016–27.
135. Sorkness RL, Bleecker ER, Busse WW, et al. Lung function in adults with stable but severe asthma: air trapping and incomplete reversal of obstruction with bronchodilation. J Appl Physiol 2008;104:394–403.
136. Little SA, Sproule MW, Cowan MD, et al. High resolution computed tomographic assessment of airway wall thickness in chronic asthma: reproducibility and relationship with lung function and severity. Thorax 2002;57:247–53.
137. Mitsunobu F, Ashida K, Hosaki Y, et al. Decreased computed tomographic lung density during exacerbation of asthma. Eur Respir J 2003;22:106–12.
138. Busacker A, Newell JD Jr, Keefe T, et al. A multivariate analysis of risk factors for the air-trapping asthmatic phenotype as measured by quantitative CT analysis. Chest 2009;135:48–56.
139. de Lange EE, Altes TA, Patrie JT, et al. Evaluation of asthma with hyperpolarized helium-3 MRI: correlation with clinical severity and spirometry. Chest 2006;130:1055–62.

Asthma Diagnosis in Otolaryngology Practice
Pulmonary Function Testing

John H. Krouse, MD, PhD[a],*, Helene J. Krouse, PhD, APN-BC, CORLN[b]

KEYWORDS

- Spirometry • Asthma • Flow-volume loop • Pulmonary function testing
- Allergic rhinitis

KEY POINTS

- Current evidence-based guidelines strongly recommend the use of objective testing in the diagnosis and treatment of patients with asthma.
- Spirometry provides an easy, readily available, and inexpensive methodology that can be used in the otolaryngology office.
- Peak flow measurement can be used by patients at home to monitor their symptoms and disease status.

As previously discussed in this issue, the diagnosis of asthma is based on a comprehensive assessment of patient symptoms and signs from physical examination. In addition, there are several standardized instruments that can assist in clarifying the diagnosis and assessing the severity of the disease. Current National Heart, Lung and Blood Institute guidelines[1] recommend the use of these elements to confirm an initial diagnosis and evaluate response to therapy.

Although assessing clinical symptoms and signs can be useful in patient management, these factors can be less reliable and objective than desired, especially in their ability to quantify the physiologic expression of the disease. Because asthma represents a disease of airflow obstruction in the small bronchioles, an objective assessment of the degree of obstruction is useful in determining the degree of direct impact on pulmonary function and following both the progression of the disease and the response to medical intervention. To assist with physiologic measurement of lung function, several specific methods have been developed that can reliably and accurately assessment the impact of asthma on respiratory physiology.

This article originally appeared in Otolaryngologic Clinics of North America, Volume 47, Issue 1, February 2014.

[a] Department of Otolaryngology-Head and Neck Surgery, Temple University School of Medicine, 3440 North Broad Street, Kresge West #300, Philadelphia, PA 19140, USA; [b] College of Nursing, Wayne State University, 5557 Cass Avenue, Detroit, MI 48202, USA
* Corresponding author.
E-mail address: jkrouse@temple.edu

PEAK FLOW MEASUREMENT

Peak flow meters are small, inexpensive devices that are simple to use and ideal for home assessment of pulmonary function. They primarily measure airflow through the larger portions of the airway, and are therefore less sensitive to small changes in the distal bronchioles. Their major value is for following lung function at home on a daily or twice daily basis to detect sequential changes over time. Although peak flow testing can be useful as a gross assessment of function, results are dependent on patient effort so education on proper technique is essential to obtain accurate results. In addition, beneficial use requires consistent measurement and recording on a regular basis, with poor patient or parent adherence compromising maximal benefit.

PULMONARY FUNCTION TESTING

The primary method used to assess respiratory physiology and status in patients diagnosed with or suspected of having asthma is pulmonary function testing (PFT). PFTs represent an integral portion of the diagnosis and therapeutic management of patients with asthma, and serve 3 core functions in practice: (1) to assess the presence and severity of asthma; (2) to establish reversibility of airway obstruction; and (3) to measure response to therapy. PFTs play an essential role in the management of patients suspected of having respiratory dysfunction, and can be considered an objective assessment of lung function much as audiometry represents an objective assessment of auditory function.

PFTs are important in differentiating specific pulmonary pathophysiology based on whether the disease is obstructive or restrictive, and whether obstruction is reversible or irreversible. PFTs also establish a reliable and valid baseline for establishing an initial diagnosis and for monitoring changes over time, with or without specific treatment. Because of advancements in measurement and computing technology, small, portable, inexpensive, and automated devices are now widely available for in-office use.

Physiologic testing of lung function involves several specific testing methodologies to assess components of normal pulmonary physiology, including mechanics of the lungs and ventilatory function, the ventilation-perfusion relationship, diffusion and gas exchange, and muscular strength. Full battery PFTs can include a variety of these procedures, although in the diagnosis of asthma not all components of the testing battery are necessary. The 4 primary procedures in common use include: (1) measurement of lung volume; (2) measurement of diffusing capacity; (3) spirometry; and (4) bronchoprovocation. The first of these 2 procedures is briefly reviewed here; spirometry and bronchoprovocation are discussed in greater detail.

Spirometry

Spirometry is the most commonly performed lung function study, and is often sufficient to confirm a diagnosis of asthma without more specialized testing. It can be easily and quickly performed in the office setting under the guidance and supervision of a trained technician or health care provider. Spirometry measures air flow in the lungs, which involves assessing how much air can move in and out of the lungs as well as how fast the air in the lungs can be exhaled. The indications for spirometry include the diagnosis and monitoring of suspected diseases of lung function, including asthma, chronic obstructive pulmonary disease, and other common and uncommon pulmonary conditions.

Spirometry involves a maneuver in which the patient voluntarily inhales maximally and then rapidly and forcefully exhales to the fullest extent possible. At full inspiration, the patient has filled the lungs with air, and at full expiration some air remains in the lungs, defined as the residual volume. This rapid and forceful exhalation of air generates forced vital capacity (FVC), or the largest volume of air that can be exhaled from the lungs, not including the residual volume left behind. Tracings obtained from this inhalation and exhalation during spirometry form the flow-volume loop, a graphical representation of lung function that can be useful as a diagnostic metric (**Fig. 1**).

The volume of air that can be exhaled forcefully in the first second of exhalation is known as the forced expiratory volume-first second (FEV_1), and is the most widely used parameter in measuring the mechanical properties of the lungs. In normal individuals, the FEV_1 represents about 75% to 85% of the FVC and the ratio of these 2 volumes can assist in differentiating obstructive from restrictive diseases. Lower FEV_1 values indicate more significant obstructive lung disease. In asthma, the FVC is generally conserved and is near normal whereas the FEV_1 is reduced. This reduced FEV_1/FVC ratio is characteristic of the patient with asthma.

Spirometry is often performed both before and after bronchodilator use to assess reversibility of airway obstruction. In this procedure, after the standard spirometry is completed, in the case of an abnormally reduced FEV_1, a short-acting β-2 agonist such as albuterol is administered via inhaler and the test repeated after several minutes. In patients with asthma, which is characterized by a reversible airway obstruction, the FEV_1 generally improves. Improvement of the FEV_1 by 12% or greater is generally diagnostic of asthma.

Spirometry values are based on referenced norms according to patient age, gender, race, height, and weight. This information is entered into the spirometer before conducting the test. As with peak flow meters, the accuracy of the test results is highly dependent on patient effort during the test. Therefore proper coaching throughout the test is essential to obtain maximal effort and results (**Table 1**). The patient is instructed to take a deep breath and blow out as hard and fast as possible and to take in a deep breath so to complete the flow-volume loop. The patient performs 3 tests or blows to get the best results (**Fig. 2**).

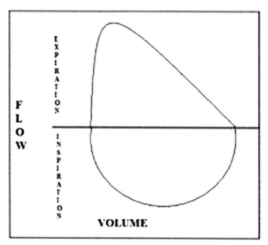

Fig. 1. Normal flow-volume loop. (*From* National Library of Medicine. Available at: http://openi.nlm.nih.gov/detailedresult.php?img=1297597_cc3516-6&req=4. Accessed September 6, 2013.)

Table 1
Questions to ask before baseline spirometry testing

How are you feeling today?	If the person has acute respiratory symptoms or illness, postpone testing for 3–5 d
Have you smoked any cigarettes, cigars, or pipes (including hookah/argileh) within the past hour?	If yes, postpone testing for 1 h
Have you used any inhaled medications within the past hour?	If yes, postpone testing for 1 h
Have you had any surgery in the past 4 wk (specifically abdominal; eye surgery; oral surgery)?	Cancel test and do not reschedule at this time

Bronchoprovocation

In patients with suspected asthma who have normal spirometry, testing is often done by stimulation of the airways with a bronchoconstrictive agent to assess the degree of bronchial hyperreactivity. Patients with mild asthma often have underlying subacute bronchial irritability and respond with a decline in FEV_1 during inhalational challenge with a bronchoconstrictor. Methacholine and histamine are the most commonly used agents for inhalational challenge, although methacholine is more widely used. It is considered safe and free from systemic side effects.

In performing inhalational challenges, increasing concentrations of methacholine are administered via a dosimeter through aerosolized inhalation. Five increasing

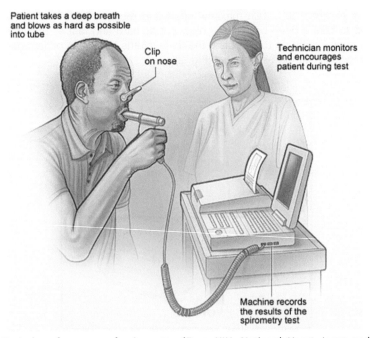

Fig. 2. Typical performance of spirometry. (*From* NIH, National Heart, Lung and Blood Institute. Available at: http://www.nhlbi.nih.gov/health/health-topics/topics/lft/types.html. Accessed July 3, 2013.)

concentrations are generally used. When there is a 20% drop in FEV_1 to inhalation, the test is terminated and is considered to be a positive indication of clinically significant airway hyperreactivity. The dosage required to trigger this reduction is known as the PC_{20FEV1}. If the FEV_1 does not drop by 20% at the highest concentration, then the test is considered negative. A PC_{20FEV1} of less than 8 mg/mL is interpreted as demonstrating clinically important airway hyperreactivity and would suggest a diagnosis of asthma.

Diffusing Capacity

Various pulmonary diseases can affect the ability of oxygen to diffuse from the alveolus into the capillary system in the lungs. Diseases that affect the lung parenchyma such as emphysema and cystic fibrosis can result in thickened alveolar-capillary membranes and impair air exchange. These findings are not generally seen in asthma, and diffusing capacity is not a commonly required test in patients suspected of having asthma.

Lung Volume

Lung volume measurements can be obtained to assess the total capacity of the lungs, which represents the full volume of the lungs, including the residual air remaining after forced expiration. Calculation of total capacity may be important in assessing restrictive lung diseases but is not generally necessary in the diagnosis and management of asthma.

SUMMARY

PFT is an important diagnostic modality in the workup of patients suspected of having asthma. It is also valuable to follow response to treatment among patients initiated and sustained on asthma therapy, and to assess patients complaining of symptoms suggestive of an asthma exacerbation. Spirometry is the most useful test in patients suspected of having asthma, and can easily be performed and interpreted in the otolaryngology office with readily available, inexpensive equipment. PFT should be considered for use in all otolaryngology patients with significant rhinitis and in those suspected of having lower respiratory disease.

REFERENCE

1. National Heart, Lung and Blood Institute. Expert Panel Report 3 (EPR3): guidelines for the diagnosis and management of asthma. Bethesda (MD): NHLBI; 2007.

Asthma Diagnosis and Management

Ariana Murata, MD, Patrick M. Ling, MD, MPH*

KEYWORDS

• Asthma • Emergency • Diagnosis • Management

EPIDEMIOLOGY

Asthma is one of the most common chronic diseases in adults, affecting 300 million people worldwide.[1] Asthma affects 7% to 8% of people in North America,[2–4] including more than 24 million Americans[4] and 3 million Canadians.[2,3] The prevalence of asthma in older adults is 6% to 10%.[4,5] The number of elderly patients will increase in the future as this segment of the population continues to grow. Currently, the highest prevalence of asthma is seen in English-language countries and Latin America.[6] Asthma rates steadily increased from the 1960s to 1990s, with most ongoing gains seen in developing countries and older adults.[5,7,8] Since the late 1990s, the prevalence of asthma has been either stabilizing or declining in higher income countries.[6,7,9–12]

Asthma accounts for 2 million visits to emergency departments (EDs) annually in the United States.[13] Between 6% and 13% of those with asthma exacerbations require hospital admission.[14,15] Older adults have higher rates of hospitalization. In a large-scale study, older adults were twice as likely (14%) to be hospitalized as younger adults (7%).[16] Asthma accounts for around 4000 deaths annually in the United States[4,13] and 500 deaths in Canada.[3] Mortality from asthma has been decreasing since the 1990s.[3,17] However, mortality remains highest in elderly patients, accounting for two-thirds of deaths from asthma.[5] Asthma exacerbations are potentially fatal and should be treated seriously, although death occurs in a minority of asthmatics.[17–19]

PATHOPHYSIOLOGY

Asthma is a chronic inflammatory disorder that is characterized by bronchial hyperresponsiveness and airway obstruction.[20] Bronchospasm is the key feature of asthma, and is triggered by allergens or other stimuli. Mast cells are activated through immunoglobulin E receptors to release inflammatory mediators that directly target bronchial

This article originally appeared in Emergency Medicine Clinics of North America, Volume 30, Issue 2, May 2012.

The authors have nothing to disclose.

Division of Emergency Medicine, Royal University Hospital, University of Saskatchewan, Room 2684, 103 Hospital Drive, Saskatoon, Saskatchewan S7N 0W8, Canada

* Corresponding author.

E-mail address: patrick.ling@usask.ca

http://dx.doi.org/10.1016/j.ccol.2014.09.006

smooth muscle.[21,22] Bronchodilators are usually effective in reversing these symptoms, and are the recommended first-line treatment of asthma.[20,23,24]

Inflammation is central to the pathophysiology of asthma, and can lead to permanent changes in airway structure and pulmonary function, in a process known as airway remodelling.[25,26] Inflammatory cells involved in asthma include lymphocytes,[27,28] mast cells,[21] eosinophils,[29,30] neutrophils, dendritic cells,[31] macrophages,[32] and epithelial cells.[33] Research into the inflammatory nature of asthma is leading to advances in therapy, in areas such as immunotherapy and leukotriene receptor modulators.

HISTORY AND PHYSICAL EXAMINATION

The classic triad of asthma includes chronic cough, wheeze, and dyspnea. However, patients often present with only 1 of these symptoms, which can make diagnosis challenging. In studies of patients presenting solely with wheeze, chronic cough, or dyspnea, only 24% to 35% were eventually diagnosed with asthma.[25,34,35] Symptoms of asthma are typically worse at night or early in the morning. A personal history of atopy and family history of asthma favor the diagnosis.

Asthma symptoms are typically variable and worsen with exposure to triggers. Common precipitants include house dust mites,[36,37] animal dander, cockroaches,[36] Alternaria,[38] pollens, and molds. Air pollutants and sulfites can cause exacerbations.[39] In a recent multicenter study of 654 asthmatics, exposure to environmental tobacco smoke was associated with worse lung function, higher acuity of exacerbations, and increased health care use.[40] Viral respiratory infections are the most common causes of asthma exacerbations in children and infants.[41,42] Aspirin and other nonsteroidal antiinflammatory drugs (NSAIDs) can trigger attacks in up to 20% of asthmatics.[43] Occupational exposure to chemicals and dust should be considered.[44] Strong emotional expression,[45,46] exercise,[47] and menstrual cycles may worsen the symptoms of asthma.[48,49]

Risk factors for severe, uncontrolled asthma should be assessed, including previous intubations or intensive care admissions, 2 or more hospitalizations for asthma in the past year, 3 or more ED visits for asthma in the past year, hospitalization or ED visit for asthma in the past month, using more than 2 canisters of short-acting β-agonist monthly, and lack of a written asthma action plan.[20] Difficulty perceiving the severity of asthma symptoms is a worrisome sign.[20] Low socioeconomic status, inner-city residence, illicit drug use, and major psychosocial problems are risk factors for death from asthma.[20]

A history of compliance with medications, prehospital care, and types and doses of asthma maintenance medications should be obtained. Prolonged symptoms are more difficult to treat, given the inflammatory nature of asthma. Differential diagnoses should be ruled out by careful history taking. Comorbidities that could aggravate asthma should be identified, including allergic bronchopulmonary aspergillosis, gastroesophageal reflux disease, obesity, rhinosinusitis, obstructive sleep apnea, and depression.[20]

Asthma is often underdiagnosed and undertreated in older adults.[5,50] The elderly asthmatic suffers from the typical symptoms of asthma, but is more likely to have reduced perception of bronchoconstriction.[51–53] This may lead to delay in seeking medical care and increased risk of severe asthma attacks.[53–55] Older adults are more likely to have comorbidities or use medications (eg, β-blockers, acetylsalicylic acid, NSAIDs) that may exacerbate asthma.[43,56]

The severity of an asthma exacerbation can be assessed by quantitative measurements of lung function, such as peak expiratory flow (PEF). Patients with mild asthma

(PEF ≥70% of predicted) present with dyspnea on exertion and increased respiratory rate. They are able to speak in sentences and to lie down. Moderate wheeze may be heard on auscultation. The patient suffering from a moderate asthma exacerbation (PEF 40%–69%) has dyspnea at rest, and is more comfortable sitting than lying down. Loud wheeze is commonly heard throughout exhalation. Suprasternal retractions and use of accessory respiratory muscles are commonly seen.

Clinical signs of severe asthma (PEF <40%) include use of accessory respiratory muscles, inability to speak or lie supine because of dyspnea, and pulsus paradoxus (decrease in systolic blood pressure of ≥12 mm Hg with inspiration). In particularly severe attacks, pulsus paradoxus can be greater than 25 mm Hg. Respiratory rate is often more than 30 breaths per minute. The patient is most comfortable sitting up and can be agitated. Loud wheeze is heard throughout inspiration and expiration. Cyanosis, decreasing level of consciousness, and respiratory muscle fatigue are markers of impending respiratory arrest. Failure of severe symptoms to respond to initial treatment is particularly worrisome.

DIFFERENTIAL DIAGNOSIS

Wheezing is characteristic of asthma, but can be a presentation of many different diseases. Physicians should be aware that "all that wheezes is not asthma; all that wheezes is not obstruction." The clinical diagnosis of asthma should be confirmed by quantitative measurements of lung function.[20] Spirometry is the preferred diagnostic test, and can be done in pulmonary function laboratories, or alternatively in the primary care office. Spirometry measures the forced vital capacity (FVC; the maximal volume of air that can be exhaled from maximal expiration) and the FEV_1 (volume of air exhaled during the first second). Spirometry assesses obstruction and potential reversibility of symptoms, and can be done in patients older than 5 years of age.[20] Additional pulmonary studies, methacholine bronchoprovocation, or chest radiography may be needed if the diagnosis is in doubt. Allergy testing may be indicated. Biomarkers of inflammation, such as sputum eosinophils[57,58] and fractional exhaled nitric oxide,[59] are currently being evaluated as adjunctives for the diagnosis of asthma.

More than 50% of older adults with obstructive disease may share features of both asthma and chronic obstructive pulmonary disease (COPD).[60] Overlap syndrome of asthma and COPD is characterized by evidence of incompletely reversible airway obstruction (COPD) and increased variability of airflow. This subgroup of patients is still poorly recognized and is typically excluded from current therapeutic trials. A recent study of 1546 patients showed that those with overlap syndrome had lower quality of life than those with either disease alone.[61] These patients would benefit from further studies to clarify optimal treatment strategies **Box 1**.

ED EVALUATION

Asthma exacerbations are characterized by obstruction to expiratory airflow, and can be assessed by quantitative tests of lung function. These measurements include PEF and spirometry, and are more reliable indicators of the severity of acute asthma than clinical symptoms alone.[20] PEF is the most commonly used test in the ED to assess the degree of obstruction. PEF readings are safe, quick, and cost-effective. They can be used to monitor a patient's response to treatment over time. Normal PEF values vary with gender, height, age, and ethnicity. A value less than 200 L/min usually indicates severe obstruction. Repeated PEF or FEV_1 measurements at ED presentation and 1 hour after treatment are the strongest predictors of hospitalization in asthmatics.[62,63]

Box 1
Differential diagnosis of wheezing in adults

- Asthma
- COPD
- Congestive heart failure
- Pulmonary embolism
- Pneumonia
- Tumors
- Cough secondary to drugs (eg, angiotensin-converting enzyme [ACE] inhibitors)
- Foreign body in trachea or bronchus
- Aspiration pneumonitis
- Allergic rhinitis and sinusitis
- Postnasal drip
- Gastroesophageal reflux
- Vocal cord dysfunction
- Recurrent cough not caused by asthma

Clinicians should educate patients in the early recognition and treatment of asthma exacerbations. Patients should start immediate treatment at home with inhaled bronchodilators if they recognize symptoms or if PEF decreases to less than 80% of predicted. PEF should be reassessed after initial bronchodilator treatment (eg, up to 2 treatments 20 minutes apart of 2–6 puffs by metered-dose inhaler [MDI] or nebulizer treatments). Initial PEF or FEV_1 is used to classify the severity of asthma in patients in the ED. Signs, symptoms, and clinical course vary with the different levels of asthma severity (**Table 1**).

Pulse oximetry is a reliable way to monitor for hypoxemia in the asthmatic patient. It is recommended for patients in severe distress, PEF or FEV_1 less than 40% of normal, or if the patient cannot perform lung function measurements.[20] Arterial blood gas measurements are rarely done, and are indicated only in patients with PEF less than 25% of predicted, because this group alone is at risk for significant hypercapnia or acidosis.[64] Increased or normal arterial carbon dioxide pressure ($Paco_2$) is a worrisome sign, because it indicates that obstruction is so severe that the patient cannot respond to the increased respiratory drive that typifies acute asthma. When indicated, venous blood gases are strongly correlated with arterial blood gases and can reliably be used to measure pH and CO_2 pressure (pco_2).[65] Respiratory failure can develop from further progression of symptoms. Blood gases can also be considered in patients who are unable to perform pulmonary function tests.

Chest radiographs are generally not useful in the setting of acute asthma, and most commonly show pulmonary hyperinflation.[66] They should only be used to evaluate other suspected causes of the patient's symptoms (eg, pneumonia, pneumothorax, congestive heart failure). Electrocardiograms should be done in patients with suspected cardiac disorders.

TREATMENT

Early recognition and treatment of the asthma exacerbation is essential for success in overall management. Patients presenting to the ED with acute asthma should be

Table 1
Classifying severity of asthma exacerbations in the urgent or emergency care setting

	Symptoms and Signs	Initial PEF (or FEV₁)	Clinical Course
Mild	Dyspnea only with activity (assess tachypnea in young children)	PEF ≥70% predicted or personal best	Usually cared for at home Prompt relief with inhaled SABA Possible short course or oral systemic corticosteroids
Moderate	Dyspnea interferes with or limits usual activity	PEF 40%–69% predicted or personal best	Usually requires office or ED visit Relief from frequent inhaled SABA Oral systemic corticosteroids; some symptoms last for 1–2 d after treatment is begun
Severe	Dyspnea at rest; interferes with conversation	PEF <40% predicted or personal best	Usually requires ED visit and likely hospitalization Partial relief from frequent inhaled SABA Oral systemic corticosteroids; some symptoms last for >3 d after treatment is begun Adjunctive therapies are helpful
Subset: life threatening	Too dyspneic tospeak; perspiring	PEF <25% predicted or personal best	Requires ED/hospitalization; possible ICU Minimal or no relief from frequent inhaled SABA Intravenous corticosteroids Adjunctive therapies are helpful

Abbreviations: FEV₁, forced expiratory volume in 1 second; ICU, intensive care unit; SABA, short-acting β2-agonist.

Reproduced from National Asthma Education and Prevention Program. Expert panel report III: Guidelines for the diagnosis and management of asthma. Bethesda (MD): National Heart, Lung, and Blood Institute; 2007 (NIH publication no. 08-4051).

quickly evaluated for the adequacy of airway, breathing, and circulation. This evaluation should include a complete set of vital signs, pulse oximetry, respiratory rate, and an assessment of respiratory effort. Treatment should be started immediately.

Current recommendations are outlined in the 2007 National Asthma and Education and Prevention Program (NAEPP) Expert Panel Report (EPR-3) (coordinated by the National Heart, Lung, and Blood Institute of the National Institutes of Health) and the 2005 Canadian Asthma Consensus Guidelines.[20,23,24] Goals of therapy include correction of hypoxemia, rapid reversal of airway obstruction, and treatment of inflammation. Begin treatment by giving oxygen to keep the oxygen saturation at more than 90%. The adequacy of the patient's airway, breathing, and circulation should be carefully assessed. The offending stimulus, if known, should be removed. β-Agonists are given to achieve rapid reversal of airflow obstruction. Anticholinergics are added for the treatment of severe exacerbations. Administration of systemic corticosteroids should be considered early in the treatment of those with moderate or severe asthma exacerbations, or those who do not respond quickly and completely to β-agonists. Response to therapy should be monitored with serial measurements of lung function.[20]

β2-AGONISTS

β2-Agonists are potent bronchodilators that act on β receptors to quickly and effectively relax bronchial smooth muscle. Short-acting β-agonists are the recommended first-line therapy for the acute asthma exacerbation.[20] Albuterol is the most commonly used β2-agonist for acute asthma.

β2-Agonists can be administered in multiple forms, including MDI, nebulizer, subcutaneous injection, and intravenous injection. Traditionally, aerosolized bronchodilators have been administered by continuous-flow nebulization. However, multiple studies have found little difference in efficacy between MDI and nebulizer therapy.[67–69] Hospital admission rates are equivalent between the 2 modalities.[69] MDI is more cost-effective and time-effective than nebulizer therapy,[67,70] but must be administered with proper inhaler technique using a holding chamber or spacer device (eg, Aerochamber). MDI/spacers result in significantly shorter stays in the ED, greater improvements in PEF, and lower cumulative dose of albuterol.[67] MDIs can be administered easily in the patient's own home. An additional concern with aerosolized or nebulized medication is its potential to spread infectious agents.[71] Recommendations suggest the use of personal protective devices and N95 masks by health care providers for suspected influenzalike illnesses.[72] Barriers to widespread administration of MDI/spacers in the ED include lack of leadership for change, lack of consensus about the benefits of this modality, perceived resistance from patients and parents, and perceived increased in cost and workload.[73,74]

For acute asthma, 2 to 6 inhalations of albuterol are given with MDI and spacer device. Therapy is repeated every 20 minutes for up to 4 hours until there is maximal improvement in respiratory symptoms. Alternatively, if MDI is unavailable or if the patient is unable to use proper techniques, 2.5 to 5.0 mg of nebulized albuterol is given every 20 minutes to a total of 3 doses (maximum of 15 mg in one hour). Albuterol can also be given as a continuous nebulization at a rate of 10 to 15 mg over 1 hour. A Cochrane Review reported a number needed to treat (NNT) of 10 for the use of continuous versus intermittent β-agonists in the treatment of acute asthma to prevent 1 hospital admission.[75] Therapy should be titrated to an objective measure of airflow obstruction (eg, FEV_1 or PEF) and clinical response.

β-Agonists should only be used for relief of acute symptoms. If used on a chronic basis, they can cause desensitization and tolerance. Adverse effects associated with β-agonists include tremor, tachycardia, palpitations, hyperglycemia, and hypokalemia.

Current evidence does not support the use of intravenous β2-agonists for the treatment of acute severe asthma.[76] Long-acting β-agonists (LABAs) have no role in acute asthma management. LABAs can be used in combination with inhaled corticosteroids for long-term treatment of moderate or severe persistent asthma. They should not be used as monotherapy.[20]

Short-term side effects of β-agonists include tachycardia and hypokalemia. Long-term adverse effects include sinus and ventricular tachycardia, syncope, atrial fibrillation, congestive heart failure, myocardial infarction, cardiac arrest, and sudden death.[77] In long-term use, compared with placebo, β-adrenergic-agonists significantly increased the risk for cardiovascular events (relative risk, 2.54; 95% confidence interval, 1.59–4.05).

ANTICHOLINERGICS

Anticholinergics block the action of acetylcholine on the parasympathetic autonomic system. They decrease vagally mediated smooth muscle contraction in the airways, leading to bronchodilation. Anticholinergics are recommended for the treatment of severe asthma, in combination with short-acting β-agonists.[20,78] The synergistic effects of these 2 agents decrease hospitalization rates and improve lung function.[78–80] Ipratropium bromide is the most commonly used anticholinergic agent for the treatment of asthma.

Ipratropium has a slow onset of action, reaching its peak effect in 90 minutes. In contrast, the onset of action for albuterol is less than 5 minutes. In addition, ipratropium is not as potent a bronchodilator as albuterol. For these reasons, ipratropium should not be used alone for acute asthma management. For the acute exacerbation, 0.5 mg of ipratropium is given by nebulization every 20 minutes for 3 doses. Alternatively, 8 puffs with MDI and spacer can be given every 20 minutes for up to 3 hours.

A recent study showed the benefit of a multiple-dose protocol of ipratropium combined with albuterol in patients with severe asthma exacerbations (FEV <50%). Both medications were administered through MDI every 10 minutes for 3 hours. Patients had significant improvements in pulmonary function and decreased admission rates. The most benefit was seen in those with more severe obstruction (FEV ≤30%) and long duration of symptoms (≥24 hours before ED presentation).[80] In a 2008 Cochrane Review, the addition of multiple doses of anticholinergics to β2-agonists decreased the risk of hospital admission by 25% in children with moderate and severe asthma. The NNT using multiple additional doses of anticholinergics plus β-agonists for the treatment of asthma exacerbation to prevent 1 hospital admission is 12.[78]

Anticholinergics are not recommended for hospitalized patients.[20] Two randomized controlled trials did not show significant benefit from ipratropium for hospitalized patients with severe asthma.[81,82]

CORTICOSTEROIDS

Acute asthma is characterized by airway edema, mucus hypersecretion, and cellular infiltration, in addition to bronchospasm. This inflammatory reaction can lead to persistent airway obstruction, and is the target of corticosteroids. Corticosteroids are the most potent and effective antiinflammatory agents available for the treatment of asthma. Their onset of action can take up to 6 hours to become clinically apparent.[83]

Early systemic corticosteroids in the ED are recommended for moderate or severe asthma, or if β-agonists do not fully correct the decline in pulmonary function.[20] A 2001 Cochrane Review of 863 patients showed a significant reduction in hospital admission rates when corticosteroids were given within 1 hour of ED presentation; absolute risk reduction was 12.5% (NNT of 8).[84] In addition, a short course of corticosteroids for asthma exacerbations significantly decreases relapse rates and use of short-acting β2-agonist.[85] Current guidelines recommend that systemic corticosteroids be added immediately if there is an incomplete (PEF 50%–79% of best or predicted) or poor (<50% PEF) response to β-agonist therapy. The patient's response to β-agonists is established by administering up to 2 treatments 20 minutes apart, either by MDI or nebulizer. Systemic corticosteroids can also be considered in those with a good (≥80% PEF) response to short-acting β2-agonists (SABAs).[20] Following ED discharge, a course of corticosteroids should be given for 3 to 10 days to prevent relapse.[20,85]

Systemic corticosteroids come in multiple forms, including oral, intravenous, and intramuscular. The efficacy of oral corticosteroids is equivalent to the intravenous form.[86–88] Oral steroids are preferred, because they are less invasive.[20] Prednisone is administered orally at a dose of 40 to 60 mg. A recent randomized controlled trial showed that adults treated in the ED with 2 days of dexamethasone (16 mg daily) had equivalent outcomes to those treated with 5 days of prednisone (50 mg daily). In this study, 104 subjects receiving dexamethasone and 96 subjects receiving prednisone were assessed. The outcomes measured included return to normal level of activity and prevention of relapse.[89]

Intravenous corticosteroids are recommended for critically ill patients and those intolerant of the oral form.[20] Hospitalized patients are given 40 to 60 mg of methylprednisolone intravenously every 12 to 24 hours. For patients who require critical care admission, higher doses of 60 to 80 mg of methylprednisolone are given every 12 hours. Several studies have shown that intramuscular corticosteroids are as effective as oral treatment.[85,90] A randomized controlled trial of 190 adult patients in the ED showed that subjects treated with a single dose of 160 mg intramuscular methylprednisolone had similar relapse rates to those treated with 160 mg of oral methylprednisolone tapered over 8 days.[90]

Long-term use of systemic corticosteroids should be avoided; it is indicated only for the most severe cases of asthma. Side effects of chronic corticosteroid use can be significant, and include immune suppression, adrenal suppression, growth suppression, Cushing syndrome, cataracts, and glucose imbalances.[20] Conversely, inhaled corticosteroids are the recommended first-line therapy for long-term treatment of mild, moderate, and severe persistent asthma.[20,23,24] They are absorbed locally and have a minimal side effect profile.

MAGNESIUM SULFATE

There is evidence that magnesium inhibits the influx of calcium into smooth muscle cells, causing bronchodilation.[91] In addition, magnesium acts on neutrophils to decrease inflammation.[92] A 2009 Cochrane Review found that intravenous magnesium sulfate significantly improved pulmonary function and decreased hospital admission rates in patients suffering from severe asthma. There was no significant effect noted for all asthmatics in general.[93] Side effects of intravenous magnesium were minimal.

Current guidelines recommend that magnesium be given for life-threatening exacerbations of acute asthma, or if the exacerbation remains severe (PEF <40%) after 1 hour of conventional therapy.[20] For these indications, 2 g of intravenous magnesium sulfate should be administered.

Limited studies have shown variable efficacy of nebulized inhaled magnesium in combination with β2-agonists for the treatment of acute asthma. The benefit seems to be greatest in the subgroup of severe asthma.[94] More data are needed to support definitive conclusions.

HELIOX

Heliox is a blend of 70% to 80% helium and 20% to 30% oxygen, which has a lower gas density than air. Heliox can potentially decrease resistance to airflow and enhance delivery of nebulized bronchodilators.[95,96] The role of heliox in asthma management remains unclear. Currently, it is not recommended as an initial treatment of asthma.[20,97] There have been few controlled studies and the optimal duration of heliox treatment is unknown. Current guidelines recommend that heliox-driven albuterol nebulization should be given for life-threatening exacerbations or if the exacerbation remains severe (PEF <40%) after 1 hour of conventional therapy.[20]

A 2006 Cochrane Review concluded that heliox improved pulmonary function only in the subgroup of patients with the most severe obstruction. However, this conclusion was based on a small number of studies.[97] A recent randomized trial of 59 adults with severe asthma found significant improvements in FEV_1 in those treated with nebulized bronchodilators with heliox. The largest gains were in those who sat upright and leaned the trunk forward at an angle of 50° to –60°.[98] A randomized controlled trial of 80 adults showed the greatest benefit in older adults and those with the lower pretreatment PEFs.[99] A randomized controlled trial of 30 children with moderate to severe asthma showed a greater degree of clinical improvement in those treated with heliox-driven albuterol nebulization. Eleven patients (73%) in the heliox group were discharged in less than 12 hours, compared with 5 (33%) in the control group.[100]

Since the 2006 Cochrane Review, 2 small studies have been conducted in children with moderate to severe asthma comparing heliox-powered albuterol therapy versus controls; these did not show a statistical difference in clinically important outcomes (admission rate, need for intubation, hospital length of stay).[101,102]

LEUKOTRIENE MODIFIERS

Leukotrienes are potent inflammatory mediators. Leukotriene modifiers improve lung function and decrease asthma exacerbations.[103,104] Three leukotriene modifiers are currently available for long-term therapy for asthma: montelukast, zafirlukast, and zileuton. However, many studies have found that overall efficacy of inhaled corticosteroids is superior to that of leukotriene modifiers for the long-term control of asthma.[103,104] Leukotriene modifiers are an alternative chronic treatment of patients with mild persistent asthma, who are unable to use inhaled corticosteroids.[20]

Leukotriene modifiers have not been used traditionally in the emergent setting. However, promising new research shows that leukotriene modifiers may have a future role in the ED. A randomized multicenter trial evaluated the effects of oral zafirlukast in 641 acute asthmatics. Those receiving zafirlukast in the ED had significant improvement in dyspnea and FEV_1, decreased risk of relapse, and decreased need for extended hospital care.[105] Intravenous leukotriene modifiers have also shown promise in the setting of acute asthma. A randomized controlled trial of 201 asthmatics showed significant improvements in FEV_1 in the first 20 minutes after treatment with intravenous montelukast.[106]

IMMUNOTHERAPY

Immunotherapy is an emerging area of asthma treatment that targets allergen triggers of asthma. It is the only treatment modality that modifies the underlying disease process. Immunotherapy has no role in the acute management of asthma but can be used for long-term maintenance therapy. Injection immunotherapy should be considered when the allergic component is well documented, and when asthma control remains inadequate.[23,24,107]

METHYLXANTHINES

Theophylline and aminophylline are widely prescribed for asthma worldwide, and have been used for more than 50 years. However, current evidence shows that this medication class does not produce additional bronchodilation when combined with standard β-agonist therapy, and results in more adverse effects.[108] Currently, the methylxanthines are not recommended as therapy for the acute exacerbation of asthma. Sustained-release theophylline can be considered for the treatment of mild persistent asthma.[20]

CROMOLYN SODIUM AND NEDOCROMIL

Cromolyn sodium and nedocromil are alternative treatments for mild persistent asthma. These medications block chloride channels and modulate mast cell mediator release.[109] They can be used as preventive treatment before exercise or allergen exposure.[20] These agents have no role in the acute management of asthma.

MANAGEMENT OF STATUS ASTHMATICUS

Status asthmaticus is an acute, severe exacerbation of asthma that does not respond to conventional treatment. It can progress to respiratory failure and death. All patients presenting to the ED with severe asthma should be started on early intensive therapy. This therapy includes β2-agonists, anticholinergics, and systemic corticosteroids. If patients fail to respond to initial therapy, they should be moved to a more closely monitored setting.

Heliox-driven nebulization of bronchodilators and intravenous magnesium sulfate are recommended adjunctive treatments for life-threatening asthma exacerbations, or for severe exacerbations that fail to respond to conventional therapy within the first hour.[20] Subcutaneous epinephrine (0.01 mg/kg to maximum dose of 0.3–0.5 mg) or nebulized epinephrine can be considered. A meta-analysis of 6 studies (including 161 adults and 121 children and adolescents) compared the efficacy of nebulized epinephrine with nebulized β2-agonists. Patients receiving nebulized epinephrine had a nonsignificant improvement in lung function.[110]

Ketamine is a dissociative agent that dilates bronchial smooth muscle and increases circulating catecholamines. Ketamine reduces bronchospasm and can help delay the need for intubation.[111,112] Several case reports of patients with status asthmaticus treated with intravenous ketamine have shown promising results. In these studies, ketamine was given as an intravenous bolus of 0.5 to 1 mg/kg, then as an infusion of 0.5 to 2 mg/kg over 1 hour. These patients failed to improve with conventional therapies, but responded successfully to ketamine.[113,114] However a double-blind randomized controlled trial comparing ketamine bolus and infusion with placebo in moderately severe asthma exacerbations in children did not show improvement in pulmonary index score.[115]

If the patient continues to deteriorate despite maximal medical therapy, noninvasive ventilation or endotracheal intubation with mechanical ventilation should be considered.

NONINVASIVE VENTILATION

Noninvasive ventilation is a promising area of acute asthma treatment. The goal of this modality is to support and reduce the patient's respiratory effort, giving enough time to allow other treatments to take effect and possibly avoid intubation.[116] Small studies have supported its use for acute asthma.[117,118] Noninvasive ventilation can be considered for the stable asthmatic who is tiring from the high respiratory demand, and who is expected to recover in the next few hours.[116] A recent Cochrane Review and guidelines do not support the routine use of noninvasive ventilator support.[119–122]

INTUBATION AND MECHANICAL VENTILATION

A minority of severe asthmatics require invasive ventilation in a critical care setting. Endotracheal intubation should be considered in the patient with impending respiratory failure, despite maximal medical therapy. Risk factors for death from asthma include previous intubations or intensive care admissions, or recent history of poorly controlled asthma.[123–127] Four percent of patients hospitalized for asthma require endotracheal intubation and mechanical ventilation.[128]

Mortality among those requiring ventilation is around 8%.[129] Death is multifactorial, and can be caused by severe obstruction, extreme hyperinflation, complications of acute asthma, failure by the patient or clinician to appreciate the severity of the disease, and failure to optimally control asthma.

Warning signs that a patient will need intubation include decreasing level of consciousness, cyanosis, deterioration of FEV_1 or PEF, inability to maintain oxygenation by mask, respiratory muscle fatigue, and cardiac instability.[116] There is no evidence to support a specific pH or Pco_2 for intubation, and the decision should be made on clinical grounds. Intubation should be done by the most experienced clinician available, ideally with a large-bore endotracheal tube ($\geq$8.0 mm).[20] Rapid-sequence intubation (RSI) is the preferred approach, because the patient is typically exhausted with little physiologic reserve. The clinician should anticipate rapid oxygen desaturation with RSI, and use preoxygenation or positive pressure ventilation to optimize respiratory status.

Ketamine is the induction agent of choice for sedation and intubation of an asthmatic patient, because of its bronchodilating properties.[111,112] Intravenous ketamine is given at a dose of 1 to 2 mg/kg at a rate of 0.5 mg/kg/min and results in general anesthesia without respiratory depression.[130] Propofol induces bronchodilation and is an alternative induction agent, but can cause hypotension.[131,132]

Ventilator settings should be adjusted to minimize the risk of dynamic hyperinflation, caused by air trapping because of insufficient time for exhalation. Dynamic hyperinflation can lead to cardiovascular collapse and barotrauma. Asthmatics are particularly at risk for this complication, because the nature of the disease causes airflow obstruction that significantly affects expiratory flow. Respiratory rate settings should be decreased to give the patient more time to exhale. Initial tidal volume should be set at less than 8 mL/kg, to decrease the risk of lung inflation.[133]

Bronchodilators and systemic corticosteroids can be administered to the ventilated patient. For the intubated patient with refractory asthma, intravenous ketamine or inhaled isoflurane can be useful adjuncts. Heliox and extracorporeal life support can also be considered.

ASTHMA AND PREGNANCY

Asthma affects 3% to 8% of pregnant women and has a variable clinical course.[134–137] Clinical symptoms improve in one-third of pregnancies, worsen in one-third, and remain unchanged in one-third.[133,138] Clinical severity of asthma during pregnancy seems to follow severity before pregnancy.[139,140] Asthma exacerbations occur in 20% to 36% of pregnancies, most frequently between weeks 14 and 24. Poorly controlled asthma during pregnancy has been linked with increased risk of prematurity, cesarean delivery, preeclampsia, and growth restriction.[135,141–143]

The treatment of asthma during pregnancy can be challenging. The goal of asthma treatment during pregnancy should be to optimize the outcome of both mother and fetus. SABAs, anticholinergics, and inhaled corticosteroids seem to be safe during pregnancy. Budesonide is the long treatment of choice, because it has been extensively studied in pregnancy.[20] Systemic corticosteroids have been linked with prematurity, low birth weight, preeclampsia, congenital malformations, and cerebral palsy, and should be used with caution.[144–147] A meta-analysis of mothers treated with oral corticosteroids in the first trimester showed a significant increase in the risk of oral clefts in their offspring.[146] A recent large-scale study of antenatal steroids showed no difference in body size or survival free of major neurosensory disability in children at 2 years of age.[148] Epinephrine should be avoided during pregnancy, except in cases of anaphylaxis.

DISPOSITION

The goal for discharge from the ED is an FEV_1 or PEF greater than or equal to 70% of predicted, and a response that is sustained for 60 minutes after last treatment. Patient education is a key component to successful asthma management, and should be initiated in the ED.[20] Medications and inhaler techniques should be reviewed. A written asthma action plan that describes early recognition and self-management of exacerbations should be started or reviewed.[20] Patients should be counseled to avoid allergens or other triggers of asthma. Cigarette smoking in asthma is associated with increased disease severity, more frequent hospital admissions, and accelerated lung function decline.[149] Counseling for smoking cessation should be an essential component of asthma management.[150] Patients should seek follow-up asthma care within 1 to 4 weeks.[20]

β-Agonists and corticosteroids should be included in the discharge plan. Many studies have shown that a short course of corticosteroids significantly reduces early relapse rates after treatment of acute asthma in the ED.[151,152] In mild to moderate asthma exacerbations, inhaled corticosteroids and oral corticosteroids were similarly effective in preventing relapse. Patients with significant asthma exacerbations should receive a course of oral corticosteroids for 3 to 10 days. Intramuscular injection of long-acting methylprednisolone can be considered in patients at high risk of medical noncompliance.[90] Compared with oral, intramuscular corticosteroids are equally effective in terms of rates of relapse. A combination inhaled and oral corticosteroids regimen compared with oral corticosteroid treatment alone showed a trend toward reduced asthma relapse rates.[153]

Patients with FEV_1 or PEF 40% to 69% of predicted despite intensive therapy require continued treatment in the ED or hospital admission. Patients with FEV_1 or PEF less than 40% should be admitted to the intensive care unit. Adjunctive therapies and mechanical ventilation should be considered for these patients. Patients who continue to have features of severe exacerbation after initial treatment require admission. Patients who show greater than 75% PEF following one hour of initial treatment are suitable candidates for discharge from the ED.[121]

SUMMARY

Asthma is a chronic inflammatory disease that is commonly encountered in the ED. Early signs of worsening asthma should be recognized and immediate treatment given. β-Agonists, anticholinergics, and corticosteroids are mainstays of treatment of the asthma exacerbation. Magnesium sulfate, epinephrine, and heliox can be considered for life-threatening presentations of asthma. Control of environmental triggers, improvements in daily maintenance therapy for asthma, and increasing patient education should help to reduce the severity and frequency of asthma exacerbations seen in the ED.

REFERENCES

1. Masoli M, Fabian D, Holt S, et al. The global burden of asthma: executive summary of the GINA Dissemination Committee Report. Allergy 2004;59: 469–78.

2. Statistics Canada. Asthma by sex, provinces and territories 2010. Available at: http://www40.statcan.ca/l01/cst01/HEALTH50A-eng.htm. Accessed October 27, 2011.
3. Public Health Agency of Canada. Life and breath: respiratory disease in Canada. 2007. Available at: http://www.phac-aspc.gc.ca/publicat/2007/lbrdc-vsmrc/index-eng.php#tphp. Accessed October 27, 2011.
4. Centers for Disease Control and Prevention. National Health Interview Survey: Asthma. 2009. Available at: http://www.cdc.gov/asthma/default.htm. Accessed October 27, 2011.
5. Gibson P, McDonald V, Marks G. Asthma in older adults. Lancet 2010; 376(9743):803–13.
6. Lai CKW, Beasley R, Crane J, et al. Global variation in the prevalence and severity of asthma symptoms: Phase Three of the International Study of Asthma and Allergies in Childhood (ISAAC). Thorax 2009;64:476–83.
7. Eder W, Ege MJ, von Mutius E. The asthma epidemic. N Engl J Med 2006;355: 2226–35.
8. Bjorksten B, Clayton T, Ellwood P, et al, ISAAC Phase III Study Group. Worldwide trends for symptoms of rhinitis and conjunctivitis: phase III of the International Study of Asthma and Allergies in Childhood. Pediatr Allergy Immunol 2008;19: 110–24.
9. Asher MI, Montefort S, Bjorksten B, et al, ISAAC Phase Three Study Group. Worldwide time trends in the prevalence of symptoms of asthma, allergic rhino-conjunctivitis, and eczema in childhood: ISAAC Phases One and Three repeat multicountry cross-sectional surveys. Lancet 2006;368:733–43.
10. Senthilselvan A, Lawson J, Rennie DC, et al. Stabilization of an increasing trend in physician-diagnosed asthma prevalence in Saskatchewan, 1991 to 1998. Chest 2003;124(2):438–48.
11. Braun-Fahrlander C, Gassner M, Grize L, et al. No further increase in asthma, hay fever and atopic sensitisation in adolescents living in Switzerland. Eur Respir J 2004;23(3):407–13.
12. Ronchetti R, Villa MP, Barreto M, et al. Is the increase in childhood asthma coming to an end? Findings from three surveys of schoolchildren in Rome, Italy. Eur Respir J 2001;17(5):881–6.
13. Moorman JE, Rudd RA, Johnson CA. National surveillance for asthma–United States, 1980-2004. MMWR Surveill Summ 2007;56:1–54.
14. Rowe BH, Bota G, Clark S. Comparison of Canadian versus American emergency department visits for acute asthma. Can Respir J 2007;14:331–7.
15. Lougheed MD, Garvey N, Chapman KR. The Ontario Asthma Regional Variation Study: emergency department visit rates and the relation to hospitalization rates. Chest 2006;129:909–17.
16. Diette G, Krishnan JA, Dominici F, et al. Asthma in older adults: factors associated with hospitalization. Arch Intern Med 2002;162(10):1123–32.
17. Chen Y, Johansen H, Thillaiampalam S, et al. "Asthma". Health Reports. Statistics Canada Catalogue 2005;no. 82-003.16(2):43–6.
18. Restrepo RD, Peters J. Near-fatal asthma: recognition and management. Curr Opin Pulm Med 2008;14(1):13–23.
19. Romagnoli M, Caramori G, Braccioni F, et al. Near-fatal asthma phenotype in the ENFUMOSA Cohort. Clin Exp Allergy 2007;37(4):552–7.
20. National Asthma Education and Prevention Program. Expert panel report III: guidelines for the diagnosis and management of asthma. Bethesda (MD): National Heart, Lung, and Blood Institute; 2007 (NIH publication no. 08-4051).

21. Boyce JA. Mast cells: beyond IgE. J Allergy Clin Immunol 2003;111(1):24–32.
22. Brightling CE, Bradding P, Symon FA, et al. Mast-cell infiltration of airway smooth muscle in asthma. N Engl J Med 2002;346(22):1699–705.
23. Becker A, Lemiere C, Bérubé D, et al. Summary and recommendations from the Canadian Asthma Consensus Guidelines, 2003. CMAJ 2005;173:S3–11.
24. Becker A, Berube D, Chad Z, et al. Canadian Pediatric Asthma Consensus Guidelines, 2003 (updated to December 2004): introduction. CMAJ 2005;173: S12–4.
25. Pratter MR, Curley FJ, Dubois J, et al. Cause and evaluation of chronic dyspnea in a pulmonary disease clinic. Arch Intern Med 1989;149(10):2277–82.
26. Busse WW, Lemanske RF. Asthma. N Engl J Med 2001;344(5):350–62.
27. Cohn L, Elias JA, Chupp GL. Asthma: mechanisms of disease progression and persistence. Annu Rev Immunol 2004;22:789–815.
28. Akbari O, Faul JL, Hoyte EG, et al. CD4+ invariant T-cell–receptor+ natural killer T cells in bronchial asthma. N Engl J Med 2006;354(11):1117–29.
29. Williams TJ. The eosinophil enigma. J Clin Invest 2004;113(4):507–9.
30. Chu HW, Martin RJ. Are eosinophils still important in asthma? Clin Exp Allergy 2001;31(4):525–8.
31. Kuipers H, Lambrecht BN. The interplay of dendritic cells, Th2 cells and regulatory T cells in asthma. Curr Opin Immunol 2004;16(6):702–8.
32. Peters-Golden M. The alveolar macrophage: the forgotten cell in asthma. Am J Respir Cell Mol Biol 2004;31(1):3–7.
33. Polito AJ, Proud D. Epithelial cells as regulators of airway inflammation. J Allergy Clin Immunol 1998;102(5):714–8.
34. Pratter MR, Hingston DM, Irwin RS. Diagnosis of bronchial asthma by clinical evaluation. An unreliable method. Chest 1983;84(1):42–7.
35. Irwin R, Curley FJ, French CL. Chronic cough. The spectrum and frequency of causes, key components of the diagnostic evaluation, and outcome of specific therapy. Am Rev Respir Dis 1990;141:640–7.
36. Huss K, Adkinson NF Jr, Eggleston PA, et al. House dust mite and cockroach exposure are strong risk factors for positive allergy skin test responses in the Childhood Asthma Management Program. J Allergy Clin Immunol 2001; 107(1):48–54.
37. Htut T, Higgenbottam TW, Gill GW, et al. Eradication of house dust mites from homes of atopic asthmatic subjects: a double-blind trial. J Allergy Clin Immunol 2001;107(1):55–60.
38. Bush RK, Prochnau JJ. Alternaria-induced asthma. J Allergy Clin Immunol 2004; 113(2):227–34.
39. Taylor SL, Bush RK, Selner JC, et al. Sensitivity to sulfited foods among sulfite-sensitive subjects with asthma. J Allergy Clin Immunol 1988;81(6):1159–67.
40. Comhair SA, Gaston BM, Ricci KS, et al, National Heart Lung Blood Institute Severe Asthma Research Program (SARP). Detrimental effects of environmental tobacco smoke in relation to asthma severity. PLoS One 2011;6(5):e18574.
41. Johnston SL, Pattemore PK, Sanderson G, et al. Community study of role of viral infections in exacerbations of asthma in 9-11 year old children. BMJ 1995; 310(6989):1225–9.
42. Martinez FD, Wright AL, Taussig LM, et al. Asthma and wheezing in the first six years of life. N Engl J Med 1995;332(3):133–8.
43. Jenkins C, Costello J, Hodge L. Systematic review of prevalence of aspirin induced asthma and its implications for clinical practice. BMJ 2004; 328(7437):434.

44. Quirce S, Sastre J. New causes of occupational asthma. Curr Opin Allergy Clin Immunol 2011;11:80–5.
45. Furgał M, Nowobilski R, Pulka G, et al. Dyspnea is related to family functioning in adult asthmatics. J Asthma 2009;46(3):280–3.
46. Rosenkranz MA, Davidson RJ. Affective neural circuitry and mind-body influences in asthma. Neuroimage 2009;47(3):972–80.
47. Randolph C. An update on exercise-induced bronchoconstriction with and without asthma. Curr Allergy Asthma Rep 2009;9(6):433–8.
48. Macsali F, Real FG, Plana E, et al. Early age at menarche, lung function, and adult asthma. Am J Respir Crit Care Med 2011;183(1):8–14.
49. Martinez-Moragon E, Plaza V, Serrano J, et al. Near-fatal asthma related to menstruation. J Allergy Clin Immunol 2004;113(2):242–4.
50. Jones SC, Iverson D, Burns P, et al. Asthma and ageing: an end user's perspective - the perception and problems with the management of asthma in the elderly. Clin Exp Allergy 2011;41(4):471–81.
51. Cuttitta G, Cibella F, Bellia V, et al. Changes in FVC during methacholine-induced bronchoconstriction in elderly patients with asthma: bronchial hyperresponsiveness and aging. Chest 2001;119(6):1685–90.
52. Quadrelli SA, Roncorini A. Features of asthma in the elderly. J Asthma 2001;38(5):377–89.
53. Ekici M, Apan A, Ekici A, et al. Perception of bronchoconstriction in elderly asthmatics. J Asthma 2001;38(8):691–6.
54. Kikuchi Y, Okabe S, Tamura G, et al. Chemosensitivity and perception of dyspnea in patients with a history of near-fatal asthma. N Engl J Med 1994;330(19):1329–34.
55. Bijl-Hofland ID, Cloosterman SG, Folgering HT, et al. Relation of the perception of airway obstruction to the severity of asthma. Thorax 1999;54(1):15–9.
56. Brooks TW, Creekmore FM, Young DC, et al. Rates of hospitalizations and emergency department visits in patients with asthma and chronic obstructive pulmonary disease taking beta-blockers. Pharmacotherapy 2007;27(5):684–90.
57. Deykin A, Lazarus SC, Fahy JV, et al, Asthma Clinic Research Network, National Heart, Lung and Blood Institute/NIH. Sputum eosinophil counts predict asthma control after discontinuation of inhaled corticosteroids. J Allergy Clin Immunol 2005;115(4):720–7.
58. Green RH, Brightling CE, McKenna S, et al. Asthma exacerbations and sputum eosinophil counts: a randomised controlled trial. Lancet 2002;360(9347):1715–21.
59. Smith AD, Cowan JO, Brassett KP, et al. Use of exhaled nitric oxide measurements to guide treatment in chronic asthma. N Engl J Med 2005;352(21):2163–73.
60. Gibson PG, Simpson JL. The overlap syndrome of asthma and COPD: what are its features and how important is it? Thorax 2009;64(8):728–35.
61. Kauppi P, Kupiainen H, Lindqvist A, et al. Overlap syndrome of asthma and COPD predicts low quality of life. J Asthma 2011;48(3):279–85.
62. Karras DJ, Sammon ME, Terregino CA, et al. Clinically meaningful changes in quantitative measurements of asthma severity. Acad Emerg Med 2000;7(4):327–34.
63. Kelly AM, Kerr D, Powell C. Is severity assessment after one hour of treatment better for predicting the need for admission in acute asthma? Respir Med 2004;98(8):777–81.

64. Martin TG, Elenbaas RM, Pingleton SH. Use of peak expiratory flow rates to eliminated unnecessary arterial blood gases in acute asthma. Ann Emerg Med 1982;11(20):70–3.
65. Rang LC, Murray HE, Wells GA, et al. Can peripheral venous blood gases replace arterial blood gases in emergency department patients? CJEM 2002; 4(1):7–15.
66. Tsai TW, Gallagher EJ, Lombardi G, et al. Guidelines for the selective ordering of admission chest radiography in adult obstructive airway disease. Ann Emerg Med 1993;22(12):1854–8.
67. Newman KB, Milne S, Hamilton C, et al. A comparison of albuterol administered by metered-dose inhaler and spacer with albuterol by nebulizer in adults presenting to an urban emergency department with acute asthma. Chest 2002; 121(4):1036–41.
68. Idris AH, McDermott MF, Raucci JC, et al. Emergency department treatment of severe asthma. Metered-dose inhaler plus holding chamber is equivalent in effectiveness to nebulizer. Chest 1993;103(3):665–72.
69. Cates CJ, Crilly JA, Rowe BH. Holding chambers (spacers) versus nebulisers for beta-agonist treatment of acute asthma. Cochrane Database Syst Rev 2009:CD000052.
70. Burrows T, Connett GJ. The relative benefits and acceptability of metered dose inhalers and nebulisers to treat acute asthma in preschool children [abstract]. Thorax 2004;59(Suppl 2):ii20.
71. Davies A, Thomson G, Walker J, et al. A review of the risks and disease transmission associated with aerosol generating medical procedures. J Infect Prev 2009;10(4):122–6.
72. Bahadori K, Doyle-Waters MM, Marra C, et al. Economic burden of asthma: a systematic review. BMC Pulm Med 2009;9:24.
73. Scott SD, Osmond MH, O'Leary KA, et al, Pediatric Emergency Research Canada (PERC) MDI/spacer Study Group. Barriers and supports to implementation of MDI/spacer use in nine Canadian pediatric emergency departments: a qualitative study. Implement Sci 2009;4:65.
74. Osmond MH, Gazarian M, Henry RL, et al, PERC Spacer Study Group. Barriers to metered-dose inhaler/spacer use in Canadian emergency departments: a national survey. Acad Emerg Med 2007;14(11):1106–13.
75. Camargo CA Jr, Spooner CH, Rowe BH. Continuous versus intermittent beta-agonists for acute asthma. Cochrane Database Syst Rev 2009:CD001115.
76. Travers AA, Jones AP, Kelly KD, et al. Intravenous beta2-agonists for acute asthma in the emergency department. Cochrane Database Syst Rev 2009: CD002988.
77. Salpeter SR, Ormiston TM, Salpeter EE. Cardiovascular effects of β-agonists in patients with asthma and COPD: A meta-analysis. Chest 2004;125(6): 2309–21.
78. Plotnick L, Ducharme F. Combined inhaled anticholinergics and beta2-agonists for initial treatment of acute asthma in children. Cochrane Database Syst Rev 2008:CD000060.
79. Rodrigo GJ, Castro-Rodriguez JA. Anticholinergics in the treatment of children and adults with acute asthma: a systematic review with meta-analysis. Thorax 2005;60(9):740–6.
80. Rodrigo GJ, Rodrigo C. First-line therapy for adult patients with acute asthma receiving a multiple-dose protocol of ipratropium bromide plus albuterol in the emergency department. Am J Respir Crit Care Med 2000;161(6):1862–8.

81. Craven D, Kercsmar CM, Myers TR, et al. Ipratropium bromide plus nebulized albuterol for the treatment of hospitalized children with acute asthma. J Pediatr 2001;138(1):51–8.
82. Goggin N, Macarthur C, Parkin PC. Randomized trial of the addition of ipratropium bromide to albuterol and corticosteroid therapy in children hospitalized because of an acute asthma exacerbation. Arch Pediatr Adolesc Med 2001; 155(12):1329–34.
83. Hood PP, Cotter TP, Costello JE, et al. Effect of intravenous corticosteroid on ex vivo leukotriene generation by blood leucocyctes of normal and asthmatic patients. Thorax 1999;54(12):1075–82.
84. Rowe BH, Spooner CH, Ducharme FM, et al. Early emergency department treatment of acute asthma with systemic corticosteroids. Cochrane Database Syst Rev 2001;1:CD002178.
85. Rowe BH, Spooner CH, Ducharme FM, et al. Corticosteroids for preventing relapse following acute exacerbations of asthma. Cochrane Database Syst Rev 2007;3:CD000195.
86. Becker JM, Arora A, Scarfone RJ, et al. Oral versus intravenous corticosteroids for children hospitalized with asthma. J Allergy Clin Immunol 2005;103(4):586–90.
87. Barnett PL, Caputo GL, Baskin M, et al. Intravenous versus oral corticosteroids in the management of acute asthma in children. Ann Emerg Med 1997;30(3): 355–6.
88. Ratto D, Alfaro C, Sipsey J, et al. Are intravenous corticosteroids required in status asthmaticus? JAMA 1988;260(4):527–9.
89. Kravitz J, Dominici P, Ufberg J, et al. Two days of dexamethasone versus 5 days of prednisone in the treatment of acute asthma: a randomized controlled trial. Ann Emerg Med 2011;58(2):200–4.
90. Lahn M, Bijur P, Gallagher EJ. Randomized clinical trial of intramuscular vs oral methylprednisolone in the treatment of asthma exacerbations following discharge from an emergency department. Chest 2004;126(2):362–8.
91. Gourgoulianis KI, Chatziparasidis G, Chatziefthimiou A, et al. Magnesium as a relaxing factor of airway smooth muscles. J Aerosol Med 2001;14(3):301–7.
92. Cairns CB, Kraft M. Magnesium attenuates the neutrophil respiratory burst in adult asthmatic patients. Acad Emerg Med 1996;3:1093–7.
93. Rowe BH, Bretzlaff JA, Bourdon C, et al. Magnesium sulfate for treating acute exacerbations of acute asthma in the emergency department. Cochrane Database Syst Rev 2009:CD001490.
94. Blitz M, Blitz S, Beasely R, et al. Inhaled magnesium sulfate in the treatment of acute asthma. Cochrane Database Syst Rev 2009:CD003898.
95. Goode ML, Fink JB, Dhand R, et al. Improvement in aerosol with helium-oxygen mixtures during mechanical ventilation. Am J Med 2001;163:109–14.
96. Kress JP, Noth I, Gehlbach BK, et al. The utility of albuterol nebulized with heliox during acute asthma exacerbations. Am J Respir Crit Care Med 2002;165(9): 1317–21.
97. Rodrigo GJ, Pollack C, Rodrigo C, et al. Heliox for non-intubated acute asthma patients. Cochrane Database Syst Rev 2010:CD002884.
98. Brandão DC, Britto MC, Pessoa MF, et al. Heliox and forward-leaning posture improve the efficacy of nebulized bronchodilator in acute asthma: a randomized trial. Respir Care 2011;56(7):947–52.
99. Lee DL, Hsu CW, Lee H, et al. Beneficial effects of albuterol therapy driven by heliox versus by oxygen in severe asthma exacerbation. Acad Emerg Med 2005;12(9):820–7.

100. Kim IK, Phrampus E, Venkataraman S, et al. Helium/oxygen-driven albuterol nebulization in the treatment of children with moderate to severe asthma exacerbations: a randomized, controlled trial. Pediatrics 2005;116(5):1127–33.
101. Rivera ML, Kim TY, Stewart GM, et al. Albuterol nebulized in heliox in the initial ED treatment of pediatric asthma: a blinded, randomized controlled trial. Am J Emerg Med 2006;24(1):38–42.
102. Bigham MT, Jacobs BR, Monaco MA, et al. Helium/oxygen-driven albuterol nebulization in the management of children with status asthmaticus: a randomized, placebo-controlled trial. Pediatr Crit Care Med 2010;11(3):356–61.
103. Garcia-Garcia ML, Wahn U, Gilles L, et al. Montelukast, compared with fluticasone, for control of asthma among 6- to 14-year-old patients with mild asthma: the MOSAIC study. Pediatrics 2005;116(2):360–9.
104. Ostrom NK, Decotiis BA, Lincourt WR, et al. Comparative safety and efficacy of low-dose fluticasone propionate and montelukast in children with persistent asthma. J Pediatr 2005;147(2):213–20.
105. Silverman RA, Nowak RM, Korenblat PE, et al. Zafirlukast treatment for acute asthma: evaluation in a randomized, double-blind, multicenter trial. Chest 2004;126(5):1480–9.
106. Camargo CA Jr, Smithline HA, Malice MP, et al. A randomized controlled trial of intravenous montelukast in acute asthma. Am J Respir Crit Care Med 2003; 167(4):528–33.
107. Abramson MJ, Puy RM, Weiner JM. Injection allergen immunotherapy for asthma. Cochrane Database Syst Rev 2010:CD001186.
108. Parameswaran K, Belda J, Rowe BH. Addition of intravenous aminophylline to beta2-agonists in adults with acute asthma. Cochrane Database Syst Rev 2009:CD002742.
109. Alton EW, Norris AA. Chloride transport and the actions of nedocromil sodium and cromolyn sodium in asthma. J Allergy Clin Immunol 1996;98(5 Pt 2): S102–5.
110. Rodrigo GJ, Nannini LJ. Comparison between nebulized adrenaline and beta2 agonists for the treatment of acute asthma. A meta-analysis of randomized trials. Am J Emerg Med 2006;24(2):217–22.
111. L'Hommedieu CS, Arens JJ. The use of ketamine for the emergency intubation of patients with status asthmaticus. Ann Emerg Med 1987;16(5):568–71.
112. Hemmingsen C, Nielsen PK, Odorico J. Ketamine in the treatment of bronchospasm during mechanical ventilation. Am J Emerg Med 1994;12(4): 417–20.
113. Denmark TK, Crane HA, Brown L. Ketamine to avoid mechanical ventilation in severe pediatric asthma. J Emerg Med 2006;30(2):163–6.
114. Shlamovitz GZ, Hawthorne T. Intravenous ketamine in a dissociating dose as a temporizing measure to avoid mechanical ventilation in adult patient with severe asthma exacerbation. J Emerg Med 2011;41(5):492–4.
115. Allen JY, Macias CG. The efficacy of ketamine in pediatric emergency department patients who present with acute severe asthma. Ann Emerg Med 2005; 46(1):43–50.
116. Hodder R, Lougheed D, FitzGerald M, et al. Management of acute asthma in adults in the emergency department: assisted ventilation. CMAJ 2010;182(3): 265–72.
117. Murase K, Tomii K, Chin K, et al. The use of non-invasive ventilation for life-threatening asthma attacks: changes in the need for intubation. Respirology 2010;15(4):714–20.

118. Soroksy S, Stav D, Shpirer I. A pilot prospective, randomized, placebo-controlled trial of bilevel positive airway pressure in acute asthmatic attack. Chest 2003;123:1018–25.
119. Ram FS, Wellington S, Rowe BH, et al. Non-invasive positive pressure ventilation for treatment of respiratory failure due to severe acute exacerbations of asthma. Cochrane Database Syst Rev 2005;1:CD004360.
120. Bateman ED, Hurd SS, Barnes PJ, et al. Global strategy for asthma management and prevention: GINA executive summary. Eur Respir J 2008;31(1): 143–78.
121. Douglas G, Higgins B, Barnes N, et al. British guideline on the management of asthma: a national clinical guideline. Thorax 2008;63(Suppl 4):iv1–121.
122. Sutton L. Is NIV an effective intervention for patients with acute exacerbations of asthma? BestBETS, 2009. Available at: http://www.bestbets.org/bets/bet. php?id=15529. Accessed October 27, 2011.
123. Dhuper S, Maggiore D, Chung V, et al. Profile of near-fatal asthma in an inner-city hospital. Chest 2003;124(5):1880–4.
124. Mitchell I, Tough SC, Semple LK, et al. Near-fatal asthma: a population-based study of risk factors. Chest 2002;121(5):1407–13.
125. Eisner MD, Lieu TA, Chi F, et al. Beta agonists, inhaled steroids, and the risk of intensive care unit admission for asthma. Eur Respir J 2001;17(2): 233–40.
126. Malmstrom K, Kaila M, Kajosaari M, et al. Fatal asthma in Finnish children and adolescents 1976-1998: validity of death certificates and a clinical description. Pediatr Pulmonol 2007;42(3):210–5.
127. Turner MO, Noertjojo K, Vedal S, et al. Risk factors for near-fatal asthma. A case-control study in hospitalized patients with asthma. Am J Respir Crit Care Med 1998;157(6 Pt 1):1804–9.
128. Krishnan V, Diette GB, Rand CS, et al. Mortality in patients hospitalized for asthma exacerbations in the United States. Am J Respir Crit Care Med 2006; 174(6):633–8.
129. McFadden ER Jr. Acute severe asthma. Am J Respir Crit Care Med 2003;168: 740–59.
130. Papiris S, Kotanidou A, Malagari K, et al. Clinical review: severe asthma. Crit Care 2002;6(1):30–44.
131. Conti G, Ferretti A, Tellan G, et al. Propofol induces bronchodilation in a patient mechanically ventilated for status asthmaticus. Intensive Care Med 1993;19(5): 305.
132. Zaloga G, Todd M, Levit P, et al. Propofol-induced bronchodilation in patients with status asthmaticus. Internet J Emerg Intensive Care Med 2001;5(1).
133. Brenner B, Corbridge T, Kazzi A. Intubation and mechanical ventilation of the asthmatic patient in respiratory failure. J Allergy Clin Immunol 2009; 124(Suppl 2):S19–28.
134. Murphy VE, Gibson PG, Smith R, et al. Asthma during pregnancy: mechanisms and treatment implications. Eur Respir J 2005;25(4):731–50.
135. Namazy JA, Schatz M. Pregnancy and asthma: recent developments. Curr Opin Pulm Med 2005;11(1):56–60.
136. Liccardi G, Cazzola M, Canonica GW, et al. General strategy for the management of bronchial asthma in pregnancy. Respir Med 2003;97(7):778–89.
137. Kwon HL, Belanger K, Bracken MB. Asthma prevalence among pregnant and childbearing-aged women in the United States: estimates from national health surveys. Ann Epidemiol 2003;13(5):317–24.

138. Gluck JC. The change of asthma course during pregnancy. Clin Rev Allergy Immunol 2004;26(3):171–80.

139. Schatz M, Dombrowski MP, Wise R, et al. Asthma morbidity during pregnancy can be predicted by severity classification. J Allergy Clin Immunol 2003; 112(2):283–8.

140. Murphy VE, Gibson P, Talbot PI, et al. Severe asthma exacerbations during pregnancy. Obstet Gynecol 2005;106(5 Pt 1):1046–54.

141. Dombrowski MP, Schatz M. Asthma in pregnancy. Clin Obstet Gynecol 2010; 53(2):301–10.

142. Bakhireva LN, Schatz M, Jones KL, et al, Organization of Teratology Information Specialists Collaborative Research Group. Asthma control during pregnancy and the risk of preterm delivery or impaired fetal growth. Ann Allergy Asthma Immunol 2008;101(2):137–43.

143. Murphy VE, Clifton VL, Gibson PG. Asthma exacerbations during pregnancy. Thorax 2006;61(2):169–76.

144. Schatz M, Dombrowski MP, Wise R, et al, Maternal-Fetal Medicine Units Network, The National Institute of Child Health and Development; National Heart, Lung and Blood Institute. The relationship of asthma medication use to perinatal outcomes. J Allergy Clin Immunol 2004;113(6):1040–5.

145. Schatz M, Zeiger RS, Harden K, et al. The safety of asthma and allergy medications during pregnancy. J Allergy Clin Immunol 1997;100(3):301–6.

146. Park-Wyllie L, Mazzotta P, Pastuszak A, et al. Birth defects after maternal exposure to corticosteroids: prospective cohort study and meta-analysis of epidemiological studies. Teratology 2000;62(6):385–92.

147. Wapner RJ, Sorokin Y, Mele L, et al, National Institute of Child Health and Human Development Maternal-Fetal Medicine Units Network. Long-term outcomes after repeat doses of antenatal corticosteroids. N Engl J Med 2007;357(12):1190–8.

148. Crowther CA, Doyle LW, Haslam RR, et al, ACTORDS Study Group. Outcomes at 2 years of age after repeat doses of antenatal corticosteroids. N Engl J Med 2007;357(12):1179–89.

149. Fattahi F, Hylkema MN, Melgert BN, et al. Smoking and nonsmoking asthma: differences in clinical outcome and pathogenesis. Expert Rev Respir Med 2011; 5(1):93–105.

150. Jang AS, Park SW, Kim DJ, et al. Effects of smoking cessation on airflow obstruction and quality of life in asthmatic smokers. Allergy Asthma Immunol Res 2010;2(4):254–9.

151. Chapman KR, Verbeek PR, White JG, et al. Effect of a short course of prednisone in the prevention of early relapse after the emergency room treatment of acute asthma. N Engl J Med 1991;324(12):788–94.

152. Fiel SB, Swartz MA, Glanz K, et al. Efficacy of short-term corticosteroid therapy in outpatient treatment of acute bronchial asthma. Am J Med 1983;75(2): 259–62.

153. Krishnan JA, Nowak R, Davis SQ, et al. Anti-inflammatory treatment after discharge home from the emergency department in adults with acute asthma. J Allergy Clin Immunol 2009;124(Suppl 2):S29–34.

Stepwise Treatment of Asthma

John A. Fornadley, MD

KEYWORDS

- Bronchospasm • Intermittent bronchospasm • Persistent bronchospasm

KEY POINTS

- Asthma management is based on severity of disease.
- Overmedication or undermedication of asthma is a concern.
- Uncontrolled asthma may lead to irreversible lung disease.

Step therapy for treatment of asthma has proven a successful means of guiding practitioners through marked changes in management strategy and of gaining better control over this difficult disease process.

In the middle to late twentieth century, asthma therapy was not providing satisfactory control of the disease. Physician visits, self-reported reactive airway disease prevalence, and deaths due to asthma increased between 1960 and 1990.[1–4] Even more troubling was that a percentage of the deaths were attributed to the bronchodilator therapy, specifically exacerbations of disease related to long-acting beta2-agonist (LABA) use. Even without these concerns, bronchodilator therapy did not seem to be the definitive therapy to manage asthma.

Scientific work in the 1960s included the discovery of IgE and a better delineation of the role of inflammation in reversible airway disease.[5] In combination with recently developed inhaled corticosteroids, this provided a better understanding of the disease as well as a pathway that could make a substantial positive impact on the quality of life for a patient with asthma.

Several challenges surrounded the acceptance of this radical algorithm change. The first was the need to educate and change practice patterns of the wide range of practitioners treating asthma, which required informing them and gaining their acceptance of the strategy. Unlike a new medication or adjunctive therapy, the concept of inflammation-based therapy for asthma represented a marked philosophic change. Because physicians tend to gather their continuing education from the medical journals and societies related to their specific field, there was a need to reach out to several disparate societies and journals to get information to the practitioners regarding changes in the therapy of asthma.

This article originally appeared in Otolaryngologic Clinics of North America, Volume 47, Issue 1, February 2014.
Department of Surgery, Penn State University, 500 University Drive, Hershey, PA 17036, USA
E-mail address: entshop@aol.com

Asthma therapy is also complicated by the variability of the disease from life-threatening exacerbations to a completely normal quality of life between episodes. This disease process does not lend itself to simply starting a medication and continuing it routinely for years, as in the case of hypertension or types of cardiac disease. There is a legitimate concern among physicians and patients about overmedication or undermedication of asthma. Without guidelines, it was unclear when it would be most appropriate to start medications. Unfortunately, with the medications involved, there were side effect profiles that made overuse undesirable. Steroid therapy, which represented a critical new role in asthma care, is known to have side effects that include growth retardation, decreased immunocompetence, and multiple system-based complications. All branches of medicine recognize a strong desire to limit steroid use, which complicates acceptance of the new regimen. In asthma, these limitations must be balanced against the risk of progression of disease and the inability to stabilize the airway by other means.

Beta agonists have a somewhat diminished but still vital role in the more modern therapy approach. These agents also suffer from reported complications, including electrolyte disorders, cardiac dysrhythmias, and sudden death.[2,4]

This change in asthma management occurred at a time when clinical practice guidelines were less well understood and certainly less trusted. Current data on the value of evidence-based guidelines were obviously not available and the physicians of the time were concerned that guidelines were intended to restrict testing and control medical practices for the benefit of third-party payers.

It was in this medical environment that the National Asthma Education and Prevention Program (NAEPP), under the auspices of the National Heart, Lung, and Blood Institute, performed a thorough literature review and created a guideline pathway for asthma that was published in 1991.[6] The guidelines have been revised in 1997, 2002, and most recently in 2007. The guideline divided asthma into categories of intermittent or persistent, with the latter category being subdivided into mild, moderate, or severe. This categorization then provided the clinician with a step therapy based on the severity of the asthma. These pathways have largely succeeded in changing the way asthma is managed, starting in the last decade of the twentieth century. The intervening time has allowed statistical analysis to identify actual improvement in asthma management as measured by fewer emergency visits and deaths.

From 1991 to 2006, progress in the field, new medications, and updated data resulted in the need for changes to the asthma management algorithm. The stepwise approach has grown necessarily more complicated, but the overall principles remain. The guideline continues to provide some rigidity but allows physician judgment and insight. In the current version, the guidelines include patient education and some patient responsibilities. Although some of the elegant simplicity of the 1991 algorithm is lost, the present update allows better active consideration of allergic components of the disease. In addition, there are more options for effectively allowing medication use to step up when needed and step down when possible.

The now-familiar four categories of asthma remain unchanged. The step approach for asthma therapy has increased these to six steps. The care recommendations are stratified for patient ages of 0 to 4 years, 5 to 11 years, and 12-plus years to allow for better treatment of pediatric medication variances.

The initial step, as before, is the diagnosis of asthma. The goal is to identify asthma, evaluate and exclude other diagnoses, and determine the severity of the disease. Patient history, spirometry (in patients older than 5 years), and the exclusion of other diagnoses is important in arriving at the correct diagnosis. The severity of the disease is important in determining how to initiate therapy. The control aspect of disease is vital in monitoring and controlling therapy. Severity is defined as the intrinsic intensity of the disease process. This parameter is important for the initiation of therapy (**Table 1**).

The initial assessment is the first and arguably the most critical step, because it has a role in both diagnosis and the direction of initial therapy. The steps of the initial assessment are illustrated in **Table 1**. Note that the diagnosis includes a history of symptoms and types of precipitating factors, not only spirometry. Spirometry is nevertheless required in patients 5 years and older. These historical data combined with the results of spirometry assist the clinician in making the diagnosis of asthma and provides for patient stratification into a defined level of asthma severity.

Because this clinical information is vital to the correct categorization of the patient's level of asthma, the clinician should be familiar with **Table 1** when taking the asthma history. In addition to categorization into intermittent versus persistent, and as mild, moderate, or severe, the patients are also grouped according to age. Based on the level of findings, the clinician is directed to a subsequent algorithm that indicates the recommended medical therapeutic selection (**Table 2**).

CRITICAL CHANGES IN THE THIRD REVISION

The updated guidelines reflect a identified need to monitor the control of asthma. Whereas the initial evaluation of the patient with asthma is to determine at which step to initiate therapy, the reassessments are geared to determine the control of therapy and the need to adjust medications. The evaluation with ongoing therapy is to assess whether the patient's quality of life has improved by the control of symptoms as outlined in the written physician-patient plan. The evaluation should allow a determination of whether medication use should increase (step up) or decrease (step down). This permits the best quality of life with minimal medication use.

In addition to the medication therapy, the guidelines make education a central component to therapy. This includes assuring that the patient understands self-monitoring of asthma control and can identify signs of acute exacerbation or generalized worsening of disease. Education also encompasses the correct way of physically taking the medications and the decision process for the use of rescue medications. Finally, education extends to the lifestyle changes vital to minimizing asthmatic episodes.

Emphasis is placed on a written asthma plan, which is to be created individually for the patient and reviewed regularly between the patient and physician.

Allergic disease also receives recognition and therapeutic recommendations in the 2007 version of the guidelines.[7] The second expert panel acknowledged the inflammatory component of asthma and the genetic disposition to atopic disease as a major factor. However, the most recent guideline takes the singular step of advocating allergy immunotherapy in cases where a clear connection exists "between symptoms and exposure to an allergen to which the patient is sensitive."[8] This is an important comment for several reasons. Patients with asthma have a higher risk of adverse response to immunotherapy. There have been questions in the literature about whether allergy immunotherapy is sufficiently helpful in the control of asthma to make it worth the risks of adverse reaction. The inclusion of immunotherapy by the expert panel seems to address these concerns, approving the use of immunotherapy in mild to moderate persistent disease, at least in cases in which a direct link to asthma can be appreciated.[9]

Recommendations that are more specific are possible when patients are grouped into 0 to 4 year olds and 5 to 11 year olds. The latter group was represented as a portion of the adult recommendations in earlier versions of the expert panel recommendations.

Table 1
Initial visit: classifying asthma severity and initiating therapy (in patients who are not currently taking long-term control medications)

Components of Severity	Intermittent 0–4 y	Intermittent 5–11 y	Intermittent ≥12 y	Mild 0–4 y	Mild 5–11 y	Mild ≥12 y	Moderate 0–4 y	Moderate 5–11 y	Moderate ≥12 y	Severe 0–4 y	Severe 5–11 y	Severe ≥12 y
Impairment												
Symptoms	≤2 d/wk	≤2 d/wk	≤2 d/wk	>2 d/wk but not daily	>2 d/wk but not daily	>2 d/wk but not daily	Daily	Daily	Daily	Throughout the day	Throughout the day	Throughout the day
Nighttime awakenings	0	≤2x/mo	≤2x/mo	1–2x/mo	3–4x/mo	3–4x/mo	3–4x/mo	>1x/wk but not nightly	>1x/wk but not nightly	>1x/wk	Often 7x/wk	Often 7x/wk
SABA use for symptom control (not to prevent EIB)	≤2 d/wk	≤2 d/wk	≤2 d/wk	>2 d/wk but not daily	>2 d/wk but not daily and not more than once on any day	>2 d/wk but not daily and not more than once on any day	Daily	Daily	Daily	Several times per day	Several times per day	Several times per day
Interference with normal activity	None	None	None	Minor limitation	Minor limitation	Minor limitation	Some limitation	Some limitation	Some limitation	Extremely limited	Extremely limited	Extremely limited
Lung function — FEV$_1$ (% predicted)	Not applicable	Normal FEV$_1$ between exacerbations >80%	Normal FEV$_1$ between exacerbations >80%	Not applicable	>80%	>80%	Not applicable	60%–80%	60%–80%	Not applicable	<60%	<60%
Lung function — FEV$_1$/FVC	Not applicable	>85%	Normal[a]	Not applicable	>80%	Normal[a]	Not applicable	75%–80%	75%–80%	Not applicable	<75%	Reduced >5%[a]
Risk												
Asthma exacerbations requiring oral systemic corticosteroids[b]	0–1/y	0–1/y	0–1/y	≥2 exacerb. in 6 mo, or wheezing >4x per y lasting >1 d AND risk factors for persistent asthma	≥2/y	≥2/y						
Recommended Step for Initiating Therapy (See "Stepwise Approach for Managing Asthma Long Term".)	Step 1	Step 1	Step 1	Step 2	Step 2	Step 2	Step 3	Step 3 medium-dose ICS option	Step 3	Step 3	Step 3 medium-dose ICS option or Step 4	Step 4 or 5

Generally, more frequent and intense events indicate greater severity.

Relative annual risk of exacerbations may be related to FEV$_1$.

Consider severity and interval since last asthma exacerbation. Frequency and severity may fluctuate over time for patients in any severity category.

The stepwise approach is meant to help, not replace, the clinical decisionmaking needed to meet individual patient needs.

[b] Consider short course of oral systemic corticosteroids.

In 2–6 wk, depending on severity, assess level of asthma control achieved and adjust therapy as needed.

For children 0–4 y old, if no clear benefit is observed in 4–6 wk, consider adjusting therapy or alternate diagnoses.

Level of severity (columns 2–5) is determined by events listed in column 1 for both impairment (frequency and intensity of symptoms and functional limitations) and risk (of exacerbations). Assess impairment by patient's or caregiver's recall of events during the previous 2 to 4 weeks; assess risk over the last year. Recommendations for initiating therapy based on level of severity are presented in the last row.

Abbreviations: EIB, exercise-induced bronchospasm; FEV$_1$, forced expiratory volume in 1 second; FVC, forced vital capacity; ICS, inhaled corticosteroid; SABA, short-acting beta2-agonist.

[a] Normal FEV$_1$/FVC by age: 8–19 y, 85%; 20–39 y, 80%; 40–59 y, 75%; 60–80 y, 70%.

[b] Data are insufficient to link frequencies of exacerbations with different levels of asthma severity. Generally, more frequent and intense exacerbations (eg, requiring urgent care, hospital or intensive care admission, and/or oral corticosteroids) indicate greater underlying disease severity. For treatment purposes, patients with ≥2 exacerbations may be considered to have persistent asthma, even in the absence of impairment levels consistent with persistent asthma.

From National Heart, Lung, and Blood Institute. Asthma care quick reference. Available at: http://www.nhlbi.nih.gov/guidelines/asthma/asthma_qrg.pdf. Accessed September 17, 2013.

Table 2
Stepwise approach for managing asthma long-term

ASSESS CONTROL:

STEP UP IF NEEDED (first, check medication adherence, inhaler technique, environmental control, and comorbidities)

STEP DOWN IF POSSIBLE (and asthma is well controlled for at least 3 mo)

At each step: Patient education, environmental control, and management of comorbidities

0–4 y of age

	STEP 1	STEP 2	STEP 3	STEP 4	STEP 5	STEP 6
	Intermittent Asthma	Persistent Asthma: Daily Medication — Consult with asthma specialist if step 3 care or higher is required. Consider consultation at step 2.				
Preferred Treatment[a]	SABA as needed	low-dose ICS	medium-dose ICS	medium-dose ICS + either LABA or montelukast	high-dose ICS + either LABA or montelukast	high-dose ICS + either LABA or montelukast + oral corticosteroids
Alternative Treatment[a,b]		cromolyn or montelukast				

If clear benefit is not observed in 4–6 wk, and medication technique and adherence are satisfactory, consider adjusting therapy or alternate diagnoses.

Quick-Relief Medication
- SABA as needed for symptoms; intensity of treatment depends on severity of symptoms.
- With viral respiratory symptoms: SABA every 4–6 h up to 24 h (longer with physician consult). Consider short course of oral systemic corticosteroids if asthma exacerbation is severe or patient has history of severe exacerbations.
- Caution: Frequent use of SABA may indicate the need to step up treatment.

5–11 y of age

	STEP 1	STEP 2	STEP 3	STEP 4	STEP 5	STEP 6
	Intermittent Asthma	Persistent Asthma: Daily Medication — Consult with asthma specialist if step 4 care or higher is required. Consider consultation at step 3.				
Preferred Treatment[a]	SABA as needed	low-dose ICS	low-dose ICS + either LABA, LTRA, or theophylline[b] OR medium-dose ICS	medium-dose ICS + LABA	high-dose ICS + LABA	high-dose ICS + LABA + oral corticosteroids
Alternative Treatment[a,b]		cromolyn, LTRA, or theophylline[c]		medium-dose ICS + either LTRA or theophylline[c]	high-dose ICS + either LTRA or theophylline[c]	high-dose ICS + either LTRA or theophylline[c] + oral corticosteroids

Consider subcutaneous allergen immunotherapy for patients who have persistent, allergic asthma.

Quick-Relief Medication
- SABA as needed for symptoms. The intensity of treatment depends on severity of symptoms: up to 3 treatments every 20 min as needed. Short course of oral systemic corticosteroids may be needed.
- Caution: Increasing use of SABA or use >2 d/wk for symptom relief (not to prevent EIB) generally indicates inadequate control and the need to step up treatment.

≥12 y of age

	STEP 1	STEP 2	STEP 3	STEP 4	STEP 5	STEP 6
	Intermittent Asthma	Persistent Asthma: Daily Medication — Consult with asthma specialist if step 4 care or higher is required. Consider consultation at step 3.				
Preferred Treatment[a]	SABA as needed	low-dose ICS	low-dose ICS + LABA OR medium-dose ICS	medium-dose ICS + LABA	high-dose ICS + LABA AND consider omalizumab for patients who have allergies[e]	high-dose ICS + LABA + oral corticosteroid[f] AND consider omalizumab for patients who have allergies[e]
Alternative Treatment[a,b]		cromolyn, LTRA, or theophylline[c]	low-dose ICS + either LTRA, theophylline,[c] or zileuton[d]	medium-dose ICS + either LTRA, theophylline,[c] or zileuton[d]		

Consider subcutaneous allergen immunotherapy for patients who have persistent, allergic asthma.

Quick-Relief Medication
- SABA as needed for symptoms. The intensity of treatment depends on severity of symptoms: up to 3 treatments every 20 min as needed. Short course of oral systemic corticosteroids may be needed.
- Caution: Use of SABA >2 d/wk for symptom relief (not to prevent EIB) generally indicates inadequate control and the need to step up treatment.

The stepwise approach tailors the selection of medication to the level of asthma severity or asthma control. The stepwise approach is meant to help, not replace, the clinical decision making needed to meet individual patient needs.

Abbreviations: EIB, exercise-induced bronchospasm; ICS, inhaled corticosteroid; LTRA, leukotriene receptor antagonist; SABA, short-acting beta2-agonist (inhaled).

[a] Treatment options are listed in alphabetical order, if more than one.

[b] If alternative treatment is used and response is inadequate, discontinue and use preferred treatment before stepping up.

[c] Theophylline is a less desirable alternative because of the need to monitor serum concentration levels. Based on evidence for dust mites, animal dander, and pollen; evidence is weak or lacking for molds and cockroaches. Evidence is strongest for immunotherapy with single allergens. The role of allergy in asthma is greater in children than in adults.

[d] Zileuton is less desirable because of limited studies as adjunctive therapy and the need to monitor liver function.

[e] Clinicians who administer immunotherapy or omalizumab should be prepared to treat anaphylaxis that may occur.

[f] Before oral corticosteroids are introduced, a trial of high-dose ICS + LABA + either LTRA, theophylline, or zileuton, may be considered, although this approach has not been studied in clinical trials.

From National Heart, Lung, and Blood Institute. Asthma care quick reference. Available at: http://www.nhlbi.nih.gov/guidelines/asthma/asthma_qrg.pdf. Accessed September 17, 2013.

STEPPING THROUGH THE PROCESS OF STEPWISE CARE
The Asthma Diagnosis

The frequency of symptoms, nighttime awakenings, and use of short-acting beta2-agonists (SABA) combined with spirometry data are the first level used to categorize the severity of asthma. Next it is categorized by intermittent versus persistent. The persistent category is subdivided into mild-moderate or severe. The diagnosis of severity is based on these four categories (see **Table 1**).

Once asthma severity is categorized, the clinician has guidelines to choose from six levels of therapy. Having more levels of therapy than categories of severity allows a different starting point for pediatric and adult patients. It also provides more flexibility in stepping up and down the regimen for patients who require only subtle changes in therapy. Alternative therapies are noted as appropriate (see **Table 2**).

In all age groups, intermittent asthma is managed with step 1 therapy. This primary level therapy is the use of a SABA on an as-needed basis. There is no alternative treatment needed or appropriate at this level.

Mild persistent asthma is the second category. At this level, alternative therapies can be considered. Essentially, the primary or recommended therapy is low-dose inhaled corticosteroids. An alternative therapy includes cromolyn, leukotriene receptor antagonists, or (5 years and older) theophylline. This provides the option to withhold inhaled corticosteroids if there is a strong patient or parental concern. Although these two alternative therapies are considered equivalent for the management of mild intermittent asthma, studies indicate that inhaled corticosteroids may better prevent inflammation, and decrease risk of exacerbation and subsequent airway remodeling. Step 2 is also the first level at which subcutaneous allergen immunotherapy should be considered for patients with allergic disease that clearly relates to asthma exacerbations. The data are considered stronger for allergy exacerbating asthma in children and the best evidence seems to support allergy against dust mites, animal dander, and pollen.[9]

Moderate persistent asthma is initially treated with step 3 therapy. This involves the use of low-dose inhaled corticosteroids plus an LABA or the use of medium-dose inhaled corticosteroids alone. An alternative for adults is to avoid the LABA by substituting leukotriene receptor antagonists or theophylline. A similar option exists for children 5 to 11 years old. The youngest children requiring step 3 therapy are managed using medium-dose inhaled corticosteroids alone.

Severe persistent asthma is managed in adults using medium dose inhaled corticosteroids and LABA. An alternative of medium dose inhaled corticosteroids with theophylline or a leukotriene receptor antagonist is also an option. Some adults may exhibit such a severe level of asthma that they require initiation with therapy above step 4 care. Step 5 is high-dose inhaled corticosteroids, combined with LABA, with consideration given to the use of oral steroids. Once step 5 or step 6 is reached, allergy immunotherapy is no longer a recommendation. At this level of asthma, the risk of triggering a significant exacerbation outweighs the benefits of allergy immunotherapy. At this level of severity in the allergic population, omalizumab may be used as replacement for allergy immunotherapy for step 5 and 6 care.[10]

Step 6 is not used as a starting level, but has been added to the guidelines to provide a rational increased level of care for patients experiencing incomplete control on follow-up visits. Step 6 includes oral corticosteroids in all age groups in addition to high-dose inhaled corticosteroids. LABA is recommended all age groups at level 6.

As previously noted, patient's should leave the initial visit with medical therapy based on the severity of the disease. They should receive education about the disease

Table 3
Follow-up visits: assessing asthma control and adjusting therapy

Components of Control	Well Controlled			Not Well Controlled			Very Poorly Controlled		
	Ages 0–4 y	Ages 5–11 y	Ages ≥12 y	Ages 0–4 y	Ages 5–11 y	Ages ≥12 y	Ages 0–4 y	Ages 5–11 y	Ages ≥12 y
Impairment									
Symptoms	≤2 d/wk	≤2 d/wk but not more than once on each day	≤2 d/wk	>2 d/wk	>2 d/wk or multiple times on ≤2 d/wk	>2 d/wk	Throughout the day	Throughout the day	Throughout the day
Nighttime awakenings	≤1x/mo	≤1x/mo	≤2x/mo	>1x/mo	≥2x/mo	1–3x/wk	>1x/wk	≥2x/wk	≥4x/wk
Interference with normal activity	None	None	None	Some limitation	Some limitation	Some limitation	Extremely limited	Extremely limited	Extremely limited
SABA use for symptom control (not to prevent EIB)	≤2 d/wk	≤2 d/wk	≤2 d/wk	>2 d/wk	>2 d/wk	>2 d/wk	Several times per day	Several times per day	Several times per day
Lung function ➔ FEV₁ (% predicted) or peak flow (% personal best)	Not applicable	>80%	>80%	Not applicable	60%–80%	60%–80%	Not applicable	<60%	<60%
➔ FEV₁/FVC		>80%	Not applicable		75%–80%	Not applicable		<75%	Not applicable
Validated questionnaires[a] ➔ ATAQ ➔ ACQ ➔ ACT	Not applicable	Not applicable	0 / ≤0.75[b] / ≥20	Not applicable	Not applicable	1–2 / ≥1.5 / 16–19	Not applicable	Not applicable	3–4 / Not applicable / ≤15
Risk									
Asthma exacerbations requiring oral systemic corticosteroids[c]	0–1/y	0–1/y	0–1/y	2–3/y	≥2/y	≥2/y	>3/y	≥2/y	≥2/y
				Consider severity and interval since last asthma exacerbation.					
Reduction in lung growth/Progressive loss of lung function	Not applicable	Evaluation requires long-term follow-up care.	Evaluation requires long-term follow-up care.	Not applicable	Evaluation requires long-term follow-up care.	Evaluation requires long-term follow-up care.	Not applicable	Evaluation requires long-term follow-up care.	Evaluation requires long-term follow-up care.
Treatment-related adverse effects	Medication side effects can vary in intensity from none to very troublesome and worrisome. The level of intensity does not correlate to specific levels of control but should be considered in the overall assessment of risk.								
Recommended Action for Treatment (See "Stepwise Approach for Managing Asthma Long Term") *The stepwise approach is meant to help, not replace, the clinical decisionmaking needed to meet individual patient needs.*	*Maintain current step.* *Regular follow-up every 1–6 mo.* *Consider step down if well controlled for at least 3 mo.*			Step up 1 step	Step up at least 1 step	Step up 1 step	*Consider short course of oral systemic corticosteroids.* *Step up 1–2 steps.* *Reevaluate in 2 wk to achieve control.*		
				Reevaluate in 2–6 wk to achieve control. *For children 0–4 y, if no clear benefit observed in 4–6 wk, consider adjusting therapy or alternative diagnoses.*					
				Before step up in treatment: *Review adherence to medication, inhaler technique, and environmental control. If alternative treatment was used, discontinue and use preferred treatment for that step. For side effects, consider alternative treatment options.*					

Level of control (columns 2–4) is based on the most severe component of impairment (symptoms and functional limitations) or risk (exacerbations). Assess impairment by patient's or caregiver's recall of events listed in column 1 during the previous 2 to 4 weeks and by spirometry and/or peak flow measures. Symptom assessment for longer periods should reflect a global assessment, such as inquiring whether the patient's asthma is better or worse since the last visit. Assess risk by recall of exacerbations during the previous year and since the last visit. Recommendations for adjusting therapy based on level of control are presented in the last row.

Abbreviations: ACQ, Asthma Control Questionnaire; ACT, Asthma Control Test; ATAQ, Asthma Therapy Assessment Questionnaire; EIB, exercise-induced bronchospasm; FEV_1, forced expiratory volume in 1 second; FVC, forced vital capacity; SABA, short-acting beta2-agonist.

[a] Minimal important difference: 1.0 for the ATAQ; 0.5 for the ACQ; not determined for the ACT.

[b] ACQ values of 0.76–1.4 are indeterminate regarding well-controlled asthma.

[c] Data are insufficient to link frequencies of exacerbations with different levels of asthma control. Generally, more frequent and intense exacerbations (eg, requiring urgent care, hospital or intensive care admission, and/or oral corticosteroids) indicate poorer asthma control.

From National Heart, Lung, and Blood Institute. Asthma care quick reference. Available at: http://www.nhlbi.nih.gov/guidelines/asthma/asthma_qrg.pdf. Accessed September 17, 2013.

process and ways to monitor their process by means of either symptoms or expiratory flow measures. Lifestyle adjustment information and careful allergy history and testing as appropriate are recommended.

Once therapy has been initiated, follow-up visits are crucial to the step-wise nature of the treatment. Despite all guidelines, the best measure of success in therapy is how the patient progresses. If additional medication is needed, it is important to identify this early in the process and step up the treatment. Similarly, if satisfactory disease control is achieved, reducing medications (step down) will limit the risk of medicine side effects. During the initial phase of asthma therapy, follow-up every 2 to 6 weeks may be necessary. Ongoing asthma management can vary from 1 to 6 months, with spirometry every 1 to 2 years. Follow-up of approximately 3 months is considered most reasonable if the patient is a candidate for decreased therapy. Certainly, if control of asthma is insufficient, visits that are more frequent will be required in order to step up the therapy in a timely fashion.

Although the initial diagnosis is geared mostly to the severity of asthma, follow-up visits are mostly concerned with the level of control achieved on the given step of therapy. **Table 3** defines the asthma has well controlled, not well controlled, or very poorly controlled, based on the most severe component of the patient's impairment. The impairments include nighttime awakenings, interference with normal activity, need for rescue inhaler use (not including exercise-induced bronchospasm).

Objective measures of lung function include forced expiratory volume in 1 second (FEV_1) or peak flow as a percentage of personal best. In children ages 5 to 11 years, the FEV_1 to forced vital capacity (FVC) ratio is a helpful alternative metric.

As an example, adults who wake fewer than two times a month are considered well controlled, whereas those who wake more than four times a week are considered very poorly controlled. Normal activity should be completely free of interference in well-controlled asthma. A patient who has asthma that is not well controlled has some limitation, whereas the patient with poorly controlled asthma is extremely activity-limited. SABA therapy several times a day is an indicator of poor control, whereas more than two days a week is considered not well controlled, and fewer than twice a week defines well-controlled asthma.

At follow-up visits, a patient with well-controlled asthma maintains the same level of medication. The patient is considered for a step down to lower medical regimen if control remains satisfactory for at least 3 months. Patients whose asthma is considered not well controlled or poorly controlled should be evaluated carefully. Before simply adding medications, consideration should be given to the presence of any underlying illness or an unfavorable lifestyle adjustment that has precipitated the unfavorable change. Additionally, the clinician should assess patient compliance to medication regimen and patient understanding and use of satisfactory techniques (particularly for inhalers). Reassessment of allergic disease and the use of environmental controls should be undertaken. If there is no specific deficiency in the present therapy, and the patient is experiencing problems with control, treatment will need to move up at least one step in therapy.

When considering stepping up therapy, two schools of thought have emerged. One is to increase the therapy gradually, one step at a time, while keeping the patient under careful surveillance. This minimizes the additional use of medications and avoids overshooting the appropriate treatment endpoint. The disadvantage of this therapy is that a patient with moderate or severe asthma who is experiencing poor control might experience significant problems, including need for emergency room intervention, before satisfactory control is achieved. The other option is to advance the therapy two or three steps to a near-maximal therapy, often including oral corticosteroids.

The goal is to achieve rapid control of the asthma exacerbation, and then withdraw medical therapy down to a level that allows for a normal lifestyle. The more aggressive approach has reasonable literature support. The belief is that rapid use of additional steroids will decrease airway inflammation and eventually allow patient management at a lower level than if the medications are increased gradually (allowing airway inflammation to be present for a longer time).

SUMMARY

Therapy for asthma has undergone substantial changes in the past three decades, prompted by a better understanding of the role of inflammation in reversible airway disease. Improved therapies and a workable algorithm of step therapy guidelines have provided an improved quality of life for the patient with asthma.

REFERENCES

1. Sly RM. Mortality from asthma, 1979–1984. J Allergy Clin Immunol 1988;82(5 Pt 1): 705–17.
2. Wijesingh M, Weatherall M, Perrin K, et al. International trends in asthma mortality rates in the 5- to 34 year age group: a call for closer surveillance. Chest 2009; 135(4):1045–9.
3. Mannino DM, Homa DM, Pertowski CA, et al. Surveillance for asthma—US 1960–1995. MMWR CDC Surveill Summ 1998;47(SS-1):1–2. Available at: http://www.cdc.gov/mmwr/preview/mmwrhtml/00052262.htm.
4. Barger LW, Vollmer WM, Felt RW, et al. Further investigation into the recent increase in asthma death rates: a review of 41 asthma deaths in Oregon in 1982. Ann Allergy 1988;60(1):31–9.
5. Ishizaka T, Ishizaka K. Molecular basis of reaginic hypersensitivity. Prog Allergy 1975;19:60–121.
6. Guidelines for the diagnosis and management of asthma. National Heart, Lung and Blood Institute. National Asthma Education Program Expert Panel Report. J Allergy Clin Immunol 1991;88(3 pt 2):425–534.
7. National Asthma Education and Prevention Program. 2007 guidelines of the national heart lungs and blood institute; Expert Panel Report 3 (EPR-3): guidelines for the diagnosis and management of asthma-summary report 2007. J Allergy Clin Immunol 2007;120(Suppl 5):S94–138.
8. Hurst DS, Gordon BR, Fornadley JA, et al. Safety of home-based and office allergy immunotherapy: a multicenter prospective study. Otolaryngol Head Neck Surg 1999;121(5):553–61.
9. Lin SY, Erekosima N, Suarez-Cuervo C, et al. Allergen specific immunotherapy for the treatment of allergic rhinoconjunctivitis and/or asthma: comparative effectiveness review 111; ARHQ pub 13 EHC061-EP 2013.
10. Chapman KR, Cartier A, Hébert J, et al. The role of omalizumab in the treatment of severe allergic asthma. Can Respir J 2006;13(Suppl B):1B–9B.

Asthma Pharmacotherapy

Minka L. Schofield, MD

KEYWORDS

- Asthma • Therapy • Medications • Short acting beta agonists
- Inhaled corticosteroids • Long acting beta agonists • Anti-IgE therapy

KEY POINTS

- Inhaled SABAs are the preferred medication for intermittent asthma symptoms and acute reversal of bronchoconstriction.
- Persistent asthma symptoms are preferably managed with inhaled corticosteroids (ICSs) with or without adjunctive therapy consisting of LTRAs, zileuton, or theophylline.
- Particle size of inhalers plays a key role in lung deposition and hence effectiveness.
- Omalizumab, anti-IgE therapy injection, has been indicated as an adjunct for persistent allergic patients with asthma uncontrolled with ICS+LABA combination therapy with a low risk of anaphylaxis after injection.
- Many novel asthma therapies are being investigated that target gene expression, anti-inflammatory mechanisms, and steroid resistance.

INTRODUCTION

Asthma represents a chronic inflammatory process marked by bronchial hyperactivity, mucus hypersecretion, and airway edema that leads to airway obstruction. These changes in the airway initially are reversible, but with continued airway remodeling the extent of reversibility may vary, leading to more difficult management. The goals of asthma pharmacotherapy are to reverse the inflammatory state and airway obstruction. The National Asthma Education and Prevention Program (NAEPP) Expert Panel has devised evidence-based guidelines for asthma care, including recommendations for therapy based on asthma severity (**Fig. 1**).[1]

BETA-2 AGONISTS
Short-Acting Beta-2 Agonists

Short-acting beta-2 agonists (SABAs), such as albuterol and levalbuterol, are recommended for intermittent asthma symptoms and serve to immediately reverse

This article originally appeared in Otolaryngologic Clinics of North America, Volume 47, Issue 1, February 2014.
Disclosures: None.
Division of Sinus and Allergy, Department of Otolaryngology-Head and Neck Surgery, The Eye and Ear Institute, Wexner Medical Center, The Ohio State University, 915 Olentangy River Road, Suite 4000, Columbus, OH 43212, USA
E-mail address: minka.schofield@osumc.edu

Clinics Collections 2 (2014) 87–96
http://dx.doi.org/10.1016/j.ccol.2014.09.008

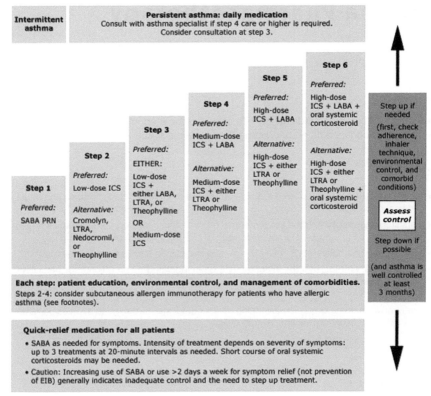

Fig. 1. NAEPP expert panel guidelines for asthma care. (*From* National Heart, Lung, and Blood Institute. Full Report 2007, guidelines for the diagnosis and management of asthma. Available at: www.nhlbi.nih.gov/guidelines/asthma. Accessed September 10, 2013.)

bronchoconstriction via potent bronchodilation. The mechanism of action is via a selective interaction on beta-2 receptors of bronchial smooth muscle to achieve bronchodilation. SABAs are the preferred medication for acute asthma exacerbations as a rescue inhaler due to the quick onset of bronchodilation. Regular use of SABAs is not recommended because of the development of tachyphylaxis and increased hyper responsiveness.

Long-Acting Beta-2 Agonists

Long-acting beta-2 agonists (LABAs), salmeterol and formoterol, provide approximately 12 hours of bronchodilation. The mechanism by which LABAs provide long-acting effects has not been clearly delineated. Multiple mechanisms have been described in the development of once-daily ultra- LABA preparations, including partitioning of the drug into lipophilic compartments after inhalation forming small depots of the drug, the presence of small lipid rafts in airway smooth muscle, and the tight binding to beta-2 adrenoreceptor and formation of ternary complexes.[2]

Since 2005, LABAs are no longer recommended as sole agents for the management of asthma. In 1993, Castle and colleagues,[3] in a study using salmeterol, showed convincing evidence that mortality increased threefold in patients with asthma, which led to a study influenced by the Food and Drug Administration (FDA), the Salmeterol

Multicentre Asthma Research Trial (SMART) study in 1996.[4] The study was aborted due to increased exacerbations and mortality. Subsequent studies using formoterol in higher doses demonstrated increased exacerbations as well.[5]

LABAs are currently recommended as a combination therapy with corticosteroids based on an FDA 2008 meta-analysis showing no significant safety risks.[6] Per NAEPP guidelines, the use of LABAs + inhaled corticosteroids (ICSs) is indicated in persistent asthma uncontrolled with ICSs alone. Three preparations are available: budesonide/formoterol, mometasone/formoterol, and fluticasone/salmeterol.

A 2011 meta-analysis comparing fluticasone/salmeterol with budesonide/formoterol showed no significant difference between the 2 preparations as it relates to oral steroid requirements, hospital admissions, rescue inhaler use, and lung function.[7] Another comparison study demonstrated that the odds of bronchodilation within 5 minutes was almost 4 times higher with fluticasone/formeterol over fluticasone/salmeterol, suggesting that this benefit may influence patient compliance with medication.[8] In an effort to manage patients with asthma using the lowest effective dose of ICS/LABA, Hojo and colleagues[9] proposed a step-down protocol to avoid asthma exacerbations. Patients were controlled on budesonide/formoterol at 640/18 μg (4 puffs/day) followed by step-down to 320/9 μg/day (2 puffs/day) when either the forced expired nitric oxide (FeNO) decreased to 28 or lower while the asthma control test (ACT) was 22 or higher or the ACT was 24 points or higher at 3 consecutive visits. After a 48-week study period, asthma control was stable based on SABA use and the number of acute exacerbations.

The selectivity of beta-2 agonists over alpha and beta-1 receptors results in fewer cardiac side effects, such as tachycardia and palpitations. Levalbuterol is an entamer of albuterol associated with even fewer cardiac side effects. Use of beta-2 agonists in diabetic patients is cautioned because of the risk of ketoacidosis related to induction of liver glycogenolysis via beta-adrenoreceptor. Other adverse reactions include hypokalemia, tremor, irritation, or anxiety after use.

ANTICHOLINERGICS

Anticholinergic agents, primarily ipratroprium, also function as bronchodilators by inhibiting the vagal muscarinic receptors on smooth muscle. These agents can be effective especially in patients who do not tolerate SABAs. Tiotropium, a long-acting antimuscarinic, has been shown to be an effective bronchodilator in chronic obstructive pulmonary disease (COPD) and investigators have also shown tiotropium to be effective in asthma. Kerstjens and colleagues[10] demonstrated in 2 randomized controlled trials that tiotropium improved asthma control in patients with poorly controlled asthma on ICSs and LABAs. Tiotropium was administered as 2 puffs of 2.5 μg via mist inhaler in addition to any previous asthma medications before the trial. After a 48-week trial period, the investigators observed an improvement in forced expiratory volume in 1 second (FEV1) in the first 24 weeks with an overall reduction in the risk of a severe exacerbation by 21% compared with placebo.

CORTICOSTEROIDS

The mechanism of action of corticosteroids is complex, involving cellular and molecular mechanisms having direct and indirect influences on the airway. In general, corticosteroids have been shown to enhance the beta-adrenergic response that relieves muscle spasm, reverse edema by decreasing vascular permeability and the inhibition of leukotriene C4 (LTC4) and LTD4, decrease mucus by inhibiting macrophage release of secretagogue, and inhibit chemotaxis to reverse inflammatory response.[11] The binding of glucocorticoid receptors triggers multiple genes involved in regulating airway inflammation (**Box 1**).[12]

ICS

ICSs have become the preferred long-term treatment recommendation for patients classified as having persistent asthma. Steroids are effective during the late phase

---

Box 1
Effect of corticosteroids on gene transcription

Increased transcription

Annexin-1 (lipocortin-1, phospholipase A_2 inhibitor)

Beta-2 adrenoceptors

Clara cell protein (CC10, phospholipase A_2 inhibitor)

Glucocorticoid-induced leucine zipper protein

IL-1 receptor antagonist

IL-1 receptor 2 (decoy receptor)

Inhibitor of NF-κB (IκB-α)

IL-10

Mitogen-activated protein kinase phosphatase-1

Secretory leukoprotease inhibitor

Decreased transcription

Cytokines

   IL-1, IL-2, IL-3, IL-4, IL-5, IL-6, IL-9, IL-11, IL-12, IL-13, IL-16, IL-17, IL-18, TNFα, GM-CSF, stem cell factor

Chemokines

   IL-8, RANTES, MIP-1α, MCP-1, MCP-3, MCP-4, eotaxins

Adhesion molecules

   E-selectin, ICAM-1, VCAM-1

Inflammatory enzymes

   Cytoplasmic phospholipase A_2

   Inducible cyclooxygenase (COX-2)

   Inducible nitric oxide synthase

Inflammatory receptors

   Bradykinin Beta-2 receptors

   Tachykinin NK_1-receptors, NK_2-receptors

Peptides

   Endothelin-1

Abbreviations: GM-CSF, granulocyte-macrophage colony stimulating factor; ICAM, intercellular adhesion molecule; IL, interleukin; MCP, monocyte chemoattractant protein; MIP, macrophage inflammatory protein; RANTES, released by normal activated T cells expressed and secreted; TNF, tumor necrosis factor; VCAM, vascular-endothelial cell adhesion molecule.

From Jang A. Steroid response in refractory asthmatics. Korean J Intern Med 2012;27:143–8; with permission.

of the hypersensitivity response; hence, are not indicated for acute reversal of bronchoconstriction during the immediate hypersensitivity reaction like SABAs. Instead, these agents function to decrease the inflammation and edema associated with asthma through continual use of the medication.

ICSs also have a direct anti-inflammatory effect on the airway, demonstrated in a study randomizing patients with asthma on placebo, oral steroid, and inhaled steroid.[13] The ICS group demonstrated better asthma control with no systemic steroid detected, suggesting that the anti-inflammatory effects of the ICS is direct or via topical effects on lung steroid receptors.

The effectiveness of these agents seems to be related to particle size and the ability to pass into the distal airway. The formulation of the agent greatly plays a role in the particle size. With the banning of chloroflourocarbons (CFCs), newly developed hydroflouroalkanes (HFAs) were developed with some companies altering the particle sizes. Metered dose inhalers (MDIs) were similarly altered to decrease particle size with solution MDIs resulting in smaller more aerosolized particles with inhalation. Overall, it appears that dry powder inhaler (DPI) steroids, suspension CFCs, and suspension HFA MDI inhalers have greater particle sizes than solution HFA MDIs (**Table 1**).[14] The smaller particle size of solution HFA MDIs has increased lung deposition from 20% to greater than 50%. Many studies have confirmed greater lung deposition in smaller particle formulations in addition to lower oropharyngeal and laryngeal deposition, lessening oral candidiasis and dysphonia side effects associated with ICSs.[15]

A 2013 Cochrane review of 6 studies comparing ciclesonide, which is a new small-particle ICS, to other ICSs in children did not demonstrate superior benefit over other fluticasones or budesonide.[16] The lung deposition of combination therapy HFA fluticasone/salmeterol compared with HFA beclomethasone was investigated by Leach and colleagues.[17] The smaller-particle HFA beclomethasone (0.7 μm) was found to have 58% of its particles deposited into the lungs compared with 16% of HFA fluticasone/salmeterol (2.7 μm) implying greater potential efficacy and fewer dosing intervals.

The effectiveness of ICS therapy has also been linked to patient compliance factors. ICSs are prescribed at daily dosing intervals of once or twice daily, with most patients achieving control at low doses. Some patients with asthma take ICSs only during periods of asthma exacerbations or worsening symptoms. A 2013 study looking at the

Table 1 Lung deposition and particle size comparison of steroid inhalers		
Inhaled Steroid	**MMAD (μm)**	**Lung Deposition Value (%)**
Fluticasone DPI	~4.0	15
Triamcinolone	4.5	14
CFC-flunisolide	3.8	19
CFC-beclomethasone	3.5	8
CFC-fluticasone	2.6	13
HFA-flunisolide solution	1.2	68
HFA-beclomethasone solution	1.1	56
HFA-ciclesonide solution	1.0	52

Abbreviations: CFC, chlorofluorocarbon; DPI, dry powder inhaler; HFA, hydrofluoroalkane; MMAD, median mass aerodynamic diameter.
From Leach C, Colice GL, Luskin AC. Particle size of inhaled corticosteroids: does it matter? J Allergy Clin Immunol 2009;124(Suppl 6):S88–93; with permission.

outcomes of intermittent versus daily ICS use in children and adults found no significant difference in overall asthma attacks.[18] However, increased frequency of rescue inhaler use, fewer symptom-free days, and decreased lung function were observed in those taking the medication only intermittently. Furthermore, it has been demonstrated that patients who stop routine use of ICSs have an increased risk of asthma exacerbation with decreased FEV1, decreased peak flow, and increased asthma symptom scores.[19]

Steroid therapy and the effects on growth rate has been a concern particularly in the pediatric population with asthma. At lower doses, there is minimal systemic absorption of ICSs. Higher doses of ICSs have been shown to retard growth in children and result in adrenal suppression. Other side effects with long-term use at high doses include osteoporosis, dermal thinning, periodontal disease, cataracts, and glaucoma.

Oral Corticosteroids

Oral corticosteroids are indicated for patients with severe persistent asthma despite management with high-dose ICSs or LABA. Oral corticosteroids are also used in cases of asthma exacerbations. The mechanism of action is similar to that outlined with ICSs; however, greater risk of systemic adverse side effects are observed with chronic use of oral corticosteroids.

LEUKOTRIENE MODIFIERS

LTRAs are recommended as a sole or adjunct therapy for patients with mild persistent asthma to decrease airway edema, bronchoconstriction, and inflammation. The mechanism of action of these agents is through the eicosanoid pathway by inhibiting the binding of cysteinyl leukotrienes (LTC4, LTD4, LTE4) from binding to cysteinyl receptors located on inflammatory cells and airway smooth muscle. Montelukast binds selectively to the cystLT1 receptor predominantly affecting the binding of LTD4. Zafirkulast selectively and competitively binds to receptors for LTD4 and LTE4 influencing both early and late phase hypersensitivity responses. Zileuton is an inhibitor of 5-lipoxygenase, thus affecting the production of LTB4, LTC4, LTD4, and LTE4. Current use of this medication is for ages 12 and older and per NAEPP recommendation is not a preferred agent due to limited studies and need to monitor liver function.

A 2012 Cochrane review comparing leukotriene modifiers to ICS suggested that antileukotrienes may have fewer adverse side effects, but as a monotherapy were not as effective as ICSs.[20]

THEOPHYLLINE

Theophylline is a methylxanthine, indicated as a sole agent for mild persistent asthma or as an adjunct therapy in more severe persistent patients with asthma with ICS. Its mechanism of action is through nonselective phosphodiesterase inhibition. Theophylline serves as a bronchodilator that can be used as an alternative to LABA. The serum concentration of theophylline must be monitored because of the narrow therapeutic index, variable hepatic clearance, and subsequent risk of cardiac arrhythmias and seizures. Diet, cardiac disease, liver disease, tobacco use, and medications that influence the cytochrome P450 system can modify the half-life of theophylline.

MAST CELL STABILIZERS

Mast cell stabilizers, such as inhaled cromolyn sodium, are primarily recommended as an alternative therapy to SABAs and LTRAs for exercise-induced bronchospasm or patients with mild persistent asthma. These agents prevent degranulation of mast cells by preventing calcium uptake into the cell, thereby playing a role in acute and late-phase responses. Netzer and colleagues,[21] after review of the literature, suggested the potential role of cromolyn sodium in the management of asthma, despite current guidelines, because of its potent anti-inflammatory effects, few side effects, and acceptable dosing making it a viable initial option for the control of asthma.

ANTI–IMMUNOGLOBULIN E THERAPY

Omalizumab is a monoclonal anti–immunoglobulin E (anti-IgE) antibody administered as a subcutaneous injection indicated for patients with severe persistent asthma who are 12 years or older and who have demonstrated underlying IgE-mediated allergies. Omalizumab selectively binds to the high-affinity IgE receptor region on IgE preventing its binding to IgE surface receptors on cells ultimately forming immune complexes that decrease available free IgE. It has also been shown to downregulate the expression of high-affinity receptors on inflammatory cells.[22] By inhibiting IgE from binding to its receptors leads to inhibition of the allergic response through inhibition of degranulation of mast cells and basophils, decreased response to antigen challenges, and a decrease in IgE-switching cytokines interleukin (IL)-4 and IL-13. The immune complexes formed by omalizumab can also bind allergens resulting in neutralization of antigen stimulus.

Reported side effects of omalizumab have included the risk of anaphylaxis of about 0.09% based on the Omalizumab Joint Task Force investigations.[22]

Most of these reactions were within the first 2 to 3 hours of the initial 3 injections and within 30 minutes after later injections. All patients responded to anaphylaxis treatment without any fatalities. Other reports of adverse effects include the risk of malignancy; however, it has been concluded that there is no increased risk of malignancy. Other reported adverse reactions include skin reactions, upper respiratory infection, and sinusitis.

In patients with severe allergic asthma uncontrolled with ICS and LABAs, evidence has shown an increased benefit when adding omalizumab to the treatment regimen. Hanania and colleagues,[23] in a randomized, double-blind placebo-controlled trial showed in a 48-week study of patients with uncontrolled allergic asthma that omalizumab reduced asthma exacerbations, albuterol rescue inhaler use, and overall quality of life.

SPECIFIC IMMUNOTHERAPY

Specific immunotherapy (SIT) has been shown to be effective as an adjunctive treatment in managing asthma. Data have consistently shown that immunotherapy decreases medication usage, and reduces asthma symptoms and airway hyperresponsiveness. A recent 2013 review of randomized control trials found that single-allergen subcutaneous immunotherapy (SCIT) improved asthma symptoms and medication usage compared with placebo and pharmacotherapy, suggesting that there may not be a role for multiple allergen immunotherapy.[24] The review also included sublingual immunotherapy (SLIT), which demonstrated an even stronger improvement in asthma symptoms compared with placebo, with most studies evaluating dust mite single-allergen therapy. Randomized controlled trials comparing the efficacy of SCIT to SLIT in improving asthma symptoms are limited and variable. Overall, SIT has been shown to be safe, with most reactions being minor local reactions. In comparison, SLIT appears to have a better safety profile than SCIT. The disadvantages of this line of therapy include the cost, time commitment, and the potential for initial worsening in asthma symptoms.

FUTURE THERAPY

The allergic reaction represents a TH2-dominant response and has been demonstrated in allergic asthma. One novel therapy serves to shift the response to a TH1-mediated protective response by injecting a Toll-like receptor 9 agonist, QbG10. Beeh and colleagues,[25] in a double-blind randomized trial, investigated its role in controlling mild to moderate persistent allergic asthma over a 12-week period compared with placebo. At the completion of the study, two-thirds of QbG10 patients had well-controlled asthma compared with one-third in the placebo group. Additionally, the FEV1 clinically worsened in the placebo group. Side effects to injections were mainly local skin reactions. Other anti-inflammatory therapies with promising results are targeting cytokines, such as IL-4 receptors, IL-5 monoclonal antibody (mepolizumab), anti-IL-9, resiquimod targeting IL-12, anti-IL-13, and MMP-12–specific inhibitor.[26–29]

Steroid resistance has been described in patients with severe persistent asthma and in patients with asthma who smoke. Several molecular mechanisms for steroid resistance have been identified, including a genetic susceptibility or familial glucocorticoid resistance. Other mechanisms include glucocorticoid receptor (GR) modifications, increased GR-beta expression, increased proinflammatory transcription factors, immune mechanisms, and defective histone acetylation via histone deacetylase (HDAC2). Delineation of these mechanisms has become a target for alternative therapies in patients with steroid-resistant asthma and patients with COPD.[30] Oral roflumilast is a phosphodiesterase-4 inhibitor that is the first anti-inflammatory marketed for COPD. P38MAPK inhibitors are being developed to suppress inflammation in patients with asthma and patients with COPD by affecting the mitogen-activated protein kinase (MAPK) pathways normally inhibited by steroids. Reversing steroid resistance by increasing HDAC2 expression, thereby lessening oxidative stress, has also been demonstrated in patients with COPD. Several drugs increase HDAC2, including theophylline and nortriptyline. LABAs also appear to reverse steroid resistance via multiple mechanisms.

Some investigations aim to provide a more personalized approach to asthma management. One such study investigated children carrying the β2- adrenoreceptor gene Arg 16 polymorphism. Patients with this gene appeared to respond better to ICS and LTRA over ICS/LABA suggesting a role for genotyping patients with asthma.[31] Asthmatic patients expressing certain polymorphisms for nitric oxide synthase enzyme appear to have greater response to ICS/LABA combination therapy.[32]

SUMMARY

The NAEPP has provided evidence-based guidelines for the management of asthma. These guidelines allow for standardization of therapy in an effort to improve asthma outcomes. In patients with persistent asthma symptoms, ICS alone or in combination with LABAs have shown to significantly reduce asthma symptoms. Unfortunately, some patients remain refractory to this treatment, requiring more advanced therapy, such as anti-IgE therapy. Other novel therapies are being investigated to treat these refractory patients targeting steroid resistance, genetic, and anti-inflammatory mechanisms.

REFERENCES

1. National Asthma Education and Prevention Program. Expert panel report 3: guidelines for the diagnosis and management of asthma. NIH Publication; 2007. 07–4051.

2. Cazzola M, Page CP, Rogliani P, et al. β2-agonist therapy in lung disease. Am J Respir Crit Care Med 2013;187(7):690–6.
3. Castle W, Fuller R, Hall J, et al. Serevent nationwide surveillance study: comparison of salmeterol with salbutamol in asthmatic patients who require regular bronchodilator treatment. BMJ 1993;306:1034–7.
4. Nelson HS, Weiss ST, Bleecker ER, et al. The salmeterol multicenter asthma research trial: a comparison of usual pharmacotherapy for asthma or usual pharmacotherapy plus salmeterol. Chest 2006;129:15–26.
5. Mann M, Chowdhury B, Sullivan E, et al. Serious asthma exacerbations in asthmatics treated with high-dose formoterol. Chest 2003;124:70–4.
6. Chowdhury BA, Dal Pan G. The FDA and safe use of long acting beta agonists in the treatment of asthma. N Engl J Med 2010;362:1169–71.
7. Lasserson TJ, Ferrara G, Casali L. Combination fluticasone and salmeterol versus fixed dose combination budesonide and formoterol for chronic asthma in adults and children. Cochrane Database Syst Rev 2011;(12):CD004106.
8. Aalbers R, Brusselle G, McIver T, et al. Onset of bronchodilation with fluticasone/formoterol combination versus fluticasone/sameterol in an open-label, randomized study. Adv Ther 2012;29(11):958–69.
9. Hojo M, Mizutani T, Iikura M, et al. Asthma control can be maintained after fixed-dose, budesonide/formoterol combination inhaler therapy is stepped down from medium to low dose. Allergol Int 2013;62:91–8.
10. Kerstjens HA, Engel M, Dahl R, et al. Tiotropium in asthma poorly controlled with standard combination therapy. N Engl J Med 2012;367:1198–207.
11. Townley RG, Suliaman F. The mechanism of corticosteroids in treating asthma. Ann Allergy 1987;58(1):1–6.
12. Jang A. Steroid response in refractory asthmatics. Korean J Intern Med 2012;27:143–8.
13. Lawrence M, Wolfe J, Webb DR, et al. Efficacy of inhaled fluticasone propionate in asthma results from topical and not from systemic activity. Am J Respir Crit Care Med 1997;156:744–51.
14. Leach C, Colice GL, Luskin AC. Particle size of inhaled corticosteroids: does it matter? J Allergy Clin Immunol 2009;124(Suppl 6):S88–93.
15. van den Berge M, ten Hacken NH, van der Wiel E, et al. Treatment of the bronchial tree from beginning to end: targeting small airway inflammation in asthma. Allergy 2013;68:16–26.
16. Kramer S, Rottier BL, Scholten RJ, et al. Ciclesonide versus other inhaled corticosteroids for chronic asthma in children. Cochrane Database Syst Rev 2013;(2):CD010352.
17. Leach CL, Kuehl PJ, Ramesh C, et al. Characterization of respiratory deposition of fluticasone-salmeterol hydrofluoroalkane-134a and hydroflouroalkane-134a beclomethasone in asthmatic patients. Ann Allergy Asthma Immunol 2012;108:135–200.
18. Chauhan BF, Chartrand C, Ducharme FM. Intermittent versus daily inhaled corticosteroids for persistent asthma in children and adults. Cochrane Database Syst Rev 2013;(2):CD009611.
19. Rank MA, Hagan JB, Park MA, et al. The risk of asthma exacerbation after stopping low-dose inhaled corticosteroids: a systematic review and meta-analysis of randomized control trials. J Allergy Clin Immunol 2013;131:724–9.
20. Chauhan BF, Ducharme FM. Anti-leukotriene agents compared to inhaled corticosteroids in the management of recurrent and/or chronic asthma in adults and children. Cochrane Database Syst Rev 2012;(5):CD002314.

21. Netzer NC, Küpper T, Voss HW, et al. The actual role of sodium cromoglycate in the treatment of asthma—a critical review. Sleep Breath 2012;16:1027–32.
22. Pelaia G, Gallelli L, Renda T, et al. Update on optimal use of omalizumab in management of asthma. J Asthma Allergy 2011;4:49–59.
23. Hanania NA, Alpan O, Hamilos DL, et al. Omalizumab in severe allergic asthma inadequately controlled with standard therapy: a randomized trial. Ann Intern Med 2011;154(9):573–82.
24. Kim JM, Lin SY, Suarez-Cuervo C, et al. Allergen-specific immunotherapy for pediatric asthma and rhinoconjunctivitis: a systematic review. Pediatrics 2013;131: 1155–67.
25. Beeh K, Kanniess F, Wagner F, et al. The novel TLR-9 agonist QbG10 shows clinical efficacy in persistent allergic asthma. J Allergy Clin Immunol 2013;131: 866–74.
26. Chang C. Asthma in children and adolescents: a comprehensive approach to diagnosis and management. Clin Rev Allergy Immunol 2012;43:98–137.
27. Hansbro PM, Scott GV, Essilfie A, et al. Th2 cytokine antagonists: potential treatments for severe asthma. Expert Opin Investig Drugs 2013;22(1):49–69.
28. Ingram JL, Krat M. IL-13 in asthma and allergic disease: asthma phenotypes and targeted therapies. J Allergy Clin Immunol 2012;130:829–42.
29. Pavord ID, Korn S, Howarth P, et al. Mepolizumab for severe eosinophilic asthma (DREAM): a multicentre, double-blind, placebo controlled trial. Lancet 2012;380: 651–9.
30. Barnes PJ. Corticosteroid resistance in patients with asthma and chronic obstructive pulmonary disease. J Allergy Clin Immunol 2013;131:636–45.
31. Lipworth BJ, Basu K, Donald HP, et al. Tailored second line therapy in asthmatic children with the Arg 16 genotype. Clin Sci (Lond) 2013;124:521–8.
32. Iordanidou M, Paraskakis E, Tavridou A, et al. G894T polymorphism of eNOS gene is a predictor of response t combination of inhaled corticosteroids with long-lasting β2- agonist in asthmatic children. Pharmacogenomics 2012;13(12): 1363–72.

A Guideline-based Approach to Asthma Management

Catherine "Casey" S. Jones, PhD, RN, ANP-C, AE-C[a],*,
Ellen A. Becker, PhD, RRT-NPS, RPFT, AE-C[b],
Catherine D. Catrambone, PhD, RN[c], Molly A. Martin, MD, MAPP[d]

KEYWORDS

- Asthma • Asthma guidelines • Asthma severity • Asthma control
- Guideline adherence

KEY POINTS

- Clinical guidelines are available for the diagnosis and management of asthma.
- Asthma assessment includes an evaluation of asthma severity and asthma control.
- Asthma severity and control include assessments of impairment and risk.
- Strategies to improve guideline adherence should include a multidimensional system-based approach.

INTRODUCTION

Despite an increased understanding of asthma mechanisms and improved treatment approaches, asthma prevalence and morbidity remain high both nationally[1] and internationally.[2] Clinical practice guidelines have evolved to disseminate best practice diagnosis and treatment recommendations to clinicians with the goal of improving asthma care and the quality of life for persons with asthma.[2,3] Guidelines have been available since 1992[4] and provide evidence to support their efficacy in improving outcomes for persons with asthma; however there remains a notable gap between guideline-recommended care and current care practices.[5–9] The failure to fully adopt and implement guidelines is partially attributed to providers. Physician adherence is affected by physician workflow and awareness of asthma guideline structure and content,[10] lack of outcome expectancy, and poor provider self-efficacy.[9] Communication, training and workload[11] and factors at the individual, organizational and

This article originally appeared in Nursing Clinics of North America, Volume 48, Issue 1, March 2013.

[a] Texas Pulmonary and Critical Care Consultants, PA, Texas Woman's University, Suite 403, 1604 Hospital Parkway, Bedford, TX 76022, USA; [b] Respiratory Care, Rush University College of Health Professions, 600 S. Paulina, 750 Armour Academic Center, Chicago, IL 60612, USA; [c] Adult Health and Gerontological Nursing, Rush University College of Nursing, 600 S. Paulina, 1064B Armour Academic Center, Chicago, IL 60612, USA; [d] Department of Preventive Medicine, Rush University Medical Center, 1700 W Van Buren, Suite 470, Chicago, IL 60612, USA
* Corresponding author.
E-mail address: cjones29@twu.edu

environmental levels[12] were identified as barriers influencing nursing adherence to practice guidelines.

The National Asthma Education Prevention Program (NAEPP) of the National Heart, Lung, and Blood Institute (NHLBI) convened three Expert Panels to prepare the most recent guidelines for the diagnosis and management of asthma. The 2007 Expert Panel Report 3: *Guidelines for the Diagnosis and Management of Asthma* (EPR-3)[3] centers around four components of effective asthma management including asthma severity and control; environmental factors and comorbid conditions affecting asthma; education for patient/provider partnership in asthma care; and pharmacologic therapy. The purpose of this article is to provide an overview of the EPR-3 guidelines for asthma management. Emphasis will be on the assessment of asthma severity and control using a case-based approach and strategies to improve guideline adherence.

CASE STUDY

Ms Jenkins is a 27-year-old female who has been struggling with wheezing, cough and chest tightness intermittently for the last two months. She has not been exposed to anyone who has been ill. She notes that she has been waking up at night due to short-ness of breath for the last three nights, and that she has had difficulty climbing stairs at work for weeks. This last week she has been having symptoms on a daily basis. She was prescribed an albuterol inhaler last year due to an episode of "bronchitis" and has been using this inhaler twice a day for the last week.

The clinician's first task is to establish that Ms Jenkins has asthma, at which time the *severity* of her asthma will be determined. *Treatment* will then be initiated. Over time, *control* will be assessed and treatment modified. In the EPR-3 guidelines,[3] the concepts of severity and control guide the comprehensive assessment required for asthma management. The overall goals of asthma therapy are to reduce impairment and reduce risk. The EPR-3 guidelines contain specific tables that address severity, control, and the step-wise approach for managing asthma. These tools are classified according to age; youths ≥12 years of age to adults (**Figs. 1–3**), children 5–11 years of age, and children 0–4 years of age.

Spirometry is performed in the clinician's office and the results are provided in **Table 1**. The pre-bronchodilator spirometry results suggest moderate obstruction, while post-bronchodilator spirometry normalized after two puffs of albuterol, a short-acting β_2-agonist (SABA). Her FEV_1 increased 26% after using albuterol. To make a diagnosis of asthma, we must demonstrate both a 12% increase in FEV_1 and 200 mL increase in FEV_1. Ms Jenkins' spirometry results reveal that she has achieved both criteria and therefore has asthma.

SEVERITY

Severity refers to the intrinsic characteristics of asthma for an individual. Asthma severity is subdivided into intermittent or persistent, and persistent disease is further divided into mild, moderate, or severe persistent. The EPR-3 guidelines recommend that initial medical management for patients taking no inhaled corticosteroid medications be based upon the patient's severity classification. In Ms Jenkins' case, she has daily symptoms, she uses albuterol twice a day for symptom relief, she has difficulty climbing stairs at work, and an FEV_1 pre-bronchodilator spirometry value that was 65% predicted. This categorizes her severity as moderate persistent (see **Fig. 1**). She also has been waking up at night due to asthma symptoms for three nights in the past month which is consistent with mild persistent asthma. When symptoms and test results fall into more than one category, as with Ms Jenkins, the highest

Classification of Asthma Severity (≥12 years of age)

Components of Severity		Intermittent	Persistent		
			Mild	**Moderate**	**Severe**
Impairment Normal FEV_1/FVC: 8-19 yr 85% 20-39 yr 80% 40-59 yr 75% 60-80 yr 70%	Symptoms	≤2 days/week	>2 days/week but not daily	Daily	Throughout the day
	Nighttime awakenings	≤2x/month	3-4x/month	>1x/week but not nightly	Often 7x/week
	Short-acting beta$_2$-agonist use for symptom control (not prevention of EIB)	≤2 days/week	>2 days/week but not daily, and not more than 1x on any day	Daily	Several times per day
	Interference with normal activity	None	Minor limitation	Some limitation	Extremely limited
	Lung function	• Normal FEV_1 between exacerbations • FEV_1 >80% predicted • FEV_1/FVC normal	• FEV_1 >80% predicted • FEV_1/FVC normal	• FEV_1 >60% but <80% predicted • FEV_1/FVC reduced 5%	• FEV_1 <60% predicted • FEV_1/FVC reduced >5%
Risk	Exacerbations requiring oral systemic corticosteroids	0-1/year (see note)	≥ 2/year (see note)		
		Consider severity and interval since last exacerbation. Frequency and severity may fluctuate over time for patients in any severity category Relative annual risk of exacerbations may be related to FEV_1			
Recommended Step for Initiating Treatment		Step 1	Step 2	Step 3	Step 4 or 5
				and consider short course of oral systemic corticosteroids	
		In 2-6 weeks, evaluate level of asthma control that is achieved and adjust therapy accordingly			

Fig. 1. Classifying asthma severity and initiating treatment in youths ≥12 years of age and adults. Assessing severity and initiating treatment for patients who are not currently taking long-term control medications. The stepwise approach is meant to assist, not replace the clinical decision-making required to meet individual patient needs. Level of severity is determined by assessment of both impairment and risk. Assess impairment domain by patient's/caregiver's recall of previous 2–4 weeks and spirometry. Assign severity to the most severe category in which any feature occurs. At present, there are inadequate data to correspond frequencies of exacerbations with different levels of asthma severity. In general, more frequent and intense exacerbations (eg, requiring urgent, unscheduled care, hospitalization, or ICU admission) indicate greater underlying disease severity. For treatment purposes, patients who had ≥2 exacerbations requiring oral systemic corticosteroids in the past year may be considered the same as patients who have persistent asthma, even in the absence of impairment levels consistent with persistent asthma.[3]

Components of Control		Classification of Asthma Control (≥12 years of age)		
		Well Controlled	Not Well Controlled	Very Poorly Controlled
Impairment	Symptoms	≤2 days/week	>2 days/week	Throughout the day
	Nighttime awakenings	≤2x/month	1-3x/week	≥4x/week
	Interference with normal activity	None	Some limitation	Extremely limited
	Short-acting beta $_2$-agonist use for symptom control (not prevention of EIB)	≤2 days/week	>2 days/week	Several times per day
	FEV $_1$ or peak flow	>80% predicted/personal best	60-80% predicted/personal best	<60% predicted/personal best
	Validated Questionnaires ATAQ ACQ ACT	0 ≤0.75* ≥20	1-2 ≥1.5 16-19	3-4 N/A ≤15
Risk	Exacerbations requiring oral systemic corticosteroids	0-1/year	≥2/year (see note)	
		Consider severity and interval since last exacerbation		
	Progressive loss of lung function	Evaluation requires long-term follow-up care.		
	Treatment-related adverse effects	Medication side effects can vary in intensity from none to very troublesome and worrisome. The level of intensity does not correlate to specific levels of control but should be considered in the overall assessment of risk.		
Recommended Action for Treatment		•Maintain current step. •Regular follow ups every 1-6 months to maintain control. •Consider step down if well controlled for at least 3 months.	•Step up 1 step and •Reevaluate in 2-6 weeks. •For side effects, consider alternative treatment options.	•Consider short course of oral systemic corticosteroids, •Step up 1-2 steps, and •Reevaluate in 2 weeks. •For side effects, consider alternative treatment options.

severity criterion is used. Therefore, we will categorize her asthma as moderate persistent. The asthma symptoms, nighttime awakenings, albuterol use, interference with normal activity and lung function constitute the *impairment* domain of asthma severity. While severity classification can sometimes be challenging,[13] it is an important step before developing a treatment plan.

A second domain of severity is the determination of *risk*. Risk is the potential for adverse events in the future including exacerbations, and progressive, irreversible loss of pulmonary function. A greater risk exists for patients who have required hospital admissions, intensive care unit stays, and frequent emergency department visits. Further, patients with low impairment might be at high risk for severe, even life-threatening asthma exacerbations.[14] Patients may also incur future risks from progressive loss of lung function.[3] Risk is present at every level of severity and an evaluation of the patient's risk for negative outcomes is important to assess at every visit. While Ms Jenkins' impairment domain criteria demonstrated a moderate persistent severity classification, her risk assessment is low because she had no prior exacerbations in the past year. Thus, her asthma severity remains classified as moderate persistent. If she had reported frequent exacerbations requiring oral corticosteroids, her risk would be high and we would consider elevating her severity classification to severe persistent.

Technically, we cannot classify severity in patients who are already using inhaled corticosteroid medications. These medications alter lung function and symptoms, thereby creating an inaccurate picture of intrinsic lung function. When this happens, a severity classification can be inferred from the lowest doses of medication required to control asthma symptoms.[3] Many clinicians inappropriately use the severity table with patients who are taking inhaled corticosteroid medications[15] rather than evaluate the lowest dose of medication needed to control asthma symptoms. For example, if Ms Jenkins were well controlled on a low-dose inhaled corticosteroid (ICS) plus long-acting beta$_2$-agonist (LABA) (Step 3), she would be classified as moderate persistent because Step 3 medications correlate with moderate severity (see **Fig. 1**).

Initial treatment of asthma is based upon the patient's severity classification.[3] The bottom section of the severity table (see **Fig. 1**) lists the corresponding step for starting therapy. Initial treatment for Ms Jenkins' moderate persistent asthma is Step 3. Using a stepwise approach, either a low-dose ICS plus LABA or a medium-dose ICS would be initiated (see **Fig. 3**). An alternative Step 3 therapy is also provided. The specific choice will be influenced by the dialogue that emerges from the partnership between the patient and provider. Ms Jenkins was started on a low-dose ICS and LABA to be

◀━━

Fig. 2. Assessing asthma control and adjusting therapy in youth ≥12 years of age and adults. The stepwise approach is meant to assist, not replace, the clinical decision making required to meet individual patient needs. The level of control is based on the most severe impairment or risk category. Assess impairment domain by patient's recall of previous 2–4 weeks and by spirometry/or peak flow measures. Symptom assessment for longer periods should reflect a global assessment, such as inquiring whether the patient's asthma is better or worse since the last visit. At present, there are inadequate data to correspond frequencies of exacerbations with different levels of asthma control. In general, more frequent and intense exacerbations (eg, requiring urgent, unscheduled care, hospitalization, or ICU admission) indicate poorer disease control. For treatment purposes, patients who had ≥2 exacerbations requiring oral systemic corticosteroids in the past year may be considered the same as patients who have not-well-controlled asthma, even in the absence of impairment levels consistent with not-well-controlled asthma.[3]

Step up if needed

(first, check adherence, environmental control, and comorbid conditions)

Assess control

Step down if possible

(and asthma is well controlled at least 3 months)

Persistent Asthma: Daily Medication

Consult with asthma specialist if step 4 care or higher is required. Consider consultation at step 3.

Intermittent Asthma

Step 1

Preferred:
SABA PRN

Step 2

Preferred:
Low-dose ICS

Alternative:
Cromolyn, LTRA, Nedocromil, or Theophylline

Step 3

Preferred:
Low dose ICS + LABA OR medium-dose ICS

Alternative:
low-dose ICS + either LTRA, Theophylline, or Zileuton

Step 4

Preferred:
Medium-dose ICS + LABA

Alternative:
Medium-dose ICS+either LTRA, Theophylline, or Zileuton

Step 5

Preferred:
High-dose ICS + LABA

AND

Consider Omalizumab for patients who have allergies

Step 6

Preferred:
High-dose ICS + LABA + oral corticosteroid

AND

Consider Omalizumab for patients who have allergies

Each step: Patient education, environmental control, and management of comorbidities.

Steps 2-4: Consider subcutaneous allergen immunotherapy for patients who have allergic asthma *

Quick-Relief Medication for All Patients

SABA as needed for symptoms. Intensity of treatment depends on severity of symptoms: up to 3 treatments at 20-minute intervals as needed. Short course of oral systemic corticosteroids may be needed

Caution: Increasing use of SABA or use >2 days a week for symptom relief (not prevention of EIB) generally indicates inadequate control and the need to step up treatment.

Table 1 Result of Ms Jenkins' spirometry in office		
	Pre-Bronchodilator	Post-Bronchodilator

FVC % Predicted
FVC = forced vital capacity: The total
  volume of air exhaled during a forced
  exhalation after a full inspiration.
	82%	85%

FEV$_1$ % Predicted
FEV$_1$ = forced expiratory volume in 1
  second: The volume of air exhaled in
  1 s during a forced exhalation after a
  full inspiration.
	65%	82%

FEV$_1$/FVC (%) FEV$_1$/FVC = The ratio of the individual's FEV$_1$/FVC.	66%	84%

taken daily with a SABA as needed. Asthma self-management education should also be initiated at this time and a written asthma action plan provided.[3] It is critical to explain to Ms Jenkins that she will not feel the same immediate relief from her ICS medication, but she will obtain relief from the LABA and SABA. It takes 4–8 weeks of regular use for the benefits of the ICS to be apparent. Routine use of an ICS needs to be emphasized, and teaching her proper technique with the new inhaler is essential. Patients need detailed instructions, practice, and sometimes assistive devices such as spacers for metered dose inhalers. Finally, it is critical to address potential barriers to medication adherence that Ms Jenkins may have such as an inability to pay for her medications or fears about routine use of an ICS medication.

CONTROL

Ms Jenkins returned to clinic 8 weeks later. She reported no episodes of wheezing, nighttime awakenings, or SABA use. She was able to regularly attend work. Her

Fig. 3. Stepwise approach for managing asthma in youths ≥12 years of age and adults. The stepwise approach is meant to assist, not replace, the clinical decision making required to meet individual patient needs. If alternative treatment is used and response is inadequate, discontinue it and use the preferred treatment before stepping up. Zileuton is a less desirable alternative because of limited studies as adjunctive therapy and the need to monitor liver function. Theophylline requires monitoring of serum concentration levels. In step 6, before oral systemic corticosteroids are introduced, a trial of high-dose ICS + inhaled long-acting beta$_2$ agonist (LABA) + leukotriene receptor agonist (LTRA), theophylline, or zileuton may be considered, although this approach has not been studied in clinical trials. Step 1, 2, and 3 preferred therapies are based on evidence A; step 3 alternative therapy is based on evidence A for LTRA, evidence B for theophylline, and evidence D for zileuton. Step 4 preferred therapy is based on evidence B, and alternative therapy is based on evidence B for LTRA and theophylline and evidence D for zileuton. Step 5 preferred therapy is based on evidence B. Step 6 preferred therapy is based on (EPR-2 1997) and evidence B for omalizumab. Immunotherapy for steps 2 to 4 is based on evidence B for house-dust mites, animal danders, and pollens; evidence is weak or lacking for molds and cockroaches. Evidence is strongest for immunotherapy with single allergens. The role of allergy in asthma is greater in children than in adults. Clinicians who administer immunotherapy should be prepared and equipped to identify and treat anaphylaxis that may occur.[3]

Asthma Control Test (ACT) score was 23 and FEV$_1$ was 82% predicted pre-bronchodilator. She reported taking her low-dose ICS and LABA regularly.

Once severity has been established and treatment initiated, we shift to the assessment of asthma control.[2,3] The three categories of control are well controlled, not well controlled, and very poorly controlled. An assessment of Ms Jenkins' symptoms, nighttime awakenings, SABA use, FEV$_1$ and ACT score all fell within the well controlled classification for impairment (see **Fig. 2**). Her risk assessment showed that she did not require an oral corticosteroid for her exacerbation. Although Ms Jenkins' asthma is well controlled based upon her symptoms and her FEV$_1$, her treatment requires ongoing evaluation. How often does she use her SABA inhaler? Using the SABA inhaler for symptoms (other than routine exercise) more than twice a week indicates that her asthma would not be in good control. Fortunately, Ms Jenkins has not needed to use her SABA recently. Should Ms Jenkins' medication therapy be reduced? Stepping down medication therapy should be delayed until there is at least three months of good asthma control. If in the future she requires a step up in therapy, review her exposure to environmental triggers, medication adherence and inhaler technique, elements that should be monitored at each encounter. If control cannot be obtained, other factors like allergic rhinitis, gastroesophageal reflux disease (GERD), and vocal cord dysfunction should be considered.[3] The emphasis on monitoring asthma control is a departure from the Expert Panel Report 2 guidelines released in 1997[16] which contained a single assessment, severity, and used the severity assessment to guide asthma treatment.

In summary, good asthma management includes assessment of asthma control and severity. Asthma severity classification is used to characterize the intrinsic nature of the disease in an individual and to guide treatment recommendations. The EPR-3 guidelines tables can be used to categorize symptoms and test data into impairment and risk domains, ultimately yielding a severity category. The treatment recommendation tables then can be appropriately applied. Other guidelines take a similar approach with the exception that the Global Initiative for Asthma (GINA) includes two constructs for the severity measure; treatment intensity—the treatment needed to control a patient's asthma symptoms (the severity of the underlying disease) and responsiveness to therapy.[2] After severity has been established and treatment initiated, the EPR-3 guidelines should be used to assess asthma control on a regular basis. Control will guide decisions about the need to step up or step down therapy. Although less critical for routine asthma management decisions, asthma severity plays an important role for population-based evaluations, research studies, or reevaluation of the patient's disease.[15] The features of asthma control and severity are outlined in **Table 2**.

Several validated questionnaires have been developed to standardize the assessment of asthma control. The EPR-3 guidelines refer to several of these questionnaires which include the Asthma Control Test (ACT) for adults[17] and children,[18] Asthma Control Questionnaire ©[19] and the Asthma Therapy Assessment Questionnaire © (ATAQ).[20]

GUIDELINE IMPLEMENTATION

Guideline-based care cannot improve outcomes unless they are effectively implemented. Following the release of EPR-3 guidelines, the NAEPP convened a Guidelines Implementation Panel (GIP) that published a guide to provide practical applications for the use of guidelines in the field. *Partners Putting Practice into Action*[21] emphasizes six priority EPR-3 messages that include asthma severity and control and highlight the evidence-based recommendations. In addition to the three core themes of communication, systems integration and patient/provider support, the GIP provided strategies

Table 2
Asthma control and severity characteristics

Feature	Control	Severity
Definition	Degree to which manifestations of asthma are minimized and treatment goals are met	Intrinsic intensity of the patient's asthma GINA guidelines define severity as the intensity of treatment needed to treat patient's asthma symptoms (severity of underlying disease) and responsiveness to treatment[2]
Variability	Changes more frequently	More stable, but can change over time
Functions	Maintain or adjust therapy by step up or step down	Descriptive for population studies and research Reevaluation of the patient's condition over time
Assessment frequency	Every encounter	Initial diagnosis, new to provider, suspicion that characteristics of underlying disease have changed

Data from National Asthma Education and Prevention Program. Expert panel report 3 (EPR-3): Guidelines for the diagnosis and management of asthma - Full report 2007. NIH Publication Number 08-5846; 2007.

for dynamic engagement of stakeholders and a host of implementation approaches to promote guideline use. Eleven strategies were recommended that include (p 17):

- Gathering information with respect to message barriers/solutions for identified priority audiences
- Convene knowledge brokers, influential leaders and decision makers
- Pilot test strategies
- Provide professional education and training
- Provide point-of service prompting
- Conduct quality improvement
- Provide patient-self management education
- Promote financing support systems
- Strengthen linkages between medical and community-based resources
- Collate, analyze and share data
- Disseminate and market the National Asthma Control Initiatives (NACI) activities, results and products.

These strategies can help guide system-level changes in asthma care. For example, the electronic health record (EHR) provides an effective platform to implement point-of-service prompting to improve adherence with asthma guidelines. Nkoy and colleagues[22] implemented an asthma-specific reminder and decision support (RADS) system within the EHR that improved compliance with pediatric asthma inpatient quality measures. Kowk[23] found that use of an asthma clinical assessment form and electronic decision support system resulted in improved compliance with and documentation of asthma severity and discharge management plans in the emergency department. Bell and colleagues[24] used an asthma decision support system across several pediatric primary care practices and demonstrated an increased prescription rate for controller medications, greater spirometry use, updated asthma action plans.

Other approaches to assist in the integration of guidelines into clinical practice integrate multiple strategies. Boulet and colleagues[25] outlined steps for a GINA guideline implementation program that can be applied and adopted according to local conditions, as well as a broader context. Some of the elements in this model include identifying stakeholders, performing a needs assessment, identifying care gaps and key messages to convey; and developing and prioritizing implementation strategies, metrics, resources, and detailed implementation plans. Alvanzo and colleagues[26] reported that a combination of education, motivation, and facilitation fostered successful guideline implementation.

The EPR-3 guidelines provide a comprehensive framework for managing patients with asthma. These guidelines include an ongoing assessment of asthma control and severity, stepwise medication management, environmental control, and education for a partnership in care. To tackle the barriers limiting the widespread implementation of guideline-recommended care, a systems-based approach should be used.

REFERENCES

1. Moorman JE, Akinbami LJ, Bailey CM, et al. National surveillance of asthma: United States, 2001-2010. National Center for Health Statistics. Vital Health Stats 2012;35(3).
2. Global Initiative for Asthma. Global strategy for asthma management and prevention 2012 (update). 2012. p. 128.
3. National Asthma Education and Prevention Program, Third expert panel on the diagnosis and management of asthma. Expert panel report 3: guidelines for the diagnosis and management of asthma. NIH Publication No. 07-4051; 2007.
4. Fitzgerald ST. National Asthma Education Program Expert Panel report: guidelines for the diagnosis and management of asthma. AAOHN J 1992;40(8):376–82.
5. Murphy K, Meltzer E, Blaiss M, et al. Asthma management and control in the United States: results of the 2009 Asthma Insight and Management survey. Allergy Asthma Proc 2012;33(1):54–6.
6. Rance K, O'Laughlen M, Ting S. Improving asthma care for African American children by increasing national asthma guideline adherence. J Pediatr Health Care 2011;25(4):235–49.
7. Weinstein AG. The potential of asthma adherence management to enhance asthma guidelines. Ann Allergy Asthma Immunol 2011;106(4):283–91.
8. Navaratnam P, Jayawant SS, Pedersen CA, et al. Physician adherence to the national asthma prescribing guidelines: evidence from national outpatient survey data in the United States. Ann Allergy Asthma Immunol 2008;100(3):216.
9. Wisnivesky JP, Lorenzo J, Lyn-Cook R, et al. Barriers to adherence to asthma management guidelines among inner-city primary care providers. Ann Allergy Asthma Immunol 2008;101(3):264.
10. Bracha Y, Brottman G, Carlson A. Physicians, guidelines, and cognitive tasks. Eval Health Prof 2011;34(3):309–35.
11. Abrahamson K, Fox R, Doebbeling B. Facilitators and barriers to clinical practice guideline use among nurses. Am J Nurs 2012;112(7):26–35.
12. Ploeg J, Davies B, Edwards N, et al. Factors influencing best-practice guideline implementation: lessons learned from administrators, nursing staff, and project leaders. Worldviews Evid Based Nurs 2007;4(4):210–9.
13. Graham L. Classifying asthma. Chest 2006;130(1 Suppl):13S–20S.
14. Ayres J, Jyothish D, Ninan T. Brittle asthma. Paediatr Respir Rev 2004;5(1):40–4.
15. Taylor DR, Bateman ED, Boulet L, et al. A new perspective on concepts of asthma severity and control. Eur Respir J 2008;32(3):545–54.

16. National Institutes of Health. Practical guide for the diagnosis and management of asthma. Washington, DC: US Department of Health and Human Services, National Institutes of Health; 1997. Publication no. 97–4053.
17. Nathan RA, Sorkness CA, Kosinski M, et al. Development of the asthma control test: a survey for assessing asthma control. J Allergy Clin Immunol 2004; 113(1):59–65.
18. Liu AH, Zeiger R, Sorkness C, et al. Development and cross-sectional validation of the Childhood Asthma Control Test. J Allergy Clin Immunol 2007;119(4): 817–25.
19. Juniper E, Guyatt G, Ferrie P, et al. Development and validation of a questionnaire to measure asthma control. Eur Respir J 2001;14(4):902–7.
20. Vollmer WM, Markson LE, O'connor E, et al. Association of asthma control with health care utilization and quality of life. Am J Respir Crit Care Med 1999; 160(5):1647–52.
21. U.S. Department of Health and Human Services. Guidelines implementation panel report for: expert panel report 3-guidelines for the diagnosis and management of asthma. Partners putting guidelines into action. 2008; NIH Publication No. 09–6147.
22. Nkoy F, Fassl B, Wolfe D, et al. Sustaining compliance with pediatric asthma inpatient quality measures. AMIA Annu Symp Proc 2010;2010:547–51.
23. Kwok R, Dinh M, Dinh D, et al. Improving adherence to asthma clinical guidelines and discharge documentation from emergency departments: implementation of a dynamic and integrated electronic decision support system. Emerg Med Australas 2009;21(1):31–7.
24. Bell LM, Grundmeier R, Localio R, et al. Electronic health record-based decision support to improve asthma care: a cluster-randomized trial. Pediatrics 2010; 125(4):e770–7.
25. Boulet L, FitzGerald JM, Levy M, et al. A guide to the translation of the Global Initiative for Asthma (GINA) strategy into improved care. Eur Respir J 2012; 39(5):1220–9.
26. Alvanzo AH, Cohen GM, Nettleman M. Changing physician behavior: half-empty or half-full? Clin Govern Int J 2003;8(1):69–78.

A Systematic Review of Complementary and Alternative Medicine for Asthma Self-management

Maureen George, PhD, RN, AE-C[a,b,*], Maxim Topaz, RN, MA[c,d]

KEYWORDS

- Asthma • Self-management • Patient-provider communication
- Complementary and alternative medicine • Mind-body • Natural products • Disclosure

KEY POINTS

- There is wide patient support for the use of complementary and alternative medicine (CAM) as part of a comprehensive asthma self-management plan for both children and adults.
- The most popular complementary and alternative treatments for asthma fall broadly into the domains of natural products, mind-body medicine, and manipulative and body-based practices.
- Little empiric evidence to support the use of CAM can be gleaned from this systematic review because of both the small number of studies and the methodological weaknesses of the studies.
- Most complementary approaches reported by children and adults with asthma would be classified by the National Center for Complementary and Alternative Medicine as "likely safe" and "effectiveness unknown" or "likely ineffective."
- Rare but serious side effects have been reported with CAM for asthma self-management.
- Risky behaviors associated with CAM use for asthma include the substitution of complementary therapies for both "rescue" short-acting β-2 agonists and inhaled corticosteroids. These behaviors may add to unnecessary delays in seeking timely and appropriate medical intervention, thus contributing to excessive morbidity.
- There is suboptimal patient-provider communication about CAM use because of the failure of health care professionals to inquire about use and because of patients' reluctance to disclose use.
- To address patient preference for integrative care (concomitant use of CAM and prescription therapies) will require that clinicians conduct a more comprehensive assessment of use, be better informed about safety and risk of different therapies, and create a safe environment that fosters disclosure and shared decision making.

This article originally appeared in Nursing Clinics of North America, Volume 48, Issue 1, March 2013.
Funding Sources: Mr Topaz: None; Dr George: This study was supported by the National Center for Complementary and Alternative Medicine (National Institutes of Health) 1K23AT003907-01A1.
Conflict of Interest: None.
[a] Department of Family and Community Health, University of Pennsylvania School of Nursing, 418 Curie Boulevard, Philadelphia, PA 19104, USA; [b] Center for Clinical Epidemiology and Biostatistics (CCEB), Department of Biostatistics and Epidemiology, Perelman School of Medicine, 837 Blockley Hall, 423 Guardian Drive, Philadelphia, PA 19104–6021, USA; [c] University of Haifa, The Cheryl Spencer Department of Nursing Haifa, Mount Carmel 31905, Haifa, Israel; [d] University of Pennsylvania School of Nursing, 418 Curie Boulevard, Philadelphia, PA 19104, USA
* Corresponding author.
E-mail address: mgeorge@nursing.upenn.edu

INTRODUCTION AND BACKGROUND

It has been more than 3 decades since Arthur Kleinman first reminded clinicians that individuals have more options to treat illness than just conventional biomedical approaches.[1] In fact, the health care professional is often the last resort for patients, consulted only after popular remedies and traditional healing methods have been exhausted.[2] To that end, it is estimated that as much as 80% of the world's health care is nonbiomedical.[3]

Although traditional healing is frequently integrated into the national medical system of its endemic country (eg, Ayurveda in India) and is common in places where limited access or prohibitive costs prevent the widespread adoption of biomedicine,[3] traditional healing is not an integral component of the North American health care systems. This has led to its characterization as "complementary" or "alternative" medicine. The term *complementary* describes traditional practices used in combination with conventional biomedical approaches, whereas *alternative* connotes traditional practices that replace or substitute for biomedicine.[4] The goal for many is *integrated* care in which the best treatments from conventional biomedical approaches are combined with safe and effective complementary and alternative medicine (CAM).[4]

The National Center for Complementary and Alternative Medicine (NCCAM), the leading federal CAM research agency in the United States, defines CAM as a variety of medical systems, healing traditions, and products not typically considered to be part of conventional biomedical approaches.[4] As seen in **Table 1**, CAM can be broadly characterized into domains that include whole medical systems, natural products, manipulative and body-based practices, movement therapies, traditional healers, and energy field healing. Although useful for purposes of grouping, the clinician must remember that a CAM approach may overlap with several domains.

Despite growing interest in integrated care,[5] much of CAM continues to be delivered outside of the North American health care systems at a considerable out-of-pocket cost.[6] In fact, US adults are more likely to use CAM when conventional medical care is unaffordable.[7] Despite these costs, CAM is widely used. Nationwide surveys suggest that three-quarters of US[7] and Canadian adults[5,8] have used some form of CAM in their lifetime. In addition, although there are no national data on CAM use in Mexico, a systematic review indicates high rates of indigenous Mexican CAM use among Mexican-American adults.[9]

Frequently, CAM use is reported to be highest among well-educated higher-income white adults.[7] However, this is likely a function of survey questions that focus on vitamins and herb ingestion, and body-based (massage, chiropractic care) and mind-body therapies (yoga, acupuncture) to the exclusion of folk medicine and prayer, which are CAMs more commonly used by people of color and by the poor. For example, when folk medicine (defined as a "range of remedies including prayer, healing touch or laying on of hands, charms, herbal teas or tinctures, magic rituals") was included in the 2002 National Health Interview Survey (NHIS), CAM prevalence was highest in black and Hispanic individuals and those living in poverty.[10] Nonvitamin, nonmineral natural products and deep-breathing exercises were the most commonly reported CAM[7] after prayer[10] among US adults, whereas chiropractic care, massage, relaxation techniques, and prayer were most common among Canadian adults.[5] In both groups, CAM was used for the treatment of a variety of somatic and psychiatric complaints, including neck, back, and joint discomfort; upper respiratory infections; anxiety; and depression.[5,7]

CAM is also frequently used by or for children. The 2006 Fraser Institute[5] and 2007 NHIS[7] surveys were the first comprehensive national surveys directed at

Table 1
CAM domains and examples

NCCAM Domain Definitions	CAM Type	Examples	NCCAM Definition/Description
Whole Medical Systems are complete systems of theory and practice that have evolved over time in different cultures and apart from Western medicine	Ayurveda		Developed in India, it aims to integrate the body, mind, and spirit to prevent and treat disease using herbs, diet, massage, and yoga.
	Naturopathy		Developed in Europe, naturopathy seeks to stimulate self-healing through the use of dietary and lifestyle changes used in concert with massage, herbs and joint manipulation.
	Traditional Chinese Medicine (TCM)		Developed in China, TCM is based on the belief that disease is the result of an imbalance in yin and yang and disrupted flow of qi (life force). Balance and flow can be restored through the use of herbs, acupuncture, meditation, and massage.
	Homeopathy		Developed in Europe, homeopathy seeks to stimulate self-healing through doses of highly diluted substances that in larger doses would produce the symptoms of concern ("like cures like").
Natural Products are substances produced by living organisms and built by cells from sugars, amino acids, and so forth	Botanicals	Herbs and herbal products	Products that include any plant-based component.
	Minerals	Calcium, folate, iron, magnesium, selenium, zinc	
	Specialized diets	Gluten-free, allergen-free, ketogenic, low-residue	A special diet in which foods that produce unwanted symptoms are avoided.
	Dietary supplements	Minerals, vitamins, herbs, enzymes, proteins, organ tissues, or glands and metabolites	Any product taken by mouth with the intent of supplementing the diet.
	Vitamins	A, B12, B6, C, D, E, K	
	Herbs and herbal preparations	Echinacea, St Johns wort, chamomile, ginseng	Plants with leaves, seeds, flowers, bark, or roots used for medicinal purposes.
	Probiotics	Live microorganisms (bacteria; yeast)	

(continued on next page)

Table 1
(continued)

NCCAM Domain Definitions	CAM Type	Examples	NCCAM Definition/Description
Mind-body Medicine	Meditation	Transcendental, Mindfulness	Meditation teaches an individual to focus attention, to become mindful of thoughts, feelings, and sensations and to observe them in a nonjudgmental way. Meditation is performed to achieve calmness, relaxation, and psychological balance.
	Tai chi		Developed in China as a martial art, tai chi is a "moving meditation" in which practitioners move their bodies slowly, gently, and with awareness, while breathing deeply.
	Guided imagery	Mental imagery, visualization	In guided imagery, the individual focuses on pleasant images or is led through storytelling or visualizations to replace negative or stressful feelings for the purpose of promoting relaxation.
	Relaxation	Progressive muscle relaxation, passive muscle relaxation, relaxation breathing	In this practice, the individual focuses on tightening and relaxing each muscle group. It is often combined with guided imagery and breathing exercises.
	Hypnosis		Phrases or nonverbal cues (called a "suggestion") produce relaxation to relieve pain and anxiety.
	Qi gong		Similar to tai chi.
	Yoga	Hatha, Iyengar, Ashtanga, Vinyasa, Bikram	Originating in ancient Indian philosophy, yoga combines physical postures, breathing techniques, and meditation or relaxation.
	Art therapy		Art-making as a therapeutic process.
	Cognitive behavioral therapy		Psychotherapeutic method to reduce stress and anxiety.
	Acupuncture		Part of traditional Chinese medicine (TCM), acupuncture aims to restore and maintain health through the stimulation of specific points on the body to encourage the flow of qi through channels called meridians.
	Biofeedback		Electronic devices are used to teach individuals to consciously reduce stress.
	Breathing retraining	Buteyko breathing exercises	Nasal breathing, reduced breathing, and relaxation are used to "normalize" breathing.
	Journaling		Writing therapy.

Category	Type	Description
	Music therapy	Use of music to promote well-being or promote relaxation.
	Humoral balance	Ancient theory that disease results from an imbalance of 4 "humors." Application of hot-cold therapies can be traced to this belief system.
	Deep breathing	Conscious slowing of breathing by focusing on taking regular and deep breaths to promote relaxation.
Manipulative and Body-based Practices focus primarily on the structures and systems of the body	Spinal manipulation — Chiropractic care, Craniosacral therapy (cranial osteopathy)	The application of a controlled force to the joint by use of hands or a device with the intent of reducing pain and/or improving physical functioning.
	Massage — Swedish, shiatsu, Acupressure, Trager, Craniosacral therapy (cranial osteopathy)	Blood flow and oxygen are increased to the massaged area by pressing, rubbing, and moving soft tissues with the hands and fingers. The intent of massage is to reduce pain and stress and enhance relaxation, mood, and general well-being.
Movement Therapies include Eastern and Western movement-based practices to promote physical, mental, emotional, and spiritual well-being	Pilates	A physical fitness approach to core training that uses apparatuses to apply resistance as well as props, such as weighted balls.
	Rolfing	Deep fascial tissue manipulation and movement used to reduce stress by bringing the body into proper alignment with gravity.
	Alexander technique (AT)	This technique aims to teach individuals to stand and move free of tension. AT is not an exercise or relaxation program.
Traditional Healers use indigenous and religious knowledge, beliefs, and experiences to treat disease and promote health	Shaman, Curandero, Santero, Houngan, Mambos	Healing power is passed down through generations via oral transmission and apprenticeships. Its use is generally reserved for members of a regional or cultural community.
Energy Field Healing involves the manipulation of the subtle energy fields imbued in humans	Magnet therapy — Reiki (Energy-field manipulation)	Magnets produce magnetic fields that are proposed to reduce pain. Healing of the body and the spirit can be facilitated by the practitioner's transmitting universal energy to the person from a distance or from placing their hands on or near the individual.
	Light therapy, Therapeutic touch	Exposure to green and blue wavelength light to promote sleep. Manipulation of energy fields by placing hands on, or near, an individual.

Abbreviations: CAM, complementary and alternative medicine; NCCAM, National Center for Complementary and Alternative Medicine.

understanding CAM use among North American children. Caregivers of children aged 0 to 17 were interviewed about the child's CAM use. Twelve percent of US[7] and 15% of Canadian youth[5] reported CAM use in the prior 12 months to treat neck and back pain, anxiety, and attention deficit and hyperactivity disorders, as well as head and chest colds.[7] Children were most likely to use nonvitamin, nonmineral natural products, chiropractic care,[5,7] homeopathy, and acupuncture.[11] CAM use was fivefold higher in children who had a CAM-using parent compared with children who did not.[7]

Complementary and Alternative Medicine for Asthma

Although CAM is commonly used to maintain wellness, national surveys have demonstrated their extensive use in treating common chronic medical conditions, including lung and digestive disorders, heart disease, hypertension, and diabetes.[5,7] Lung problems generally[5] and asthma and allergies specifically[5,7,10] rank in the top 15 most common medical conditions for which CAM is used for both children and adults. Unfortunately, there is a lack of recent literature summarizing the rates of CAM use among children and adults with asthma. Moreover, there is a critical need to compile and summarize the growing body of evidence on the most prevalent CAM modalities used, CAM effectiveness, and its possible side effects. This summary is crucial for allopathic and CAM practitioners treating patients with asthma, as well as individuals with asthma and their families who are engaged in decision making regarding asthma self-management practices.

The aim of this systematic review was twofold. First, we aimed to quantitatively summarize the existing body of research on CAM use for asthma among children and adults. Second, we wanted to reflect on the most frequent CAM modalities used, the methodological quality and patterns presented in CAM studies, and the potential benefits and dangers of CAM use in asthma.

METHODS

A systematic review of the literature[12] was conducted using the following databases: PubMed, PyscINFO, and SCOPUS. The following search terms were used: "asthma" AND "complementary medicine," "alternative medicine," "complementary and alternative medicine," "herbs," "diet," "dietary supplements," "vitamins," "acupuncture," "breathing (Buteyko) exercises," "relaxation," "mind-body," "homeopathy," "ayurveda," "traditional Chinese medicine," "colon cleansing," "music," "chiropractic," "massage," "art therapy," "aromatherapy," "yoga," "tai-chi." Search terms were determined after reviewing existing CAM literature, reviewing information from NCCAM and compiling associated keywords and subject headings. **Table 1** summarizes the different CAM domains and examples.

The place of publication was limited to North America (Canada, Mexico, and the United States). Publications were also limited to English, Spanish, and French languages. We did not limit the age of publications. Manuscripts were included if they (1) presented primary or original research and (2) were focused on CAM use among children and adults with asthma. Manuscripts were excluded if they were duplicates from different databases or did not present original research on CAM use among individuals with asthma.

Data Collection and Analyses

The two authors (M.T. and M.G.) independently reviewed the abstracts and articles for inclusion with 100% interrater reliability. Data were extracted using a standardized template developed by the researchers to capture all relevant data. The template was reviewed by the authors and consensus reached through discussion between the authors.

STUDY FINDINGS
Search Results

A total of 1960 abstracts were identified from the initial review, of which 904 were duplicates. After a detailed review, 984 additional articles were excluded because they did not meet the inclusion criteria: 322 articles did not directly focus on CAM use among individuals with asthma; 214 manuscripts did not present original research; and 448 of the studies were conducted outside of the United States, Canada, or Mexico. As a result, 72 articles were included in the review. See **Fig. 1** for the detailed description of the search process and findings and **Table 2** presenting qualitative summary of the reviewed articles.

In general, there is an increasing body of research on the use of different CAM modalities among individuals with asthma. As presented in **Fig. 2**, the number of articles on the topic remained low until the mid 1990s and then grew steadily, especially through the past decade.

Methodological Issues

Overall, the reviewed literature includes studies conducted using diverse designs and methodological techniques, ranging from randomized controlled trials (RCTs) to

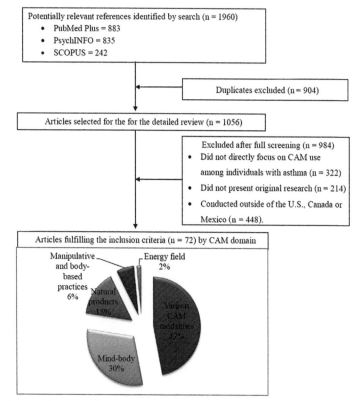

Fig. 1. Distinct phases in the process of collecting relevant publications on CAM use for asthma and their results.

Table 2
Summary of included articles: CAM use in asthma

Authors, Primary	Design	Population	Results	Conclusions	Categories/Domain
Knoeller et al,[15] 2012	Survey, correlational	27,927 employed adults with current work-related asthma (WRA) as presented in the 2006–2008 Behavioral Risk Factor Surveillance System Asthma Call-Back Survey from 37 states and the District of Columbia.	An estimated 56.6% of individuals with WRA reported using CAM compared with 27.9% of those with non-WRA (PR = 2.0). People with WRA were more likely than those with non-WRA to have adverse asthma events including an asthma attack in the past month (PR = 1.43), urgent treatment for worsening asthma (PR = 1.74), emergency room visit (PR = 1.95), overnight hospital stay (PR = 2.49), and poorly controlled asthma (PR = 1.27). The associations of WRA with adverse asthma events remained after stratifying for CAM use.	Individuals with WRA were more likely to use CAM to control their asthma. However, there was no evidence that the use of CAM modified the association of WRA with adverse asthma events.	Adults; various CAM modalities

| Luberto et al,[60] 2012 | Survey, correlational | 282 adolescents (Time 1: n = 151, Time 2: n = 131) completed self-report measures | Participants (M(age) = 15.8, SD = 1.85) were primarily African American (n = 129 [85%]) and female (n = 91 [60%]) adolescents with asthma. High and low CAM users differed significantly in terms of several psychosocial health outcomes, both cross-sectionally and longitudinally. In cross-sectional multivariable analyses, greater frequency of praying was associated with better psychosocial health-related quality of life. No longitudinal relationships remained significant in multivariable analyses. | Specific CAM techniques are differentially associated with psychosocial outcomes, indicating the importance of examining CAM modalities individually. When controlling for key covariates, CAM use was not associated with psychosocial outcomes over time. Further research should examine the effects of CAM use in controlled research settings. | Adolescents; various CAM modalities |

(continued on next page)

Table 2
(continued)

Authors, Primary	Design	Population	Results	Conclusions	Categories/Domain
Philp et al,[105] 2012	Survey, correlational (retrospective cohort study)	187 children prescribed daily medications for all 3 y of the study	Patients had high rates of adherence. The mean percent missed asthma daily controller medication doses per week was 7.7% (SD = 14.2%). Medication Adherence Scale scores (range: 4–20, with lower scores reflecting higher adherence) had an overall mean of 7.5 (SD = 2.9). In multivariate analyses, controlling for demographic factors and asthma severity, initiation of CAM use was not associated with subsequent adherence (P>.05).	The data from this study suggest that CAM use is not necessarily "competitive" with conventional asthma therapies; families may incorporate different health belief systems simultaneously in their asthma management. As CAM use becomes more prevalent, it is important for physicians to ask about CAM use in a nonjudgmental fashion.	Adolescent; Children; various CAM modalities

| Shen and Oraka,[16] 2012 | Survey, correlational | 5435 children from the Asthma Call Back Survey (ACBS) 2006–2008, were included in this analysis. | Overall, 26.7% of children with current asthma reported CAM use in the previous 12 mo. Among them, the 3 most commonly used therapies were breathing techniques, vitamins, and herbal products. Multivariate analysis of CAM use revealed higher adjusted odds ratios (aOR) among children who experienced cost barriers to conventional health care compared with children with no cost barrier (aOR = 1.8). Children with poorly controlled asthma were most likely to use all types of CAM when compared with their counterparts with well-controlled asthma: aOR = 2.3 for any CAM; aOR = 1.7, for self-care based CAM; and aOR = 4.4 for practitioner-based CAM. | Children with poorly controlled asthma are more likely to use CAM; this likelihood persists after controlling for other factors (including parent's education, barriers to conventional health care, and controller medication use). CAM is also more commonly used by children who experienced cost barriers to conventional asthma care. CAM use could be a marker to identify patients who need patient/family education and support and thus facilitate improved asthma control. | Children; various CAM modalities |

(continued on next page)

Table 2
(continued)

Authors, Primary	Design	Population	Results	Conclusions	Categories/Domain
Cotton et al,[33] 2011	Survey, correlational	151 adolescents with asthma recruited from a children's hospital completed questionnaires addressing demographic and clinical variables and 10 CAM modalities.	Participants' mean age was 15.8 (SD = 1.8), 60% were female, and 85% were African American. Seventy-one percent reported using CAM for symptom management in the past month. Relaxation (64%) and prayer (61%) were the most frequently reported modalities and were perceived to be the most efficacious. Adolescents most commonly reported considering using relaxation (85%) and prayer (80%) for future symptom management. Participants were most likely to disclose their use of yoga (59%) and diet (57%), and least likely to disclose prayer (33%) and guided	Many urban adolescents used and would consider using CAM, specifically relaxation and prayer, for asthma symptom management. African Americans, older adolescents, and those with more frequent symptoms were more likely to use and/or consider using CAM. Providers caring for urban adolescents with asthma should discuss CAM with patients, particularly those identified as likely to use CAM. Future studies should examine relationships between CAM use and health outcomes.	Adolescents; various CAM modalities

			Results	Conclusion	Details
			imagery (36%) to providers. In multivariable analyses, older adolescents (OR = 1.27, $P<.05$) and African Americans (OR = 2.76, $P<.05$) were more likely to use relaxation. Adolescents with more frequent asthma symptoms (OR = 0.98, $P<.05$) were more likely to use prayer. African Americans were more likely to report using prayer (OR = 3.47, $P<.05$) and consider using prayer (OR = 7.98, $P<.01$) in the future for symptom management.		
Kligler et al,[23] 2011	Prospective parallel group repeated measurement randomized study	154 patients were randomized and included in the intention-to-treat analysis (77 control, 77 treatment).	Treatment participants showed greater improvement than controls at 6 mo for the Asthma Quality of Life Questionnaire total score ($P<.001$) and for 3 subscales, Activity ($P<.001$), Symptoms ($P = .02$), and Emotion ($P<.001$).	A low-cost group-oriented integrative medicine intervention can lead to significant improvement in quality of life in adults with asthma.	Adults; yoga (mind-body); dietary supplements (natural products); journaling (mind-body)

(continued on next page)

Table 2
(continued)

Authors, Primary	Design	Population	Results	Conclusions	Categories/Domain
Long et al,[63] 2011	Intervention trial (feasibility study with 2 intervention groups)	Cohort 1 (n = 11) was recruited from the community and attended intervention sessions at an urban university. Cohort 2 (n = 7) was school based and recruited from an African American charter school.	The intervention was rated as highly acceptable by participating families. Feasibility was much stronger for the school-based than the university-based recruitment mechanism. Initial efficacy data suggest that both cohorts showed preintervention to postintervention improvements in lung function, perceived stress, and depressed mood.	Findings provide evidence for the feasibility of offering asthma-related stress-management training in a school setting. Initial findings offer support for future, large-scale efficacy studies.	Children; relaxation and biofeedback (mind-body)

| Mithani and Monteleone,[109] 2011 | Survey, descriptive (pilot) | 181 individuals with asthma filled out the survey | Over a period of 14 mo, 18% of the patients completing a survey reported using alternative therapies to treat asthma. The most common alternative therapy used was exercise/massage; the least popular was homeopathy. The highest users were women (59%), ages 41–50 (31%), white ethnicity (63%), higher education (56%), and higher annual household income (84%). The major reasons for usage were having more control of their health, personal beliefs, and concern over side effects of conventional medication. | The rate of alternative therapy use in patients with asthma in central New Jersey was lower than in some other studies. It is important for physicians to take CAM therapies into account to develop a health care plan consistent with patients' beliefs and expectations. | Adults; various CAM modalities |

(continued on next page)

Table 2
(continued)

Authors, Primary	Design	Population	Results	Conclusions	Categories/Domain
Wechsler et al,[80] 2011	Randomized controlled trial (pilot)	46 patients with asthma were randomized to active treatment with an albuterol inhaler, a placebo inhaler, sham acupuncture, or no intervention.	Albuterol resulted in a 20% increase in FEV(1), as compared with approximately 7% with each of the other 3 interventions ($P<.001$). However, patients' reports of improvement after the intervention did not differ significantly for the albuterol inhaler (50% improvement), placebo inhaler (45%), or sham acupuncture (46%), but the subjective improvement with all 3 of these interventions was significantly greater than that with the no-intervention control (21%) ($P<.001$).	Although albuterol, but not the 2 placebo interventions, improved FEV(1) in these patients with asthma, albuterol provided no incremental benefit with respect to the self-reported outcomes. Placebo effects can be clinically meaningful and can rival the effects of active medication in patients with asthma. However, from a clinical-management and research-design perspective, patient self-reports can be unreliable. An assessment of untreated responses in asthma may be essential in evaluating patient-reported outcomes.	Adults; acupuncture (mind-body)

| Zayas et al,[47] 2011 | Qualitative, semistructured individual interviews | 30 Puerto Rican adults who had asthma or were caregivers of children with asthma were interviewed in person. | Participants identified 75 ethnomedical treatments for asthma. Behavioral strategies that included conventional care (environmental remediation) and folk beliefs (chihuahuas in the home cure/control asthma) were significantly more likely to be used or perceived effective compared with ingested and topical remedies ($P<.001$). Among information sources for ingested and topical remedies, those recommended by community members were significantly less likely to be used or perceived to be effective ($P<.001$) compared with other sources. | Study sample of Puerto Rican subjects with a regular source of medical care was significantly more likely to use or perceive as effective behavioral strategies compared with ingested and topical remedies. Allopathic clinicians should ask Puerto Rican patients about their use of ethnomedical therapies for asthma to better understand their health beliefs and to integrate ethnomedical therapies with allopathic medicine. | Adults and caregivers of children with asthma; ethnomedical therapies; various CAM modalities |

(continued on next page)

Table 2
(continued)

Authors, Primary	Design	Population	Results	Conclusions	Categories/Domain
Beebe et al,[71] 2010	Randomized controlled trial	22 children with asthma were randomized to an active art therapy or wait-list control group.	Score changes from baseline to completion of art therapy indicated (1) improved problem-solving and affect drawing scores; (2) improved worry, communication, and total quality of life scores; and (3) improved Beck anxiety and self-concept scores in the active group relative to the control group. At 6 mo, the active group maintained some positive changes relative to the control group, including (1) drawing affect scores, (2) the worry and quality of life scores, and (3) the Beck anxiety score. Frequency of asthma exacerbations before and after the 6-mo study interval did not differ between the 2 groups.	This was the first randomized trial demonstrating that children with asthma receive benefit from art therapy that includes decreased anxiety and increased quality of life.	Children; art therapy

| Covar et al,[24] 2010 | Randomized controlled trial | 43 children with mild to moderate persistent asthma were randomized to receive daily novel nutritional formula (n = 23) or control formula (n = 20) for 12 wk. | Daily consumption of either NNF (a nutritional supplement composed of antioxidants, omega-3 and omega-6 fatty acids) or a control formula showed improvement in asthma-free days over time but there was no difference between groups. However, the NNF group had lower exhaled nitric oxide levels compared with the control group at weeks 4, 8, and 12 ($P<.05$). An overall group difference in log FEV(1) PC 20 ($P = .05$) was found in favor of the NNF group as well. Significantly higher levels of EPA in plasma ($P<.01$) and peripheral blood mononuclear cell (PBMC) ($P<.01$) phospholipids in the NNF group compared with the control group within 2 wk indicated good adherence with daily NNF intake. There were no differences in adverse events for NNF vs control groups after 12 wk. | Both NNF and control groups demonstrated improvement in asthma-free days. The NNF-treated group had reduced biomarkers of disease activity. Rapid PBMC fatty acid composition changes reflected an anti-inflammatory profile. Dietary supplementation with NNF was safe and well tolerated. | Children; dietary supplements (natural products) |

(continued on next page)

Table 2
(continued)

Authors, Primary	Design	Population	Results	Conclusions	Categories/Domain
Joubert et al,[13] 2010	Survey, correlational study	3327 responses of those ever having asthma as presented in National Health Interview Survey (NHIS) were analyzed	Overall CAM use differed significantly by asthma status, with 49% of those with asthma episodes using CAM compared with 42% of those who did not have an episode in the past year. Self-care–based therapies were more likely to be used than practitioner-based therapies by individuals with a single comorbid condition compared with those with 2 or more comorbidities.	Although this study supports previous work indicating that disease severity (in this instance, asthma within the past year) is significantly associated with CAM use, it did not support studies showing greater CAM use in the presence of a greater number of comorbidities, suggesting that disease burden is a limiting factor when it comes to self-care–based CAM use.	Adults; various CAM modalities
Kapoor et al,[65] 2010	Intervention-follow-up trial	3 participants	At the onset of the intervention, it was found that lung functioning, particularly FEV(1) increased in all 3 participants, with effect sizes ranging from −0.32 to −2.48. FEF25–75 improved in one of the participants. In addition, a positive	School-based relaxation and guided imagery intervention improved anxiety and lung functioning.	Children; relaxation and guided imagery (mind-body)

			impact was also seen in the lowering of anxiety scores across all 3 participants, with effect sizes ranging from 0.12 to 1.69.		
Kazaks et al,[50] 2010	Randomized controlled trial	55 males and females aged 21–55 y with mild to moderate asthma according to the 2002 National Heart, Lung, and Blood Institute (NHLBI) and Asthma Education and Prevention Program (NAEPP) guidelines and who used only beta-agonists or inhaled corticosteroids (ICS) as asthma medications.	The concentration of methacholine required to cause a 20% drop in FEV(1) increased significantly from baseline to month 6 within the Mg group. Peak expiratory flow rate (PEFR) showed a 5.8% predicted improvement over time ($P = .03$) in those consuming the Mg. There was significant improvement in AQLQ mean score units ($P<.01$) and in overall ACQ score only in the Mg group ($P = .05$) after 6.5 mo of supplementation. Despite these improvements, there were no significant changes in any of the markers of Mg status.	Adults who received oral Mg supplements showed improvement in objective measures of bronchial reactivity to methacholine and PEFR and in subjective measures of asthma control and quality of life.	Adults; Mg diet supplements (natural products)

(continued on next page)

Table 2
(continued)

Authors, Primary	Design	Population	Results	Conclusions	Categories/Domain
MacRedmond et al,[51] 2010	Randomized controlled study	28 adult subjects with mild asthma were randomized to conjugated linoleic acid (CLA) 4.5 g/d or placebo for 12 wk in addition to usual treatment.	Subjects in the CLA (omega-6 fatty acid) group had a significant improvement in airway hyperresponsiveness at week 12 compared with week 0 (PC 20 6.6 [2.1] mg/mL vs 2.2 [0.7] mg/mL; $P<.05$). The CLA group had a significant reduction in weight and BMI compared with placebo and this was associated with a reduction in leptin/adiponectin ratio. There were no differences in systemic cytokine levels, induced sputum cell counts, quality-of-life scores, or adverse events.	Omega-6 fatty acid treatment as an adjunct to usual care in overweight mildly and moderately severe adults with asthma was well tolerated and was associated with improvements in airway hyperresponsiveness and BMI.	Adults; conjugated linoleic acid (natural products)

| Marino and Shen,[17] 2010 | Survey, correlational | 7352 responses from the 2006 Behavioral Risk Factor Surveillance System (BRFSS) data from a subset of 25 states that completed the follow-up Asthma Callback Survey. | The prevalence of CAM use among adults with asthma was 39.6% (95% confidence interval [CI] = 36.9–42.3). There was no significant association with CAM use by sex, race/ethnicity, age, education, or geographic region. After adjusting for demographics and region, CAM use was significantly higher among persons with (1) financial barriers to asthma care (odds ratio [OR] = 2.8, 95% CI = 1.9–4.1); (2) an emergency room (ER) visit due to asthma (OR = 1.7 95% CI = 1.1–2.6); and (3) ≥ 14 asthma-associated disability days during the previous year (OR = 2.1, 95% CI = 1.4–3.1). | CAM use is common among adults with asthma. It is associated with financial barriers to asthma care and poor asthma control. Physicians should discuss CAM use with their asthma patients. | Adults; various CAM modalities |

(continued on next page)

Table 2
(continued)

Authors, Primary	Design	Population	Results	Conclusions	Categories/Domain
Metcalfe et al,[8] 2010	Survey, correlational study	400,055 Canadians aged ≥12 between 2001–2005 as presented in the Canadian Community Health Survey	Weighted estimates show that 12.4% (95% CI: 12.2–12.5) of Canadians visited a CAM practitioner in the year they were surveyed; this rate was significantly higher for those with asthma 15.1% (95% CI: 14.5–15.7) and migraine 19.0% (95% CI: 18.4–19.6), and	A large proportion of Canadians use CAM services. Physicians should be aware that their patients may be accessing other services and should be prepared to ask and answer questions about the risks and benefits of CAM services in conjunction with standard medical care.	Adults; various CAM modalities

significantly lower for those with diabetes 8.0% (95% CI: 7.4–8.6), whereas the rate in those with epilepsy (10.3%, 95% CI: 8.4–12.2) was not significantly different from the general population.

(continued on next page)

Table 2
(continued)

Authors, Primary	Design	Population	Results	Conclusions	Categories/Domain
Sidora-Arcoleo et al,[119] 2010	Tool validation study	337 parents of children with asthma from Bronx and Rochester, NY.	Bronx parents were more likely to perceive their child's asthma to be moderate or severe than the Rochester parents. Bronx children were older and had longer duration of asthma and reported more acute health care visits (past year). Bronx parents reported total Asthma Illness Representation Scale scores more closely aligned with the lay model than Rochester parents. The Asthma Illness Representation Scale instrument demonstrated acceptable internal reliability among the Bronx sample (total score alpha = 0.82) and the Asthma Illness Representation Scale (AIRS) subscale Cronbach alpha coefficients were remarkably similar to	The AIRS instrument exhibited good internal reliability, external validity, and differentiated parents based on ethnicity, poverty, and education. Assessment of asthma IRs during the health care visit will allow the HCP and parent to discuss and negotiate a shared asthma management plan for the child, which will hopefully lead to improved medication adherence and asthma health outcomes.	Children; various CAM modalities

those obtained from the original validation study (range = 0.54–0.83). Poor parents and those with less than a high school education had lower total AIRS scores than their counterparts. White parents had AIRS scores more closely aligned with the professional model compared with each of the ethnic subgroups. A perception of less severe asthma, fewer reports of asthma and somatization symptoms, and a positive HCP relationship were associated with IRs congruent with the professional model. IRs aligned with the professional model were associated with fewer acute asthma-related health care visits.

(continued on next page)

Table 2
(continued)

Authors, Primary	Design	Population	Results	Conclusions	Categories/Domain
Torres-Llenza et al,[11] 2010	Survey, correlational	2027 children with asthma.	The median age of the 2027 children surveyed was 6.1 y (interquartile range 3.3–10.5 y); 58% were male and 59% of children had persistent asthma. The prevalence of CAM use was 13% (95% CI 12%–15%). Supplemental vitamins (24%), homeopathy (18%), and acupuncture (11%) were the most commonly reported CAMs. Multivariable logistic regression analysis confirmed the association of CAM use with age younger than 6 y (OR 1.86; 95% CI 1.20–2.96), Asian ethnicity (OR 1.89; 95% CI 1.01–3.52), episodic asthma (OR 1.88; 95% CI 1.08–3.28), and poor asthma control (OR 1.98; 95% CI 1.80–3.31).	The prevalence of reported CAM use among Quebec children with asthma remained modest (13%), with vitamins, homeopathy and acupuncture being the most popular modalities. CAM use was associated with preschool age, Asian ethnicity, episodic asthma, and poor asthma control.	Children; various CAM modalities

| Roy et al,[59] 2010 | Survey, correlational | 326 adults with persistent asthma who received care at 2 inner-city outpatient clinics. | Overall, 25.4% of patients reported herbal remedy use. Univariate analyses showed that herbal remedy use was associated with decreased ICS adherence and increased asthma morbidity. In multivariable analysis, herbal remedy use was associated with lower ICS adherence (OR, 0.4; 95%) after adjusting for confounders. Herbal remedy users were also more likely to worry about the adverse effects of ICS ($P = .01$). | The use of herbal remedies was associated with lower adherence to ICS and worse outcomes among inner-city asthmatic patients. Medication beliefs, such as worry about ICS adverse effects, may in part mediate this relationship. Physicians should routinely ask patients with asthma about CAM use, especially those whose asthma is poorly controlled. | Adults; herbs (natural products) |

(continued on next page)

Table 2
(continued)

Authors, Primary	Design	Population	Results	Conclusions	Categories/Domain
Birdee et al,[18] 2009	Survey, correlational	31,044 responses from the 2002 National Health Interview Survey (NHIS) Alternative Medicine Supplement.	We found that neither age nor sex was associated with T'ai chi and qigong use. T'ai chi and qigong users were more likely than nonusers to be Asian than white (OR 2.02, 95% CI 1.30–3.15), college educated (OR 2.44, 95% CI 1.97–3.03), and less likely to live in the Midwest (OR 0.64, 95% CI 0.42–0.96) or the southern United	In the United States, T'ai chi and qigong is practiced for health by a diverse population, and users report benefits for maintaining health.	Adults; T'ai chi (mind body); qigong (energy field)

States (OR 0.51, 95% CI 0.36–0.72) than the West. T'ai chi and qigong use was associated independently with higher reports of musculoskeletal conditions (OR 1.43, 95% CI 1.11–1.83), severe sprains (OR 1.65, 95% CI 1.14–2.40), and asthma (OR 1.50, 95% CI 1.08–2.10).

(continued on next page)

Table 2
(continued)

Authors, Primary	Design	Population	Results	Conclusions	Categories/Domain
George et al,[37] 2009	Qualitative, semi-structured individual interviews	25 adults (92% female; 76% African American; mean age 39)	Only 1 subject had received asthma self-management training and only 10 (40%) used short-acting beta-(2) agonist-based (SABA) self-management protocols for the early treatment of acute asthma. No subject used a peak flow meter or an asthma action plan. Most (52%) chose to initially treat acute asthma with CAM despite the availability of SABAs. Importantly, 21 (84%) preferred an integrated approach using both conventional and CAM treatments. Four themes associated with acute asthma	All patents' acute asthma self-management strategies should be evaluated for their timeliness and appropriateness. This would be of particular importance for vulnerable populations who bear a disproportionate burden of the disease and who have the fewest resources.	Adults; various CAM modalities

self-management emerged from the qualitative analysis. The first theme, safety, reflected subjects' perception that CAM was safer than SABA. Severity addressed the calculation that subjects made in determining if SABA or CAM was indicated based on the degree of symptoms they were experiencing. The third theme, speed and strength of the combination, described subjects' belief in the superiority of integrating CAM and SABA for acute asthma self-management. The final theme, sense of identity, spoke to the ability of CAM to provide a customized self-management strategy that subjects desired.

(continued on next page)

Table 2
(continued)

Authors, Primary	Design	Population	Results	Conclusions	Categories/Domain
Post-White et al,[35] 2009	Survey, descriptive	281 respondents participated in the survey	CAM use was higher in children with epilepsy (61.9%), cancer (59%), asthma (50.7%), and sickle cell disease (47.4%) than in general pediatrics (36%). Children most often used prayer (60.5%), massage (27.9%), specialty vitamins (27.2%), chiropractic care (25.9%), and dietary supplements (21.8%). Parents who used CAM for themselves (68.7%) were more likely to access CAM for their child. Most parents (62.6%) disclosed some or all of their child's use of CAM to providers.	Within the same geographic region, children with chronic and life-threatening illness use more CAM therapies than children seen in primary care clinics.	Children; various CAM modalities
Cabana et al,[32] 2008	Survey, correlational	1322 parents of children with asthma	Eleven percent (141/1322) of children used CAM. Parents of children on daily medications who were perceived to have poor asthma control were almost 3 times more likely to use CAM than parents of	Parent perception of asthma control is significantly associated with CAM use. It is important for providers to elicit information regarding CAM use in the clinic, as this may imply that the asthma	Children; various CAM modalities

				Adults; Buteyko (mind-body)
Cowie et al,[79] 2008	Randomized controlled trial	129 individuals with asthma were randomized to 2 groups	Both groups showed substantial and similar improvement and a high proportion with asthma control 6 mo after completion of the intervention. In the Buteyko group the proportion with asthma control increased from 40% to 79% and in the control group from 44% to 72%. In addition, the Buteyko group had significantly reduced their ICS therapy compared with the control group ($P = .02$). None of the other differences between the groups at 6 mo were significant.	Six months after completion of the interventions, a large majority of subjects in each group displayed control of their asthma with the additional benefit of reduction in ICS use in the Buteyko group. The Buteyko technique or an intensive program delivered by a chest physiotherapist appear to provide additional benefit for adult patients with asthma who are being treated with ICS.
			children on no daily medications who were perceived to have high asthma control (risk ratio: = 2.81; CI: 1.72–4.60); age, gender, race, income, and education level were not significant independent predictors.	symptoms may not be well controlled.

(continued on next page)

Table 2
(continued)

Authors, Primary	Design	Population	Results	Conclusions	Categories/Domain
Freidin and Timmermans,[28] 2008	Qualitative, open-ended individual interviews	50 mothers of children with asthma	The experience with biomedical treatments, social influence in mother's network of care, concerns about adverse and long-term effects of prescription asthma medicines, health care providers' responsiveness to such concerns, and familiarity with alternative treatments explain why some families rely on alternative medicine and others do not.	Rather than constituting vastly different demographic user profiles or reflecting diverging health beliefs, the incorporation of alternative treatments in asthma care follows a decision-making process in which experiences with prescribed drugs are socially validated and evaluated.	Children; various CAM modalities
Sidora-Arcoleo et al,[107] 2008	Qualitative, structured individual interviews	228 parents of 5- to 12-y-old children with asthma	Seventy-one percent of parents reported using CAM and/or over-the-counter medication for children's asthma management, and 54% of those parents did not disclose usage. Seventy-five percent "did not think" to discuss it. Better parent-health care provider relationship led to increased disclosure.	Health care providers can play an important role in creating an environment where parents feel comfortable sharing information about their children's asthma management strategies in order to arrive at a shared asthma management plan for the child, leading to improved asthma health outcomes.	Children; various CAM modalities

Mehl-Madrona et al,[25] 2007	Randomized controlled trial	89 individuals with asthma were randomly assignment to 1 of 5 groups: acupuncture, craniosacral therapy, acupuncture and craniosacral, attention control, and waiting list control	When treatment was compared with the control group, statistically treatment was significantly better than the control group in improving asthma quality of life, whereas reducing medication use with pulmonary function test results remained the same. However, the combination of acupuncture and craniosacral treatment was not superior to each therapy alone. In fact, although all active patients received 12 treatment sessions, those who received all treatments from one practitioner had statistically significant reductions in anxiety when compared with those receiving the same number of treatments from multiple practitioners. No effects on depression were found.	Acupuncture and/or craniosacral therapy are potentially useful adjuncts to the conventional care of adults with asthma, but the combination of the two does not provide additional benefit over each therapy alone.	Adults; acupuncture (mind-body); craniosacral therapy (manipulative and body-based practices)

(continued on next page)

Table 2
(continued)

Authors, Primary	Design	Population	Results	Conclusions	Categories/Domain
Sawni and Thomas,[106] 2007	Survey, descriptive	648 pediatricians responded to the survey	More than 96% of pediatricians responding believed their patients were using CAM. Discussions of CAM use were initiated by the family (70%) and only 37% of pediatricians asked about CAM use as part of routine medical history. Most (84%) said more CME courses should be offered on CAM and 71% said they would consider referring patients to CAM practitioners. Medical conditions referred for CAM included chronic problems (headaches, pain management,	Pediatricians have a positive attitude toward CAM. Most believe that their patients are using CAM, that asking about CAM should be part of routine medical history, would consider referring to a CAM practitioner and want more education on CAM.	Pediatricians; various CAM modalities

| | | | asthma, backaches) (86%), diseases with no known cure (55.5%) or failure of conventional therapies (56%), behavioral problems (49%), and psychiatric disorders (47%). American-born, US medical school graduates, general pediatricians, and pediatricians who ask/talk about CAM were most likely to believe their patients used CAM (P<.01). | | |
| Sidora-Arcoleo et al,[34] 2007 | Survey, correlational | 228 parents and their 5 to12-y-old children with asthma | 65% of parents reported using CAM. Usage was highest among black, poor, less educated parents and children with persistent symptoms. Types of CAM differed by poverty and a trend for differences by race and education emerged. | Health care providers who educate themselves on CAM therapies that parents use for asthma can then discuss the implications of using these therapies and potentially improve adherence to the prescribed medication regimen. | Children; various CAM modalities |

(continued on next page)

Table 2
(continued)

Authors, Primary	Design	Population	Results	Conclusions	Categories/Domain
George et al,[29] 2006	Qualitative, in-depth interviews	28 individuals who self-identified as being African Americans, low income, and an inner-city resident	Sixty-four percent of participants held biologically correct causal models of asthma, although 100% reported the use of at least 1 CAM for asthma. Biologically based therapies, humoral balance, and prayer were the most popular CAM. Although most subjects trusted prescription asthma medicine, there was a preference for integration of CAM with conventional asthma treatment. CAM was considered natural, effective, and potentially curative. Sixty-three percent of participants reported nonadherence to conventional therapies in the 2 wk before the research interview. Neither CAM nor nonmedical causal models altered most individuals' (93%) willingness to use prescription	Clinicians should be aware of patient-generated causal models of asthma and use of CAM in this population. Discussing patients' desire for an integrated approach to asthma management and involving social networks are 2 strategies that may enhance patient provider partnerships and treatment fidelity.	Adults; various CAM modalities

Mickleborough et al,[52] 2006	Randomized controlled trial	16 asthmatic patients with documented exercise-induced bronchoconstriction participated in the study	medication. Three possibly dangerous CAM were identified. On the normal and placebo diet, subjects exhibited EIB; however, the fish oil diet improved pulmonary function to below the diagnostic exercise-induced bronchoconstriction threshold, with a concurrent reduction in bronchodilator use. Induced sputum differential cell count percentage and concentrations of LTC 4-LTE4, PGD2, IL-1, and TNF were significantly reduced before and following exercise on the fish oil diet compared with the normal and placebo diets. There was a significant reduction in LTB4 and a significant increase in LTB5 generation from activated PMNLs on the fish oil diet compared to the normal and placebo diets.	Data suggest that fish oil supplementation may represent a potentially beneficial nonpharmacologic intervention for exercise-induced bronchoconstriction.	Adults; fish oil (natural products)

(continued on next page)

Table 2
(continued)

Authors, Primary	Design	Population	Results	Conclusions	Categories/Domain
Nahin et al,[45] 2006	Survey, descriptive	3072 ambulatory individuals aged 75 and older	In logistic regression models, multivitamin use was associated with female sex, a higher income, a higher modified Mini-Mental State Examination score, difficulty with mobility, and asthma history; use of any other vitamin or mineral was associated with female sex, white race, nonsmoking, more years of schooling, difficulty walking, a history of osteoporosis, and reading health and senior magazines.	There were substantial differences between individuals who used vitamins and minerals and those who used NVNMDS. These data require that trial investigators pay close attention to participant use of off-protocol dietary supplements. In addition, these findings may help identify elderly individuals likely to combine nonvitamin/ nonmineral dietary supplement and prescription drugs.	Older adults; nonvitamin/ nonmineral dietary supplement (natural products)

| Aboussafy et al,[82] 2005 | Intervention trial | 31 adults with asthma participated in the study | The cold pressor test, asthma interview, and progressive muscle relaxation produced significant decreases in airflow compared with the baseline period. The cold pressor test and progressive muscle relaxation produced significant, complementary increases in vagal tone. | These results suggest that passive coping stressors and other stimuli (eg, certain forms of relaxation) that elicit increased vagal tone may be associated with poorer asthma control, a view consistent with a significant negative correlation between the participant's mean vagal tone response to the tasks and score on a measure of asthma self-efficacy. | Adults; progressive muscle relaxation (mind-body) |

(continued on next page)

Table 2
(continued)

Authors, Primary	Design	Population	Results	Conclusions	Categories/Domain
Ang et al,[36] 2005	Survey, correlational	152 subjects were interviewed on the use of CAM for their children.	Compared with parents of the healthy and asthma groups, parents of the HIV group were less likely to be employed, were less likely to have private insurance, were less likely to have a high school or college education, and were more likely to be black. Interestingly, 38% of the healthy children parents used CAM in their children compared with 22% in the HIV group and 25% in the asthma group. More than 80% of all three groups paid out of pocket for their use of CAM in their	This study revealed a relatively high rate of CAM usage by parents of all three study groups. Although parents of children with HIV infection were more likely to want CAM as part of their children's medical care, their rate of CAM usage was not higher than that in well children. This may be related to their socioeconomic factors. A larger and more diverse study population may provide more information on factors contributing to CAM usage in chronically ill and well children.	Children; various CAM modalities

			children. Within these groups, HIV parents were more likely to want CAM as part of their child's medical care and were more likely to believe that CAM was expensive.		
Dobson et al,[66] 2005	Intervention trial	4 children participants	Results demonstrated that relaxation and guided imagery significantly improved the lung functioning of 3 of 4 participants in the study. Furthermore, overall happiness improved for 1 participant in the study, state anxiety decreased for 2 of the 4 participants, and trait anxiety decreased for all 4 participants.	Relaxation and guided imagery were found to be effective in improving the lung functioning of 3 of the 4 study participants included.	Children; relaxation and guided imagery (mind-body)

(continued on next page)

Table 2
(continued)

Authors, Primary	Design	Population	Results	Conclusions	Categories/Domain
Klein et al,[104] 2005	Qualitative, focus groups	81 adolescents: suburban adolescents, urban minority adolescents, adolescents with chronic illness, (asthma, eating disorders, and diabetes), and patients of complementary/ alternative practitioners in Monroe County, NY	Most adolescents are familiar with "herbal medicine," "herbal remedies," or "nutritional supplements," and are able to name specific products or CAM therapies; however, many are unfamiliar with the term "alternative medicine." Adolescents are more familiar with remedies or CAM therapies commonly used by people from their own cultural or ethnic background. Older	Most adolescents are familiar with culturally based herbal products and nutritional supplements, used for treatment of illnesses, and not for preventive care. Providers and researchers should consider chronic illness status and culture/ family tradition, and clarify terms, when asking adolescents about self-care, over-the-counter, or CAM.	Children; various CAM modalities (natural products)

		suburban females and those with chronic illnesses are more familiar with herbs and supplements than other adolescents. Most supplement use is conceptually linked with treating illness rather than with preventive care.	
Sabina et al,[26] 2005	Randomized controlled trial (pilot)	62 participants with asthma	Intention-to-treat analysis was performed. Significant within-group differences in post bronchodilator FEV(1) and morning symptom scores were apparent in both groups at 4 and 16 wk; however, no significant differences between groups were observed on any outcome measures.	Iyengar yoga conferred no appreciable benefit in mild-to-moderate asthma. Circumstances under which yoga is of benefit in asthma management, if any, remain to be determined.	Adults; Yoga (mind-body)

(continued on next page)

Table 2
(continued)

Authors, Primary	Design	Population	Results	Conclusions	Categories/Domain
Epstein et al,[75] 2004	Randomized controlled trial (pilot)	68 adults with symptomatic asthma	There was little evidence of statistical change in this feasibility study; yet, valuable lessons were learned. Paired t tests indicated there was a significant difference in the total power scores in the imagery group, and in the expected direction and the choices subscale of the power instrument from weeks 1 to 16 of the study. Eight (47%) of 17 participants in the mental imagery group reduced or	Findings related to major outcome measures must be viewed with caution because of the small sample size resulting from attrition related to labor intensiveness and, therefore, low statistical power. However, the study did provide significant data to plan a larger scale study of the use of mental imagery with adults with asthma. The study also demonstrated that imagery is inexpensive,	Adults; mental imagery (mind-body)

discontinued their medications. Three of 16 (19%) participants in the control group reduced their medications; none discontinued. Chi-square indicated differences between groups. Persons who reduced or discontinued their medications showed neither an increase in pulmonary function before medication discontinuation, nor a fall in these parameters following discontinuation.

safe and, with training, can be used as an adjunct therapy by patients themselves. Its efficacy needs additional exploration. Further research for adults with asthma who practice imagery is important, as current treatments are not entirely efficacious. Lessons learned in this study may facilitate improvement in research designs.

(continued on next page)

Table 2
(continued)

Authors, Primary	Design	Population	Results	Conclusions	Categories/Domain
Handelman et al,[43] 2004	Qualitative, explanatory models	19 children with 17 mothers from a variety of cultural backgrounds were interviewed	Among children, contagion was the primary explanatory model for asthma etiology (53%). Twenty-five percent of children reported fear of dying from asthma, whereas fear of their child dying from asthma was reported by 76% of mothers. Mothers reported a variety of explanatory models, some culturally specific, but most reported biomedical concepts of etiology, pathophysiology, and triggers. Although 76% of mothers knew the	The traditional focus of asthma education is not sufficient to ensure adherence. Asthma education for children should address their views of etiology and fears about dying from asthma. Conversations with parents about their explanatory models and beliefs about medications and alternative therapies could assist in understanding and responding to parental concerns and choices about medications and help achieve better adherence.	Children; various CAM modalities

names of more than one of their children's medications, 47% thought their child's medications all had similar functions. Thirty-five percent of families used herbal treatments and 35% incorporated religion into asthma treatment. Seventy-one percent of families had discontinued medications and 23% reported currently not giving anti-inflammatory medication. Reasons for discontinuing daily medications included fears of unknown side effects (53%), addiction (18%), tachyphylaxis (18%), and feeling that their child was being given too much medicine (23%).

(continued on next page)

Table 2
(continued)

Authors, Primary	Design	Population	Results	Conclusions	Categories/Domain
Lehrer et al,[27] 2004	Randomized controlled trial	94 adult outpatient volunteers with asthma	Compared with the 2 control groups, subjects in both of the 2 heart rate variability biofeedback groups were prescribed less medication, with minimal differences between the 2 active treatments. Improvements averaged 1 full level of asthma severity. Measures from forced oscillation pneumography similarly showed improvement in pulmonary function. A placebo effect influenced an improvement in asthma symptoms, but not in pulmonary function. Groups did not differ in the occurrence of severe asthma flares.	The results suggest that heart rate variability biofeedback may prove to be a useful adjunct to asthma treatment and may help to reduce dependence on steroid medications. Further evaluation of this method is warranted.	Adults; biofeedback (mind-body)
Milner et al,[42] 2004	Survey, correlational (longitudinal cohort survey study)	There were 8000 total patients in the study. The cohort data were taken from the National Center for Health Statistics 1988 National Maternal-	The overall incidence of asthma was 10.5% and of food allergy was 4.9%. In univariate analysis, male gender, smoker in the household, child care,	Early vitamin supplementation is associated with increased risk for asthma in black children and food allergies in exclusively	Children; Vitamins (natural products)

Infant Health Survey, which followed pregnant women and their newborns, and the 1991 Longitudinal Follow-up of the same patients.

prematurity (<37 wk), being black, no history of breastfeeding, lower income, and lower education were associated with higher risk for asthma. Child care, higher levels of education, income, and history of breastfeeding were associated with a higher risk for food allergies. In multivariate logistic analyses, a history of vitamin use within the first 6 mo of life was associated with a higher risk for asthma in black infants (OR: 1.27). Early vitamin use was also associated with a higher risk for food allergies in the exclusively formula-fed population (OR: 1.63). Vitamin use at 3 y of age was associated with increased risk for food allergies but not asthma in both breastfed (OR: 1.62; 95% CI: 1.19–2.21) and exclusively formula-fed infants (OR: 1.39; 95% CI: 1.03–1.88).

formula-fed children. Additional study is warranted to examine which components most strongly contribute to this risk.

(continued on next page)

Table 2
(continued)

Authors, Primary	Design	Population	Results	Conclusions	Categories/Domain
Lanski et al,[44] 2003	Survey, descriptive	142 families participated in the study	Forty-five percent of caregivers reported giving their child an herbal product, and 88% of these caregivers had at least 1 y of college education. Of the children receiving these therapies, 53% had been given 1 type and 27% were given 3 or more in the past year. The most common therapies reportedly used were aloe plant/juice (44%), *Echinacea* (33%), and sweet oil (25%). The most dangerous potential herbal and prescription medication combination reported was ephedra and albuterol in an adolescent with asthma. The most unusual products reportedly used included turpentine, pine needles, and cowchips. Of all people	Herbal and home therapies are commonly used in this pediatric population. An unexpectedly wide variety of products were reportedly given to this patient population. Caregivers reported limited knowledge regarding potential adverse medication interactions and side effects. Limited discussions with the child's primary health care provider were reported. It is therefore important for health care providers to have knowledge about herbal medications, to inquire about their use, and to educate families about the risk/benefit as well as potential interactions these products may have with over-the-counter and prescription medications.	Children; Herbs (natural products)

| | | | interviewed, 77% did not believe or were uncertain if herbal products had any side effects and only 27% could name a potential side effect. Sixty-six percent were unsure or thought that herbal products did not interact with other medications and only 2 people correctly named a drug interaction. Of the people who used these therapies, 80% reported either friends or relatives as their primary source of information. Only 45% of those giving their children herbal products report discussing the use with their child's primary health care provider. | | |
| Peck et al,[67] 2003 | Intervention trial | 4 children with asthma | With the introduction of the intervention, it was found that FEV(1) improved and anxiety decreased in all students. FEF25–75 improved in 3 of the 4 participants. | Relaxation and guided imagery improved asthma outcomes | Children; relaxation and guided imagery (mind-body) |

(continued on next page)

Table 2
(continued)

Authors, Primary	Design	Population	Results	Conclusions	Categories/Domain
Anbar,[69] 2002	Intervention trial	303 patients with pulmonary symptoms attributable to psychological issues, discomfort due to medications, or fear of procedures	Hypnotherapy was associated with improvement in 80% of patients with persistent asthma, chest pain/ pressure, habit cough, hyperventilation, shortness of breath, sighing, and vocal cord dysfunction. When improvement was reported, in some cases symptoms resolved immediately after hypnotherapy was first used. For the others, improvement was achieved after hypnosis was used for a few weeks. No patients' symptoms worsened and no new symptoms emerged following hypnotherapy.	Patients described in this report were unlikely to have achieved rapid improvement in their symptoms without the use of hypnotherapy. Therefore, hypnotherapy can be an important complementary therapy for patients in a pediatric practice.	Children; hypnosis (mind-body)
Baldwin et al,[38] 2002	Survey, correlational	508 military veterans randomly selected from Southern Arizona Veterans	Of the 508 subjects, 252 (49.6%) reported CAM use. Military veteran CAM users were	Ethnicity, education, income, and several chronic health complaints are	Adults; various CAM modalities

Administration Health Care System (Tucson) primary care patient lists

significantly more likely to be non-Hispanic white, earn more than $50 000 per year (both $P<.05$), and have more than 12 y of education ($P<.01$). Current high daily stress, perceived negative impact of military life on physical or mental health, and physician-diagnosed chronic illnesses (eg, gastrointestinal problems, insomnia, and asthma) were statistically associated with CAM use. Regression analysis provided adjusted odds ratios and indicated that ethnicity (non-Hispanic white), higher education, greater current daily stress, and overseas military experience were significant predictors of CAM use by these veterans (each $P<.05$).

consistent with civilian CAM use. Findings also suggest, however, that physicians providing conventional medical care need to be aware of experiences unique to CAM-using military veterans.

(continued on next page)

Table 2
(continued)

Authors, Primary	Design	Population	Results	Conclusions	Categories/Domain
Hockemeyer and Smyth,[78] 2002	Randomized controlled trial (between-groups, prospective experimental design)	60 college students with asthma	The treatment group showed significant improvement in measures of lung function compared with the placebo group, but analysis revealed no differences in measures of perceived stress.	These findings provide initial support for the feasibility of self-administered manual-based interventions and some evidence that they can produce health benefits in individuals with asthma and, perhaps, other chronic conditions.	Adults, relaxation, cognitive-behavioral treatment (mind-body)
Reznik et al,[30] 2002	Survey, correlational	200 children with asthma	Overall, 80% of participants reported using CAM for asthma. The most commonly reported CAM included rubs (74%), herbal teas (39%), prayer (37%), massage (36%), and Jarabe 7 syrup (24%).	Most adolescents with asthma in this study used CAM. The prevalence of CAM use in this study population was twice the national average for adults.	Children; various CAM modalities

			Subjects with daily or weekly symptoms were more likely to use CAM for each episode of asthma (72% vs 51%; $P = .005$). The 61% of subjects who had a family member who used CAM were more likely to use CAM again (84% vs 39%; $P<.001$). Of the respondents, 59% reported that CAM was effective.	
Wade,[72] 2002	Intervention trial	9 children with asthma	Results indicate that the participants showed an increase or maintenance of lung functioning after singing, whereas results were not consistent following the relaxation condition.	Singing might have a positive effect on children with asthma. Children; music therapy; relaxation (mind-body)

(continued on next page)

Table 2
(continued)

Authors, Primary	Design	Population	Results	Conclusions	Categories/Domain
Blanc et al,[48] 2001	Survey, correlational	300 adults with self-report of a physician diagnosis of asthma (n = 125) or rhinosinusitis without concomitant asthma (n = 175).	Any alternative practice was reported by 127 subjects (42%; 95% CI, 36%–48%). Of these, 33 subjects (26%; 95% CI, 21%–31%) were not current prescription medication users. Herbal use was reported by 72 subjects (24%), caffeine treatment by 54	Alternative treatments are frequent among adults with asthma or rhinosinusitis and should be taken into account by health-care providers and public health and policy analysts.	Adult; various CAM modalities

subjects (18%), and other alternative treatments by 66 subjects (22%). Taking into account demographic variables, subjects with asthma were more likely than those with rhinitis alone to report caffeine self-treatment for their condition (OR, 2.5; 95% CI, 1.4%–4.8%), but herbal use and other alternative treatments did not differ significantly by condition group.

(continued on next page)

Table 2
(continued)

Authors, Primary	Design	Population	Results	Conclusions	Categories/Domain
Bronfort et al,[93] 2001	Feasibility study of conducting a full-scale, randomized clinical trial	36 patients aged 6–17 y with mild and moderate persistent asthma were admitted to the study.	It is possible to blind the participants to the nature of the spinal manipulative therapy intervention, and a full-scale trial with the described design is feasible to conduct. At the end of the 12-wk intervention phase, objective lung function tests and patient-rated day and nighttime symptoms based on diary recordings showed little or no change. Of the patient-rated measures, a reduction of approximately 20% in beta(2) bronchodilator use was seen (P = .10). The quality-of-life scores improved by 10%–28% (P <.01), with	After 3 mo of combining chiropractic spinal manipulative therapy with optimal medical management for pediatric asthma, the children rated their quality of life substantially higher and their asthma severity substantially lower. These improvements were maintained at the 1-y follow-up assessment. There were no important changes in lung function or hyperresponsiveness at any time. The observed improvements are unlikely as a result of the specific effects of chiropractic spinal manipulative therapy	Children; spinal manipulation (manipulative and body-based practices)

the activity scale showing the most change. Asthma severity ratings showed a reduction of 39% (P<.001), and there was an overall improvement rating corresponding to 50%–75%. The pulmonologist-rated improvement was small. Similarly, the improvements in parent-rated or guardian-rated outcomes were mostly small and not statistically significant. The changes in patient-rated severity and the improvement rating remained unchanged at 12-mo posttreatment follow-up as assessed by a brief postal questionnaire.

alone, but other aspects of the clinical encounter that should not be dismissed readily. Further research is needed to assess which components of the chiropractic encounter are responsible for important improvements in patient-oriented outcomes so that they may be incorporated into the care of all patients with asthma.

(continued on next page)

Table 2
(continued)

Authors, Primary	Design	Population	Results	Conclusions	Categories/Domain
Loera et al,[19] 2001	Survey, correlational	2734 responses from the Hispanic Established Populations for the Epidemiologic Study of the Elderly (Hispanic-EPESE) 1993–1994 were analyzed	The use of herbal medicine in the 2 wk before the interview was reported by 9.8% of the sample. Chamomile and mint were the 2 most commonly used herbs. Users of herbal medicines were more likely to be women, born in Mexico, older than 75, living alone, and experiencing some financial strain. Having arthritis, urinary incontinence, asthma,	Herbal medication use is common among older Mexican Americans, particularly among those with chronic medical conditions, those who experience financial strain, and those who are very frequent users of formal health care services.	Adults; herbs (natural products)

and hip fracture were also associated with an elevated use of herbal medicines, whereas heart attacks were not. Herbal medicine use was substantially higher among individuals reporting any disability in activities of daily living, poor self-reported health, and depressive symptoms. Herbal medicine use was associated with the use of over-the-counter medications but not with prescription medications. Herbal medicine use was particularly high among respondents who had more than 24 physician visits during the year before the interview.

(continued on next page)

Table 2
(continued)

Authors, Primary	Design	Population	Results	Conclusions	Categories/Domain
Ottolini et al,[31] 2001	Survey, cross-sectional	348 parents of children completed surveys.	Forty percent (138) of parents were CAM users themselves, whereas 21% (72) had treated their child with CAM over the past year. Factors positively associated with child CAM use included parents' use of CAM ($P<.0001$); greater parent age ($P = .0005$); greater child age ($P = .001$); and complaints of frequent respiratory illnesses, asthma, headaches, and nosebleeds. Ethnicity and parental education were not associated with child CAM use. More than 50% of pediatric CAM users reported specific vitamin supplementation, whereas 25% used other nutritional supplements or elimination diets, and more than 40% used	Treatment of children with CAM is common and is frequently undertaken by parents without the knowledge or advice of their pediatrician.	Children; various CAM modalities

			herbal therapies. Thirty-two percent of CAM users had visited a CAM practitioner; 81% of pediatric CAM users would have liked to discuss it with their pediatrician, but only 36% did so.		
Smyth et al,[74] 2001	Intervention trial	20 adults with asthma	Relaxation training was successful, but did not lead to the hypothesized reduction in overall cortisol levels. Participants using corticosteroid medication showed increases in cortisol after relaxation, whereas those not using corticosteroids showed decreases in cortisol ($P<.05$). Relaxation altered the cortisol reactivity to stress ($P = .007$; before relaxation training, cortisol levels increased after a stressor, whereas following relaxation training, cortisol levels decreased after a stressor.	This study suggests that relaxation training can influence cortisol secretion in individuals with asthma, but that these effects differ from those observed in healthy individuals and may be influenced by corticosteroid medication use.	Adults; breathing relaxation (mind-body)

(continued on next page)

Table 2
(continued)

Authors, Primary	Design	Population	Results	Conclusions	Categories/Domain
Hailemaskel et al,[46] 2001	Survey, descriptive	100 prospective adult customers visiting a health food store during a consecutive 5-day period completed a 20-item questionnaire	The 4 most common diseases reported were allergies, high blood pressure, depression, and asthma. The top 4 herbals used were St John's Wort, *Echinacea*, ginseng, and golden seal. Results identified 6 cases with potential herbal-drug interactions, 5 cases with potential herb-disease interactions, and 19% with potential adverse drug reactions.	The data from this survey suggest that although the use of herbals is widespread and commonly accepted, it is necessary to educate consumers about the potential risks involved in such unmonitored use.	Adults; herbs (natural products)
Smyth et al,[73] 1999	Intervention trial (pilot)	22 community residents with asthma	Listening to a 20-min audiotaped relaxation training program led to decreased negative mood and stressor report, but was unrelated to positive mood. The report of asthma symptoms decreased over time following relaxation training, and peak expiratory flow rate was significantly increased by relaxation training.	This study provides evidence that a brief, inexpensive, tape-recorded relaxation intervention can improve well-being, decrease symptom report, and improve peak expiratory flow rate in asthma. The relatively inexpensive and low-risk nature of the treatment, as well as its benefit to quality of life, support its utility as a supplemental treatment.	Adults; breathing relaxation (mind-body)

| Balon et al,[94] 1998 | Randomized controlled trial | 91 children who had continuing symptoms of asthma despite usual medical therapy | Eighty children (38 in the active-treatment group and 42 in the simulated-treatment group) had outcome data that could be evaluated. There were small increases (7–12 L per minute) in peak expiratory flow in the morning and the evening in both treatment groups, with no significant differences between the groups in the degree of change from base line (morning peak expiratory flow, $P = .49$ at 2 months and $P = .82$ at 4 months). Symptoms of asthma and use of 3-agonists decreased and the quality of life increased in both groups, with no significant differences between the groups. There were no significant changes in spirometric measurements or airway responsiveness. | In children with mild or moderate asthma, the addition of chiropractic spinal manipulation to usual medical care provided no benefit. | Children; spinal manipulation (manipulative and body-based practices) |

(continued on next page)

Table 2
(continued)

Authors, Primary	Design	Population	Results	Conclusions	Categories/Domain
Davis et al,[108] 1998	Survey, correlational	564 participants have completed the study surveys	The survey population was 46% male and 43% female; 11% did not specify gender. They ranged in age from younger than 31 y to older than 70. The largest group (37%) of respondents held degrees as medical doctors, 27% held doctorates in CAM-related disciplines, 11% had registered nursing degrees, 4% were acupuncturists, and 18% did not specify their training. Practice characteristics between MD and non-MD asthma care providers did not differ. Most had general practices (75%) seeing all ages of patients. MDs were less likely to use CAM techniques for asthma	The predominance of diet and nutrition supplementation used by MDs and non-MDs suggests that further attention and research efforts should be directed toward this area of CAM practice. Other CAM practices, such as botanicals, meditation, and homeopathy appear to warrant research efforts. Differences between MDs and non-MDs in their use of such therapies may reflect different philosophies as well as training.	Adults; various CAM modalities

compared with non-MDs. Both groups identified dietary and nutritional approaches as their most prevalent and useful asthma treatment option. Use of botanicals, meditation, and homeopathy were frequently cited; statistically significant differences appeared in the rankings of treatment usefulness and prevalence between MDs and non-MDs. Non-MD asthma care providers were more likely to ask patients about their use of CAM treatments for asthma than MDs (92% vs 70%), whereas both groups showed statistically significant increases in their levels of patient inquiries compared with 2 y previously (up 9% and 8% for MDs and non-MDs respectively).

(continued on next page)

Table 2
(continued)

Authors, Primary	Design	Population	Results	Conclusions	Categories/Domain
Field et al,[92] 1998	Randomized controlled trial	32 children with asthma	The younger children who received massage therapy showed an immediate decrease in behavioral anxiety and cortisol levels after massage. Also, their attitude toward asthma and their peak air flow and other pulmonary functions improved over the course of the study. The older children who received massage therapy reported lower anxiety after the massage. Their attitude toward asthma also improved over the study, but only one measure of pulmonary function (FEF 25%–75%) improved.	The reason for the smaller therapeutic benefit in the older children is unknown; however, it appears that daily massage improves airway caliber and control of asthma.	Children; massage (manipulative and body-based practices); relaxation (mind body)
Vedanthan et al,[76] 1998	Randomized controlled trial	17 adults with asthma	Analysis of the data showed that the subjects in the yoga group reported a significant degree of	Yoga techniques seem beneficial as an adjunct to the medical management of asthma.	Adults; yoga (mind-body)

			relaxation, positive attitude, and better yoga exercise tolerance. There was also a tendency toward lesser usage of beta adrenergic inhalers. The pulmonary functions did not vary significantly between yoga and control groups.		Adults; herbs (natural products)
Blanc et al,[49] 1997	Survey, correlational	601 adults with asthma recruited from a random sample of pulmonary and allergy specialists.	Herbal asthma self-treatment was reported by 46 (8%); coffee or black tea self-treatment by 36 (6%), epinephrine or ephedrine OTC use by 36 (6%), and any of the 3 practices by 98 subjects (16%). Adjusting for demographic and illness covariates, herbal use (OR 2.5) and coffee or black tea use (OR 3.1) were associated with asthma hospitalization; OTC use was not (OR 0.8).	Even among adults with access to specialty care for asthma, self-treatment with nonprescription products was common and was associated with increased risk of reported hospitalization. This association does not appear to be accounted for by illness severity or other disease covariates. It may reflect delay in utilization of more efficacious treatments.	

(continued on next page)

Table 2
(continued)

Authors, Primary	Design	Population	Results	Conclusions	Categories/Domain
Kohen and Wynne,[70] 1997	Intervention trial	25 children with asthma and their parent(s)	Following participation in the Preschool Asthma Program, physician visits for asthma were reduced ($P = .0013$) and parents reported increased confidence in self-management skills. Symptom severity scores improved significantly after participation ($P<.001$). A possible association was noted between participation in the program and parental expectations or projections of future outcome ($.05<P<.1$). No changes were observed in the frequency of asthma episodes or in pulmonary function tests before and after the program.	With the hypnotherapeutic approach of imagery, preschoolers developed new cooperation in asthma-care skills, including cooperative and consistent performance of peak flow measurements.	Children; hypnosis (mind-body)
Lehrer et al,[83] 1997	Intervention trial	87 adults with asthma	Changes in forced expiratory volume/forced vital capacity were negatively correlated with those in cardiac interbeat interval. Contrary to	Results suggest that the immediate effects of generalized relaxation instruction can be associated with a parasympathetic rebound, which, in	Adults; progressive muscle relaxation (mind-body)

the theory of a vagal-trigeminal reflex as mediator for relaxation-induced improvement in asthma, decreases in pulmonary function occurred during relaxation sessions, accompanied by increases in cardiovagal activity, and within-session changes in frontal EMG in the 1st session of training were positively associated with changes in forced expiratory volume/forced vital capacity. However, consistent with this hypothesis, first-session frontalis EMG changes were positively associated with changes in respiratory sinus arrhythmia, and last-session changes in cardiac interbeat interval were positively associated with changes in forced expiratory volume/forced vital capacity.

turn, may induce countertherapeutic changes in asthma.

(continued on next page)

Table 2
(continued)

Authors, Primary	Design	Population	Results	Conclusions	Categories/Domain
Coen et al,[68] 1996	Randomized controlled (pilot) study	20 participants, aged 12–22 y, with nonsteroid-dependent reactive airway disease participated.	Results showed decreased asthma severity and decreased facial muscle tension in the experimental group but not in the control group. Improvements in asthma severity were correlated with decreases in facial muscle tension. No effects on pulmonary function were seen. Data on immune measures revealed significant decreases in immunoglobulins in both groups related to seasonal change. Increases in CD4 and CD8 lymphocyte counts were observed more frequently in the experimental group than in the controls.	The findings suggest that biofeedback-assisted relaxation training has potential for improvement of asthma severity and immune function in young individuals with asthma.	Children; adults; biofeedback-assisted relaxation (mind-body)
Lehrer et al,[84] 1994	Randomized controlled trial	106 medically prestabilized adults with asthma	Relaxation-group subjects reported feeling the most deeply relaxed and produced the greatest improvement in FEF during the last presession assessment	Listening to music produced greater decreases in peaks of tension than progressive muscle relaxation, and it produced greater compliance with	Adults; music therapy; progressive muscle relaxation (mind-body)

			period. All groups evidenced decreases in asthma symptoms. All groups showed decreases in pulmonary function immediately after relaxation sessions. None of the changes in pulmonary function reached levels that are accepted in drug trials to be of clinical significance, and the therapeutic changes occurred only in the situation where training was rendered.	relaxation practice, but it did not produce any specific therapeutic effects on asthma.	
Kotses et al,[64] 1991	Randomized controlled trial	29 children with asthma	As compared with the facial stability subjects, the facial relaxation subjects exhibited higher pulmonary scores, more positive attitudes toward asthma, and lower chronic anxiety during the follow-up period. Subjects in the 2 groups, however, did not differ on self-rated asthma severity, medication usage, frequency of asthma attacks, or self-concept.	Based on the improvements we observed in pulmonary, attitude, and anxiety measures, we concluded that biofeedback training for facial relaxation contributes to the self-control of asthma and would be a valuable addition to asthma self-management programs.	Children; biofeedback-assisted relaxation (mind-body)

(continued on next page)

Table 2
(*continued*)

Authors, Primary	Design	Population	Results	Conclusions	Categories/Domain
Murphy et al,[120] 1989	Survey, correlational	12 adults with asthma	Hypnotic susceptibility measures appeared to be related to several measures of improvement in asthma symptoms, and this relationship was similar in both relaxation and placebo treatments.	Findings indicate that hypnotic susceptibility and suggestive processes play similar roles in both interventions and that hypnotic susceptibility may be a useful predictor of response to psychological treatment in asthma.	Adults; hypnosis (mind-body)
Tashkin et al,[81] 1985	Randomized controlled	25 patients with moderate to severe asthma	Two-way analysis of variance failed to reveal a significant effect of either form of acupuncture on symptoms, medication use, or lung function measurements. Similarly, no significant acute effect of acupuncture on lung function, self-ratings of efficacy, or physician's physical findings was found by covariance analysis or the	The findings failed to demonstrate any short-term or long-term benefit of acupuncture therapy in the management of moderate to severe asthma.	Adults; acupuncture (mind-body)

			Wilcoxon signed-rank test. When data during the entire course of the study were examined on an individual basis by analysis of variance with repeated measures, only two subjects demonstrated significantly favorable responses to real vs placebo acupuncture, but one subject demonstrated the reverse, suggesting that these responses were not specifically related to acupuncture therapy.			
Alexander et al,[61] 1979	Intervention trial	14 children with chronic and severe asthma	Heart rate, and to some extent, muscle tension results confirm the attainment of relaxed states. However, the lung function results fail to substantiate the previous, preliminary findings of a clinically meaningful change in pulmonary function following relaxation.	Relaxation did not have significant effect on lung function	Children; relaxation (mind-body)

(continued on next page)

Table 2
(continued)

Authors, Primary	Design	Population	Results	Conclusions	Categories/Domain
Wilson et al,[77] 1975	Intervention trial	21 adults with asthma	As compared with the initial values recorded before intervention, significant improvement in forced expiratory volume, peak expiratory flow rate, and airway resistance was noted.	The results indicated that transcendental meditation is a useful adjunct in treating asthma.	Adults; meditation (mind-body)
Alexander et al,[62] 1972	Randomized controlled trial	44 children with asthma	Results show that relaxation subjects manifested a significant mean increase in peak expiratory flow rate over sessions, compared with a nonsignificant mean peak expiratory flow decrease for controls.	Relaxation was effective to increase the peak expiratory flow rate.	Children; relaxation (mind-body)

Abbreviations: ACQ, Asthma Control Questionnaire; AQLQ, Asthma Quality of Life Questionnaire; BMI, body mass index; CAM, complementary and alternative medicine; EIB, Exercise induced bronchoconstriction; EMG, electromyogram; FEF, forced expiratory flow; FEV(1), forced expiratory volume in 1 second; HCP, health care provider; IL, interleukin; LTB, Leukotriene B4 and B5; OTC, over the counter; PC 20, provocative concentration of a substance (methacholine) causing a 20% fall in the Forced Expiratory Volume in 1 Second; PMNL, Polymorphonuclear Leukocyte; PR, Prevalence Ratio; TNF, tumor necrosis factor.

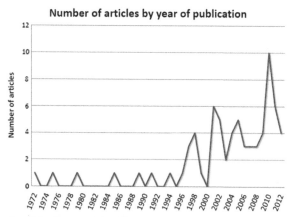

Fig. 2. Number of articles by year of publication.

qualitative research using in-depth interviews. Specifically, 42% of the reviewed articles (n = 30, see **Table 2** for details) reported results of surveys, using either descriptive or correlational designs. Most of these used secondary data from large-scale, comprehensively developed and thoroughly conducted national US surveys. For example, Joubert and colleagues[13] analyzed data from the National Health Interview Survey (NHIS), the principal source of information on the health of the civilian noninstitutionalized US population. The NHIS is one of the major US data-collection programs.[14] Using secondary NHIS data, the researchers were able to analyze 3327 responses of individuals with asthma across the United States to identify the association between asthma episodes in the past 12 months and CAM use, controlling for comorbid conditions. Several other investigators using similar survey designs were able to identify significant patterns of CAM use and its affects in the United States[15–19] and in Canada.[8,11]

Only one-third of the reviewed studies (n = 21) were RCTs despite RCTs being considered the "gold-standard" design when causal relationships between the treatments and health outcomes need to be established.[20] Further, there were several issues related to the quality of several of the RCT studies identified from this review. One example is an application of a technique that addresses the problems associated with incomplete data because of participant withdrawal, described as "intention-to-treat" analysis (ITT). In the ITT approach, all the participants are retained in study data analyses regardless of their path through the trial and completion of the study.[21,22] Participants are retained in the treatment group they are randomized to ("as randomized"), rather than being classified according to the actual treatment they received ("as treated"). In general, ITT analysis produces an unbiased estimate of treatment effectiveness.[22] One fundamental assumption of the ITT method is that missing data and participant withdrawal are not related to the unobserved outcome. ITT also assumes that compliance among those who remain in the trial and those who withdraw is equivalent. Sensitivity analysis and other statistical methods were developed to validate this assumption.[21] In our review, 24% of the RCT studies used the ITT approach in their analysis[23–27]; however, some of the researchers did not mention whether the assumptions about the missing data and adherence were validated and if sensitivity analysis was performed.[23,24] This lack of information significantly limits the interpretation of the results of the reviewed RCTs.

Thirteen of the reviewed studies (18%) were conducted using quasi-experimental designs (mostly a 1-group pretest posttest design). This type of studies is important, especially when experimental methods are impractical or unethical to use; however, it is challenging to make definitive causal inferences using results of these studies. Several statistical methods were recently developed to enhance the causality conclusions of quasi-experimental studies, for example propensity scoring that reduces the confounding effects of covariates. Unfortunately, we did not identify that these methods were used in the reviewed manuscripts. In addition, it was noted that the number of quasi-experimental studies has decreased over time, with only 2 articles using this methodology published since 2005.

The balance of the reviewed studies (10%) used qualitative methods for the data analysis. Application of qualitative methods helps researchers to glean important personal information that is usually inaccessible otherwise. For example, Freidin and Timmermans[28] used open-ended questions to understand the experience with biomedical treatments, social influences, and concerns about adverse and long-term effects of prescription asthma medicines among mothers of children with asthma. In another study, George and colleagues[29] used in-depth interviews to identify causal models of asthma and the context of conventional prescription versus CAM use in low-income African American adults with asthma. More studies using qualitative methods are needed to further understand factors related to asthma medication adherence, possible adverse effects of CAM therapies, and other issues.

Patterns of CAM Use for Asthma

High CAM prevalence rates have been reported for both children and adults with asthma. Pediatric use has been reported to be as high as 80% when folk medicine (which includes prayer) is included in the broad definition of what constitutes a CAM practice.[30] Approximately one-quarter of children reported CAM use for asthma in the past year[16,31] and use is highest in those children with poorer asthma control,[11,32] financial barriers to conventional care,[16] greater severity,[16] more symptoms,[30,33,34] or a CAM-using parent.[7,30,31,35] As much as 80% of pediatric CAM care required an out-of-pocket expenditure.[36]

Similarly, CAM use for adult asthma is extremely high (96%–100%) when survey questions include folk medicine/prayer.[29,37] More than 70% report CAM for symptom management in the past month[33] and prevalence is higher in adults with work-related asthma,[15] financial obstacles to accessing care,[17,19] more symptoms,[17,33] more stress,[38] and more frequent attacks.[13]

CAM Domains

Fig. 1 presents the reviewed articles by CAM domain. Almost half (47%) of the reviewed articles focused on multiple CAM modalities, with 30% concentrated solely on mind-body CAM approaches, 15% on natural products, and the remainder on manipulative and body-based practices (6%) or energy-field healing (2%).

Natural Products

As seen in **Table 1**, natural products encompass a wide variety of ingestible goods that include herbs, vitamins, minerals, specialized diets, dietary supplements, and botanicals. Unfortunately, much of what we know about their use is limited to prevalence surveys; few experimental studies have been conducted.

Unlike prescription drugs, manufacturers do not have to prove either the safety or the effectiveness of natural products. In fact, labels such as "safe," "standardized," "verified," or "certified" do not guarantee quality or consistency.[39] For example, herbal therapies may contain more than one herb, the wrong species of herb, a higher or lower dose of active ingredient than listed on the label, or contaminants, such as other herbs, prescription medicine, pesticides, and heavy metals.[40] In addition, natural products are not inert and may interfere with prescription drugs to cause unintended side effects.[41]

Natural Products for Pediatric Asthma

Although vitamin supplementation is commonly used for pediatric asthma,[16,31,35] a large longitudinal cohort survey study suggests that early vitamin supplementation may actually increase risk for asthma and food allergies in certain vulnerable populations.[42] High use of herbal therapies is also reported,[16,30,31,43,44] including over-the-counter (OTC) topical chest rubs made with camphor, eucalyptus oil and menthol,[30] herbal teas,[30] aloe plant juice,[44] Echinacea,[44] sweet oil (eg, olive, rapeseed, almond),[44] and an herbal cough syrup sold in *botanicas* containing sweet almond oil, castor oil, tolu (tree resin), wild cherry, licorice, cocillana (grape bark), and honey.[30] Atypical products reported include ephedra, turpentine, pine needles, and dried cow dung.[44]

Children with asthma also use dietary supplements,[35] nutritional supplements, and elimination diets[31] without scientific evaluation of their safety or effectiveness.[4] In one study, Covar and colleagues[24] randomized children with asthma to either a nutritional formula composed of antioxidants, omega-3 and omega-6 fatty acids, or a control formula; there were no differences in asthma-free days between groups, although inflammatory biomarkers decreased in the children receiving the nutritional formula.

Natural Products for Adult Asthma

Multivitamin use is associated with asthma in older adults[45] and herbal products are widely used (93%) by the general adult asthma population.[29,46] Commonly used herbal therapies include chamomile, mint, and Echinacea.[19,29,47–49] In addition, OTC ephedra products, as well as coffee and tea (which contain natural methylxanthines), are widely used to supplement, or replace, short-acting β-2 agonists (SABAs) for "rescue" treatment of acute asthma.[29,48,49] Adults also report the use of home remedies to augment asthma self-management, such as Hall's lozenge-infused tea (Mondelēz International Three Parkway North Deerfield, IL, USA), OTC chest rubs, and the ingestion of onion tonics, spicy foods (eg, horseradish), or cold drinks.[29] Importantly, a small number of individuals report oral ingestion of topical camphor products (eg, Vicks VapoRub [Proctor and Gamble, Cincinnati, Ohio, USA]).[29] Although few of these products have been scientifically evaluated, there are several studies of dietary supplements. These include studies of magnesium,[50] fish oil alone[51,52] or in combination with Vitamin C, and a standardized hops extract.[23] Asthma quality-of-life scores improved in those who received long-term magnesium supplementation[50] and the combined nutritional supplement (fish oil, Vitamin C, and hops).[23] However, there was no attention control group in the combination supplement study, making it impossible to attribute improvements to the supplement.[23] Other markers of asthma control, such as reduced bronchial hyperreactivity, pulmonary function, and inflammatory biomarkers improved with magnesium and fish oils.[50,51]

Potential Dangers of Natural Products for Pediatric and Adult Asthma

Several innocuous-appearing natural and OTC products have the potential for serious side effects, including death. For example, Echinacea (cone flower daisy) and chamomile are members of the Compositae or ragweed family. Worsening asthma may result if a ragweed-sensitive individual uses products derived from the daisy family, which includes honey made from the plants or pollens of Compositae.[53]

In addition, OTC natural ephedra (found in *ma huang*, a Traditional Chinese Medicine herb), can have a synergistic cardiovascular effect when used with albuterol.[54] Black licorice made from the glycyrrhiza root can prolong the half-life of cortisone, potentiating systemic steroid effects.[55] Further, the recommended dose of Hall's is 1 to 2 lozenges every 2 hours, which delivers a total dose of 6 to 20 mg of menthol; some adults used large quantities of lozenges (10) in a single serving of tea,[29] which may be harmful.[56]

Of greatest concern, however, were the reports of turpentine oil and Vicks VapoRub ingestion[29,44] and risky behaviors associated with natural product use. First, ingesting turpentine oil[57] and OTC topical chest rubs can be fatal in children and may pose some risk for adults.[58] Second, even when natural product use is not in and of itself harmful, its use may contribute to risky health behaviors. For example, herbal product use is associated with decreased inhaled corticosteroid adherence.[59] Further, substituting caffeinated products (tea and coffee) for SABAs translates to the use of less potent natural therapies for more rapid-acting and effective prescription therapies during acute asthma episodes.[37] This may lead to less effective reversal of bronchospasm and contribute to delays in seeking appropriate medical intervention, placing the individual at increased risk for near-fatal or fatal asthma.[41]

Mind-body Medicine

Mind-body medicine encompasses a wide variety of practices that seek to use the mind to enhance physical functioning and health and are generally considered safe in healthy people when practiced.[90] **Table 1** provides detailed information about many mind-body practices.

Mind-body Medicine for Pediatric Asthma

Breathing exercises (59%),[16] prayer (70%–80%),[33,60] and relaxation (85%) are the most popular mind-body approaches used by children with asthma.[33] Relaxation training may be taught as a stand-alone therapy[61,62] or paired with biofeedback[63,64] or guided imagery.[65–67] Although early studies suggested that relaxation might improve lung function,[62] these findings were not replicated in larger trials.[61] However, in several small feasibility studies without a control condition, biofeedback-induced relaxation was associated with improvement in lung function,[63,65,68] stress,[63] depression,[63] and anxiety,[65] whereas relaxation coupled with guided imagery improved lung function and anxiety.[66,67] Although one small RCT of biofeedback and relaxation demonstrated improved pulmonary function, anxiety, and attitudes toward asthma, there was no difference between groups in asthma medication use, number of asthma attacks, or self-concept.[64]

Hypnosis has also been examined in 2 pediatric asthma studies using a pre-post design. Reductions in symptoms[69] and severity scores without concomitant improvement in the number of asthma episodes or in pulmonary function tests were reported.[70] Further, a small RCT of an art therapy intervention (compared with a wait-list control) reported decreased anxiety and increased quality of life,[71] whereas music therapy (singing) was associated with maintenance or improvement of lung function compared with relaxation.[72]

Mind-body Medicine for Adult Asthma

Mind-body approaches are very popular among adults with asthma, including qi gong, tai chi,[11] prayer, humoral balance, and relaxation.[29,37] Intervention studies of relaxation have demonstrated improvement in well-being and pulmonary function, as well as reduced symptoms[73] without a reduction in cortisol after training.[74] Subjects enrolled in biofeedback[27] or guided (mental) imagery[75] interventions required less asthma medicine[27,75] and demonstrated improved lung function without concomitant improvement in the number of asthma flares[27] compared with a control group.

Other mind-body approaches studied included yoga, meditation, and music therapy. In a small controlled trial of yoga instruction that included postures (*yogasanas*), breathing exercises (*pranayamas*), and meditation, intervention subjects reported enhanced relaxation and less SABA use compared with control subjects, although objective measures of lung function remained unchanged.[76] Further, a randomized, controlled, double-masked clinical trial of Iyengar yoga failed to demonstrate any between-group differences in asthma quality of life, SABA use, spirometry, symptoms, or health care utilization for asthma.[26] In addition, small intervention studies of transcendental meditation,[77] music therapy, and progressive muscle relaxation[27] improved lung function, although the small increases in function were not considered to be of clinical significance.[27]

Two studies used multiple CAM interventions. In the first RCT, yoga, journaling, and nutritional manipulation (elimination diet coupled with supplements of fish oil, Vitamin C, and a standardized hops extract) were given to the intervention group with subsequent improvements in their asthma quality of life scores. These results should be viewed cautiously, however, because of the lack of a control group and the confounding of multiple interventions.[23] In the second study, patients with asthma received training on multiple mind-body approaches, including deep-breathing relaxation, a cognitive-behavioral intervention, and journaling. When compared with an attention control group, the intervention group experienced improved lung function.[78]

Single studies of Buteyko breathing and hypnotic susceptibility in adults have also been conducted. In an RCT of Buteyko, intervention subjects demonstrated improved asthma control with less medication use up to 6 months after training compared with the control condition.[79] Moreover, a correlational study identified that higher hypnotic susceptibility scores were associated with less airway hyperreactivity.[79]

Finally, several RCTs of acupuncture have been conducted in adults with asthma with mixed results. Treatment was associated with improved asthma quality of life[25] and reports of improved asthma[80] although acupuncture did not demonstrate improved lung function,[80,81] reduced need for medications,[25,81] or reduced symptoms.[81]

Potential Dangers of Mind-Body Medicine for Pediatric and Adult Asthma

NCCAM classifies most of the mind-body interventions as "safe"; however, there is small risk associated with some approaches. For example, progressive muscle relaxation has been associated with decreased airflow[82–84] and increased heart rate variability[82,83] in patients with asthma. In addition, there are case reports of untoward effects of mind-body therapies in the general population. For example, case reports describe complications related to yogic postures, including nerve or spinal damage,[85] worsened glaucoma,[86] and stroke.[87] There are also reports of yoga breathing causing pneumothorax.[88] Rare but serious complications may also result from acupuncture, including blood-borne illnesses, punctured organs, and vascular damage.[89] There are also reports of intensification of mania and distress after meditation[90] and hypnosis[91] in patients with mental illness.

Manipulative and Body-based Practices

Spinal manipulation and massage are the 2 primary manipulative and body-based approaches. As described further in **Table 1**, practitioners manipulate joints and massage soft tissue to reduce pain and stress and to facilitate relaxation.

Manipulative and Body-based Practices for Pediatric Asthma

There are very few studies of manipulative and body-based practices despite a high rate of use by children with asthma.[35] A small RCT demonstrated that massage therapy reduced anxiety and cortisol levels immediately after treatment and improved attitudes toward asthma and lung function over time compared with the control condition (progressive muscle relaxation). These findings were more pronounced in younger children compared with older children.[92] In a study by Bronfort and colleagues,[93] chiropractic spinal manipulative therapy improved asthma quality-of-life scores but failed to demonstrate any important changes in lung function or airway hyperreactivity compared with a sham chiropractic treatment. In an RCT of a spinal manipulation intervention, chiropractic care provided no additional benefit over usual medical care in children with mild to moderate asthma.[94]

Manipulative and Body-based Practices for Adult Asthma

Only one study of manipulative therapy (craniosacral treatment) for adults with asthma was identified in this review.[25] In this investigation, 89 subjects were randomized to 1 of 5 groups: acupuncture alone, craniosacral therapy alone, acupuncture and craniosacral therapy together, attention control, or usual care/wait list. Asthma quality-of-life scores improved in all 3 of the active intervention groups, although the combination of acupuncture and craniosacral treatment was not superior to either therapy alone. Medication use and pulmonary function were unchanged.[25]

Potential Dangers of Manipulative and Body-based Practices for Pediatric and Adult Asthma

When provided by a trained therapist, there are relatively few serious risks associated with massage or spinal manipulation for children or adults with asthma. Before massage therapy is initiated, a health care professional should provide medical clearance for individuals with concomitant conditions, such as pregnancy, propensity for bleeding (bleeding disorders, anticoagulant therapy), solid tumor cancers, blood clots, fractures, open wounds, skin infections, osteoporosis, or recent surgery.[95] Most serious side effects associated with spinal manipulation involve treatment of the cervical area and may include vertebrobasilar artery stroke and cauda equina syndrome.[96]

Whole Medical Systems for Asthma

Whole medical systems are complete systems of theory and practice that have evolved over time in different cultures and apart from Western medicine.[4] They include Traditional Chinese Medicine from China, Ayurveda from India, and homeopathy and naturopathy from Europe (see **Table 1**). Although these systems are widely used for asthma, no adult or pediatric studies were identified in this review.

Potential Dangers of Whole Medical Systems for Asthma

Mind-body medicine, manipulative approaches, and natural products are often essential components of whole medical systems approach to treating asthma. Therefore, the previous caution about their use is operative when patients seek such treatment; however, a particular point should be made about homeopathy. Because homeopathic treatments traditionally involve the ingestion of natural products, clinicians may be concerned about interactions or adverse side effects. Generally, plant material used in the preparation of homeopathic products is diluted to such infinitesimally small doses that not even one single active biologic molecule may remain in the "mother tincture," thus rendering the product harmless.[97] However, nasal zinc is an exception to this rule. Reports of permanent loss of smell forced the Food and Drug Administration to recall this homeopathic cold remedy, which was not neither dilute nor orally ingested.[98]

Energy Field Healing

As described in **Table 1**, magnets, Reiki, and therapeutic touch are the most commonly used energy-field healing practices. No adult or pediatric studies of energy healing were identified in this review.

Potential Dangers of Energy-Field Healing for Asthma

There is no known risk in the use of energy field healing practices such as Reiki or therapeutic touch.[99] Magnets are also safe when applied to the skin and are contraindicated only for individuals with medical devices affected by strong magnetic fields, such as pacemakers, implanted defibrillators, and insulin pumps.[100]

Movement Therapies

Pilates, Rolfing, and Alexander are common movement therapies (see detailed in **Table 1**). No adult or pediatric studies examining movement practices were identified in this review.

Potential Dangers of Movement Therapies for Asthma

Although only one scholarly article on the safety of movement therapies was located (a single case report of a spontaneous diaphragm rupture attributable to Pilates),[101] it is likely that some of the same concerns about massage may be applicable to Rolfing and that the Alexander technique might cause minor fatigue or muscle tenderness.

Traditional Healers

Mexican *Curandera*, Native American *shaman*, Puerto Rican *santeros,* and Voudoun *houngans* and *mambos* are among the many traditional healers that practice healing arts in North America (see **Table 1**). No adult or pediatric studies examining traditional healers were identified in this review.

Potential Dangers of Traditional Healers for Asthma

The use of natural products in traditional healing may cause drug-herb interactions, as previously described. In addition, some herbal preparations may be smoked as a treatment for asthma.[102] Alternatively, individuals may visit a smokehouse where poor indoor air quality has been identified as a health risk for individuals with respiratory disorders, including asthma.[103] Other potential dangers of traditional healing have not been reported.

CAM and Asthma Self-management Decisions and Behavior: Self-management Preferences, Adherence, and Patient-Provider Communication

This review uncovered important information, not only about the types and patterns of CAM use, but also about the influence of CAM on asthma self-management decisions and behaviors in children and adults with asthma. For instance, a large qualitative study found that mothers considered their child's daily asthma therapy to be optional despite it being prescribed for daily use, were strongly influenced by their social network to use CAM for their child's asthma, and were not demographically distinguishable from mothers who used conventional prescription treatment.[28] Most (77%) caregivers considered herbal therapies to be safe and did not believe that herbs interacted with medication; only 1% could correctly name a drug-herb interaction.[44]

Further, research demonstrated that adolescents were familiar with culturally relevant CAM[104] and believed CAM to be an effective part of their asthma armamentarium.[30,60] Conversely, 71% of children and their caregivers voiced concerns about the safety of prescription therapies.[43] However, self-reported adherence to daily asthma therapies did not change with the initiation of CAM.[105]

Despite the high rates of CAM use, only one-third of pediatricians asked about CAM.[106] Importantly, if asked, caregivers disclosed at relatively low rates ranging, from 36%[31] to 54%.[107] Caregivers were more comfortable disclosing yoga and dietary interventions than prayer or guided imagery.[33] As a result of this reluctance to divulge CAM use, partial disclosure was more common (62%).[35] However, 80% of caregivers reported that they wanted to tell their provider about their child's CAM use.[31]

Most adults (84%) preferred an integrated approach for asthma self-management that included CAM and prescription therapies.[37] Nurses and CAM practitioners were more likely to ask about CAM use than allopathic physicians,[108] although there are no disclosure rates available specific to adults with asthma. CAM use was associated with low rates of adherence to daily prescription medicines[37,59] and increased rates of hospitalization for life-threatening asthma.[49,59] These high rates of acute health care utilization were independent of disease severity, suggesting that the use of less potent CAM for the home management of acute asthma may unnecessarily delay professional treatment and contribute to higher hospitalization rates.[49] This is supported by qualitative studies in which patients reported that CAM was safe and effective for the initial treatment of severe attacks,[29] was safer than SABAs, worked quickly and synergistically with SABAs,[37] and allowed for the customized treatment the patients desired.[37,109]

SUMMARY

There is a growing body of evidence on the use of CAM by individuals with asthma, particularly in the domains of natural products, mind-body medicine, and manipulative and body-based practices. Natural products were the most common CAM used by both children and adults with asthma. Unfortunately, much of what is known about the effectiveness of these treatments is based primarily on prevalence surveys and a few methodologically weak intervention studies that reported mixed results. Of note, several natural OTC products have the potential for serious side effects, including death. Use of natural products was also associated with risky asthma self-management behaviors, such as decreased adherence to allopathic treatments.[59] Mind-body medicines were also frequently used for asthma with one-third of the reviewed literature focused uniquely on this CAM approach. There were also several trials of spinal manipulation and massage, examples of manipulative and body-based practices. Again, weak study designs, mixed results, and the possibility of serious side effects are concerning. Most importantly, CAM use was rarely discussed in the clinical encounter.

Many clinicians assume that patients turn to CAM only when they have received a cancer diagnosis or develop cancer treatment–related symptoms.[110,111] However, CAM is a popular treatment for asthma as well as a number of other chronic medical conditions, including diabetes,[5,6,111,112] hypertension,[5,6,113] and heart disease.[5,6,114] The desire to use CAM as a way of personalizing treatment has also been noted by other researchers.[115,116] Perhaps one of the most underappreciated risks of CAM is the failure of health care providers to inquire about CAM and patients' reluctance to disclose CAM use.[117]

There are several clinical implications of this review. First, it is important for clinicians and patients to discuss the risks associated with CAM use that include, but are not limited to, use of adulterated natural products, drug-herb interactions, and rare but serious events associated with innocuous-appearing therapies. Second, all CAM self-management strategies must be assessed for their timeliness and appropriateness, and negotiated through a shared decision-making model. For example, this review identified the risky behavior of substituting CAM for both "rescue" and daily asthma therapies. Perhaps a jointly developed plan that promotes the use of both CAM and prescription therapies at each of these events would be useful as a means of addressing patient preferences while also reducing the risk of an untoward event.

To be successful in this endeavor will require the provider to become better educated about CAM, to take the initiative in inquiring about CAM at each office visit, and to create a safe environment in which disclosure is facilitated. With this comes responsibility on the part of the health care professional to respond respectfully and professionally to disclosure. If the patient perceives that the provider is dismissive, derisive, or unsupportive, then a disruption to the therapeutic alliance can result.[118] Health care professionals need help to successfully meet these expectations. The construction and validation of research instruments that address the integral role of CAM in asthma self-management decisions is a critical first step in the systematic collection of data about patient perceptions and preferences for care.[119] Engaging in continuing education is also of paramount importance, as this training will facilitate a deeper appreciation for the reasons patients prefer CAM and will promote the acquisition of the enhanced communication skills needed to support integrative treatment as a cornerstone of patient-centered care.

In summary, this review provides clinicians with important new information: (1) CAM is widely used by both children and adults with asthma; (2) relatively little is known about the safety or effectiveness of CAM for asthma, owing to the paucity of well-designed studies; (3) patients use CAM to create a tailored asthma self-management plan; (4) CAM influences patients' prescription medication–taking behaviors, which, in turn, produces other health risks; and (5) patients and health care professionals do not talk about, or participate in, shared decision making concerning CAM use. Most importantly, this review identifies knowledge gaps that can be addressed by future research. Taken together, this new knowledge may help narrow the divide between what patients want, and what providers currently offer, for asthma self-management.

REFERENCES

1. Kleinman A, Eisenberg L, Good B. Culture, illness, and care: clinical lessons from anthropologic and cross-cultural research. Ann Intern Med 1978;88(2): 251–8.
2. Romanucci-Ross L. The hierarchy of resort in curative practices: the Admiralty Islands, Melanesia. In: Landy D, editor. Culture, disease, and healing: studies in medical anthropology. New York: Macmillan; 1977. p. 481–7.
3. World Health Organization. WHO traditional medicine strategy 2002–2005. 2002. Available at: http://elinks.library.upenn.edu/sfx_local?sid=Refworks%3AUniversity%20of%20Pennsylvani&charset=utf-8&__char_set=utf8&genre=article&aulast=World%20Health%20Organization&date=2002&volume=2012&issue=07%2F22&atitle=WHO%20traditional%20medicine%20strategy%202002%E2%80%932005.&au=World%20Health%20Organization%20&. Accessed July 22, 2012.

4. National Center for Complementary and Alternative Medicine. What is complementary and alternative medicine? 2012. Available at: http://elinks.library.upenn.edu/sfx_local?sid=Refworks%3AUniversity%20of%20Pennsylvani&charset=utf-8&__char_set=utf8&genre=article&aulast=National%20Center%20for%20Complementary%20and%20Alternative%20Medicine&date=2012&volume=2012&issue=07%2F22&atitle=What%20is%20complementary%20and%20alternative%20medicine%3F&au=National%20Center%20for%20Complementary%20and%20Alternative%20Medicine%20&. Accessed July 22, 2012.

5. Esmail N. Complementary and alternative medicine in Canada: trends in use and public attitudes 1997-2006. Public Policy Sources 2007;87:1–53.

6. Nahin RL, Barnes PM, Stussman BJ, et al. Costs of complementary and alternative medicine (CAM) and frequency of visits to CAM practitioners: United States, 2007. Natl Health Stat Report 2009;(18):1–14.

7. Barnes PM, Bloom B, Nahin RL. Complementary and alternative medicine use among adults and children: United States, 2007. Natl Health Stat Report 2008;(12):1–23.

8. Metcalfe A, Williams J, McChesney J, et al. Use of complementary and alternative medicine by those with a chronic disease and the general population—results of a national population based survey. BMC Complement Altern Med 2010;10:58.

9. Hannah L. Complementary and alternative medicine use among Mexican-Americans for general wellness and mental health. Master's thesis, Pacific University. 2010.

10. Barnes PM, Powell-Griner E, McFann K, et al. Complementary and alternative medicine use among adults: United States, 2002. Adv Data 2004;(343):1–19.

11. Torres-Llenza V, Bhogal S, Davis M, et al. Use of complementary and alternative medicine in children with asthma. Can Respir J 2010;17(4):183–7.

12. Polit D, Beck C. Nursing research: generating and assessing evidence for nursing practice. Philadelphia: Lippincott Williams & Wilkins; 2011.

13. Joubert A, Kidd-Taylor A, Christopher G, et al. Complementary and alternative medical practice: self-care preferred vs. practitioner-based care among patients with asthma. J Natl Med Assoc 2010;102(7):562–9.

14. Centers for Disease Control and Prevention. About the National Health Interview Survey. 2012. Available at: http://elinks.library.upenn.edu/sfx_local?sid=Refworks%3AUniversity%20of%20Pennsylvani&charset=utf-8&__char_set=utf8&genre=article&aulast=Centers%20for%20Disease%20Control%20and%20Prevention&date=2012&volume=2012&issue=27%2F07&atitle=About%20the%20National%20Health%20Interview%20Survey&au=Centers%20for%20Disease%20Control%20and%20Prevention%20&. Accessed July 27, 2012.

15. Knoeller GE, Mazurek JM, Moorman JE. Complementary and alternative medicine use among adults with work-related and non-work-related asthma. J Asthma 2012;49(1):107–13.

16. Shen J, Oraka E. Complementary and alternative medicine (CAM) use among children with current asthma. Prev Med 2012;54(1):27–31.

17. Marino LA, Shen J. Characteristics of complementary and alternative medicine use among adults with current asthma, 2006. J Asthma 2010;47(5):521–5.

18. Birdee GS, Wayne PM, Davis RB, et al. T'ai chi and qigong for health: patterns of use in the United States. J Altern Complement Med 2009;15(9):969–73.

19. Loera JA, Black SA, Markides KS, et al. The use of herbal medicine by older Mexican Americans. J Gerontol A Biol Sci Med Sci 2001;56(11):M714–8.

20. Bero L, Rennie D. The Cochrane Collaboration. Preparing, maintaining, and disseminating systematic reviews of the effects of health care. JAMA 1995; 274(24):1935–8.

21. Salim A, Mackinnon A, Griffiths K. Sensitivity analysis of intention-to-treat estimates when withdrawals are related to unobserved compliance status. Stat Med 2008;27(8):1164–79.

22. Lachin JL. Statistical considerations in the intent-to-treat principle. Control Clin Trials 2000;21(5):526.

23. Kligler B, Homel P, Blank AE, et al. Randomized trial of the effect of an integrative medicine approach to the management of asthma in adults on disease-related quality of life and pulmonary function. Altern Ther Health Med 2011; 17(1):10–5.

24. Covar R, Gleason M, MacOmber B, et al. Impact of a novel nutritional formula on asthma control and biomarkers of allergic airway inflammation in children. Clin Exp Allergy 2010;40(8):1163–74.

25. Mehl-Madrona L, Kligler B, Silverman S, et al. The impact of acupuncture and craniosacral therapy interventions on clinical outcomes in adults with asthma. Explore (NY) 2007;3(1):28–36.

26. Sabina AB, Williams AL, Wall HK, et al. Yoga intervention for adults with mild-to-moderate asthma: a pilot study. Ann Allergy Asthma Immunol 2005;94(5): 543–8.

27. Lehrer PM, Vaschillo E, Vaschillo B, et al. Biofeedback treatment for asthma. Chest 2004;126(2):352–61.

28. Freidin B, Timmermans S. Complementary and alternative medicine for children's asthma: satisfaction, care provider responsiveness, and networks of care. Qual Health Res 2008;18(1):43–55.

29. George M, Birck K, Hufford DJ, et al. Beliefs about asthma and complementary and alternative medicine in low-income inner-city African-American adults. J Gen Intern Med 2006;21(12):1317–24.

30. Reznik M, Ozuah PO, Franco K, et al. Use of complementary therapy by adolescents with asthma. Arch Pediatr Adolesc Med 2002;156(10):1042–4.

31. Ottolini MC, Hamburger EK, Loprieato JO, et al. Complementary and alternative medicine use among children in the Washington, DC area. Ambul Pediatr 2001; 1(2):122–5.

32. Cabana MD, Gollapudi A, Jarlsberg LG, et al. Parent perception of their child's asthma control and concurrent complementary and alternative medicine use. Pediatr Asthma Allergy Immunol 2008;21(4):167–72.

33. Cotton S, Luberto CM, Yi MS, et al. Complementary and alternative medicine behaviors and beliefs in urban adolescents with asthma. J Asthma 2011; 48(5):531–8.

34. Sidora-Arcoleo K, Yoos HL, McMullen A, et al. Complementary and alternative medicine use in children with asthma: prevalence and sociodemographic profile of users. J Asthma 2007;44(3):169–75.

35. Post-White J, Fitzgerald M, Hageness S, et al. Complementary and alternative medicine use in children with cancer and general and specialty pediatrics. J Pediatr Oncol Nurs 2009;26(1):7–15.

36. Ang JY, Ray-Mazumder S, Nachman SA, et al. Use of complementary and alternative medicine by parents of children with HIV infection and asthma and well children. South Med J 2005;98(9):869–75.

37. George M, Campbell J, Rand C. Self-management of acute asthma among low-income urban adults. J Asthma 2009;46(6):618–24.

38. Baldwin CM, Long K, Kroesen K, et al. A profile of military veterans in the south-western United States who use complementary and alternative medicine: implications for integrated care. Arch Intern Med 2002;162(15):1697–704.

39. National Center for Complementary and Alternative Medicine. Time to talk about dietary supplements: 5 things consumers need to know. 2012. Available at: http://elinks.library.upenn.edu/sfx_local?sid=Refworks%3AUniversity%20of%20Pennsylvani&charset=utf-8&__char_set=utf8&genre=article&aulast=National%20Center%20for%20Complementary%20and%20Alternative%20Medicine&date=2012&volume=2012&issue=07%2F25&atitle=Time%20To%20Talk%20About%20Dietary%20Supplements%3A5%20Things%20Consumers%20Need%20To%20Know&au=National%20Center%20for%20Complementary%20and%20Alternative%20Medicine%20&. Accessed July 25, 2012.

40. National Center for Complementary and Alternative Medicine. Using dietary supplements wisely. 2012. Available at: http://elinks.library.upenn.edu/sfx_local?sid=Refworks%3AUniversity%20of%20Pennsylvani&charset=utf-8&__char_set=utf8&genre=article&aulast=National%20Center%20for%20Complementary%20and%20Alternative%20Medicine&date=2012&volume=2012&issue=07%2F24&atitle=Using%20Dietary%20Supplements%20Wisely&au=National%20Center%20for%20Complementary%20and%20Alternative%20Medicine%20&. Accessed July 24, 2012.

41. National Center for Complementary and Alternative Medicine. Safe use of complementary health products and practices. 2012. Available at: http://elinks.library.upenn.edu/sfx_local?sid=Refworks%3AUniversity%20of%20Pennsylvani&charset=utf-8&__char_set=utf8&genre=article&aulast=National%20Center%20for%20Complementary%20and%20Alternative%20Medicine&date=2012&volume=2012&issue=07%2F25&atitle=Safe%20Use%20of%20Complementary%20Health%20Products%20and%20Practices&au=National%20Center%20for%20Complementary%20and%20Alternative%20Medicine%20&. Accessed July 25, 2012.

42. Milner JD, Stein DM, McCarter R, et al. Early infant multivitamin supplementation is associated with increased risk for food allergy and asthma. Pediatrics 2004; 114(1):27–32.

43. Handelman L, Rich M, Bridgemohan CF, et al. Understanding pediatric inner-city asthma: an explanatory model approach. J Asthma 2004;41(2):167–77.

44. Lanski SL, Greenwald M, Perkins A, et al. Herbal therapy use in a pediatric emergency department population: expect the unexpected. Pediatrics 2003; 111(5 Pt 1):981–5.

45. Nahin RL, Fitzpatrick AL, Williamson JD, et al. Use of herbal medicine and other dietary supplements in community-dwelling older people: baseline data from the Ginkgo Evaluation of Memory study. J Am Geriatr Soc 2006;54(11):1725–35.

46. Hailemaskel B, Dutta A, Wutoh A. Adverse reactions and interactions among herbal users. Issues Interdiscipl Care 2001;3(4):297–300.

47. Zayas LE, Wisniewski AM, Cadzow RB, et al. Knowledge and use of ethnomedical treatments for asthma among Puerto Ricans in an urban community. Ann Fam Med 2011;9(1):50–6.

48. Blanc PD, Trupin L, Earnest G, et al. Alternative therapies among adults with a reported diagnosis of asthma or rhinosinusitis: data from a population-based survey. Chest 2001;120(5):1461–7.

49. Blanc PD, Kuschner WG, Katz PP, et al. Use of herbal products, coffee or black tea, and over-the-counter medications as self-treatments among adults with asthma. J Allergy Clin Immunol 1997;100(6 Pt 1):789–91.

50. Kazaks AG, Uriu-Adams JY, Albertson TE, et al. Effect of oral magnesium supplementation on measures of airway resistance and subjective assessment of asthma control and quality of life in men and women with mild to moderate asthma: a randomized placebo controlled trial. J Asthma 2010;47(1):83–92.
51. MacRedmond R, Singhera G, Attridge S, et al. Conjugated linoleic acid improves airway hyper-reactivity in overweight mild asthmatics. Clin Exp Allergy 2010;40(7):1071–8.
52. Mickleborough TD, Lindley MR, Ionescu AA, et al. Protective effect of fish oil supplementation on exercise-induced bronchoconstriction in asthma. Chest 2006;129(1):39–49.
53. National Center for Complementary and Alternative Medicine. Chamomile. 2011. Available at: http://elinks.library.upenn.edu/sfx_local?sid=Refworks%3AUniversity%20of%20Pennsylvani&charset=utf-8&__char_set=utf8&genre=article&aulast=National%20Center%20for%20Complementary%20and%20Alternative%20Medicine&date=2011&volume=2012&issue=07%2F25&atitle=Chamomile&au=National%20Center%20for%20Complementary%20and%20Alternative%20Medicine%20&. Accessed July 25, 2012.
54. Newall CA, Anderson LA, Phillipson JD. Herbal medicines: a guide for health-care professionals. London: The Pharmaceutical Press; 1996.
55. National Center for Complementary and Alternative Medicine. Licorice root. 2011. Available at: http://elinks.library.upenn.edu/sfx_local?sid=Refworks%3AUniversity%20of%20Pennsylvani&charset=utf-8&__char_set=utf8&genre=article&aulast=National%20Center%20for%20Complementary%20and%20Alternative%20Medicine&date=2011&volume=2012&issue=07%2F25&atitle=Licorice%20Root&au=National%20Center%20for%20Complementary%20and%20Alternative%20Medicine%20&. Accessed July 25, 2012.
56. Michael JB, Sztajnkrycer MD. Deadly pediatric poisons: nine common agents that kill at low doses. Emerg Med Clin North Am 2004;22(4):1019–50.
57. McKenzie LB, Ahir N, Stolz U, et al. Household cleaning product-related injuries treated in US emergency departments in 1990-2006. Pediatrics 2010;126(3):509–16.
58. Nair B. Final report on the safety assessment of Mentha piperita (peppermint) oil, Mentha piperita (peppermint) leaf extract, Mentha piperita (peppermint) leaf, and Mentha piperita (peppermint) leaf water. Int J Toxicol 2001;20(Suppl 3):61–73.
59. Roy A, Lurslurchachai L, Halm EA, et al. Use of herbal remedies and adherence to inhaled corticosteroids among inner-city asthmatic patients. Ann Allergy Asthma Immunol 2010;104(2):132–8.
60. Luberto CM, Yi MS, Tsevat J, et al. Complementary and alternative medicine use and psychosocial outcomes among urban adolescents with asthma. J Asthma 2012;49(4):409–15.
61. Alexander AB, Cropp GJ, Chai H. Effects of relaxation training on pulmonary mechanics in children with asthma. J Appl Behav Anal 1979;12(1):27–35.
62. Alexander AB, Miklich DR, Hershkoff H. The immediate effects of systematic relaxation training on peak expiratory flow rates in asthmatic children. Psychosom Med 1972;34(5):388–94.
63. Long KA, Ewing LJ, Cohen S, et al. Preliminary evidence for the feasibility of a stress management intervention for 7- to 12-year-olds with asthma. J Asthma 2011;48(2):162–70.
64. Kotses H, Harver A, Segreto J, et al. Long-term effects of biofeedback-induced facial relaxation on measures of asthma severity in children. Biofeedback Self Regul 1991;16(1):1–21.

65. Kapoor GV, Bray MA, Kehle TJ. School-based intervention: relaxation and guided imagery for students with asthma and anxiety disorder. Can J Sch Psychol 2010;25(4):311–27.

66. Dobson RL, Bray MA, Kehle TJ, et al. Relaxation and guided imagery as an intervention for children with asthma: a replication. Psychol Schools 2005;42(7):707–20.

67. Peck HL, Bray MA, Kehle TJ. Relaxation and guided imagery: a school-based intervention for children with asthma. Psychol Schools 2003;40(6):657–75.

68. Coen BL, Conran PB, McGrady A, et al. Effects of biofeedback-assisted relaxation on asthma severity and immune function. Pediatr Asthma Allergy Immunol 1996;10(2):71–8.

69. Anbar RD. Hypnosis in pediatrics: applications at a pediatric pulmonary center. BMC Pediatr 2002;2:11.

70. Kohen DP, Wynne E. Applying hypnosis in a preschool family asthma education program: uses of storytelling, imagery, and relaxation. Am J Clin Hypn 1997; 39(3):169–81.

71. Beebe A, Gelfand EW, Bender B. A randomized trial to test the effectiveness of art therapy for children with asthma. J Allergy Clin Immunol 2010;126(2):263–6, 266.e1.

72. Wade LM. A comparison of the effects of vocal exercises/singing versus music-assisted relaxation on peak expiratory flow rates of children with asthma. Music Ther Perspect 2002;20(1):31–7.

73. Smyth JM, Soefer MH, Hurewitz A, et al. The effect of tape-recorded relaxation training on well-being, symptoms, and peak expiratory flow rate in adult asthmatics: a pilot study. Psychol Health 1999;14(3):487–501.

74. Smyth J, Litcher L, Hurewitz A, et al. Relaxation training and cortisol secretion in adult asthmatics. J Health Psychol 2001;6(2):217–27.

75. Epstein GN, Halper JP, Barrett EA, et al. A pilot study of mind-body changes in adults with asthma who practice mental imagery. Altern Ther Health Med 2004; 10(4):66–71.

76. Vedanthan PK, Kesavalu LN, Murthy KC, et al. Clinical study of yoga techniques in university students with asthma: a controlled study. Allergy Asthma Proc 1998; 19(1):3–9.

77. Wilson AF, Honsberger R, Chiu JT, et al. Transcendental meditation and asthma. Respiration 1975;32(1):74–80.

78. Hockemeyer J, Smyth J. Evaluating the feasibility and efficacy of a self-administered manual-based stress management intervention for individuals with asthma: results from a controlled study. Behav Med 2002;27(4):161–72.

79. Cowie RL, Conley DP, Underwood MF, et al. A randomized controlled trial of the Buteyko technique as an adjunct to conventional management of asthma. Respir Med 2008;102(5):726–32.

80. Wechsler ME, Kelley JM, Boyd IO, et al. Active albuterol or placebo, sham acupuncture, or no intervention in asthma. N Engl J Med 2011;365(2):119–26.

81. Tashkin DP, Kroening RJ, Bresler DE. A controlled trial of real and simulated acupuncture in the management of chronic asthma. J Allergy Clin Immunol 1985;76(6):855–64.

82. Aboussafy D, Campbell TS, Lavoie K, et al. Airflow and autonomic responses to stress and relaxation in asthma: the impact of stressor type. Int J Psychophysiol 2005;57(3):195–201.

83. Lehrer PM, Hochron SM, Mayne T, et al. Relationship between changes in EMG and respiratory sinus arrhythmia in a study of relaxation therapy for asthma. Appl Psychophysiol Biofeedback 1997;22(3):183–91.

84. Lehrer PM, Hochron SM, Mayne T, et al. Relaxation and music therapies for asthma among patients prestabilized on asthma medication. J Behav Med 1994;17(1):1–24.

85. Sinaki M. Yoga spinal flexion positions and vertebral compression fracture in osteopenia or osteoporosis of spine: case series. Pain Pract 2012. [Epub ahead of print].

86. Baskaran M, Raman K, Ramani KK, et al. Intraocular pressure changes and ocular biometry during Sirsasana (headstand posture) in yoga practitioners. Ophthalmology 2006;113(8):1327–32.

87. Duval EL, Van Coster R, Verstraeten K. Acute traumatic stroke: a case of bow hunter's stroke in a child. Eur J Emerg Med 1998;5(2):259–63.

88. Johnson DB, Tierney MJ, Sadighi PJ. Kapalabhati pranayama: breath of fire or cause of pneumothorax? A case report. Chest 2004;125(5):1951–2.

89. National Center for Complementary and Alternative Medicine. Acupuncture side effects, and risks. 2012. Available at: http://elinks.library.upenn.edu/sfx_local? sid=Refworks%3AUniversity%20of%20Pennsylvani&charset=utf-8&__char_set= utf8&genre=article&aulast=National%20Center%20for%20Complementary% 20and%20Alternative%20Medicine&date=2012&volume=2012&issue=07% 2F25&atitle=Acupuncture%20Side%20Effects%20and%20Risks&au=National %20Center%20for%20Complementary%20and%20Alternative%20Medicine% 20&. Accessed July 25, 2012.

90. National Center for Complementary and Alternative Medicine. Meditation: side effects and risks. 2012. Available at: http://elinks.library.upenn.edu/sfx_local? sid=Refworks%3AUniversity%20of%20Pennsylvani&charset=utf-8&__char_set= utf8&genre=article&aulast=National%20Center%20for%20Complementary% 20and%20Alternative%20Medicine&date=2012&volume=2012&issue=07%2F 25&atitle=Meditation%3A%20Side%20Effects%20and%20Risks&au=National %20Center%20for%20Complementary%20and%20Alternative%20Medicine% 20&. Accessed July 25, 2012.

91. Kluft RP. Issues in the detection of those suffering adverse effects in hypnosis training workshops. Am J Clin Hypn 2012;54(3):213–32.

92. Field T, Henteleff T, Hernandez-Reif M, et al. Children with asthma have improved pulmonary functions after massage therapy. J Pediatr 1998;132(5):854–8.

93. Bronfort G, Evans RL, Kubic P, et al. Chronic pediatric asthma and chiropractic spinal manipulation: a prospective clinical series and randomized clinical pilot study. J Manipulative Physiol Ther 2001;24(6):369–77.

94. Balon J, Aker PD, Crowther ER, et al. A comparison of active and simulated chiropractic manipulation as adjunctive treatment for childhood asthma. N Engl J Med 1998;339(15):1013–20.

95. National Center for Complementary and Alternative Medicine. Massage therapy: an introduction. 2012. Available at: http://elinks.library.upenn.edu/sfx_local? sid=Refworks%3AUniversity%20of%20Pennsylvani&charset=utf-8&__char_set= utf8&genre=article&aulast=National%20Center%20for%20Complementary%20 and%20Alternative%20Medicine&date=2012&volume=2012&issue=07%2F25 &atitle=Massage%20Therapy%3A%20An%20Introduction&au=National%20 Center%20for%20Complementary%20and%20Alternative%20Medicine%20&. Accessed July 25, 2012.

96. National Center for Complementary and Alternative Medicine. Chiropractic: an introduction. 2012. Available at: http://elinks.library.upenn.edu/sfx_local?sid= Refworks%3AUniversity%20of%20Pennsylvani&charset=utf-8&__char_set=utf8 &genre=article&aulast=National%20Center%20for%20Complementary%20and

%20Alternative%20Medicine&date=2012&volume=2012&issue=07%2F25& atitle=Chiropractic%3A%20An%20Introduction&au=National%20Center%20for %20Complementary%20and%20Alternative%20Medicine%20&. Accessed July 25, 2012.

97. National Center for Complementary and Alternative Medicine. Homeopathy: an introduction. 2012. Available at: http://elinks.library.upenn.edu/sfx_local? sid=Refworks%3AUniversity%20of%20Pennsylvani&charset=utf-8&__char_ set=utf8&genre=article&aulast=National%20Center%20for%20Complementary %20and%20Alternative%20Medicine&date=2012&volume=2012&issue=07% 2F25&atitle=Homeopathy%3A%20An%20Introduction&au=National%20Center %20for%20Complementary%20and%20Alternative%20Medicine%20&. Accessed July 25, 2012.

98. National Center for Complementary and Alternative Medicine. Time to talk about natural products for the flu and colds: what does the science say? 2012. Available at: http://elinks.library.upenn.edu/sfx_local?sid=Refworks%3AUniversity%20of% 20Pennsylvani&charset=utf-8&__char_set=utf8&genre=article&aulast=National %20Center%20for%20Complementary%20and%20Alternative%20Medicine&date= 2012&volume=2012&issue=07%2F25&atitle=Time%20To%20Talk%20About% 20Natural%20Products%20for%20the%20Flu%20and%20Colds%3AWhat% 20Does%20the%20Science%20Say%3F&au=National%20Center%20for% 20Complementary%20and%20Alternative%20Medicine%20&. Accessed July 25, 2012.

99. National Center for Complementary and Alternative Medicine. Reiki: an introduc-tion. 2012. Available at: http://elinks.library.upenn.edu/sfx_local?sid=Refworks% 3AUniversity%20of%20Pennsylvani&charset=utf-8&__char_set=utf8&genre= article&aulast=National%20Center%20for%20Complementary%20and%20Alter native%20Medicine&date=2012&volume=2012&issue=07%2F25&atitle=Reiki% 3A%20An%20Introduction&au=National%20Center%20for%20Complementary %20and%20Alternative%20Medicine%20&. Accessed July 25, 2012.

100. National Center for Complementary and Alternative Medicine. Magnets for pain. 2012. Available at: http://elinks.library.upenn.edu/sfx_local?sid=Refworks %3AUniversity%20of%20Pennsylvani&charset=utf-8&__char_set=utf8&genre= article&aulast=National%20Center%20for%20Complementary%20and%20Alter native%20Medicine&date=2012&volume=2012&issue=07%2F25&atitle=Mag nets%20for%20Pain&au=National%20Center%20for%20Complementary%20 and%20Alternative%20Medicine%20&. Accessed July 25, 2012.

101. Yang YM, Yang HB, Park JS, et al. Spontaneous diaphragmatic rupture compli-cated with perforation of the stomach during Pilates. Am J Emerg Med 2010; 28(2):259.e1–3.

102. University of Maryland Medical Center. Lobelia. 2010. Available at: http://elinks. library.upenn.edu/sfx_local?sid=Refworks%3AUniversity%20of%20Pennsylvani &charset=utf-8&__char_set=utf8&genre=article&aulast=University%20of%20 Maryland%20Medical%20Center&date=2010&volume=2012&issue=07%2F25 &atitle=Lobelia&au=University%20of%20Maryland%20Medical%20Center% 20&. Accessed July 25, 2012.

103. Flanagan ME, Zaferatos NC. Appropriate technologies in the traditional Native American smokehouse: public health considerations in tribal community devel-opment. Am Indian Cult Res J 2000;24(4):69–93.

104. Klein JD, Wilson KM, Sesselberg TS, et al. Adolescents' knowledge of and beliefs about herbs and dietary supplements: a qualitative study. J Adolesc Health 2005;37(5):409.

105. Philp JC, Maselli J, Pachter LM, et al. Complementary and alternative medicine use and adherence with pediatric asthma treatment. Pediatrics 2012;129(5):e1148–54.
106. Sawni A, Thomas R. Pediatricians' attitudes, experience and referral patterns regarding complementary/alternative medicine: a national survey. BMC Complement Altern Med 2007;7:18.
107. Sidora-Arcoleo K, Yoos HL, Kitzman H, et al. Don't ask, don't tell: parental nondisclosure of complementary and alternative medicine and over-the-counter medication use in children's asthma management. J Pediatr Health Care 2008;22(4):221–9.
108. Davis PA, Gold EB, Hackman RM, et al. The use of complementary/alternative medicine for the treatment of asthma in the United States. J Investig Allergol Clin Immunol 1998;8(2):73–7.
109. Mithani S, Monteleone C. Use of alternative therapies in patients with asthma in central New Jersey data from a pilot survey: data from a pilot survey. Journal of Asthma and Allergy Educators 2011;2(3):130–4.
110. Anderson JG, Taylor AG. Use of complementary therapies for cancer symptom management: results of the 2007 National Health Interview Survey. J Altern Complement Med 2012;18(3):235–41.
111. Vapiwala N, Mick R, Hampshire MK, et al. Patient initiation of complementary and alternative medical therapies (CAM) following cancer diagnosis. Cancer J 2006;12(6):467–74.
112. Nahas R, Moher M. Complementary and alternative medicine for the treatment of type 2 diabetes. Can Fam Physician 2009;55(6):591–6.
113. Nahas R. Complementary and alternative medicine approaches to blood pressure reduction: an evidence-based review. Can Fam Physician 2008;54(11):1529–33.
114. Greenfield S, Pattison H, Jolly K. Use of complementary and alternative medicine and self-tests by coronary heart disease patients. BMC Complement Altern Med 2008;8:47.
115. Edwards E. The role of complementary, alternative, and integrative medicine in personalized health care. Neuropsychopharmacology 2012;37(1):293–5.
116. Astin JA. Why patients use alternative medicine: results of a national study. JAMA 1998;279(19):1548–53.
117. Eisenberg DM, Kessler RC, Van Rompay MI, et al. Perceptions about complementary therapies relative to conventional therapies among adults who use both: results from a national survey. Ann Intern Med 2001;135(5):344–51.
118. Tasaki K, Maskarinec G, Shumay DM, et al. Communication between physicians and cancer patients about complementary and alternative medicine: exploring patients' perspectives. Psychooncology 2002;11(3):212–20.
119. Sidora-Arcoleo K, Feldman J, Serebrisky D, et al. Validation of the Asthma Illness Representation Scale (AIRS). J Asthma 2010;47(1):33–40.
120. Murphy AI, Lehrer PM, Karlin R, et al. Hypnotic susceptibility and its relationship to outcome in the behavioral treatment of asthma: some preliminary data. Psychol Rep 1989;65(2):691–8.

Corticosteroids
Still at the Frontline in Asthma Treatment?

Renaud Louis, MD, PhD[a],*, Florence Schleich, MD[a],
Peter J. Barnes, MD, PhD[b]

KEYWORDS

- Eosinophilic asthma • Corticosteroids • Inflammation • Mast cells
- Asthma phenotypes

KEY POINTS

- Inhaled corticosteroids (ICS) have led to considerably improved asthma control and reduced asthma mortality in the Western world over the last 2 decades, particularly in combating T-helper type 2–driven inflammation featuring mast cell and eosinophilic airway infiltration.
- Their effect on innate immunity-driven neutrophilic inflammation is rather poor and their ability to prevent airway remodeling and accelerated lung decline is highly controversial.
- Although ICS remain pivotal drugs in asthma management, research is needed to find drugs complementary to the combination ICS/long-acting β2-agonist in refractory asthma and perhaps a new class of drugs as a first-line treatment in mild to moderate noneosinophilic asthma.

INTRODUCTION

There was a time when asthmatics had their symptoms treated with a regular short-acting bronchodilator and theophylline, while reserving the use of systemic corticosteroids for severe exacerbations and for chronic maintenance treatment of the most severe patients. The emergence of corticosteroids suitable for the inhaled route in the 1970s followed by convincing clinical trials during the late 1980s has dramatically changed the picture of asthma treatment. The class of inhaled corticosteroids (ICS) has rapidly demonstrated its superiority over other classes of drugs used in asthma.[1] The first Global Initiative for Asthma consensus in the early 1990s further highlighted the importance of the role of ICS in asthma treatment.[2] There is no doubt that the

This article originally appeared in Clinics in Chest Medicine, Volume 33, Issue 3, September 2012.
[a] Deparment of Pneumology, CHU Liege, GIGAI3 Research Group, University of Liege, Liege, Belgium; [b] National Heart and Lung Institute, Imperial College, London, UK
* Corresponding author.
E-mail address: R.Louis@chu.ulg.ac.be

Clinics Collections 2 (2014) 207–221
http://dx.doi.org/10.1016/j.ccol.2014.09.011

reduced mortality and morbidity of asthma observed since the 1990s is, in a large part, related to the regular use of ICS as the mainstay of asthma treatment. Yet some studies have pointed out the variability of the response to ICS in patients with asthma, suggesting that ICS administered alone might not be the best drug for all patients.[3]

FROM EARLY PROMISE TO THE TIME OF CERTITUDE

The first studies using inhaled hydrocortisone and prednisone in asthma were disappointing. It became apparent that this was because of the inappropriate chemical structure of prednisone, which has first to be metabolized to become pharmacologically effective, and the lack of topical activity of these corticosteroids. The chemical transformation of prednisone to increase both lipophilicity and interaction with glucocorticosteroid receptor made it possible to find compounds that were suitable for the inhaled route. Early studies in the 1970s used inhaled beclomethasone dipropionate and triamcinolone acetate in moderate to severe asthma and showed that these drugs were effective in improving lung function and reducing symptoms despite tapering oral corticosteroids.[4–6] The introduction of ICS dramatically and effectively changed the conventional approach to asthma therapy. The institution of ICS made it possible to replace, in most of the patients, the chronic use of oral corticosteroids, thereby avoiding side effects that were often severe and debilitating.[7] Furthermore, it soon seemed to be an inverse relationship between the rate of hospitalization for acute asthma exacerbation and the sales of ICS. In a cohort study of more than 13,000 patients with asthma, ICS were shown to be more effective than theophylline in reducing the hospitalization rate as long as they were taken regularly.[8] In a population-based epidemiologic study it was found that the regular use of low-dose ICS was associated with a reduced risk of death from asthma.[9]

The interest of ICS in the milder form of the disease was established later. The first pivotal study proving the superiority of ICS over β2-agonists as a maintenance treatment dates back to 1991. Haahtela and colleagues[10] demonstrated that the regular use of inhaled budesonide at the dosage of 1200 μg/d was by far superior to the regular use of terbutaline in improving the day-to-day peak expiratory flow rate and reducing asthma symptoms and as-needed relief bronchodilator usage. It is also by this time that the fundamental inflammatory nature of asthma was recognized even in the mildest form of the disease.[11] Asthma has then been regarded as a chronic airway inflammatory disease featuring eosinophil and mast cell airway wall infiltration as a consequence of a T-helper type 2 (Th2)–driven inflammatory process. The role of cytokines, such as interleukin 4 (IL-4) and IL-5, were highlighted as key cytokine in immunoglobulin E (IgE) synthesis from B cells and eosinophil survival respectively.[12] The role of chemokines for eosinophils, like eotaxin, was also demonstrated in asthma.[13] Regular treatment with ICS was shown to reduce the number of T-lymphocytes, eosinophils, and mast cells[14] and restore epithelial integrity[15] in bronchial biopsies. Numerous studies showed that regular treatment with ICS sharply and quickly reduces the percentage of eosinophils contained in the sputum from patients with asthma.[16–20] Therefore, corticosteroids were thought to be effective in asthma treatment because of their ability to repress the release of Th2 cytokine from lymphocytes[21] and eotaxin from epithelial cells,[22] thereby depleting airways from eosinophils and mast cells. More recently, it has been shown that corticosteroids are highly effective in inhibiting the transcription factor GATA3, which drives Th2 cells and the release of Th2 cytokines.[23] Therefore, ICS have been regarded as the perfect treatment of asthma leading to control for the peculiar airway inflammation while minimizing the systemic side effects because of their local action. Even in the mildest form of the disease, severe exacerbations may occur and ICS were shown to be extremely effective in preventing them.[24] This important property of ICS can lead us to think of this drug class as a disease-modifying drug in asthma. However, it soon appeared that ICS, even administrated at high doses, might not treat all facets of asthma or control all patients with asthma.

CORTICOSTEROIDS AND LOSS OF LUNG FUNCTION

Accelerated lung decline is a well-known feature of chronic obstructive pulmonary disease (COPD) and it is generally accepted that ICS fails to prevent it when patients continue to smoke.[25] The recognition that patients with asthma also have an accelerated lung function decline regardless of smoking[26,27] and despite regular treatment with ICS[24,28] has questioned the role of this class of drugs as a disease-modifying agent in asthma. In contrast to what has been shown for airway inflammation, it has been extremely difficult to convincingly demonstrate an effect of corticosteroids on airway remodeling. These effects require higher doses and sustained administration to show small changes in airway structure.[29,30] On the other hand, it has been demonstrated that in some young children, there is intense airway remodeling without any inflammation.[31,32] These observations led to the concept that airway inflammation and airway remodeling may be largely independent processes and, consequently, governed by different cytokine and growth factor networks, with corticoids being essentially active against the Th2 inflammatory component.[33] The recent observation that bronchoconstriction by itself may be a trigger for airway remodeling is of great importance because it may have potential significant implications for a treatment strategy to prevent lung function decrease.[34] In this view, it would seem logical to combine corticoids and long-acting-β2-agonist (LABA) at the early stages of asthmatic disease to maximize the bronchoprotecting effect and reduce the chance to evolve toward airway remodeling.

THE RECOGNITION OF REFRACTORY ASTHMA

The Gaining Optimal Asthma Control study showed that most patients with asthma can become largely asymptomatic when regularly treated by a combination ICS/LABA.[35] This therapeutic strategy also proved to be efficient in preventing asthma exacerbation in most patients. Yet a small fraction of patients with asthma, called patients with refractory or severe asthma, escape to that treatment. Severe or refractory asthma is generally thought to affect 1% to 5% of all patients with asthma and accounts for most asthma costs.[35–39] This phenotype is defined by inadequate asthma control despite a high dose of inhaled corticosteroids or the need for oral corticosteroids, often associated with other controller medication, such as LABA, leukotriene receptor antagonist, or theophylline.[40,41] By itself, this phenotype clearly points out the inability of corticosteroids to control disease expression in some patients with asthma. Early studies showed that these patients had consistent persistent eosinophilic or neutrophilic airway inflammation despite regular antiinflammatory treatment,[42–46] indicating that corticosteroids were unable to control the underlying airway inflammation. These studies have certainly contributed to the emergence of the concept of an eosinophilic versus neutrophilic asthma phenotype, a concept that has extended beyond the sole group of refractory asthma (see later discussion). In severe asthma, this concept has proved to be useful in asthma management. It was clearly demonstrated that persistent eosinophilic inflammation may still be responsive to an increase in the dose of inhaled or systemic corticosteroids in terms of lung function and symptom improvement[47] and chiefly in terms of the reduction of exacerbation.[48,49] These important studies point to a reduced sensitivity rather than to a real resistance to eosinophilic inflammation to corticosteroids. Reduced eosinophil apoptosis in induced sputum despite a high dose of inhaled corticosteroids was shown to be related to disease severity.[50] The molecular reason why severe eosinophilic inflammation may persist despite heavy treatment with corticosteroids remains unknown, but there are several molecular mechanisms for corticosteroid resistance in asthma.[51]

THE MOLECULAR CONCEPT OF CORTICOSTEROID RESISTANCE

It has been well demonstrated that corticosteroids have a positive interaction with β2-agonists at the molecular level. Indeed, corticosteroids increase the transcription of the β2-agonist receptor, resulting in increased expression of the receptor at the cell surface.[52,53] On the other hand, there is growing evidence to show that β2-agonists enhance the action of corticosteroids, particularly through enhancing the translocation of glucocorticoid receptor (GR), therefore, increasing the binding of GR to the glucocorticoid response element at the gene level.[54] However, patients with severe asthma have a poor response to corticosteroids, even when combined to β2-agonists, which necessitates the need for high doses and a few patients are completely resistant. Patients with asthma who smoke are also relatively corticosteroid resistant and require increased doses of corticosteroids for asthma control.[55] Several molecular mechanisms have now been identified to account for corticosteroid resistance in severe asthma.[51] In smoking patients with asthma and patients with severe asthma, there is a reduction in activity and expression of the critical nuclear enzyme histone deacetylase-2, which prevents corticosteroids from switching off activated inflammatory genes.[56–58] In steroid-resistant asthma, other mechanisms may also contribute to corticosteroid insensitivity, including the reduced translocation of GR as a result of phosphorylation by p38 mitogen-activated protein (MAP) kinase[59] and abnormal histone acetylation patterns.[60] A proposed mechanism is an increase in GR-β, which prevents GR binding to DNA,[61] but there is little evidence that this would be sufficient to account for corticosteroid insensitivity because the amounts of GR-β are too low.[62] Th17 cells may be involved in driving neutrophilic inflammation in some patients with severe asthma and these cells seem to be largely corticosteroid resistant.[63,64]

COMPLEMENTARY TREATMENT TO CORTICOSTEROIDS IN REFRACTORY ASTHMA

Although abundantly used in COPD, tiotropium has been poorly validated in asthma treatment. A recent study conducted in patients with uncontrolled asthma, despite a moderate dose of inhaled beclomethasone, showed that tiotropium was at least equivalent to salmeterol in improving asthma lung function and symptoms.[65] Further studies focusing on patients with more severe asthma and looking at exacerbations as the major outcome are now warranted to validate the use of a long-acting anticholinergic in refractory asthma.

In those patients with refractory asthma, with moderately elevated total serum IgE and sensitization to a perennial allergen, omalizumab, a humanized monoclonal antibody against IgE, has proved to be effective in reducing the exacerbation rate and improving quality of life,[66,67] although part of the effect seen in clinical practice in quality-of life-improvement is likely to be caused by a placebo effect and a careful follow-up of patients inherent in the mode of drug administration.[68] Like for corticosteroids, the clinical benefit of omalizumab might be partly explained by a reduction of eosinophilic inflammation.[69,70] The major drawback of this currently available treatment is the high cost, which weakens the cost-effectiveness relationship.[71] Cost-effectiveness, however, depends on how hospitalization for exacerbation may be prevented; a drug that may reduce the hospitalization rate in high-risk patient is likely to be cost-effective.

Some studies indicate a continuous synthesis and release of Th2 cytokines, such as IL-4 and IL-5, both at a systemic[72] and airway level[73] despite the regular treatment with inhaled corticoids. Yet there is no sign of reduced activity of corticosteroids in vitro to inhibit cytokine release from circulating leukocytes in those patients with refractory asthma.[72] The importance of IL-5 in driving the persistent systemic and airway eosinophilic inflammation has recently been demonstrated by the efficacy of mepolizumab, an anti–IL-5 monoclonal antibody, to further decrease eosinophilic inflammation in those patients with refractory asthma despite a high dose of corticosteroids.[74,75] The clinical relevance of the persistent eosinophilic inflammation is demonstrated by the reduction in the exacerbation rate and the improvement in quality of life observed in those patients receiving mepolizumab,[74] even if no effect is observed on airway caliber and bronchial hyperresponsiveness,[74] which is confirmatory of earlier studies with other anti–IL-5 antibodies.[76,77] Importantly, mepolizumab made it possible to taper and sometimes suppress the use of oral corticosteroids.[75] A recent 16-week study using reslizumab, a new monoclonal antibody against IL-5, has shown a significant improvement in forced expiratory volume in the first second of expiration in patients with moderate to severe eosinophilic asthma displaying prominent reversibility to a β2-agonist.[78]

Anti–tumor necrosis factor (TNF)-α is an established treatment in chronic inflammatory diseases, like Crohn disease or rheumatoid arthritis. Despite early promising pilot studies,[79–82] treatments that target TNF-α have generally proved to be disappointing in improving asthma control in patients with refractory asthma. This finding has been demonstrated with drugs, such as golimumab[83] and etanercept.[84]

The studies focusing on neutrophilic inflammation in refractory asthma have been limited so far. One study using clarithromycin has shown a significant reduction of sputum neutrophil count and sputum elastase together with an improved quality of life.[85] However, there was no improvement in asthma control or airway caliber. On the other hand, targeting neutrophils may theoretically prove to be a dangerous strategy in patients with refractory asthma by increasing their susceptibility to infections.[86] A recent study in COPD, another disease with prominent neutrophilic inflammation,[87,88] has shown a reduction of the exacerbation rate by regular treatment with azithromycin.[89] The mechanisms by which macrolide antibiotics might be effective remain elusive. Whether it is through antiinflammatory activity or by limiting airway colonization with typical or atypical bacterial pathogens remains to be investigated.[90] Clearly, in refractory asthma, further studies conducted on a longer-term period are needed to investigate the impact of macrolides on asthma exacerbation rate. Other treatments in development, mainly for COPD, also target neutrophilic inflammation, including antagonists against the chemokine receptor CXCR2, phosphodiesterase-4 inhibitors, and p38 MAP kinase inhibitors.[91]

Bronchial thermoplasty (BT) is an innovative nonpharmacologic treatment approach to reduce the bronchoconstrictor response in asthma. Although technically demanding, BT has been shown to improve asthma control and quality of life and to be safe in patients with moderate to severe asthma.[92–94] A recent multicenter study confirmed the ability of BT to improve control and quality of life in patients with refractory asthma and showed that BT resulted in a reduced severe exacerbation rate in the posttreatment period.[95]

EMERGENCE OF THE CONCEPT OF ASTHMA PHENOTYPE IN MILD TO MODERATE ASTHMA

The development of the technique of induced sputum has been a key step in the appearance of the concept of inflammatory phenotype in asthma. Although it confirmed the eosinophilic inflammation as a prominent feature of asthma,[96] which relates to disease severity,[43,50,72] it also showed that up to 50% of patients with asthma failed to exhibit this eosinophilic phenotype.[97,98] Almost half of them are characterized by intense neutrophilic inflammation[99] but the other half fails to show any abnormal granulocytic inflammation despite excessive lung function variability. The importance of these phenotypes is that the underlying molecular mechanisms are different. Although the eosinophilic phenotype is likely to reflect ongoing adaptive immunity in response to an allergen with Th2 cytokine IL-4, IL-5, and IL-13 playing a key role, the neutrophilic phenotype is thought to reflect innate immune system activation in response to pollutants or infectious agents.[100,101] Therefore, it is conceivable that the 2 phenotypes actually require different therapeutic molecular approaches.

Exhaled nitrous oxide (NO) is increased in patients with asthma[102] and particularly in those with eosinophilic inflammation.[103] A large-scale study conducted in routine has shown that a fractional exhaled NO threshold of around 40 ppb (measured at an exhaled flow of 50 mL/s) is predictive of eosinophilic inflammation in patients with asthma even though this threshold may be decreased by smoking and a high dose of ICS. The threshold was 27 ppb in smoking asthmatics and 28 ppb in those receiving at least 1000 µg/d of fluticasone (considered as high dose ICS). Moreover the threshold can be as low as 15 ppb in a non atopic smoking patient receiving high dose of ICS.[104] However, we lack an equivalent noninvasive marker for neutrophilic inflammation. The development of breath print by chromatography and mass spectrometry is a promising tool to approach these cellular phenotypes.

PREDICTING FACTORS OF CLINICAL RESPONSE TO CORTICOSTEROIDS

The results of large, randomized controlled clinical trials have perhaps masked for too long the fact that the response of ICS is variable in patients with asthma.[105] As pointed out earlier, the response to ICS is characterized by a high intraindividual repeatability and a high interindividual variability, with up to 40% of patients showing no short-term response to the treatment.[3] The presence of a persistent airway eosinophilic inflammation seems to be a good predicting factor for a short-term response to ICS.[105–109] Alternatively, a high exhaled NO level (>47 ppb according to the studies) is predictive of a good response to ICS in patients with chronic respiratory symptoms regardless of the disease label.[110] Furthermore, the presence of a Th2 cytokine profile in the airways seems to be needed to have rapid lung function improvement with ICS.[111] Even if a convincing response may be sometimes observed[112] in those with high exhaled NO (>33 ppb),[107] noneosinophilic asthma generally exhibits a limited response to ICS[113] and the response seems to be particularly poor in those patients exhibiting intense airway neutrophilic inflammation,[99] which is reminiscent of the inability of ICS to control airway inflammation in COPD.[114,115] A recent study has highlighted the importance of the genetic background in the improvement of lung function following chronic treatment with ICS. A functional variant of glucocorticosteroid transcript 1 gene was found to be associated with a decreased response to ICS in several randomized clinical trials.[116] In the studies published so far, the corticosteroid response has been assessed either by lung function or quality-of-life improvement over a short-term period (a few weeks). There is, however, a lack of evidence to support that denying treatment with ICS over a long-term period in some patients does not place them at risk of severe exacerbation. Clearly, new long-term prospective studies with asthma exacerbation as the main outcome are needed to clarify this important point.

CORTICOSTEROIDS IN CLINICAL PRACTICE

Like in many chronic diseases, poor compliance to maintenance treatment has been shown to be a major issue in asthma.[117] Poor inhalation technique is a further impediment in achieving a successful treatment with inhaled therapies in patients with asthma.[117] Because corticosteroids do not bring acute relief for asthma symptoms, it is likely to play a role in poor compliance. Although ICS have clearly demonstrated superior efficacy to leukotriene receptor antagonists with respect to most clinical outcomes in randomized controlled trials, a recent field study conducted in the United Kingdom has not confirmed this superiority in terms of asthma control.[118] The emergence of the SMART concept (Symbicort as a maintenance and relief therapy) has been an interesting paradigm that allows patients to inhale a dose of corticosteroids whenever he or she feels the need to use a rapid-acting bronchodilator. The concept that has been extensively validated in randomized controlled clinical trials[119] has also been shown to be valid in daily clinical practice.[120] The SMART approach has been shown to be particularly efficient in reducing the rate of severe asthma exacerbation.

NEW CLASS DRUG IN DEVELOPMENT

There are several new drugs for asthma currently in development that may be suited more for patients who do not respond well to corticosteroids.[91] Several cytokines are involved in the pathophysiology of asthma, including Th2 cytokines. Anti–IL-5 antibodies (mepolizumab, reslizumab) are currently in clinical trials for severe eosinophilic asthma that is resistant to corticosteroids, as discussed earlier. IL-13 is increased in severe asthma and causes corticosteroid resistance, so it is a logical target. Currently, anti–IL-13 antibodies, such as lebrikizumab, have been disappointing with little physiologic effect and no effect on symptoms or exacerbations.[121] Blocking antibodies to other cytokines, including IL-9, IL-25, IL-33, and thymus stromal lymphopoietin, are also in development for asthma. Small molecule antagonists of inflammatory mediators have been disappointing in asthma, but there has recently been great interest in blocking prostaglandin (PG) D_2, which is released from mast cells and attracts Th2 cells and eosinophils via the receptor chemoattractant homologous receptor expressed on Th2 cells (CRTH2) (or DP_2 receptors). PGD_2 seems to be increased in patients with severe asthma who are not controlled on inhaled therapy.[122] Several oral CRTH2 antagonists are now in development and have shown some clinical benefit.[123] As discussed earlier, there are several broad-spectrum antiinflammatory treatments that target neutrophilic inflammation, so they may be effective in patients with severe asthma who do not respond well to corticosteroid therapy.[124] Mast-cell activation is found in patients with severe asthma, suggesting that mast-cell inhibitors may be useful in these patients. As discussed earlier, omalizumab is useful in some patients with severe asthma and reduces exacerbations[66,67] but cannot be used in patients with high circulating IgE concentrations, so antibodies with a higher affinity are now in development. Other drugs that target mast cells include c-kit and Syk inhibitors.

SUMMARY

There is no doubt that ICS have led to considerably improved asthma control and reduced asthma mortality in the Western world over the last 2 decades. ICS are

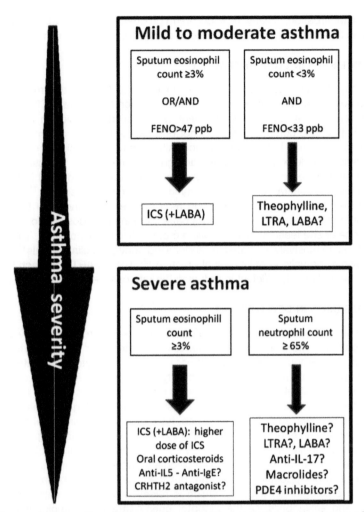

Fig. 1. Proposed strategy for asthma mainstay treatment according to the degree of severity and the sputum inflammatory phenotype. CRTH2, chemoattractant homologous receptor expressed on Th2 cells, also known as DP_2 receptor, a receptor for PGD_2; ICS, inhaled corticosteroids; LABA, long-acting β2-agonists; LTRA, leukotriene receptor antagonist; PDE4, phosphodiesterase 4 inhibitor.

particularly effective in combating Th2-driven inflammation featuring mast-cell and eosinophilic airway infiltration. Their effect on innate immunity-driven neutrophilic inflammation is poor and their ability to prevent airway remodeling and accelerated lung decline is highly controversial. Although ICS remain pivotal drugs in asthma management, research is needed to find drugs complementary to the combination ICS/LABA in refractory asthma and perhaps a new class of drugs as a first-line treatment in mild to moderate noneosinophilic asthma (**Fig. 1**).

ACKNOWLEDGMENTS

The work was supported by federal grant PAI P7/30 Aireway II. We also thank Anne Chevremont for excellent technical assistance.

REFERENCES

1. Barnes PJ. Will it be steroids for ever? Clin Exp Allergy 2005;35:843–5.
2. Global strategy for asthma management and prevention: NHLBI/WHO workshop report March 1993. National Institutes of Health; 2002. Publication number 95–36–59 issued January 1995.
3. Drazen JM, Silverman EK, Lee TH. Heterogeneity of therapeutic responses in asthma. Br Med Bull 2000;56:1054–70.
4. Brown HM, Storey G, George WH. Beclomethasone dipropionate: a new steroid aerosol for the treatment of allergic asthma. Br Med J 1972;1:585–90.
5. Gaddie J, Petrie GR, Reid IW, et al. Aerosol beclomethasone dipropionate: a dose-response study in chronic bronchial asthma. Lancet 1973;2:280–1.
6. Kriz RJ, Chmelik F, doPico G, et al. A short-term double-blind trial of aerosol triamcinolone acetonide in steroid-dependent patients with severe asthma. Chest 1976;69:455–60.
7. Gerdtham UG, Hertzman P, Jonsson B, et al. Impact of inhaled corticosteroids on acute asthma hospitalization in Sweden 1978 to 1991. Med Care 1996;34: 1188–98.
8. Blais L, Ernst P, Boivin JF, et al. Inhaled corticosteroids and the prevention of re-admission to hospital for asthma. Am J Respir Crit Care Med 1998;158:126–32.
9. Suissa S, Ernst P, Benayoun S, et al. Low-dose inhaled corticosteroids and the prevention of death from asthma. N Engl J Med 2000;343:332–6.
10. Haahtela T, Jarvinen M, Kava T, et al. Comparison of a beta 2-agonist, terbutaline, with an inhaled corticosteroid, budesonide, in newly detected asthma. N Engl J Med 1991;325:388–92.
11. Djukanovic R, Roche WR, Wilson JW, et al. Mucosal inflammation in asthma. Am Rev Respir Dis 1990;142:434–57.
12. Kay AB. Allergy and allergic diseases. First of two parts. N Engl J Med 2001; 344:30–7.
13. Corrigan C. The eotaxins in asthma and allergic inflammation: implications for therapy. Curr Opin Investig Drugs 2000;1:321–8.
14. Djukanovic R, Wilson JW, Britten KM, et al. Effect of an inhaled corticosteroid on airway inflammation and symptoms in asthma. Am Rev Respir Dis 1992;145: 669–74.
15. Laitinen LA, Laitinen A, Haahtela T. A comparative study of the effects of an inhaled corticosteroid, budesonide, and a beta 2-agonist, terbutaline, on airway inflammation in newly diagnosed asthma: a randomized, double-blind, parallel-group controlled trial. J Allergy Clin Immunol 1992;90:32–42.
16. Aldridge RE, Hancox RJ, Robin TD, et al. Effects of terbutaline and budesonide on sputum cells and bronchial hyperresponsiveness in asthma. Am J Respir Crit Care Med 2000;161:1459–64.
17. Fahy JV, Boushey HA. Effect of low-dose beclomethasone dipropionate on asthma control and airway inflammation. Eur Respir J 1998;11:1240–7.
18. Jatakanon A, Lim S, Chung KF, et al. An inhaled steroid improves markers of airway inflammation in patients with mild asthma. Eur Respir J 1998;12:1084–8.
19. van Rensen EL, Straathof KC, Veselic-Charvat MA, et al. Effect of inhaled steroids on airway hyperresponsiveness, sputum eosinophils, and exhaled nitric oxide levels in patients with asthma. Thorax 1999;54:403–8.
20. Meijer RJ, Kerstjens HA, Arends LR, et al. Effects of inhaled fluticasone and oral prednisolone on clinical and inflammatory parameters in patients with asthma. Thorax 1999;54:894–9.

21. Corrigan CJ, Haczku A, Gemou-Engesaeth V, et al. CD4 T-lymphocyte activation in asthma is accompanied by increased serum concentrations of interleukin-5. Effect of glucocorticoid therapy. Am Rev Respir Dis 1993;147:540–7.

22. Lilly CM, Nakamura H, Kesselman H, et al. Expression of eotaxin by human lung epithelial cells: induction by cytokines and inhibition by glucocorticoids. J Clin Invest 1997;99:1767–73.

23. Maneechotesuwan K, Yao X, Ito K, et al. Suppression of GATA-3 nuclear import and phosphorylation: a novel mechanism of corticosteroid action in allergic disease. PLoS Med 2009;6:e1000076.

24. Pauwels RA, Pedersen S, Busse WW, et al. Early intervention with budesonide in mild persistent asthma: a randomised, double-blind trial. Lancet 2003;361:1071–6.

25. Pauwels RA, Lofdahl CG, Laitinen LA, et al. Long-term treatment with inhaled budesonide in persons with mild chronic obstructive pulmonary disease who continue smoking. European Respiratory Society Study on Chronic Obstructive Pulmonary Disease. N Engl J Med 1999;340:1948–53.

26. James AL, Palmer LJ, Kicic E, et al. Decline in lung function in the Busselton Health Study: the effects of asthma and cigarette smoking. Am J Respir Crit Care Med 2005;171:109–14.

27. Lange P, Parner J, Vestbo J, et al. 15-year follow-up study of ventilatory function in adults with asthma. N Engl J Med 1998;339:1194–200.

28. O'Byrne PM, Pedersen S, Busse WW, et al. Effects of early intervention with inhaled budesonide on lung function in newly diagnosed asthma. Chest 2006;129:1478–85.

29. Sont JK, Willems LN, Bel EH, et al. Clinical control and histopathologic outcome of asthma when using airway hyperresponsiveness as an additional guide to long-term treatment. The AMPUL Study Group. Am J Respir Crit Care Med 1999;159:1043–51.

30. Ward C, Pais M, Bish R, et al. Airway inflammation, basement membrane thickening and bronchial hyperresponsiveness in asthma. Thorax 2002;57:309–16.

31. Cokugras H, Akcakaya N, Seckin I, et al. Ultrastructural examination of bronchial biopsy specimens from children with moderate asthma. Thorax 2001;56:25–9.

32. Jenkins HA, Cool C, Szefler SJ, et al. Histopathology of severe childhood asthma: a case series. Chest 2003;124:32–41.

33. Davies DE, Wicks J, Powell RM, et al. Airway remodeling in asthma: new insights. J Allergy Clin Immunol 2003;111:215–25.

34. Grainge CL, Lau LC, Ward JA, et al. Effect of bronchoconstriction on airway remodeling in asthma. N Engl J Med 2011;364:2006–15.

35. Bateman ED, Boushey HA, Bousquet J, et al. Can guideline-defined asthma control be achieved? The Gaining Optimal Asthma Control study. Am J Respir Crit Care Med 2004;170:836–44.

36. Antonicelli L, Bucca C, Neri M, et al. Asthma severity and medical resource utilisation. Eur Respir J 2004;23:723–9.

37. Barnes PJ, Jonsson B, Klim JB. The costs of asthma. Eur Respir J 1996;9:636–42.

38. Godard P, Chanez P, Siraudin L, et al. Costs of asthma are correlated with severity: a 1-yr prospective study. Eur Respir J 2002;19:61–7.

39. Serra-Batlles J, Plaza V, Morejon E, et al. Costs of asthma according to the degree of severity. Eur Respir J 1998;12:1322–6.

40. Proceedings of the ATS workshop on refractory asthma: current understanding, recommendations, and unanswered questions. American Thoracic Society. Am J Respir Crit Care Med 2000;162:2341–51.

41. Chanez P, Wenzel SE, Anderson GP, et al. Severe asthma in adults: what are the important questions? J Allergy Clin Immunol 2007;119:1337–48.
42. Jatakanon A, Uasuf C, Maziak W, et al. Neutrophilic inflammation in severe persistent asthma. Am J Respir Crit Care Med 1999;160:1532–9.
43. Louis R, Lau LC, Bron AO, et al. The relationship between airways inflammation and asthma severity. Am J Respir Crit Care Med 2000;161:9–16.
44. Wenzel SE, Schwartz LB, Langmack EL, et al. Evidence that severe asthma can be divided pathologically into two inflammatory subtypes with distinct physiologic and clinical characteristics. Am J Respir Crit Care Med 1999; 160:1001–8.
45. ten Brinke A, Grootendorst DC, Schmidt JT, et al. Chronic sinusitis in severe asthma is related to sputum eosinophilia. J Allergy Clin Immunol 2002;109: 621–6.
46. The ENFUMOSA cross-sectional European multicentre study of the clinical phenotype of chronic severe asthma. European Network for Understanding Mechanisms of Severe Asthma. Eur Respir J 2003;22:470–7.
47. ten Brinke A, Zwinderman AH, Sterk PJ, et al. "Refractory" eosinophilic airway inflammation in severe asthma: effect of parenteral corticosteroids. Am J Respir Crit Care Med 2004;170:601–5.
48. Green RH, Brightling CE, McKenna S, et al. Asthma exacerbations and sputum eosinophil counts: a randomised controlled trial. Lancet 2002;360:1715–21.
49. Jayaram L, Pizzichini MM, Cook RJ, et al. Determining asthma treatment by monitoring sputum cell counts: effect on exacerbations. Eur Respir J 2006;27: 483–94.
50. Duncan CJ, Lawrie A, Blaylock MG, et al. Reduced eosinophil apoptosis in induced sputum correlates with asthma severity. Eur Respir J 2003;22:484–90.
51. Barnes PJ, Adcock IM. Glucocorticoid resistance in inflammatory diseases. Lancet 2009;373:1905–17.
52. Baraniuk JN, Ali M, Brody D, et al. Glucocorticoids induce beta2-adrenergic receptor function in human nasal mucosa. Am J Respir Crit Care Med 1997; 155:704–10.
53. Mak JC, Nishikawa M, Barnes PJ. Glucocorticosteroids increase beta 2-adrenergic receptor transcription in human lung. Am J Physiol 1995;268:L41–6.
54. Roth M, Johnson PR, Rudiger JJ, et al. Interaction between glucocorticoids and beta2 agonists on bronchial airway smooth muscle cells through synchronised cellular signalling. Lancet 2002;360:1293–9.
55. Thomson NC, Spears M. The influence of smoking on the treatment response in patients with asthma. Curr Opin Allergy Clin Immunol 2005;5:57–63.
56. Barnes PJ. Reduced histone deacetylase in COPD: clinical implications. Chest 2006;129:151–5.
57. Hew M, Bhavsar P, Torrego A, et al. Relative corticosteroid insensitivity of peripheral blood mononuclear cells in severe asthma. Am J Respir Crit Care Med 2006;174:134–41.
58. Ito K, Ito M, Elliott WM, et al. Decreased histone deacetylase activity in chronic obstructive pulmonary disease. N Engl J Med 2005;352:1967–76.
59. Irusen E, Matthews JG, Takahashi A, et al. p38 mitogen-activated protein kinase-induced glucocorticoid receptor phosphorylation reduces its activity: role in steroid-insensitive asthma. J Allergy Clin Immunol 2002;109:649–57.
60. Matthews JG, Ito K, Barnes PJ, et al. Defective glucocorticoid receptor nuclear translocation and altered histone acetylation patterns in glucocorticoid-resistant patients. J Allergy Clin Immunol 2004;113:1100–8.

61. Goleva E, Li LB, Eves PT, et al. Increased glucocorticoid receptor beta alters steroid response in glucocorticoid-insensitive asthma. Am J Respir Crit Care Med 2006;173:607–16.
62. Pujols L, Mullol J, Picado C. Alpha and beta glucocorticoid receptors: relevance in airway diseases. Curr Allergy Asthma Rep 2007;7:93–9.
63. Alcorn JF, Crowe CR, Kolls JK. TH17 cells in asthma and COPD. Annu Rev Physiol 2010;72:495–516.
64. McKinley L, Alcorn JF, Peterson A, et al. TH17 cells mediate steroid-resistant airway inflammation and airway hyperresponsiveness in mice. J Immunol 2008;181:4089–97.
65. Peters SP, Kunselman SJ, Icitovic N, et al. Tiotropium bromide step-up therapy for adults with uncontrolled asthma. N Engl J Med 2010;363:1715–26.
66. Hanania NA, Alpan O, Hamilos DL, et al. Omalizumab in severe allergic asthma inadequately controlled with standard therapy: a randomized trial. Ann Intern Med 2011;154:573–82.
67. Humbert M, Beasley R, Ayres J, et al. Benefits of omalizumab as add-on therapy in patients with severe persistent asthma who are inadequately controlled despite best available therapy (GINA 2002 step 4 treatment): INNOVATE. Allergy 2005;60:309–16.
68. Louis R. Anti-IgE: a significant breakthrough in the treatment of airway allergic diseases. Allergy 2004;59:698–700.
69. Djukanovic R, Wilson SJ, Kraft M, et al. Effects of treatment with anti-immunoglobulin E antibody omalizumab on airway inflammation in allergic asthma. Am J Respir Crit Care Med 2004;170:583–93.
70. van Rensen EL, Evertse CE, van Schadewijk WA, et al. Eosinophils in bronchial mucosa of asthmatics after allergen challenge: effect of anti-IgE treatment. Allergy 2009;64:72–80.
71. Wu AC, Paltiel AD, Kuntz KM, et al. Cost-effectiveness of omalizumab in adults with severe asthma: results from the Asthma Policy Model. J Allergy Clin Immunol 2007;120:1146–52.
72. Manise M, Schleich F, Gusbin N, et al. Cytokine production from sputum cells and blood leukocytes in asthmatics according to disease severity. Allergy 2010;65:889–96.
73. Cho SH, Stanciu LA, Holgate ST, et al. Increased interleukin-4, interleukin-5, and interferon-gamma in airway CD4+ and CD8+ T cells in atopic asthma. Am J Respir Crit Care Med 2005;171:224–30.
74. Haldar P, Brightling CE, Hargadon B, et al. Mepolizumab and exacerbations of refractory eosinophilic asthma. N Engl J Med 2009;360:973–84.
75. Nair P, Pizzichini MM, Kjarsgaard M, et al. Mepolizumab for prednisone-dependent asthma with sputum eosinophilia. N Engl J Med 2009;360:985–93.
76. Kips JC, O'Connor BJ, Langley SJ, et al. Effect of SCH55700, a humanized anti-human interleukin-5 antibody, in severe persistent asthma: a pilot study. Am J Respir Crit Care Med 2003;167:1655–9.
77. Leckie MJ, ten Brinke A, Khan J, et al. Effects of an interleukin-5 blocking monoclonal antibody on eosinophils, airway hyper-responsiveness, and the late asthmatic response. Lancet 2000;356:2144–8.
78. Castro M, Mathur S, Hargreave F, et al. Reslizumab for poorly controlled, eosinophilic asthma: a randomized, placebo-controlled study. Am J Respir Crit Care Med 2011;184:1125–32.
79. Berry MA, Hargadon B, Shelley M, et al. Evidence of a role of tumor necrosis factor alpha in refractory asthma. N Engl J Med 2006;354:697–708.

80. Howarth PH, Babu KS, Arshad HS, et al. Tumour necrosis factor (TNF alpha) as a novel therapeutic target in symptomatic corticosteroid dependent asthma. Thorax 2005;60:1012–8.
81. Morjaria JB, Chauhan AJ, Babu KS, et al. The role of a soluble TNF alpha receptor fusion protein (etanercept) in corticosteroid refractory asthma: a double blind, randomised, placebo controlled trial. Thorax 2008;63:584–91.
82. Erin EM, Leaker BR, Nicholson GC, et al. The effects of a monoclonal antibody directed against tumor necrosis factor-alpha in asthma. Am J Respir Crit Care Med 2006;174:753–62.
83. Wenzel SE, Barnes PJ, Bleecker ER, et al. A randomized, double-blind, placebo-controlled study of tumor necrosis factor-alpha blockade in severe persistent asthma. Am J Respir Crit Care Med 2009;179:549–58.
84. Holgate ST, Noonan M, Chanez P, et al. Efficacy and safety of etanercept in moderate-to-severe asthma: a randomised, controlled trial. Eur Respir J 2011; 37:1352–9.
85. Simpson JL, Powell H, Boyle MJ, et al. Clarithromycin targets neutrophilic airway inflammation in refractory asthma. Am J Respir Crit Care Med 2008;177:148–55.
86. Louis R, Djukanovic R. Is the neutrophil a worthy target in severe asthma and chronic obstructive pulmonary disease? Clin Exp Allergy 2006;36:563–7.
87. Keatings VM, Barnes PJ. Granulocyte activation markers in induced sputum: comparison between chronic obstructive pulmonary disease, asthma, and normal subjects. Am J Respir Crit Care Med 1997;155:449–53.
88. Moermans C, Heinen V, Nguyen M, et al. Local and systemic cellular inflammation and cytokine release in chronic obstructive pulmonary disease. Cytokine 2011;56:298–304.
89. Albert RK, Connett J, Bailey WC, et al. Azithromycin for prevention of exacerbations of COPD. N Engl J Med 2011;365:689–98.
90. Martinez FJ, Curtis JL, Albert R. Role of macrolide therapy in chronic obstructive pulmonary disease. Int J Chron Obstruct Pulmon Dis 2008;3:331–50.
91. Barnes PJ. New therapies for asthma: is there any progress? Trends Pharmacol Sci 2010;31:335–43.
92. Cox G, Thomson NC, Rubin AS, et al. Asthma control during the year after bronchial thermoplasty. N Engl J Med 2007;356:1327–37.
93. Cox G. Bronchial thermoplasty for severe asthma. Curr Opin Pulm Med 2011;17: 34–8.
94. Pavord ID, Cox G, Thomson NC, et al. Safety and efficacy of bronchial thermoplasty in symptomatic, severe asthma. Am J Respir Crit Care Med 2007;176: 1185–91.
95. Castro M, Rubin AS, Laviolette M, et al. Effectiveness and safety of bronchial thermoplasty in the treatment of severe asthma: a multicenter, randomized, double-blind, sham-controlled clinical trial. Am J Respir Crit Care Med 2010; 181:116–24.
96. Louis R, Sele J, Henket M, et al. Sputum eosinophil count in a large population of patients with mild to moderate steroid-naive asthma: distribution and relationship with methacholine bronchial hyperresponsiveness. Allergy 2002;57: 907–12.
97. Gibson PG, Simpson JL, Saltos N. Heterogeneity of airway inflammation in persistent asthma: evidence of neutrophilic inflammation and increased sputum interleukin-8. Chest 2001;119:1329–36.
98. Simpson JL, Scott R, Boyle MJ, et al. Inflammatory subtypes in asthma: assessment and identification using induced sputum. Respirology 2006;11:54–61.

99. Green RH, Brightling CE, Woltmann G, et al. Analysis of induced sputum in adults with asthma: identification of subgroup with isolated sputum neutrophilia and poor response to inhaled corticosteroids. Thorax 2002;57:875–9.

100. Anderson GP. Endotyping asthma: new insights into key pathogenic mechanisms in a complex, heterogeneous disease. Lancet 2008;372:1107–19.

101. Douwes J, Gibson P, Pekkanen J, et al. Non-eosinophilic asthma: importance and possible mechanisms. Thorax 2002;57:643–8.

102. Kharitonov SA, Yates D, Robbins RA, et al. Increased nitric oxide in exhaled air of asthmatic patients. Lancet 1994;343:133–5.

103. Berry MA, Shaw DE, Green RH, et al. The use of exhaled nitric oxide concentration to identify eosinophilic airway inflammation: an observational study in adults with asthma. Clin Exp Allergy 2005;35:1175–9.

104. Schleich FN, Seidel L, Sele J, et al. Exhaled nitric oxide thresholds associated with a sputum eosinophil count $\geq$3% in a cohort of unselected patients with asthma. Thorax 2010;65:1039–44.

105. Szefler SJ, Martin RJ, King TS, et al. Significant variability in response to inhaled corticosteroids for persistent asthma. J Allergy Clin Immunol 2002; 109:410–8.

106. Berry M, Morgan A, Shaw DE, et al. Pathological features and inhaled corticosteroid response of eosinophilic and non-eosinophilic asthma. Thorax 2007; 62:1043–9.

107. Cowan DC, Cowan JO, Palmay R, et al. Effects of steroid therapy on inflammatory cell subtypes in asthma. Thorax 2010;65:384–90.

108. Meijer RJ, Postma DS, Kauffman HF, et al. Accuracy of eosinophils and eosinophil cationic protein to predict steroid improvement in asthma. Clin Exp Allergy 2002;32:1096–103.

109. Pavord ID, Brightling CE, Woltmann G, et al. Non-eosinophilic corticosteroid unresponsive asthma. Lancet 1999;353:2213–4.

110. Smith AD, Cowan JO, Brassett KP, et al. Exhaled nitric oxide: a predictor of steroid response. Am J Respir Crit Care Med 2005;172:453–9.

111. Woodruff PG, Modrek B, Choy DF, et al. T-helper type 2-driven inflammation defines major subphenotypes of asthma. Am J Respir Crit Care Med 2009; 180:388–95.

112. Godon P, Boulet LP, Malo JL, et al. Assessment and evaluation of symptomatic steroid-naive asthmatics without sputum eosinophilia and their response to inhaled corticosteroids. Eur Respir J 2002;20:1364–9.

113. Bacci E, Cianchetti S, Bartoli M, et al. Low sputum eosinophils predict the lack of response to beclomethasone in symptomatic asthmatic patients. Chest 2006; 129:565–72.

114. Culpitt SV, Maziak W, Loukidis S, et al. Effect of high dose inhaled steroid on cells, cytokines, and proteases in induced sputum in chronic obstructive pulmonary disease. Am J Respir Crit Care Med 1999;160:1635–9.

115. Keatings VM, Jatakanon A, Worsdell YM, et al. Effects of inhaled and oral glucocorticoids on inflammatory indices in asthma and COPD. Am J Respir Crit Care Med 1997;155:542–8.

116. Tantisira KG, Lasky-Su J, Harada M, et al. Genomewide association between GLCCI1 and response to glucocorticoid therapy in asthma. N Engl J Med 2011;365:1173–83.

117. Cochrane MG, Bala MV, Downs KE, et al. Inhaled corticosteroids for asthma therapy: patient compliance, devices, and inhalation technique. Chest 2000; 117:542–50.

118. Price D, Musgrave SD, Shepstone L, et al. Leukotriene antagonists as first-line or add-on asthma-controller therapy. N Engl J Med 2011;364:1695–707.
119. Barnes PJ. Scientific rationale for using a single inhaler for asthma control. Eur Respir J 2007;29:587–95.
120. Louis R, Joos G, Michils A, et al. A comparison of budesonide/formoterol maintenance and reliever therapy vs. conventional best practice in asthma management. Int J Clin Pract 2009;63:1479–88.
121. Corren J, Lemanske RF, Hanania NA, et al. Lebrikizumab treatment in adults with asthma. N Engl J Med 2011;365:1088–98.
122. Balzar S, Fajt ML, Comhair SA, et al. Mast cell phenotype, location, and activation in severe asthma. Data from the Severe Asthma Research Program. Am J Respir Crit Care Med 2011;183:299–309.
123. Pettipher R, Hansel TT, Armer R. Antagonism of the prostaglandin D2 receptors DP1 and CRTH2 as an approach to treat allergic diseases. Nat Rev Drug Discov 2007;6:313–25.
124. Barnes PJ. New molecular targets for the treatment of neutrophilic diseases. J Allergy Clin Immunol 2007;119:1055–62.

Childhood Asthma
Considerations for Primary Care Practice and Chronic Disease Management in the Village of Care

Michael P. Rosenthal, MD

KEYWORDS

- Asthma • Chronic disease • Care coordination • Patient-centered medical home
- Community intervention

KEY POINTS

- The example of childhood asthma can help us to understand the importance of the awareness of the many social, economic, environmental, behavioral, and cultural aspects of care that contribute to better health outcomes.
- Our ability to be more successful as primary care providers can be greatly enhanced by building connections to, integrating with, and incorporating community-based supports and approaches to care for our patients.
- Successful "community-included" approaches to childhood asthma may also serve as examples for other chronic disease care.

INTRODUCTION

Primary care practice development and related considerations for approaches to chronic disease management are significant topics in this era of rapid change in health care. The burden of chronic disease in the United States has been increasing, and there has been an increased recognition of the need for primary care to address this problem.[1] Interacting issues (the chronic disease model of care, the patient-centered medical home [PCMH], the Patient Centered Affordable Care Act) have developed during the past decade have led to an increased recognition of the need for an advanced model of primary care to improve the health of patients in the context of their families, homes, and communities.[2,3]

This article presents a practical question-oriented approach to considerations for chronic disease care, using childhood asthma as an example, to help primary care

This article originally appeared in Primary Care: Clinics in Office Practice, Volume 39, Issue 2, June 2012.

The author has nothing to disclose.

Department of Family and Community Medicine, Christiana Care Health System, 1400 North Washington Street, Suite 420, Wilmington, DE 19801, USA

E-mail address: mrosenthal@christianacare.org

http://dx.doi.org/10.1016/j.ccol.2014.09.012

providers (PCPs) appreciate the wide-ranging concept of advanced primary care. How do primary care practices develop efforts within the context of a PCMH that can be linked to community-based efforts for addressing chronic disease care? Also, specifically, how does a PCP envision the role of an individual practice in the practice neighborhood (community)?[4] There is a stated need and new emphasis for PCPs to not only consider a transformed model of care in a PCMH but also shift the paradigm from an individual practice and one-on-one care to population-based approaches, with coordination and integration of care in the medical neighborhood.[4] The neighborhood of the medical system includes specialists, health care institutions, and health care teams, and PCPs need to help patients navigate the system to ensure that plans of all entities are coordinated and work together as a whole for patients' health care needs.[4] Importantly, the neighborhood can and likely should be extended to include developing better relationships and supports through community services.[4] PCPs need to consider a new paradigm of care that includes population-based approaches, positioning their practice efforts within a broader context of health care at a community level and developing a community-included system integration model of care for chronic diseases.

However, as much as there is a developing emphasis on providing a supportive primary care environment and PCMH, it is important to recognize that the real medical home is the patient's home. In other words, using the example of childhood asthma, children and their families must be seen as central to addressing their issues in care and to making health care most effective. We need to find new and innovative ways to reach children and their families, via a potential array of community-based services and supports, and work with them to improve care.

This article highlights the value of community-based contributions to childhood asthma care and discusses how that value might be linked to evolving practice and health system needs. It underscores the concept of enhancing practice connections to local community services to build a local "village of care."

QUESTION 1: WHY DOES THIS RELATE TO MY PRACTICE AND THE CARE I PROVIDE

Traditional medical training, in both medical school and primary care residencies, has emphasized care of the individual patient. Even when the context of patient care has been expanded to the understanding of inclusion of the family within the home and the home environment, there has been a disconnection, much more often than not, from the consideration of the people living in their community, the village of care. The community has its own culture, attitudes, and beliefs about health and health care. Those attributes provide the community with an enormous potential to influence the attitudes, education, medical literacy, behaviors, and health actions of the individuals who live within it. Many community-based efforts can influence health care via community-based organizations and institutions (eg, schools, health care institutions, advocacy agencies). Furthermore, the community establishes the environment for living and health care through policies (eg, outdoor air quality, smoking in public venues, housing standards) that affect those who live within it.

QUESTION 2: WHY SHOULD WE USE CHILDHOOD ASTHMA TO CONSIDER A MODEL OF ADVANCED PRIMARY CARE

Despite a redefinition of the approach to and care for childhood asthma more than 2 decades ago (eg, routine use of anti-inflammatory medications, such as inhaled corticosteroids for persistent asthma) under the National Asthma Education and Prevention Program (NAEPP), the incidence of childhood asthma has increased to historically high levels and disparities in care remain high.[5–7] Furthermore, high rates of emergency department (ED) visits and hospitalizations indicate a lack of control of this disease from a population perspective.[5–8]

Childhood asthma presents an excellent opportunity to understand control and management of a chronic disease from a broad-based advanced primary care perspective. It has a multifactorial nature related to indoor and external environments; it produces intermittent challenges through unpredictable exacerbations; and, as a health system, we are falling short in consistently reaching and caring for those who are most at risk.

It is apparent that the burden of childhood asthma remains extraordinarily high, even in the face of a better understanding of the disease process, improved medications, and more expenditures on care in the medical system. Primary care efforts are underutilized and have not been well coordinated with EDs and hospital care.[8] Community-based services and supports may be available, but they are not routinely coordinated with practice-based efforts. Fragmentation of care in the medical system is high, and care coordination is, on the whole, lacking.[9,10] There is significant room and an imperative for improvement. An advanced model of primary care, which leads to a higher degree of patient- and family-centered support, partnerships in care, integration of health services, care coordination, and improved understanding and self-management abilities, has the potential to make an enormous difference.[2]

QUESTION 3: WHY IS IT IMPORTANT TO CONTROL CHILDHOOD ASTHMA

Childhood asthma is frequently underappreciated in terms of its effect on children, families, and the costs of health care. It is the most prevalent chronic disease in children and causes absenteeism from school (a marker for poor school performance), missed workdays for parents, and lost productivity for employers.[5–7,11–13] Costs of medical care related to unnecessary or excessive ED visits are high, as well as hospitalizations for children with uncontrolled asthma. In the United States by 2007, for all types of asthma, an estimated $56 billion was spent on medical costs, lost school days and workdays, and early deaths.[13,14]

The prevalence of asthma continues to increase.[14] Childhood asthma has also been found to be significantly higher in poor children and in those from minority populations. Among all children younger than 18 years, the prevalence in 2009 was 9.6% nationally but was highest among poor children (13.5%) and non-Hispanic black children (17%). In addition, disparities in care are apparent; mortality rates in black children are 6 times higher than that in white children.[13,15]

QUESTION 4: WHY HAS IT BEEN DIFFICULT TO CONTROL CHILDHOOD ASTHMA

Asthma is a multifactorial illness with a variety of causes and triggers. Identification and removal of triggers can be problematic. Common triggers and/or environmental irritants may include outdoor air quality (pollution, fumes), indoor air quality, environmental tobacco smoke, mold, pets, rodents, dust, and many others.[5,6,9]

Furthermore, the transient intermittent nature of childhood asthma often results in decreased understanding and underestimation of the disease or its importance.[7,11,12] Children, parents, and providers alike may be caught in the trap of lines of thought such as "this is only a mild case of asthma," "it's normal to have a little shortness of breath," or "this is just reactive airway disease, it's nothing severe." Many patients and families accept short of breath or wheezing as a normal part of having asthma. This relative lack of appreciation for the seriousness of the disease and need for control may result in lack of visits for primary care (because the asthma is perceived to be "stable") and/or decreased adherence by children/families. Costs of medications and insurance coverage for needed medications are also responsible for decreased control. In a fragmented health system with incomplete insurance coverage, many children do not have primary providers, or do not routinely see them, and their parents are often unsure of when to get assistance or where to turn during an exacerbation or attack.[5–9]

In addition, providers may be unaware that they play a role in the underappreciation and undertreatment of childhood asthma. Despite years of national recommendations and specific guidelines under the NAEPP to prescribe anti-inflammatory medications for childhood asthma beyond mild status, many providers do not do so on a routine basis.[5–7,16] Moreover, some providers are reluctant to provide a diagnosis of asthma because they do not want to label a patient, but this may actually do patients a disservice; referring to childhood asthma as multiple episodes of reactive airway disease or bronchitis may delay appropriate treatment because it builds into the belief that the patients/families are not dealing with a significant disease. In fact, it is important to improve partnerships between patients, families, and providers.[5–7,16,17] Structured provider education on caring for children with asthma has been shown to be beneficial in improving outcomes without needing to increase provider office time.[16,17] Directly communicating the diagnosis of asthma with children and families to help them appreciate the nature of the disease and accept the need for care and support, as well as providing specific clear recommendations, have been show to decrease asthma symptoms, acute office visits, ED use, and hospitalizations.[16,17]

It would be beneficial for children with asthma and their families if providers establish Asthma Action Plans (AAPs). There are several forms of AAPs that can be easily included in office practice to provide medications and document approaches at times of asthma exacerbations (**Fig. 1**).[18,19] AAPs also provide a mechanism for building patient-provider communication and partnerships; help in documentation; and, because they can "travel" with the patient, serve as a "vehicle" to build consistency among multiple providers and sites of care.[18] Importantly, AAPs are not routinely prescribed by many providers, and, even if they are, they may not be used.[14] AAPs, as part of an overall approach to education about asthma care and services, may be beneficial to improving asthma outcomes.[10,20]

QUESTION 5: HOW DOES THE AFFORDABLE CARE ACT APPLY TO THESE CONSIDERATIONS FOR CHILDHOOD ASTHMA AND CHRONIC DISEASE CARE

The Patient Protection and Affordable Care Act (ACA), signed into law in March, 2010, will have far-reaching effects for fostering change in primary care practice. Emphasis is placed on "reaching" the practice population at risk, electronic health records with "meaningful use," developing patient registries (eg, all children in a practice with asthma), coordination of care, and incentives for improved patient outcomes, and there is an expanded emphasis on community-based care. These emphases of the ACA fit into the developing concept of the PCMH.[2,3]

In many locales, care for childhood asthma, the most prevalent chronic disease in children, serves as a quality indicator for tracking and outcomes under meaningful use. Capitated rates or bundled payments from health insurers to control costs will need to include broad-based strategies for reaching children and families to keep their asthma under control and prevent unnecessary or excessive ED visits and hospitalizations. Developing effective practice strategies that are well integrated with community efforts fosters increased communication among patients and providers, more effective care coordination via integration of care and support services, improved access

Asthma Action Plan

(To be completed by Doctor/Nurse)

ALLIES AGAINST ASTHMA

Name	Birth Date	Effective Date

School	Parent/Guardian	Parent's Phone

Doctor/Nurse's Name	Doctor/Nurse's Office Phone

Emergency Contact After Parent	Contact Phone

Asthma Severity: ☐ Mild Intermittent   ☐ Mild Persistent   ☐ Moderate Persistent   ☐ Severe Persistent

Asthma Triggers: ☐ Colds   ☐ Exercise   ☐ Animals   ☐ Dust   ☐ Smoke   ☐ Food   ☐ Weather   ☐ Other: _____

TAKE THESE MEDICINES EVERYDAY (Green)

Child feels good:
- Breathing is good
- No cough or wheeze
- Can work/play
- Sleeps all night

MEDICINE:	HOW MUCH:	WHEN TO TAKE IT:

Peak flow in this area: _____ to _____

20 MINUTES BEFORE EXERCISE USE THIS MEDICINE:

IF NOT FEELING WELL   TAKE EVERYDAY MEDICINES AND (ADD) THESE RESCUE MEDICINES (Yellow)

Child has any of these:
- Cough
- Wheeze
- Tight Chest

MEDICINE:	HOW MUCH:	WHEN TO TAKE IT:

Peak flow in this area: _____ to _____

Call your doctor/nurse's office if the symptoms don't improve in 2 days OR if the flare lasts for longer than ___ days. After _____ days go back to GREEN ZONE and take everyday medications as instructed.

IF FEELING VERY SICK CALL THE DOCTOR OR NURSE NOW!   TAKE THESE MEDICINES (Red)

Child has any of these:
- Medicine not helping
- Breathing is hard and fast
- Lips and fingernails are blue
- Can't walk or talk well

MEDICINE:	HOW MUCH:	WHEN TO TAKE IT:

Peak flow below: _____

IF UNABLE TO CONTACT YOUR DOCTOR OR NURSE:
Call 911 or go to the nearest emergency room and bring this form with you!

I give permission to the doctor, nurse, health plan, and other health care providers to share information about my child's asthma to help improve the health of my child.

Parent/Guardian Signature	Date

Health Care Provider Signature

Adapted from the NYC Childhood Asthma Initiative
Adapted from the NHLBI
Printed 2004
To download additional forms go to: www.hpcpa.org

Fig. 1. Asthma Action Plan (AAP). This was developed by the Health Promotion Council (HPC) of Southeastern Pennsylvania with collaborating partners of the Philadelphia Allies Against Asthma Coalition. (*Courtesy of* Health Promotion Council, Philadelphia, PA; with permission.)

to care, more support at times of need, better asthma control, and decreased ED and hospital use.

QUESTIONS 6 AND 7: WHAT IS THE IMPORTANCE OF CHILDHOOD ASTHMA IN THE CONTEXT OF THE CHRONIC CARE MODEL AND HOW DO WE REACH THOSE WHO CANNOT BE REACHED

Plumb and colleagues in an article elsewhere in this issue discuss the importance of community-based partnerships for improving chronic disease management. The investigators emphasize the importance of expanding the Chronic Care Model developed by Wagner and colleagues to include community-based approaches to enable patients and families to become better, informed partners in care.[21–23] Furthermore, Plumb and colleagues develop the concept that the Social Ecology Model can provide the framework for integrating community partnerships and chronic disease management. Examples are provided regarding improved education and awareness and the opportunity for approaches to multiple chronic disease states.

From a PCPs' viewpoint, the considerations of working with community-based efforts may be seen as "not part of my practice" and "unrelated to my patients' care." However, if viewed in the context of the ACA, the importance of reaching an entire practice's population of patients or those with a certain disease state takes on new significance.[2,3] The provider's accountability for all patients in a practice with childhood asthma, a population-based consideration, is different from the individual accountability for the individual patient "seen in my office." Having a disease registry to identify and track patients who may not routinely visit the office implies the need to reach all patients and provide them needed care and services, but any practice may be limited by its resources and ability to bring patients to its "PCMH."

Furthermore, PCPs are often disappointed in their ability to influence their patients' care. PCPs' impact on the daily lives of patients may be limited, and they often wrestle with the difficulty of helping patients become informed partners in care. This is not surprising when considering that most patients spend a maximum of only a few hours, total, each year within a practice seeing their provider and/or staff, even in a well-developed PCMH.

Including community efforts to help patients become informed partners in care, enhanced by community-based programs and education, developed and administered in the context of people's lives, where they live and what they do, may be a great help. In addition, educators, health workers, and other health care personnel, working in the home or community, may be in an advantageous position to develop influential relationships with children and their families to improve understanding, build positive attitudes, promote healthy behaviors, and enhance self-care.

More traditional views of medical education and care may raise questions about the evidence regarding community-based approaches and how they might be helpful in achieving outcomes in care. There is a growing evidence base, however, that such community-based approaches have been beneficial in addressing the burden of childhood asthma and are important to consider in building a more comprehensive and successful approach.[5,6]

QUESTION 8: WHAT HAVE WE LEARNED FROM COMMUNITY COALITION EXAMPLES TO ADDRESS THE BURDEN OF CHILDHOOD ASTHMA

Two national multisite projects (Allies Against Asthma, Robert Wood Johnson Foundation; Merck Childhood Asthma Network [MCAN], Merck Foundation),[13,24] developed via foundation support, provide examples and considerable insight into the ability of communities to form coalitions and collaborative approaches to address the burden of childhood asthma. The key tenet for both efforts relies on the capacity of a coalition or collaborative partnership to bring many local stakeholders together to form a unique entity with infrastructure support to focus on a common health care issue. Coalitions bring many experiences and perspectives together to identify discrepancies in health care, develop innovative approaches that cross traditional boundary lines, implement creative programs that reach many difficult-to-reach individuals, address health literacy, enhance coordination of care, integrate systems, influence policy, promote education and behavior change, and lead to improved health outcomes. Even though they were part of national efforts, the community site-specific efforts (discussed later) included local coalition/partnership formation and project development specific to the local community. Each national project had a coordinating center for approach, evaluation, periodic sharing of experiences among sites via telephone conferences and annual meetings, and a national expert advisory panel.[10,11,13,24]

The Robert Wood Johnson Foundation supported the Allies Against Asthma project from 2000 to 2004. This project required 2 key goals: to form a local coalition and to address the burden of childhood asthma in the community. Through a competitive grant application process, 7 communities (Long Beach, California; Kings County/Seattle, Washington; Philadelphia, Pennsylvania; Hampton Roads, Virginia; Washington, DC; Milwaukee, Wisconsin; and, San Juan, Puerto Rico) were chosen to undergo a planning year and subsequent 3-year intervention.[11] Lead institutions were identified, and plans for coalition infrastructure and development were proposed as part of each proposal. Every coalition progressed through stages of formation to the action of addressing the burden of childhood asthma in each community.[9,25] Allies Against Asthma was coordinated via a national program office at the University of Michigan in Ann Arbor.[11,24]

Multisite evaluation showed that the Allies Against Asthma project was successful in developing system and policy changes in all sites and contributing to broad-based childhood asthma care in its communities.[26] Local change and influences included a variety of approaches, developed by each community in response to its assessment and needs. Examples of interventions ranged from legislative outdoor air policy change (Long Beach) to redesigned and integrated health care delivery (Milwaukee) to incorporation of wide-scale community health worker education and care coordinator programs (Kings County), home care assessment and education (Philadelphia), physician and nurse education (Virginia), electronic data sharing and case coordination (Washington, DC), and community health worker coordination with nurses and provider teams (Puerto Rico).[9] In total, there were 89 policy or system changes in the 7 sites during the 3-year implementation phase of the project. Asthma symptoms were reduced in children who were involved in the coalition programs of Allies Against Asthma in comparison with a group of children who were not involved.[26] In addition, the Philadelphia Allies Against Asthma program established the Child Asthma Link Line (Link Line), an interactive telephonic care coordination system with asthma educators who provided basic asthma education and administrative links to care and support services for children who were primarily seen at ED visits.[9] The Link Line intervention was designed to get appropriate and timely support services and care from children and their families. This program decreased asthma morbidity as measured by decreased ED visits and hospitalizations for those who received the Link Line intervention in comparison with a matched group who did not; it demonstrated the ability of a coalition to implement a community-wide program to affect changes in end point outcomes of care.[27]

The Merck Foundation supports the MCAN. Five sites (New York, New York; Philadelphia, Pennsylvania; Chicago, Illinois; Los Angeles, California; and, San Juan, Puerto Rico) were chosen for the initial MCAN project, which ran from 2005 through 2009.[13] The MCAN national office in Washington, DC, coordinated the project that emphasized the need for coalitions or partnerships to identify children with asthma in their communities and provide them evidence-based interventions and care.[10,13,28,29] All sites were involved in aspects of system delivery change, implementation of care coordination at a community level, and inclusion of components from evidence-based interventions such as Yes We Can (a medical-social model of asthma care for children and families), the Inner-City Asthma Study Environmental Intervention, and the National Cooperative Inner-City Asthma Study.[28] The comprehensive cross-site evaluation of the programs demonstrated that the community-based care coordination achieved via MCAN efforts improved patient/family education, enhanced the processes of care, and significantly reduced morbidity as measured by ED visits and hospitalizations.[10,29]

QUESTION 9: HOW DO THESE EXPERIENCES WITH LARGE COMMUNITY COALITIONS RELATE TO DEVELOPING INTEGRATED PRACTICE AND COMMUNITY-BASED APPROACHES IN A LOCAL COMMUNITY ON A SMALLER SCALE

The community coalition experiences described earlier indicate the ability to assess community needs and bring stakeholders together to plan effective programs for childhood asthma care and services in a variety of communities. Every primary care practice exists within the context of its own community. The people or families that any practice serves are community members who are affected by the community's circumstances, economics, institutions, structure, supports, and services. Each practice has the opportunity to consider ways to build supports for its patients' care by working with community members, organizations, or institutions.

The coalitions mentioned had funding and infrastructure support for developing interventions. An individual practice might consider it difficult to become involved in integrating practice-based care with community efforts. On the other hand, the imperative of the PCMH movement and the ACA, based on a greater focus on health care for the US population, emphasizes the need for broader practice and population-based approaches to care in local practice.[2–4]

QUESTION 10: HOW DO WE LINK COMMUNITY-BASED APPROACHES WITH PRACTICE-BASED APPROACHES TO CARE

For the provider in primary care practice, it may seem beyond the scope of care to include community-based care and services in a practice-based approach. This article is intended to encourage thought about how to consider expanding the reach of care to create a more coordinated, comprehensive, and inclusive arrangement of practice and community-based services to support children with asthma, and their families, to improve outcomes in care. As the health system moves toward a higher degree of expectation regarding each practice's responsibility for its population of patients, population-based approaches to care, including involvement of community-based organizations, institutions, and services, become increasingly important.

Community providers and practices do not have the same infrastructure and support provided by the community coalitions described earlier. On the other hand, they do not need to have that level of support to begin building the bridges necessary to overcome the gap between practice and community efforts that is commonly seen.

Each practice has to assess its own needs as well as the opportunities for increasing community-based supports in its local environment. A thoughtful, steady, and practical effort, which builds relationships and collaborations, one step at a time, is more likely to succeed than overwhelmingly complex endeavors. Straightforward considerations that intend to building partnerships among patients, their families, community supports, and primary care practices are needed. Setting common goals with partners and working together to align strategies to achieve them are also more likely to predict success.

There are many ways to consider building a bridge. The following are a few among them: discuss a need for a comprehensive approach to childhood asthma in your community with health care agencies, institutions, and hospitals; coordinate efforts with other medical providers in your community; identify and contact community-based organizations that have programs and services for childhood asthma (eg, American Lung Association, grassroots advocacy groups); connect with schools (where children spend a majority of their time), as schools have a vested interest in lower absenteeism to improve scholastic performance; coordinate care with school nurses and provide education for children with asthma and their parents; work with housing professionals, local officials, public health, and/or other health-oriented community-based organizations; obtain materials and information about creating better home and school environment for children with asthma from the US Environmental Protection Agency and the Department of Health and Human Services; provide support for patients and families with education, information, and plans for care; and enhance access and availability in community practices, so children and their families can get to the site of care when needed.

The understanding that any one model will not work in every community is essential to achieving success. The best approach includes an assessment of local community needs and opportunities that can lead to thoughtful and creative plans to improve childhood asthma care and support. Care providers should define a specific intervention and implement it. This intervention could start with something that is reasonable and achievable. PCPs should learn from it, modify it as needed, and then build from there.

Most importantly, being actively involved in the development and inclusion of new approaches to primary care, in an enhanced and advanced model, supported and integrated with community efforts, can be extremely rewarding. Creating opportunities to promote an improved local system of patient- and family-centered health care can augment providers' accomplishments and sense of satisfaction, while improving health outcomes for patients that help them achieve a better quality of life.

SUMMARY

The example of childhood asthma can help us to understand the importance of the awareness of the many social, economic, environmental, behavioral, and cultural aspects of care that contribute to better health outcomes. The care for children with asthma depends on the many factors and influences of life beyond the office time spent with the children and their families or caregivers. Our ability to be more successful as PCPs will be greatly enhanced by building connections to, integrating with, and incorporating community-based supports and approaches to care for our patients.

Some PCPs may choose to be champions and look to directly become involved in building community-based contributions to care or influencing relevant policy change. Some may not. However, every provider can be proactive in developing a PCMH that better connects to and works with the many system supports available in our communities to foster better care, health outcomes, and quality of life for those who live in our village.

ACKNOWLEDGMENTS

The author acknowledges the many colleagues and partners who participated in the Robert Wood Johnson Foundation Allies Against Asthma Coalitions and the Merck Childhood Asthma Network of the Merck Foundation. Also appreciated are the efforts of the staff of the Health Promotion Council of Southeastern Pennsylvania, which served as the infrastructure organization supporting the Philadelphia Allies Against Asthma Coalition and the Philadelphia Merck Childhood Asthma Network Project.

REFERENCES

1. Starfield B, Shi L, Macinko J. Contribution of primary care to health systems and health. Milbank Q 2005;83(3):457–502.
2. Patient-Centered Primary Care Collaborative. Available at: http://www.pcpcc.net/. Accessed March 25, 2012.
3. The Patient Protection and Affordable Care Act. Available at: http://www.healthcare.gov/law/index.html. Accessed March 25, 2012.
4. Taylor EF, Lake T, Nysenbaum J, et al. Coordinating care in the medical neighborhood. AHRQ Publication No. 11–0064, 2011. Available at: www.ahrq.gov. Accessed March 25, 2012.
5. National Asthma Education and Prevention Program. Expert Panel Report 3 (EPR-3): Guidelines for the Diagnosis and Management of Asthma—Summary Report 2007. Report of the National Asthma Education and Prevention Program of the National Heart, Lung, and Blood Institute (NHLBI) of the National Institutes of Health, US Department of Health and Human Services. Bethesda, MD, August, 2007.
6. National Asthma Education and Prevention Program. Guidelines implementation panel report for Expert Panel Report 3—Guidelines for the Diagnosis and Management of Asthma. Partners Putting Guidelines into Action. Report of the National Asthma Education and Prevention Program of the National Heart, Lung, and Blood Institute (NHLBI) of the National Institutes of Health, US Department of Health and Human Services. Bethesda, MD, December, 2008.
7. Wechsler ME. Managing asthma in primary care: putting new guideline recommendations into context. Mayo Clin Proc 2009;84(8):707–17.
8. Baren JM, Boudreaux ED, Brenner BE, et al. Randomized controlled trial of emergency department interventions to improve primary care follow-up for patients with acute asthma. Chest 2006;129:257–65.
9. Rosenthal MP, Butterfoss FD, Doctor LJ, et al. The coalition process at work: building care coordination models to control chronic disease. Health Promot Pract 2006;7(Suppl 2):117S–26S.
10. Findley S, Rosenthal M, Bryant-Stephens T, et al. Community-based care coordination: practical applications for childhood asthma. Health Promot Pract 2011;12:52S.
11. Clark NM, Doctor L, Friedman AR, et al. Community coalitions to control chronic disease: Allies Against Asthma as a model and case study. Health Promot Pract 2006;7(Suppl 2):14S–22S.
12. Gupta RS, Weiss KB. The 2007 National Asthma Education and Prevention Program Asthma Guidelines: accelerating their implementation and facilitating their impact on children with asthma. Pediatrics 2009;123(Suppl 3):S193–8.
13. Merck Childhood Asthma Network. Available at: http://www.mcanonline.org/. Accessed March 25, 2012.
14. Centers for Disease Control and Prevention (CDC). Vital signs: asthma prevalence, disease, and self-management education: United States, 2001–2009. MMWR Morb Mortal Wkly Rep 2011;60(17):547–52.
15. Akinbami LJ, Moorman JE, Garbe PL, et al. Status of childhood asthma in the United States, 1980–2007. Pediatrics 2009;123(Suppl 3):S131–45.
16. Clark NM, Cabana M, Kaciroti N, et al. Long-term outcomes of physician peer teaching. Clin Pediatr (Phila) 2008;47(9):883–90.
17. Cabana MD, Slish KK, Evans D, et al. Impact of physician care education on patient outcomes. Pediatrics 2006;117(6):2149–57.

18. Pennsylvania Asthma Partnership. Available at: http://www.paasthma.org/. Accessed March 25, 2012.
19. National Heart Lung and Blood Institute, Asthma Action Plan. Available at: http://www.nhlbi.nih.gov/health/public/lung/asthma/asthma_actplan.htm. Accessed March 25, 2012.
20. Brouwer AF, Brand PL. Asthma education and monitoring: what has been shown to work. Paediatr Respir Rev 2008;9:193–200.
21. Wagner EH, Austin BT, Davis C, et al. Improving chronic illness care: translating evidence into action. Health Aff 2001;20:64–78.
22. Bodenheimer TM, Wagner EH, Grumbach KM. Improving primary care for patients with chronic illness. JAMA 2002;288:1775–9.
23. Bodenheimer TM, Wagner EH, Grumbach KM. Improving primary care for patients with chronic illness: the Chronic Care Model, part 2. JAMA 2002;288:1909–14.
24. Allies Against Asthma: The Center for Chronic Disease Management, University of Michigan. Available at: http://cmcd.sph.umich.edu/Allies-Against-Asthma.html. Accessed March 25, 2012.
25. Butterfoss FD, Gilmore LA, Krieger JW, et al. From formation to action: how allies against asthma coalitions are getting the job done. Health Promot Pract 2006; 6(Suppl 2):34S–43S.
26. Clark NM, Lachance L, Doctor LJ, et al. Policy and system change and community coalitions: outcomes from allies against asthma. Am J Public Health 2010; 5(100):904–12.
27. Coughey K, Klein G, West C, et al. The child asthma link line: a coalition-initiated, telephone-based, care coordination intervention for childhood asthma. J Asthma 2010;47(3):303–9.
28. Lara M, Bryant-Stephens T, Damitz M, et al. Balancing "Fidelity" and community context in the adaptation of asthma evidence-based interventions in the "Real World". Health Promot Pract 2011;12(Suppl 1):63S–72S.
29. Mansfield C, Viswanathan M, Woodell C, et al. Outcomes from a cross-site evaluation of a comprehensive pediatric asthma initiative incorporating translation of evidence-based interventions. Health Promot Pract 2011;12:34S.

Childhood Asthma
A Guide for Pediatric Emergency Medicine Providers

Sarah Kline-Krammes, MD, Nirali H. Patel, MD*,
Shawn Robinson, MD

KEYWORDS

- Asthma • Pediatrics • Emergency department • Asthma exacerbation
- Treatment and management

KEY POINTS

- Although the prevalence of asthma has remained stable, the financial impact of asthma management on the healthcare system remains significant.
- Pediatric asthma scores may facilitate the assessment and management of asthma exacerbations in the emergency room setting.
- The mainstay of treatment for asthma exacerbations include short acting beta agonists, corticosteroids, and ipratropium bromide.
- Patient and family education remains a cornerstone in the prevention and management of future asthma exacerbations.

INTRODUCTION

Asthma is a chronic inflammatory disease of the airways. The immunohistopathologic features of asthma are those of inflammation, and include neutrophils, eosinophils, mast cell activation, and epithelial cell damage.[1] This inflammation causes airway obstruction that is at least partially reversible with medications.

PREVALENCE

Asthma prevalence in children increased steadily from 1980 to 1995, when it peaked at 7.5% (**Fig. 1**). Since 1997, asthma prevalence has remained stable.[2] It affects every state, although the midwest, northeast, and southeast are disproportionately more affected than other regions of the United States. In addition, asthma affects minorities at a higher rate: Hispanic people have the highest risk and are 2.4 times more likely to

This article originally appeared in Emergency Medicine Clinics of North America, Volume 31, Issue 3, August 2013.
The authors have no financial relationship or conflicts of interest to disclose.
Department of Emergency Medicine, Akron Children's Hospital, 1 Perkins Square, Akron, OH 44308, USA
* Corresponding author.
E-mail address: npatel@chmca.org

Clinics Collections 2 (2014) 235–262
http://dx.doi.org/10.1016/j.ccol.2014.09.013
2352-7986/14/$ – see front matter

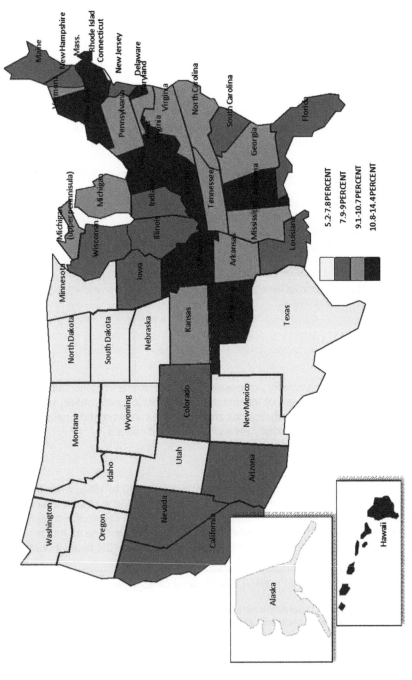

5.2-7.8 PERCENT
7.9-9.9 PERCENT
9.1-10.7 PERCENT
10.8-14.4 PERCENT

Fig. 1. United States: asthma prevalence 2007.

have asthma compared with the general pediatric population. African-Americans, Native Americans, and Native Aleutians are 1.6 and 1.3 times more likely to be affected with asthma. In addition, African-American children are 4 times more likely to die from asthma.[3]

Several theories exist to explain this discrepancy in prevalence. Children are more vulnerable to the effects of air pollution because their immune systems are still maturing and because they have increased minute ventilation per square meter of total body surface area compared with adults.[4] As air pollution of ozone, nitrogen dioxide, sulfur dioxide, and carbon monoxide increases, the odds of developing wheezing in children also increases.[5,6] In addition, the tendency for minorities to reside in densely populated urban regions and have increased exposure to higher levels of air pollution may be a contributing factor for their increase in asthma prevalence.

BURDEN OF DISEASE

The total cost to society of asthma is estimated at $56 billion dollars per year as of 2007. This cost includes morbidity productivity losses of $3.8 billion dollars and mortality productivity losses of $2.1 billion dollars.[7] In pediatrics, the cost of treating asthma is also high, especially if the child requires intubation. Nearly 50% of all children who are intubated for status asthmaticus experience a complication (most commonly aspiration pneumonia, pneumothorax, and pneumomediastinum), and these complications translate to a hospital cost of $117,000 versus $38,000 for a visit with no complications.[8] Most striking is the yearly cost of treating asthma per child. In 2005, the cost per year of health care for a child without asthma was $618. The same yearly cost of health care for a child with asthma was more than 60% higher, costing more than $1000.[9] In addition, asthma is the leading cause of missed school days.[10] Even if a child is not seeking care in a hospital setting, asthma may still affect a child's ability to participate in school and the ability to sleep.[11]

PATHOPHYSIOLOGY

Many studies have documented the relationship of histamine and/or leukotriene release with the inhalation of cold air, leading to bronchoconstriction.[12] However, this does not account for the increased prevalence of asthma in the warmer regions of the southeast United States. A study in 2012 by Hayes and colleagues[13] showed that bronchoconstriction increased among patients with asthma who inhaled hot air versus room air (112% vs 38% respectively) and was mediated by cholinergic reflexes that improved with use of ipratropium, suggesting an underlying seasonal or viral trigger.

Allergic asthma is considered to have a large inflammatory component. Allergens induce a cascade of events leading to interleukin release, mast cell degranulation, mucus hypersecretion, and neutrophilic inflammation, which ultimately contribute to steroid-resistant, severe asthma.[14]

Certain polymorphisms causing structural changes have been associated with an accelerated decrease in lung function with asthma.[15] Xiao and colleagues[16] reported that the bronchial epithelial wall in asthmatics seemed to be damaged such that allergens passed through the epithelial wall, leading to immune activation and asthma exacerbation. Likewise, Lopez-Guisa and colleagues[17] found that interleukin (IL) 3 and IL4 stimulated the production of transforming growth factor B2 and periostin, both of which promote airway remodeling.

Environment may have a contributing role in the development of asthma. Although the prevalence of asthma is increased in areas with high air pollution, a study conducted by Omland and colleagues[18] found that being born and raised on a farm with high allergen exposures reduced the risk of asthma versus being raised in rural, nonfarm environments. They also noted that exposure to dairy confinements, welding smoke, and tobacco smoke were all risk factors for asthma development. They therefore concluded that high exposure to potential allergens early in life may be protective against future development of asthma.

HISTORY

A detailed medical history is an important tool in the assessment of a wheezing child. Many children present to the emergency department (ED) with a first-time episode of wheezing. Although this is a common symptom of asthma, most of these children do not go on to develop asthma. A thorough history is essential in determining causes other than asthma in a first-time wheezing patient. Questions include age of patient, onset of symptoms, and associated symptoms. Sudden onset in symptoms may indicate foreign body aspiration (more common in toddlers with associated choking, cyanosis) or anaphylaxis (with associated urticaria, stridor, and hypotension). Fever with cough or congestion may indicate bronchiolitis (<2 years with first-time wheezing) or lower airway tract infection. More chronic symptoms such as failure to thrive, difficulty feeding, persistent wheezing, or failure to respond to short-acting beta agonists (SABAs) should concern the medical provider for underlying gastroesophageal reflux, cardiac disease/failure, thoracic masses, or cystic fibrosis. Historical clues that help distinguish those that are more suggestive of asthma are included in **Box 1**.[19,20] Patients with a congenital cause for wheezing (vascular rings, cystic lung malformations) usually have a history of wheezing since birth without response to traditional asthma therapies like SABAs and corticosteroids.[21]

When a patient with a history of asthma presents with wheezing, certain historical data can help characterize the underlying severity of asthma. This classification of asthma is based on current symptoms, use of SABAs, and interference with daily activity (**Table 1**).[1]

Common symptoms of an asthma exacerbation include cough, wheezing, and some degree of respiratory distress. Young children may manifest shortness of breath as decreased activity or vocalizations. To help determine the severity of the exacerbation, it is important to ascertain the current usage of SABAs; compliance with controller medications; and the delivery mode of the medications, including spacer use. Assessment of risk factors of near-fatal asthma is critical because this may change the management of the current exacerbation (**Box 2**).[22]

Predictors of severe asthma exacerbation remain multifactorial. A study in 2011 noted that experiencing persistent symptoms from asthma was related to having severe exacerbations; receiving inhaled corticosteroids (ICSs) was protective against a severe exacerbation. However, some predictors of a severe exacerbation were independent of persistent symptoms. These factors included young age, history of ED

Box 1
History suggestive of asthma

More than 1 episode of wheezing per month

Triggers for wheezing (allergen, exercise, smoke, upper respiratory illness)

Previous bronchodilator use including response to therapy

Family history of asthma (especially in first-degree relative)

Atopy (allergic rhinitis, atopic dermatitis, or food allergy)

visits or hospitalizations in the past year, and history of greater than or equal to 3 days of oral steroids in the prior 3 months. Thus, it is important to assess the underlying severity of disease as well as the risk of having a severe exacerbation.[23]

Recent studies have assessed the factors that may be associated with pediatric asthma-related ED visits. Previous studies indicated that age, race, insurance status, and average household income all played a role in predicting ED visits. However, a recent study showed that, after controlling for all variables, the only statistically significant predictor of a pediatric asthma-related ED visit was a previous asthma-related ED visit.[24]

PHYSICAL EXAMINATION

The physical examination of children with asthma brought to the ED begins with a rapid 30-second cardiopulmonary assessment as described by the American Heart Association.[25] This assessment helps with a quick determination of general appearance, airway patency, effectiveness of respiratory effort, and adequacy of circulation. Vitals signs are also helpful in assessment of severity of exacerbation. Children presenting with hypoxia (less than 92%) are more likely to require aggressive treatment and require hospital admission. Severe exacerbations cause tachypnea, tachycardia, and sometimes pulsus paradoxus. Accessory muscle usage is more likely to indicate a severe exacerbation. Severe retractions, especially supraclavicular retractions, indicate a forced expiratory volume less than 50% of predicted. Poor air movement found on chest auscultation is a sign of impending respiratory failure. Patients presenting with agitation or depressed mental status may be approaching respiratory failure.[21,22]

Wheezing is the most common symptom associated with asthma in children aged 5 years and younger. Cough caused by asthma may be recurrent and/or persistent and is usually accompanied by wheezing episodes and breathing difficulties. Shortness of breath that is recurrent or occurs during exercise increases the likelihood of asthma.[19] Cough-variant asthma can present as a dry harsh cough, usually worse at night; these patients often do not wheeze at all.

Physical examination findings can also help distinguish between other causes of cough and wheezing in children. Foreign body aspiration can present as unilateral wheezing. Wheezing secondary to a cardiac cause has hepatomegaly as an associated physical finding. Wheezing along with urticaria and uvular edema suggests anaphylaxis as the cause of wheezing. Wheezing along with signs of upper airway tract infection and fever indicates bronchiolitis.

ASTHMA SCORES

Pediatric asthma scores have been used to help classify severity of exacerbation. Most scores assess suprasternal retractions, air entry, and wheezing, and most also add respiratory rate and oxygen saturation. A study in 2008 showed that the Preschool Respiratory Assessment Measure (PRAM) was applicable to children between 2 and 17 years of age and was a feasible, reliable, valid, and responsive tool to measure asthma severity in a busy pediatric ED.[26] Another tool, the Pediatric Asthma Severity Score (PASS) is a valid, reliable tool to measure asthma in the acute setting in children aged 1 to 18 years in a pediatric ED. The PASS score is limited because it only assesses 3 clinical measures: wheezing, prolonged expiration, and work of breathing. The Pediatric Asthma Score (PAS) is another measurement tool that includes measures of respiratory rate, oxygen saturation, auscultatory findings, retractions, and dyspnea. Kelly and colleagues[27] in 2000 showed that the PAS showed good interobserver agreement and excellent face validity in the ED setting. The PAS allowed providers to have an objective understanding of the severity of each patient being cared

Table 1
Determination of asthma severity in children

Classifying Asthma Severity and Initiating Therapy in Children

		Intermittent		Mild		Persistent Moderate		Severe	
Components of Severity		Ages 0–4 y	Ages 5–11 y	Ages 0–4 y	Ages 5–11 y	Ages 0–4 y	Ages 5–11 y	Ages 0–4 y	Ages 5–11 y
Impairment	Symptoms	<2 d/wk		>2 d/wk but not daily		Daily		Throughout the day	
	Nighttime awakenings	0	≤2/mo	1–2/mo	3–4/mo	3–4/mo	>1/wk but not nightly	>1/wk	Often 7/wk
	Short-acting beta-2 agonist use for symptom control	≤2 d/wk		>2 d/wk but not daily		Daily		Several times per day	
	Interference with normal activity	None		Minor limitation		Some limitation		Extremely limited	
	Lung Function	N/A	Normal FEV$_1$ between exacerbations >80%	N/A	—	N/A	—	N/A	—
	FEV$_1$ (predicted) or peak flow (personal best)		>80%		>80%		60%–80%		<60%
	FEV$_1$/FVC		>85%		>80%		75%–80%		<75%

Risk	Exacerbations requiring oral systemic corticosteroids (consider severity and interval since last exacerbation)	0–1/y (see notes)	≥2 exacerbations in 6 mo requiring oral systemic corticosteroids, or ≥4 wheezing episodes in 1 y lasting >1 d and risk factors for persistent asthma	>2/y (see notes) Relative annual risk may be related to FEV_1	—
			—	—	—

Notes:

Level of severity is determined by both impairment and risk. Assess impairment domain by caregiver's recall of previous 2 to 4 weeks. Assign severity to the most severe category in which any feature occurs.

Frequency and severity of exacerbations may fluctuate over time for patients in any severity category. There are currently inadequate data to correlate frequencies of exacerbations with different levels of asthma severity. In general, more frequent and severe exacerbations (eg, requiring urgent, unscheduled care; hospitalization; or ICU admission) indicate greater underlying disease severity. For treatment purposes, patients with 2 or more exacerbations described may be considered the same as patients who have persistent asthma, even in the absence of impairment levels consistent with persistent asthma.

Abbreviations: FEV_1, forced expiratory volume in 1 second; FVC, forced vital capacity; ICS, inhaled corticosteroids; ICU, intensive care unit; N/A, not applicable.

From National Heart, Lung, and Blood Institute. Expert panel report 3: guidelines for the diagnosis and management of asthma. US Department of Health and Human Services, National Institutes of Health, National Heart, Lung, and Blood Institute. 2007. NIH Publication Number 08-5486.

Box 2
Characteristics of near-fatal asthma

Characteristics of a near-fatal asthma exacerbation

Doubling of beta agonist usage or using 1 or more metered-dose inhaler canister per month

African-American race

Adolescents

Hospital admission within the past year for asthma

Intensive care unit admission for asthma

Multiple ED visits within the last year for asthma

Oxygen saturations less than 91%

Psychological or psychosocial problems

Difficulty perceiving symptoms of a severe exacerbation

---

for with an asthma exacerbation. This scoring system and corresponding clinical pathway resulted in a decreased length of stay, cost of hospitalization, and improved quality of care when used on the inpatient floors. In the same study, ED nurses preferred the PAS to peak flow measurements.

The PAS has been adapted for use in our institution including the ED, inpatient floors, pediatric intensive care unit (PICU), and transport settings (**Table 2**).

DIFFERENTIAL DIAGNOSIS

Asthma is the most common cause of chronic cough in children, although symptoms of cough, wheeze, and dyspnea can be the presenting symptoms for other diagnoses.

The differential diagnosis for first-time wheezing is broad and requires a thorough history and physical to make the appropriate diagnosis. Although the list can be extensive, it is important for the emergency medicine physician to initially consider and address life-threatening causes of wheezing as well as recognize causes that may need further evaluation. Partial airway obstruction from foreign body aspiration must be considered in toddlers with first-time wheezing that is of sudden onset, with a history of choking or gagging, and findings of unilateral wheezing. Although sudden in onset, anaphylaxis may have associated urticaria as well as a history of exposure to a possible allergen. Respiratory symptoms associated with first-time wheezing in infants may suggest bronchiolitis. History of inhalant use or exposure may indicate a chemical pneumonitis, whereas a history of hemoptysis may indicate pulmonary hemorrhage. Other life-threatening causes of first-time wheezing include cardiac disease and malformation, thoracic masses, or mediastinal masses. These patients often have a history of failure to thrive, feeding difficulties, and physical examination findings of murmur and hepatomegaly in cardiac failure. Wheezing secondary to structural anomalies may present with wheezing since birth, failure of improvement in symptoms following standard asthma treatment, and symptom severity that is associated with positional changes. Tracheomalacia or bronchomalacia caused by tracheal or main stem bronchi collapse manifests as cough and wheezing. In addition, symptoms caused by tracheomalacia improve with prone positioning and worsen with agitation or excitement because of increase in intrathoracic pressures. Right-sided aortic arch also causes mechanical compression of the airway resulting in wheezing.

Table 2 PAS and interpretation			
	1	**2**	**3**
Respiratory rate (breaths/minute)			
Age 1–3 y	$\leq$34	35–39	$\geq$40
Age 4–5 y	$\leq$30	31–35	$\geq$36
Age 6–12 y	$\leq$26	27–31	$\geq$31
>12 y	$\leq$23	24–27	$\geq$28
Oxygen requirement (%)	>95 on room air	90–95 on room air	<90 on room air or requiring any amount of O_2
Retractions	None or intercostal	Intercostal and substernal, or nasal flaring (infants)	Intercostal, substernal, and supraclavicular; or nasal flaring and head bobbing (infants)
Dyspnea 1–4 y	Normal feeding, vocalization, and play	Decreased appetite, coughing after play, hyperactivity	Stops eating or drinking, stops playing; or drowsy and confused and/or grunting
Dyspnea >5 y	Counts to $\geq$10 in 1 breath; or speaks in complete sentences	Counts to 4–6 in 1 breath; or speaks in partial sentences	Counts to $\leq$3 in 1 breath; or speaks in single words; or grunts
Auscultation	Normal breath sounds, end-expiratory wheezes	Expiratory wheezing	Inspiratory and expiratory wheezing to diminished breath sounds
Total PAS	Mild 5–7	Moderate 8–11	Severe 12–15

Courtesy of Akron Children's Hosptal, Akron, OH.

Gastroesophageal reflux in infants can present as wheezing that is exacerbated by feedings or infant positioning.

Patients who present with chronic cough or wheezing that does not improve with traditional asthma therapy also require a thoughtful differential diagnosis to ensure that the diagnosis is correct. Underlying congenital, immunologic, and infectious causes must be considered. Patients presenting with chronic cough along with multiple respiratory infections and symptoms of malabsorption should be evaluated for cystic fibrosis, primary ciliary dyskinesia, and cardiac disease. Chronic cough may be the presenting symptom of infectious causes such as pertussis or tuberculosis.

Parents often confuse other symptoms for wheezing. Patients with upper airway noises or stridor suggest a viral upper respiratory tract infection or croup as the cause. Vocal cord dysfunction is most common in adolescents and can be misdiagnosed as wheezing, although it is inspiratory stridor associated with chest or throat tightness. Habit cough may present as chronic cough not improving with traditional asthma therapy. Hyperventilation causes dyspnea that can be confused with asthma. Anxiety can also give the sensation of chest tightness resulting in a misdiagnosis of asthma.[28,29] **Box 3** summarizes important differential diagnoses to consider during the presentation of wheezing in the ED.

The distinguishing characteristic of asthma is the response to bronchodilator or corticosteroids when symptomatic. Knowledge of the natural history of asthma and

---

Box 3
Differential diagnosis of wheezing

Congenital	Cystic fibrosis
	Lobar emphysema
	Tracheobronchomalacia
	Tracheal or bronchial stenosis
	Tracheoesophageal fistula
	Vascular ring
	Alpha 1 antitrypsin deficiency
Allergic	Anaphylaxis
	Asthma
Acquired	Foreign body aspiration
	Bronchopulmonary dysplasia
	Mediastinal bronchial compression
	Recurrent aspiration
Infectious	Bronchiolitis
	Viral or bacterial pneumonia
Cardiac	Congestive heart failure
	Pulmonary edema

---

response to treatment can guide clinicians in determining when to consider alternative diagnoses. Diagnostic testing or chest imaging may be required to help exclude other causes of wheezing or cough.

DIAGNOSTIC EVALUATION

Few diagnostic tools exist that help determine the diagnosis of asthma in the ED setting. In children, asthma is a clinical diagnosis. Diagnostic studies are used to help exclude other causes of wheezing or cough, to help recognize atypical presentations of asthma, and evaluate those patients who do not respond as expected to traditional asthma therapy.

Pulse Oximetry

The clinical assessment of hypoxemia relies on many factors. Under optimal conditions, an arterial blood saturation of approximately 75% is needed before central cyanosis is clinically detectable. Oxygen saturation is a sensitive indicator of disease severity in conditions associated with ventilation/perfusion mismatch like asthma. Oxygen saturations can be used to assess severity of disease and response to treatment. Mild asthma exacerbations are associated with oxygen saturations greater than 95%. Oxygen saturations less than 92% 1 hour after treatment correlate with an increased need for hospitalization.[30] Therefore, pulse oximetry may be a useful tool during the management and disposition planning of an patient with asthma.

Chest Radiograph

For a child with known asthma who is responding as expected to traditional therapy, there is no evidence showing that chest radiographs change the management of asthma in children. Further, they are not helpful as a routine work-up of asthma in children in the ED.[31] Children with an acute asthma exacerbation often have abnormal chest radiographs including hyperinflation, atelectasis, peribronchial thickening, and increased extravascular fluid. These findings do not play a role in directing patient management or assessing severity of exacerbation. A study in 2000 analyzed the clinical predictors of focal infiltrate on chest radiograph. Grunting and pulse oximetry less than or equal to 93% was highly specific when diagnosing pneumonia in a wheezing infant and toddler. First-time wheezing, tachypnea, and fever were not associated with findings of infiltrate on chest radiograph.[32]

Chest radiographs can be used to help exclude other diagnoses of wheezing or cough, especially in patients with first-time wheezing. Acute-onset, unilateral wheezing suggests foreign body aspiration, and patients may show hyperinflation on chest radiographs. Chest radiographs may show a structural abnormality or mass in a patient with chronic wheezing that fails to respond to bronchodilator therapy. Chest radiograph in patients who present in extremis or with impending respiratory failure may help rule out complications from asthma such as pneumothorax or pneumomediastinum as well as other contributing causes for respiratory distress such as superimposed infection or cardiac disease. Although no clear guidelines exist, chest radiographs should be considered in the following instances: asymmetric wheezing, wheezing that fails to respond to bronchodilator therapy, or patients who present in extremis or with impending respiratory failure.

Peak Expiratory Flow Measurements

National guidelines for the treatment of asthma call for measures of peak expiratory flow rate as a valid and reproducible measure of airway obstruction and a guide for treatment plans. They are infrequently done in the ED setting and a 2004 study showed that only 64% of children eligible for peak flow measurements had it attempted in the ED. Most reports state that children less than 5 years old cannot reliably perform this maneuver, which is effort dependent and requires a significant degree of coordination. In the same study, less than half of the patients had a pre–peak flow and post–peak flow measurement obtained with bronchodilator treatment. Children with a more severe exacerbation as judged by asthma score or need for admission were less likely to be judged able to obtain a peak flow measurement.[33]

Peak flow measurements are predicted based on the patient's age, height, and gender. Patients who regularly perform peak flow measurements at home may know their personal best. Peak flow measurements correlate with the forced expiratory volume in 1 second (FEV_1), although there is more variability in peak flow measurements. A peak flow greater than 70% of expected is classified as a mild exacerbation. A peak flow between 40% and 70% is a moderate exacerbation, and less than 40% predicts a severe exacerbation. Both initial peak flow measurement and follow-up measures can help direct management and response to treatments. Patients with a peak flow less than 60% of predicted best after ED treatment are more likely to relapse in the outpatient setting. These measurements add to objective measures of severity of asthma exacerbation but are infrequently performed in the ED.[33]

MANAGEMENT

Children with acute exacerbations should be rapidly assessed and triaged to a location in the ED where observation and frequent reassessment can be performed by medical and nursing staff. Reassessment of patients after each round of treatment is the most important aspect in the management of acute asthma exacerbations.[20] Most children seen in the ED for asthma do not require hospital admission.[21] In 2004, 754,000 children in the United States visited the ED for asthma and approximately 198,000 required hospital admissions.[34] Regardless of disposition, the mainstay of asthma exacerbation treatment in the emergency room are SABAs, systemic corticosteroids, and ipratropium bromide. A summary of medication recommendations established by the National Heart, Lung, and Blood Institute (NHLBI) guidelines are shown in **Table 3**.

Table 3
Drug dosages in asthma exacerbation

Medication	Dosages		Comments
	Child Dose[a]	Adult Dose	
Inhaled SABAs			
Albuterol			
Nebulizer solution (0.63 mg/3 mL, 1.25 mg/3 mL, 2.5 mg/3 mL, 5.0 mg/mL)	0.15 mg/kg (minimum dose 2.5 mg) every 20 min for 3 doses then 0.15–0.3 mg/kg up to 10 mg every 1–4 h as needed, or 0.5 mg/kg/h by continuous nebulization	2.5–5 mg every 20 min for 3 doses, then 2.5–10 mg every 1–4 h as needed, or 10–15 mg/h continuously	Only selective beta-2 agonists are recommended. For optimal delivery, dilute aerosols to minimum of 3 mL at gas flow of 6–8 L/min. Use large-volume nebulizers for continuous administration. May mix with ipratropium nebulizer solution
MDI (90 µg/puff)	4–8 puffs every 20 min for 3 doses, then every 1–4 h inhalation maneuver as needed. Use VHC; add mask in children <4 y old	4–8 puffs every 20 min up to 4 h, then every 1–4 h as needed	In mild to moderate exacerbations, MDI plus VHC is as effective as nebulized therapy with appropriate administration technique and coaching by trained personnel
Bitolterol			
Nebulizer solution (2 mg/mL)	See albuterol dose; thought to be half as potent as albuterol on mg basis	See albuterol dose	Has not been studied in severe asthma exacerbations. Do not mix with other drugs
MDI (370 µg/puff)	See albuterol MDI dose	See albuterol MDI dose	Has not been studied in severe asthma exacerbations
Levalbuterol (R-Albuterol)			
Nebulizer solution (0.63 mg/3 mL, 1.25 mg/0.5 mL, 1.25 mg/3 mL)	0.075 mg/kg (minimum dose 1.25 mg) every 20 min for 3 doses, then 0.075–0.15 mg/kg up to 5 mg every 1–4 h as needed	1.25–2.5 mg every 20 min for 3 doses, then 1.25–5 mg every 1–4 h as needed	Levalbuterol administered in one-half the mg dose of albuterol provides comparable efficacy and safety. Has not been evaluated by continuous nebulization

MDI (45 μg/puff)	See albuterol MDI dose	See albuterol MDI dose	—
Pirbuterol			
MDI (200 μg/puff)	See albuterol MDI dose; thought to be half as potent as albuterol on a mg basis	See albuterol MDI dose	Has not been studied in severe asthma exacerbations
Systemic (Injected) Beta-2 Agonists			
Epinephrine 1:1000 (1 mg/mL)	0.01 mg/kg up to 0.3–0.5 mg every 20 min for 3 doses sq	0.3–0.5 mg every 20 min for 3 doses sq	No proven advantage of systemic therapy compared with aerosol
Terbutaline (1 mg/mL)	0.01 mg/kg every 20 min for 3 doses then every 2–6 h as needed sq	0.25 mg every 20 min for 3 doses sq	No proven advantage of systemic therapy compared with aerosol
Anticholinergics			
Ipratropium Bromide			
Nebulizer solution (0.25 mg/mL)	0.25–0.5 mg every 20 min for 3 doses, then as needed	0.5 mg every 20 min for 3 doses then as needed	May mix in same nebulizer with albuterol. Should not be used as first-line therapy; should be added to SABA therapy for severe exacerbations. The addition of ipratropium has not been shown to provide further benefit once the patient is hospitalized
MDI (18 μg/puff)	4–8 puffs every 20 min as needed up to 3 h	8 puffs every 20 min as needed up to 3 h	Should use with VHC and face mask for children <4 y old. Studies have examined ipratropium bromide MDI for up to 3 h
Ipratropium with Albuterol			
Nebulizer solution (each 3-mL vial contains 0.5 mg ipratropium bromide and 2.5 mg albuterol)	1.5–3 mL every 20 min for 3 doses, then as needed	3 mL every 20 min for 3 doses, then as needed	May be used for up to 3 h in the initial management of severe exacerbations. The addition of ipratropium to albuterol has not been shown to provide further benefit once the patient is hospitalized

(continued on next page)

Table 3
(continued)

Medication	Dosages		Comments
	Child Dose[a]	Adult Dose	
MDI (each puff contains 18 μg ipratropium bromide and 90 μg of albuterol)	4–8 puffs every 20 min as needed up to 3 h	8 puffs every 20 min as needed up to 3 h	Should use with VHC and face mask for children <4 y old
Systemic Corticosteroids			
Prednisone Methylprednisolone Prednisolone	1–2 mg/kg in 2 divided doses (maximum 60 mg/d) until PEF is 70% of predicted or personal best	40–80 mg/d in 1 or 2 divided doses until PEF reaches 70% of predicted or personal best	For outpatient "burst," use 40–60 mg in single or 2 divided doses for total of 5–10 d in adults (children, 1–2 mg/kg/d maximum 60 mg/d for 3–10 d)

Notes:
There is no known advantage for higher doses of corticosteroids in severe asthma exacerbations, nor is there any advantage for intravenous administration compared with oral therapy provided gastrointestinal transit time or absorption is not impaired.

The total course of systemic corticosteroids for an asthma exacerbation requiring an ED visit or hospitalization may last from 3 to 10 days. For corticosteroid courses of less than 1 week, there is no need to taper the dose. For slightly longer courses (eg, up to 10 days), there probably is no need to taper, especially if patients are concurrently taking ICSs.

ICSs can be started at any point in the treatment of an asthma exacerbation.

Abbreviations: MDI, metered-dose inhaler; PEF, peak expiratory flow; sq, subcutaneous; VHC, valved holding chamber.

[a] Children ≤12 years of age.

From National Heart, Lung, and Blood Institute. Expert panel report 3: guidelines for the diagnosis and management of asthma. US Department of Health and Human Services, National Institutes of Health, National Heart, Lung, and Blood Institute. 2007. NIH Publication Number 08-5486.

OXYGEN

Children, and especially infants, are at risk for respiratory failure and develop hypoxemia more rapidly than adults. Therefore, monitoring of oxygen saturation is necessary.[1,20,35] NHLBI guidelines recommend oxygen administration to maintain saturations greater than 90% (greater than 95% in pregnant women and in patients who have coexistent heart disease). Sao_2 is to be monitored until a clear response to bronchodilator therapy has occurred.[1] Indiscriminate high-flow oxygen despite good saturations can lead to poorer outcomes.[20,36]

SABAS

SABA is the most effective treatment of relieving bronchospasm and reversing airway obstruction. The most commonly used SABA in the United States is the beta-2 selective drug albuterol.[37] Through its sympathomimetic effects, it exerts bronchodilating effects by relaxing airway smooth muscle and thus relieving bronchospasm. Secondary effects are enhancement of water output from bronchial mucous glands and improvement of mucociliary clearance.

Albuterol is available in 2 forms: albuterol or levalbuterol. Albuterol is a 50:50 mixture of R-enantiomers and S-enantiomers. The R-enantiomer is pharmacologically active and shows more potent binding to beta-2 receptors than the S-enantiomer. The S-enantiomer is pharmacologically inactive, has a longer elimination half-life, and may induce paradoxical bronchospasm, contributing to airway irritation.[20] Levalbuterol consists solely of the R-enantiomer and is thought to provide maximum bronchodilating benefits and to minimize adverse side effects, including tachycardia and hypokalemia.[20,38,39] Studies have shown mixed results, with some trials showing benefits in pulmonary function, reduction in hospital admission rate, and reduced side effects, whereas other studies have shown no difference.[20,39–45] Current guidelines do not recommend using one rather than the other.

Albuterol has 2 common mechanisms of delivery: a metered-dose inhaler (MDI) with a spacer or nebulized solution typically via small-volume constant output jet nebulizers (SVN). A newer mechanism of delivery is breath-actuated nebulizer treatments, which are nebulizers that initiate aerosol production with the onset of inhalation, limiting the loss of aerosol during exhalation. A randomized control study conducted in the ED found that a breath-actuated nebulizer improved clinical asthma score, decreased respiratory rate, and decreased hospital admissions, but did not significantly affect length of stay in the ED.[46] In mild to moderate asthma, an MDI with spacer has been shown to be at least equivalent, if not better, in efficacy to a nebulizer and is more cost-effective.[20,47–51] Factors that influence delivery mechanism include patient cooperation, response to treatment via MDI, severity of exacerbation, and local protocols.[20] Children less than 24 months old are thought to have a more difficult time with MDI and spacer. However, a double-blind, randomized, placebo-controlled clinical trial by Delgado and colleagues[52] showed that MDI with spacers may be as efficacious as nebulizers in the ED treatment of wheezing in children from 2 to 24 months of age. Another double-blind, randomized equivalence trial of MDI with spacer versus nebulizer treatment in children 12 to 60 months of age found that the efficacy of albuterol administered via MDI and spacer was equivalent to nebulizer.[53] The type of delivery system used may be determined by institution policy as well as provider preference and comfort.

Albuterol can be given as intermittent therapy every 20 minutes (up to 3 doses) or continuously for an hour depending on severity. Response to medication on reevaluation determines further frequency. Following reassessment, SABA can be administered by MDI and spacer, 2 to 4 puffs, continuous or spaced to hourly based on severity (**Fig. 2**) or asthma score. Albuterol administered via nebulizer can be given at 0.15 to 0.3 mg/kg with a minimum of 2.5 mg and a maximum of 5 mg. The volume of albuterol is then diluted with normal saline for a total of 5 mL fluid per nebulized mask.[20] With continuous nebulization, the recommended dose of albuterol is 0.5 mg/kg/h with the total hourly dose not to exceed 10 to 15 mg/h.[1,20] Approximately 2% to 10% of albuterol given by nebulized treatment

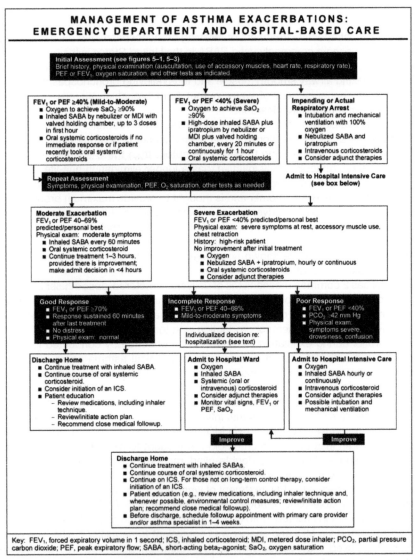

Fig. 2. ED evaluation and management of asthma exacerbation. (*From* National Heart, Lung, and Blood Institute. Expert panel report 3: guidelines for the diagnosis and management of asthma. US Department of Health and Human Services, National Institutes of Health, National Heart, Lung, and Blood Institute. 2007. NIH Publication Number 08-5486.)

reaches the lung. An MDI gives 90 μg/puff, but the delivery is considered to be more efficient.[37]

Side effects of albuterol are common, but minor in severity. Sinus tachycardia is the most common side effect, but rarely causes serious problems. Other cardiovascular-related effects include palpitations, hypertension, and, rarely, ventricular dysrhythmias. Central nervous system side effects are secondary to stimulation and include tremors, hyperactivity, and nausea with vomiting. Metabolic side effects include hypokalemia and hyperglycemia. Periodic serum potassium levels should be monitored with long-term continuous use of SABA treatment.

SYSTEMIC CORTICOSTEROIDS

The overriding physiologic derangement in asthma is airway inflammation and corticosteroids are among the mainstays of treatment. Glucocorticoids suppress cytokine production, granulocyte-macrophage colony-stimulating factor, and inducible nitric oxide synthase activation (all important components of the underlying inflammatory cells), decrease airway mucous production, and attenuate microvascular permeability.[21] The guidelines indicate use of steroid in asthma exacerbation when the patient does not completely respond to one inhaled beta agonist treatment, even if the patient is having a mild exacerbation.[1] Systemic corticosteroids have been shown to decrease the need for hospital admission as well as the length of stay.[20,54–56] A time series controlled trial on nurse initiation of oral systemic steroids in triage for moderate to severe asthma exacerbation in children 2 to 17 years of age showed earlier clinical improvement, decreased hospital admission rates, and earlier time to discharge in triage-administered steroids compared with systemic oral corticosteroid administration following physician assessment.[57]

Systemic corticosteroids may be given either orally or intravenously. Studies have showed that the effects of oral and intravenous (IV) steroids are equivalent.[37,58] Advantages of oral dosing include ease of administration and decreased cost. IV steroids are indicated when a patient cannot tolerate oral medication, is too ill to take oral medication, or has intestinal issues affecting absorption of medication.[1,20,35] Patients who vomit within 30 minutes of an oral dose should have dosing repeated.[37] Side effects of systemic corticosteroids are more prevalent in the critically ill child because of duration and dose of medication, and include hyperglycemia, hypertension, and occasionally agitation related to steroid-induced psychosis.

Systemic corticosteroids begin to exert their effect in 1 to 3 hours and reach maximal effect within 4 to 8 hours.[21] Oral prednisone or prednisolone is administered at a dose of 1 to 2 mg/kg once daily (maximum of 60 mg/d),[20,59,60] typically for 3 to 5 days. The total course of systemic corticosteroids for an asthma exacerbation requiring an ED visit of hospitalization may last longer. For corticosteroid courses of less than 1 week, there is no need to taper the dose. For slightly longer courses (eg, up to 10 days), there probably is no need to taper, especially if patients are concurrently taking ICSs.[1] IV steroids can be given as methylprednisolone, 2 mg/kg/d.[21] An alternative to prednisone is dexamethasone. Dexamethasone is well absorbed orally and has the same bioavailability as when given parenterally, with the action lasting up to 72 hours after a single dose.[61] Studies suggest that a 2-day course of oral dexamethasone at a dose of 0.6 mg/kg daily (maximum 16 mg) is as effective and well tolerated as a 5-day course of oral prednisone in adults and children.[20,62–64] In addition, Qureshi and colleagues[65] found that 2 doses of oral dexamethasone had fewer side effects with similar efficacy and better compliance compared with 5 doses of oral prednisone in children with acute asthma. High doses of ICS may be considered in conjunction with oral corticosteroids in the ED. The data on ICS use in children are inconsistent and may be a result of dosing inconsistency.[1,66] One trial reporting greater efficacy for oral corticosteroids used a single high dose of an ICS (2 mg fluticasone), whereas a trial giving multiple doses of budesonide (1.2 mg total) reported increased efficacy for the inhaled route.[67,68] Although the data are suggestive, a meta-analysis concluded that evidence was insufficient for firm conclusions.[69] ICSs in the ED management of acute asthma exacerbations are currently not recommended as a replacement for oral systemic corticosteroids because of lack of efficacy when used alone.[37,54,55,67,69–71]

IPRATROPIUM BROMIDE

Ipratropium bromide, an anticholinergic agent, is also used in the treatment of severe asthma exacerbation. Ipratropium promotes bronchodilation without inhibiting mucociliary clearance, as with atropine. It also acts as a parasympatholytic, antagonizing acetylcholine effects and ultimately impairing bronchial smooth muscle contraction.[21] Adding multiple high doses of ipratropium bromide (0.5 mg nebulizer solution or 8 puffs by MDI in adults; 0.25–0.5 mg nebulizer solution or 4–8 puffs by MDI in children) to a selective SABA produces additional bronchodilation, resulting in fewer hospital admissions, particularly in patients who have severe airflow obstruction.[1,72,73] It can be administered every 30 minutes for up to 3 doses. The most common adverse effects are dry mouth, bitter taste, flushing, tachycardia, and dizziness.[21] However, because of inability to cross membranes from the lung to the systemic circulation, there is no significant effect on the systemic system, including heart rate, even at high doses.[37,74]

IV FLUIDS

Children presenting with severe or life-threatening asthma exacerbation are often dehydrated secondary to poor oral intake as well as increased insensible losses from increased minute ventilation. Appropriate fluid resuscitation is necessary; however, care should be used in avoiding overhydration, which may place these children at risk for pulmonary edema secondary to microvascular permeability, increased left ventricular afterload, and alveolar fluid migration associated with the inflammatory lung process.[21] Oral routes of hydration are preferable except in exacerbations with the possibility of noninvasive ventilator support or endotracheal intubation.[1]

MAGNESIUM SULFATE

Magnesium sulfate is a bronchodilator that should be used in severe asthma. Magnesium sulfate acts through its role as a calcium channel blocker, ultimately inhibiting calcium-mediated smooth muscle contraction and facilitating bronchodilation.[21] Recommendations for use of IV magnesium sulfate include those whose FEV_1 fails to improve to more than 60% of predicted in 1 hour following therapy,[60] exacerbations that remain in the severe category after 1 hour of intensive conventional therapy, or life-threatening asthma.[1] It has shown improved clinical asthma scores with minimal side effects.[20,75,76] It is also inexpensive, easily administered intravenously, and well tolerated.[37] A randomized control study also showed that IV magnesium sulfate therapy within the first hour of hospitalization in children aged 2 to 15 years classified as acute severe asthma had a reduced requirement for mechanical ventilation support and had a statistically significant shorter PICU and hospital stay.[77] However, not all individual studies have found positive results.[1,78–80] The treatment has no apparent value in patients who have exacerbations of lesser severity, and one study found that IV magnesium sulfate improved pulmonary function only in patients whose initial FEV_1 was less than 25% predicted, and the treatment did not improve hospital admission rates.[81] If administered, a single IV dose of 25 to 75 mg/kg (maximum of 2 g) magnesium sulfate can be given over 20 to 30 minutes.[1,20,35]

Nebulized magnesium is also available. A recent meta-analysis of 6 trials suggests that the use of nebulized magnesium sulfate in combination with SABA may result in further improvements in pulmonary function. A Cochrane Review found that 1 study from 3 trials suggested possible improvement in pulmonary function in those with severe exacerbations (FEV_1 <50% predicted). However, heterogeneity among the trials precluded definite conclusions. In addition, there is currently no good evidence that inhaled $MgSO_4$ can be used as a substitute for inhaled SABA. When used in addition to inhaled SABA (with or without inhaled ipratropium), there is currently no overall clear evidence of improved pulmonary function or reduced hospital admissions.[82] Inhaled magnesium sulfate may be used as a diluent in place of normal saline (usually 2.5 mL of a 250 mmol/L solution) combined with albuterol and ipratropium bromide in the same mask.[20,82] Magnesium levels do not need to be monitored if a 1 time dose is given, but may be followed if repeated doses are considered.[37] Side effects include hypotension, central nervous system depression, muscle weakness, and flushing. More serious side effects include cardiac arrhythmias, including complete heart block, respiratory failure caused by severe muscle weakness, and sudden cardiopulmonary arrest, but these are usually in the setting of very high serum magnesium levels.[21]

IV BETA AGONIST

IV and subcutaneous administration of beta agonists in the management of acute severe asthma are controversial. It has been postulated that children presenting with acute severe asthma exacerbation do not optimally benefit from inhaled SABA therapy because of the inability of the medication to penetrate constricted airways.[83] Systemic administration of a beta agonist may help dilate obstructed airways and improve the efficacy of inhaled beta agonist in severe asthma exacerbations. A double-blind, randomized controlled study in Australia showed more rapid improvement in patients who received a single bolus of IV albuterol in addition to nebulized albuterol than in those who received nebulized albuterol alone.[37,84]

IV terbutaline, a selective beta-2 agonist, is available in the United States for IV or subcutaneous administration. It may be used in children with no IV access as an adjunct to inhaled SABA. Subcutaneous dosing is 0.01 mg/kg/dose with a maximum dose of 0.3 mg. This dose may be repeated every 15 to 20 minutes for up to 3 doses. IV terbutaline is started with a loading dose of 10 μg/kg over 10 min followed by continuous infusion at 0.1 to 10 μg/kg/min. The side effects include a risk of myocardial ischemia caused by selective beta agonist activity. Between 10% and 50% of asthmatics can have increased troponin I levels during terbutaline therapy. However, data are limited and monitoring cardiac-specific enzymes (creatine phosphokinase or troponin) may be of value in children who receive more than 1 dose of terbutaline.[21]

Nonselective beta agonists such as ephedrine, epinephrine, and isoproterenol are rarely used because of their high side effect profile and availability of more selective IV or subcutaneous agents.[21] The NHLBI guidelines do not recommend use of IV isoproterenol in the treatment of asthma because of the danger of myocardial toxicity.[85]

At present, the NHLBI guidelines do not consider systemic beta agonist therapy to have advantage compared with inhaled SABA.[1] A meta-analysis addressing this issue concluded that there was no evidence supporting the use of IV beta agonists compared with aerosol administration in the treatment of acute severe asthma.[86] Data are also sparse on the benefit of adding an IV beta-2 agonist to high-dose nebulized therapy.[84] Systemic beta-2 agonists should be only considered in patients with life-threatening asthma exacerbations who have failed to respond to maximal inhaled therapy and systemic corticosteroids.[37]

LEUKOTRIENE RECEPTOR ANTAGONISTS

Leukotriene receptor antagonists (LTRAs) (montelukast, zafirlukast) have been shown to decrease symptoms of mild to moderate asthma exacerbations.[20] Leukotriene pathways are activated in acute asthma, as shown in increases of urinary leukotriene excretion.[87–89] LTRAs block the production of these natural mediators that are involved in bronchoconstriction.[37] LTRAs are considered to have potential additive benefit in combination with inhaled SABA and corticosteroids. There is some evidence in the adult literature that IV administration may be effective in acute, severe asthma[20,87] and this may be another route of rapid bronchodilation in life-threatening asthma.[1] A randomized, double-blind, parallel-group pilot study of IV montelukast versus placebo in adults with moderate to severe asthma exacerbation showed significant improvement in FEV_1 within 10 minutes of administration of montelukast. There was also a trend toward reduction of inhaled beta agonist use compared with the placebo.[87] Although its role in acute asthma is now being explored, there are insufficient data to recommend it as a possible adjunct treatment.[1]

HELIOX

Heliox, a blend of helium and oxygen (80% helium/20% oxygen), is less dense than air and improves air flow resistance in small airways by reducing turbulent flow and enhancing laminar gas flow,[90] increasing carbon dioxide elimination, increasing expiratory flow, decreasing work of breathing, and enhancing particle deposition of aerosolized medication in distal lung segments.[91–93] However, hypoxemia is one of the limits of this therapy.[37] A Cochrane Review concluded that existing evidence did not support the therapeutic use of heliox-driven albuterol in all patients presenting to the ED with status asthmaticus. However, the review only included 3 pediatric trials with a total of 82 patients.[94] Of these, a prospective, randomized controlled, single-blind study conducted by Kim and colleagues[95] in children 2 to 18 years of age with moderate to severe asthma showed that continuously nebulized albuterol delivery by heliox early in the course of care was associated with a greater degree of clinical improvement than delivery by oxygen. There was also a statistically significant difference in discharge rates at the 12-hour treatment point between the two groups. However, there was no statistically significant difference in ED discharge or PICU admission rates. Other pediatric studies have shown that there was no clinical benefit compared with standard therapy in the initial treatment of moderate to severe asthma in the ED,[91] nor was there decreased length of hospital stay or time to clinical improvement.[90] At this time, heliox is to be considered in patients with life-threatening asthma or those who are considered to have severe asthma after 1 hour of conventional therapy.[1]

NONINVASIVE MECHANICAL VENTILATION

Mortality in mechanically ventilated children with life-threatening asthma is increased compared with children who do not need mechanical ventilation. Noninvasive positive pressure ventilation (NIPPV) is an alternative to conventional mechanical ventilation and is used in 3% to 5% of critically ill asthmatic children.[21] NIPPV is considered to be a temporizing measure that may help avoid intubation and improve outcomes in children with status asthmaticus.[20,96–100] A Cochrane Review highlighted one trial that showed the benefit of NIPPV in hospitalization rates, number of patients discharged, FEV$_1$, forced vital capacity, and respiratory rates compared with medical therapy alone. However, they still concluded that data were insufficient and that NIPPV was still controversial therapy in severe asthma.[101] More recently, multiple pediatric trials have shown NIPPV to be well tolerated, safe, and to have minimal complications in pediatric patients.[97,102,103] A recent study also showed that bilevel positive airway pressure ventilation, a form of NIPPV, was well tolerated in pediatric patients weighing less than 20 kg with no major complications, including death or pneumothorax.[104] NIPPV in the pediatric patient does require pediatric specific equipment (mask, ventilator), and pediatric respiratory therapists who can monitor the circuit.[104] If NIPPV is available, a trial may be warranted before the institution of conventional mechanical ventilation.

INTUBATION

Tracheal intubation in the management of asthma exacerbation is absolutely indicated for patients who present with apnea or coma.[1] However, intubation should be strongly considered for the following conditions: refractory hypoxemia, significant respiratory acidosis unresponsive to pharmacotherapy,[21] worsening mental status,[37] and exhaustion.[1] Ventilation goals should include maintaining adequate oxygenation, allowing for permissive hypercarbia (moderate respiratory acidosis), and minute ventilation adjustment (peak pressure, tidal volume, and rate) to maintain an arterial pH of 7.2. Strategies should attempt to minimize hyperinflation and air trapping, which can be accomplished by using slow ventilator rates with prolonged expiratory phase, minimal end-expiratory pressure, and short inspiratory time. In addition, adjustment to ventilator rate, inspiratory and expiratory time, or positive end-expiratory pressure can be made to facilitate full expiration between breaths.[21]

DISPOSITION

Adequate evaluation of the severity of asthma exacerbation is important for the initial management of patients, as well as for assessing the clinical response[105] and subsequent disposition. Clinicians often have varying degrees of experience in determining the severity of an asthma exacerbation. More objective tools such as peak flow and spirometry require trained personnel as well as a patient who has adequate coordination and comprehension.[105] This requirement makes such tools more difficult to use in the pediatric population, especially in infants and toddlers. To standardize asthma management in the ED, the PAS score has been used. The authors' institution's PAS-based management is shown in **Fig. 3** for reference.

No single measure is best for assessing severity or predicting hospital admission. Lung function measures (FEV$_1$ or peak expiratory flow) may be useful for children 5 years of age, but these measures may not be obtainable during an exacerbation. Pulse oximetry may be useful for assessing the initial severity; a repeated measure of pulse oximetry of less than 92% to 94% after 1 hour predicts the need for hospitalization. Children who have signs and symptoms after 1 to 2 hours of initial treatment and who continue to meet the criteria for a moderate or severe exacerbation have greater than an 84% chance of requiring hospitalization.[1] If patients are being discharged, a written asthma action plan should be considered. Most guidelines

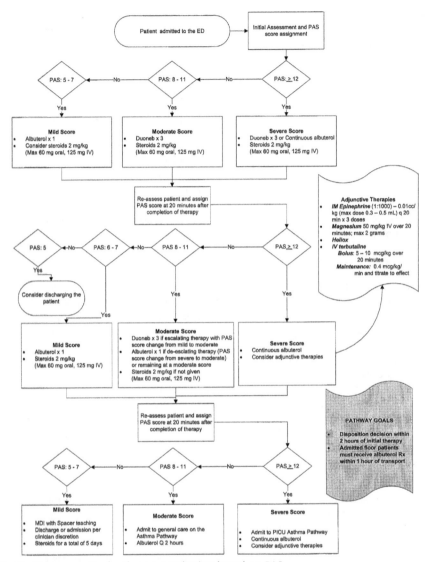

Fig. 3. Management of asthma exacerbation based on PAS.

recommend the provision of a written discharge plan with instructions for medication and follow-up.[1,26,60,106] Although there are limited data to firmly conclude that provision of an action plan is superior to none, there is clear evidence suggesting that symptom-based plans are superior to peak flow–based plans in children and adolescents.[107] Use of written action plans significantly reduced acute care visits per child compared with control subjects. Children using plans also missed less school, had less nocturnal awakening, and had improved symptom scores.

Patients who have severe exacerbations and are slow to respond to therapy may benefit from admission to an intensive care unit (ICU), where they can be monitored closely and intubated if indicated.[1,21]

SUMMARY

Pediatric asthma plays a significant role in health care costs as well as quality of life. Early treatment of asthma exacerbation is the best strategy for management and includes patient education, an asthma action plan, early recognition of worsening symptoms, and intensification of treatment. Despite this, asthma exacerbations may require urgent medical attention. In these cases, beta agonists, systemic corticosteroids, and ipratropium bromide remain the cornerstones of treatment. With life-threatening asthma, various adjunct therapy including IV magnesium, IV beta agonists, heliox, and NIPPV may be considered. Although morbidity secondary to asthma is significant, overall mortality remains low.

REFERENCES

1. National Heart, Lung, and Blood Institute. Expert panel report 3: guidelines for the diagnosis and management of asthma. Washington, DC: US Department of Health and Human Services, National Institutes of Health, National Heart, Lung, and Blood Institute; 2007. NIH Publication Number 08-5486.
2. Akinbami LJ, Moorman JE, Garbe PL, et al. Status of childhood asthma in the United States, 1980-2007. Pediatrics 2009;123(Suppl 3):S131–45.
3. Mayrides M, Levy R. Ethnic disparities in the burden and treatment of asthma. Reston (VA): Allergy and Asthma Foundation of America and the National Pharmaceutical Council; 2005.
4. Moya J, Bearer CF, Etzel RA. Children's behavior and physiology and how it affects exposure to environmental contaminants. Pediatrics 2004;113(Suppl 4):996–1006.
5. Kim BJ, Kwon JW, Seo JH, et al. Association of ozone exposure with asthma, allergic rhinitis, and allergic sensitization. Ann Allergy Asthma Immunol 2011; 107(3). 214–9.e1.
6. McConnell R, Berhane K, Gilliland F, et al. Asthma in exercising children exposed to ozone: a cohort study. Lancet 2002;359(9304):386–91.
7. Barnett SB, Nurmagambetov TA. Costs of asthma in the United States: 2002–2007. J Allergy Clin Immunol 2011;127(1):145–52.
8. Carroll CL, Zucker AR. The increased cost of complications in children with status asthmaticus. Pediatr Pulmonol 2007;42(10):914–9.
9. Wang LY, Zhong Y, Wheeler L. Direct and indirect costs of asthma in school-age children. Prev Chronic Dis 2005;2(1):A11.
10. Asthma's impact on children and adolescents. Atlanta (GA): National Center for Environmental Health Centers for Disease Control and Prevention; 2005.
11. Merkle SL, Wheeler LS, Gerald LB, et al. Introduction: learning from each other about managing asthma in schools. J Sch Health 2006;76(6):202–4.
12. Anderson SD, Daviskas E. The mechanism of exercise-induced asthma is.... J Allergy Clin Immunol 2000;106(3):453–9.
13. Hayes D Jr, Collins PB, Khosravi M, et al. Bronchoconstriction triggered by breathing hot humid air in patients with asthma: role of cholinergic reflex. Am J Respir Crit Care Med 2012;185(11):1190–6.
14. Levine SJ, Wenzel SE. Narrative review: the role of Th2 immune pathway modulation in the treatment of severe asthma and its phenotypes. Ann Intern Med 2010;152(4):232–7.
15. Koppelman GH, Sayers I. Evidence of a genetic contribution to lung function decline in asthma. J Allergy Clin Immunol 2011;128(3):479–84.
16. Xiao C, Puddicombe SM, Field S, et al. Defective epithelial barrier function in asthma. J Allergy Clin Immunol 2011;128(3). 549–56.e1–12.

17. Lopez-Guisa JM, Powers C, File D, et al. Airway epithelial cells from asthmatic children differentially express proremodeling factors. J Allergy Clin Immunol 2012;129(4). 990–7.e6.
18. Omland O, Hjort C, Pedersen OF, et al. New-onset asthma and the effect of environment and occupation among farming and nonfarming rural subjects. J Allergy Clin Immunol 2011;128(4):761–5.
19. Pedersen SE, Hurd SS, Lemanske RF, et al. Global strategy for the diagnosis and management of asthma in children 5 years and younger. Pediatr Pulmonol 2011;46(1):1–17.
20. Choi J, Lee GL. Common pediatric respiratory emergencies. Emerg Med Clin North Am 2012;30(2):529–63, x.
21. Bigham M. Status asthmacticus. In: Rogers M, Nichols D, editors. Textbook of pediatric intensive care. 4th edition. Philadelphia: Williams & Wilkins; 2012.
22. Partridge R, Abramo T. Acute asthma in the pediatric emergency department. Pediatric Emergency Medicine Practice. Available at: ebmedicine.net. 2008. Accessed October 22, 2012.
23. Wu AC, Tantisira K, Li L, et al. Predictors of symptoms are different from predictors of severe exacerbations from asthma in children. Chest 2011;140(1):100–7.
24. Tolomeo C, Savrin C, Heinzer M, et al. Predictors of asthma-related pediatric emergency department visits and hospitalizations. J Asthma 2009;46(8):829–34.
25. Chameides L, editor. Pediatric Advanced Life Support Manual. Dallas (TX): American Heart Association; 2011.
26. Ducharme FM, Chalut D, Plotnick L, et al. The pediatric respiratory assessment measure: a valid clinical score for assessing acute asthma severity from toddlers to teenagers. J Pediatr 2008;152(4):476–80, 480.e1.
27. Kelly CS, Andersen CL, Pestian JP, et al. Improved outcomes for hospitalized asthmatic children using a clinical pathway. Ann Allergy Asthma Immunol 2000;84(5):509–16.
28. Slaughter MC. Not quite asthma: differential diagnosis of dyspnea, cough, and wheezing. Allergy Asthma Proc 2007;28(3):271–81.
29. Weinberger M, Abu-Hasan M. Pseudo-asthma: when cough, wheezing, and dyspnea are not asthma. Pediatrics 2007;120(4):855–64.
30. Fouzas S, Priftis KN, Anthracopoulos MB. Pulse oximetry in pediatric practice. Pediatrics 2011;128(4):740–52.
31. Hederos CA, Janson S, Andersson H, et al. Chest X-ray investigation in newly discovered asthma. Pediatr Allergy Immunol 2004;15(2):163–5.
32. Mahabee-Gittens EM, Dowd MD, Beck JA, et al. Clinical factors associated with focal infiltrates in wheezing infants and toddlers. Clin Pediatr (Phila) 2000;39(7):387–93.
33. Gorelick MH, Stevens MW, Schultz T, et al. Difficulty in obtaining peak expiratory flow measurements in children with acute asthma. Pediatr Emerg Care 2004;20(1):22–6.
34. Akinbami L. Asthma prevalence, health care use and mortality 2003-2005. Available at: http://www.cdc.gov/nchs/data/hestat/asthma03-05/asthma03-05.htm. Accessed October 22, 2012.
35. British Thoracic Society Scottish Intercollegiate Guidelines Network. British guideline on the management of asthma. Thorax 2008;63(Suppl 4):iv1–121.
36. Rodrigo GJ, Rodriquez Verde M, Peregalli V, et al. Effects of short-term 28% and 100% oxygen on $PaCO_2$ and peak expiratory flow rate in acute asthma: a randomized trial. Chest 2003;124(4):1312–7.

37. Baren JM, Zorc JJ. Contemporary approach to the emergency department management of pediatric asthma. Emerg Med Clin North Am 2002;20:115–38.
38. Asmus MJ, Hendeles L. Levalbuterol nebulizer solution: is it worth five times the cost of albuterol? Pharmacotherapy 2000;20(2):123–9.
39. Milgrom H, Skoner DP, Bensch G, et al. Low-dose levalbuterol in children with asthma: safety and efficacy in comparison with placebo and racemic albuterol. J Allergy Clin Immunol 2001;108(6):938–45.
40. Nelson HS, Bensch G, Pleskow WW, et al. Improved bronchodilation with levalbuterol compared with racemic albuterol in patients with asthma. J Allergy Clin Immunol 1998;102(6 Pt 1):943–52.
41. Gawchik SM, Saccar CL, Noonan M, et al. The safety and efficacy of nebulized levalbuterol compared with racemic albuterol and placebo in the treatment of asthma in pediatric patients. J Allergy Clin Immunol 1999;103(4):615–21.
42. Carl JC, Myers TR, Kirchner HL, et al. Comparison of racemic albuterol and levalbuterol for treatment of acute asthma. J Pediatr 2003;143(6):731–6.
43. Tripp K, McVicar WK, Nair P, et al. A cumulative dose study of levalbuterol and racemic albuterol administered by hydrofluoroalkane-134a metered-dose inhaler in asthmatic subjects. J Allergy Clin Immunol 2008;122(3):544–9.
44. Lam S, Chen J. Changes in heart rate associated with nebulized racemic albuterol and levalbuterol in intensive care patients. Am J Health Syst Pharm 2003; 60(19):1971–5.
45. Wilkinson M, Bulloch B, Garcia-Filion P, et al. Efficacy of racemic albuterol versus levalbuterol used as a continuous nebulization for the treatment of acute asthma exacerbations: a randomized, double-blind, clinical trial. J Asthma 2011;48(2):188–93.
46. Sabato K, Ward P, Hawk W, et al. Randomized controlled trial of a breath-actuated nebulizer in pediatric asthma patients in the emergency department. Respir Care 2011;56(6):761–70.
47. Cates CJ, Crilly JA, Rowe BH. Holding chambers (spacers) versus nebulisers for beta-agonist treatment of acute asthma. Cochrane Database Syst Rev 2006;(2):CD000052.
48. Closa RM, Ceballos JM, Gómez-Papí A, et al. Efficacy of bronchodilators administered by nebulizers versus spacer devices in infants with acute wheezing. Pediatr Pulmonol 1998;26(5):344–8.
49. Wildhaber JH, Devadason SG, Hayden MJ, et al. Aerosol delivery to wheezy infants: a comparison between a nebulizer and two small volume spacers. Pediatr Pulmonol 1997;23(3):212–6.
50. Rubilar L, Castro-Rodriguez JA, Girardi G. Randomized trial of salbutamol via metered-dose inhaler with spacer versus nebulizer for acute wheezing in children less than 2 years of age. Pediatr Pulmonol 2000;29(4):264–9.
51. Doan Q, Shefrin A, Johnson D. Cost-effectiveness of metered-dose inhalers for asthma exacerbations in the pediatric emergency department. Pediatrics 2011; 127(5):e1105–11.
52. Delgado A, Chou KJ, Silver EJ, et al. Nebulizers vs metered-dose inhalers with spacers for bronchodilator therapy to treat wheezing in children aged 2 to 24 months in a pediatric emergency department. Arch Pediatr Adolesc Med 2003;157(1):76–80.
53. Ploin D, Chapuis FR, Stamm D, et al. High-dose albuterol by metered-dose inhaler plus a spacer device versus nebulization in preschool children with recurrent wheezing: a double-blind, randomized equivalence trial. Pediatrics 2000;106(2 Pt 1):311–7.

54. Row B, Edmonds M, Spooner C, et al. Corticosteroid therapy for acute asthma. Respir Med 2004;43(5):321–31.
55. Fiel SB, Vincken W. Systemic corticosteroid therapy for acute asthma exacerbations. J Asthma 2006;43(5):321–31.
56. Smith M, Iqbal S, Elliott TM, et al. Corticosteroids for hospitalised children with acute asthma. Cochrane Database Syst Rev 2003;(2):CD002886.
57. Zemek R, Plint A, Osmond MH, et al. Triage nurse initiation of corticosteroids in pediatric asthma is associated with improved emergency department efficiency. Pediatrics 2012;129(4):671–80.
58. Rowe BH, Keller JL, Oxman AD. Effectiveness of steroid therapy in acute exacerbations of asthma: a meta-analysis. Am J Emerg Med 1992;10(4):301–10.
59. American Lung Association EaSU. Trends in asthma morbidity and mortality. Available at: http://www.lung.org/finding-cures/our-research/trend-reports/asthma-trend-report.pdf. Accessed October 22, 2012.
60. Global Initiative for Asthma. Global strategy for asthma management and prevention. Bethesda (MD): Global Initiative for Asthma; 2010.
61. Derendorf H, Hochhaus G, Möllmann H, et al. Receptor-based pharmacokinetic-pharmacodynamic analysis of corticosteroids. J Clin Pharmacol 1993;33(2):115–23.
62. Kravitz J, Dominici P, Ufberg J, et al. Two days of dexamethasone versus 5 days of prednisone in the treatment of acute asthma: a randomized controlled trial. Ann Emerg Med 2011;58(2):200–4.
63. Greenberg RA, Kerby G, Roosevelt GE. A comparison of oral dexamethasone with oral prednisone in pediatric asthma exacerbations treated in the emergency department. Clin Pediatr (Phila) 2008;47(8):817–23.
64. Shefrin AE, Goldman RD. Use of dexamethasone and prednisone in acute asthma exacerbations in pediatric patients. Can Fam Physician 2009;55(7):704–6.
65. Qureshi F, Zaritsky A, Poirier MP. Comparative efficacy of oral dexamethasone versus oral prednisone in acute pediatric asthma. J Pediatr 2001;139(1):20–6.
66. Rowe BH, Bota GW, Fabris L, et al. Inhaled budesonide in addition to oral corticosteroids to prevent asthma relapse following discharge from the emergency department: a randomized controlled trial. JAMA 1999;281(22):2119–26.
67. Schuh S, Reisman J, Alshehri M, et al. A comparison of inhaled fluticasone and oral prednisone for children with severe acute asthma. N Engl J Med 2000;343(10):689–94.
68. Singhi S, Banerjee S, Nanjundaswamy H. Inhaled budesonide in acute asthma. J Paediatr Child Health 1999;35(5):483–7.
69. Edmonds ML, Camargo CA, Pollack CV, et al. Early use of inhaled corticosteroids in the emergency department treatment of acute asthma. Cochrane Database Syst Rev 2003;(3):CD002308.
70. FitzGerald JM, Becker A, Sears MR, et al. Doubling the dose of budesonide versus maintenance treatment in asthma exacerbations. Thorax 2004;59(7):550–6.
71. Schuh S, Dick PT, Stephens D, et al. High-dose inhaled fluticasone does not replace oral prednisolone in children with mild to moderate acute asthma. Pediatrics 2006;118(2):644–50.
72. Rodrigo GJ, Castro-Rodriguez JA. Anticholinergics in the treatment of children and adults with acute asthma: a systematic review with meta-analysis. Thorax 2005;60(9):740–6.
73. Plotnick LH, Ducharme FM. Combined inhaled anticholinergics and beta2-agonists for initial treatment of acute asthma in children. Cochrane Database Syst Rev 2000;(4):CD000060.

74. Anderson W. Hemodynamic and nonbronchial effects of ipratropium bromide. Am J Med 1986;81:45–52.
75. Rowe BH, Bretzlaff JA, Bourdon C, et al. Intravenous magnesium sulfate treatment for acute asthma in the emergency department: a systematic review of the literature. Ann Emerg Med 2000;36(3):181–90.
76. Rowe BH, Bretzlaff JA, Bourdon C, et al. Magnesium sulfate for treating exacerbations of acute asthma in the emergency department. Cochrane Database Syst Rev 2000;(2):CD001490.
77. Torres S, Sticco N, Bosch JJ, et al. Effectiveness of magnesium sulfate as initial treatment of acute severe asthma in children, conducted in a tertiary-level university hospital: a randomized, controlled trial. Arch Argent Pediatr 2012; 110(4):291–6.
78. Boonyavorakul C, Thakkinstian A, Charoenpan P. Intravenous magnesium sulfate in acute severe asthma. Respirology 2000;5(3):221–5.
79. Porter RS, Nester BA, Braitman LE, et al. Intravenous magnesium is ineffective in adult asthma, a randomized trial. Eur J Emerg Med 2001;8(1):9–15.
80. Scarfone RJ, Loiselle JM, Joffe MD, et al. A randomized trial of magnesium in the emergency department treatment of children with asthma. Ann Emerg Med 2000;36(6):572–8.
81. Silverman RA, Osborn H, Runge J, et al. IV magnesium sulfate in the treatment of acute severe asthma: a multicenter randomized controlled trial. Chest 2002; 122(2):489–97.
82. Blitz M, Blitz S, Hughes R, et al. Aerosolized magnesium sulfate for acute asthma: a systematic review. Chest 2005;128(1):337–44.
83. Bogie AL, Towne D, Luckett PM, et al. Comparison of intravenous terbutaline versus normal saline in pediatric patients on continuous high-dose nebulized albuterol for status asthmaticus. Pediatr Emerg Care 2007;23(6):355–61.
84. Browne GJ, Penna AS, Phung X, et al. Randomised trial of intravenous salbutamol in early management of acute severe asthma in children. Lancet 1997; 349(9048):301–5.
85. Maguire JF, O'Rourke PP, Colan SD, et al. Cardiotoxicity during treatment of severe childhood asthma. Pediatrics 1991;88(6):1180–6.
86. Travers A, Jones AP, Kelly K, et al. Intravenous beta2-agonists for acute asthma in the emergency department. Cochrane Database Syst Rev 2001;(2):CD002988.
87. Camargo CA, Smithline HA, Malice MP, et al. A randomized controlled trial of intravenous montelukast in acute asthma. Am J Respir Crit Care Med 2003; 167(4):528–33.
88. Drazen JM, O'Brien J, Sparrow D, et al. Recovery of leukotriene E4 from the urine of patients with airway obstruction. Am Rev Respir Dis 1992;146(1): 104–8.
89. Sampson AP, Castling DP, Green CP, et al. Persistent increase in plasma and urinary leukotrienes after acute asthma. Arch Dis Child 1995;73(3):221–5.
90. Bigham MT, Jacobs BR, Monaco MA, et al. Helium/oxygen-driven albuterol nebulization in the management of children with status asthmaticus: a randomized, placebo-controlled trial. Pediatr Crit Care Med 2010;11(3):356–61.
91. Rivera ML, Kim TY, Stewart GM, et al. Albuterol nebulized in heliox in the initial ED treatment of pediatric asthma: a blinded, randomized controlled trial. Am J Emerg Med 2006;24(1):38–42.
92. Berkenbosch J, Grueber R, Graff G, et al. Patterns of helium-oxygen (heliox) usage in the critical care environment. J Intensive Care Med 2004;19(6): 335–44.

93. Kudukis TM, Manthous CA, Schmidt GA, et al. Inhaled helium-oxygen revisited: effect of inhaled helium-oxygen during the treatment of status asthmaticus in children. J Pediatr 1997;130(2):217–24.

94. Rodrigo G, Pollack C, Rodrigo C, et al. Heliox for nonintubated acute asthma patients. Cochrane Database Syst Rev 2006;(4):CD002884.

95. Kim IK, Phrampus E, Venkataraman S, et al. Helium/oxygen-driven albuterol nebulization in the treatment of children with moderate to severe asthma exacerbations: a randomized, controlled trial. Pediatrics 2005;116(5):1127–33.

96. Bernet V, Hug MI, Frey B. Predictive factors for the success of noninvasive mask ventilation in infants and children with acute respiratory failure. Pediatr Crit Care Med 2005;6(6):660–4.

97. Carroll CL, Schramm CM. Noninvasive positive pressure ventilation for the treatment of status asthmaticus in children. Ann Allergy Asthma Immunol 2006;96(3): 454–9.

98. Essouri S, Chevret L, Durand P, et al. Noninvasive positive pressure ventilation: five years of experience in a pediatric intensive care unit. Pediatr Crit Care Med 2006;7(4):329–34.

99. Padman R, Lawless ST, Kettrick RG. Noninvasive ventilation via bilevel positive airway pressure support in pediatric practice. Crit Care Med 1998;26(1): 169–73.

100. Thill PJ, McGuire JK, Baden HP, et al. Noninvasive positive-pressure ventilation in children with lower airway obstruction. Pediatr Crit Care Med 2004;5(4): 337–42.

101. Ram FS, Wellington S, Rowe BH, et al. Non-invasive positive pressure ventilation for treatment of respiratory failure due to severe acute exacerbations of asthma. Cochrane Database Syst Rev 2005;(1):CD004360.

102. Mayordomo-Colunga J, Medina A, Rey C, et al. Non-invasive ventilation in pediatric status asthmaticus: a prospective observational study. Pediatr Pulmonol 2011;46(10):949–55.

103. Beers SL, Abramo TJ, Bracken A, et al. Bilevel positive airway pressure in the treatment of status asthmaticus in pediatrics. Am J Emerg Med 2007;25(1):6–9.

104. Williams AM, Abramo TJ, Shah MV, et al. Safety and clinical findings of BiPAP utilization in children 20 kg or less for asthma exacerbations. Intensive Care Med 2011;37(8):1338–43.

105. Gouin S, Robidas I, Gravel J, et al. Prospective evaluation of two clinical scores for acute asthma in children 18 months to 7 years of age. Acad Emerg Med 2010;17(6):598–603.

106. Ducharme FM, Zemek RL, Chalut D, et al. Written action plan in pediatric emergency room improves asthma prescribing, adherence, and control. Am J Respir Crit Care Med 2011;183(2):195–203.

107. Zemek RL, Bhogal SK, Ducharme FM. Systematic review of randomized controlled trials examining written action plans in children: what is the plan? Arch Pediatr Adolesc Med 2008;162(2):157–63.

Management of Pediatric Asthma at Home and in School

Linda Sue Van Roeyen, MS, CSN, CCRP, FNP-BC

KEYWORDS

- Asthma • Pediatrics • Chronic inflammatory disorder • Shortness of breath

KEY POINTS

- The incidence of pediatric asthma in the United States creates a huge financial burden to the economy as well as a negative impact on child health.
- The management of asthma in the home and school is positively impacted through improved education for children, their families, and all those who care for them.
- Identification and elimination of asthma triggers are helpful in reducing asthma exacerbations.
- The incidence of asthma is higher in African American and underserved populations.
- Improved management of pediatric asthma leads to improved school performance, improved mental health, and general well-being.

Asthma is a chronic inflammatory disorder of the airways affecting adults and children of all ages. Asthma symptoms include shortness of breath, wheezing, coughing, and chest tightness. The single greatest risk factor for developing asthma in infants and children is the genetic predisposition for allergic diseases that includes atopic dermatitis and allergies. The Tucson Birth Cohort[1] identified the existence of eczema as a major risk factor in predicting the likelihood of persistent disease. Viral illnesses and previous infection with respiratory syncytial virus are also known to be risk factors. The asthma predictive index was developed from the Tucson Birth Cohort and provides major and minor criteria for the asthma predictive index. Major risk factors include parental asthma and physician-diagnosed atopic dermatitis. Minor risk factors include physician-diagnosed allergic rhinitis, wheezing unrelated to colds, and blood eosinophilia (>4%).[1]

According to the summary data from the 2010 National Health Institute Survey,[2] currently 7 million children or 9.6% of the pediatric population (less than 18 years of age) in the United States suffer from asthma. Asthma incidence is higher in the

This article originally appeared in Nursing Clinics of North America, Volume 48, Issue 1, March 2013.

Ann & Robert H. Lurie Children's Hospital of Chicago, Pulmonary Habilitation Program, Box 246, 225 East Chicago Avenue, Chicago, IL 60611, USA

E-mail address: Lvanroeyen@luriechildrens.org

northeast and midwest United States geographically and, among women and children, African Americans, and persons with income below the level of poverty.[2,3]

Medical costs, hospitalizations, and emergency room visits for asthma are estimated at $50.1 billion per year.[3] Some costs include $3.8 billion in loss of productivity resulting from missed days of school or work, and $2.1 billion from lost productivity due to premature death.[4] In 2008 persons with acute asthma exacerbations missed an average of 4.5 days of school or work per year.[5] According to Healthy People 2020, 132.7 emergency room visits for asthma per 10,000 children less than the age of 5 occurred in 2005 to 2007 and 41.4 hospitalizations for asthma per 10,000 children less than the age of 5 occurred in 2007. The goals of Healthy People 2020 include promotion of respiratory health through better prevention, detection, treatment, and education efforts. The Healthy People 2020 goals related to asthma include the following: reduce asthma-related deaths, reduce asthma-related hospitalizations, reduce emergency department visits for asthma, reduce the proportion of persons who miss work or school days, and increase the proportion of persons with current asthma who receive appropriate asthma care according to National Asthma Education and Prevention Program Expert Panel Review 3 guidelines.[6] Established in 2007, the Expert Panel Review 3 guidelines focus on 4 areas of asthma care aimed at improving the quality of care and health outcomes. These guidelines include assessment and monitoring, patient education, control of factors contributing to asthma severity, and medical treatment. The guidelines report that inhaled corticosteroids are the most consistently effective long-term control medications for asthma management.[7] Pediatric health management of asthma requires coordination between a child's health care providers, school, and home. Children with asthma receive care in multiple settings from multiple persons: parents, caregivers, coaches, and teachers, who have variable knowledge and skills in asthma recognition and management. Children spend 7 hours or more per day in school. Therefore, it is extremely important to provide tools for the caregivers and teachers to assist in asthma management. The quality of life in children with asthma causes a negative impact on how they see themselves and how they interact with their peers and environment. Educational programs aimed at home and school management provide an excellent opportunity to decrease the rates of morbidity and mortality related to pediatric asthma.

ASTHMA IN THE HOME

The environmental triggers in the home significantly impact the quality of life of a child with asthma. Eliminating asthma triggers can be a key factor in decreasing exacerbations. Motivated and educated parents can learn to identify and eliminate or modify exposure to triggers and decrease the incidence of asthma flare-ups in their children. Commoon triggers include the following: exposure to cold air, viral illnesses, exercise, food allergies, pet dander, house dust mites, cockroaches, tobacco smoke, air pollution, perfumes, cleaning fluids, lead-based paints, mold, and pollen. Bronchoconstriction and increased airway inflammation are a result of the increased immunoglobulin E (in response to allergen exposure), which activates the release of mast cells. Repeated exposure to allergens can lead to worsening symptoms.[7] Parents should be taught to eliminate, to the extent possible, the triggers causing exacerbations. Elimination of triggers may include more frequent cleaning in the home with nonirritating chemicals. Pets may be confined to common family areas, and removed from the bedrooms, to provide decreased exposure for at least 8 to 10 hours per day. Pillowcases and mattress covers made to decrease allergens also assist in decreasing the effect of dust mites. Identification of food allergies for children greater than 2 years of age can be obtained through skin testing by a pediatric allergist and may assist in an avoidance of food allergy triggers. Identification and subsequent avoidance of food allergies are helpful in decreasing asthma symptoms. Promoting a clean, smoke-free environment, with the least amount of irritants, is helpful for the child with asthma.

CASE MANAGEMENT

Case management is another approach in promoting guideline care for asthma. In 2011 a study investigated the implementation of nurse case management and housing interventions to reduce allergen exposures. This study, known as the Milwaukee Randomized Controlled Trial,[8] included 121 children with asthma. The control group (n = 64) received a visual assessment, asthma education, bed/pillow dust mite encasings, and treatment of lead-based paint hazards. In addition, the interventions group (n = 57) received the following: nurse case management, which consisted of a tailored, individual asthma action plan; minor home repairs; home cleaning using special vacuuming and wet washing; and integrated pest management. The study concluded that nurse case management and home environmental interventions, while increasing collaboration between health and housing professionals, were effective in decreasing exposures to allergens such as settled dust; however, it was difficult to change home behavior related to food storage and disposal of food debris.[8] The use of case management in managing children with asthma and their home environmental condition has proven to be helpful. The use of emergency visits for pediatric patients was evaluated in 2010.[9] In this study, children with asthma received a home environmental assessment as recommended by a pediatric allergist as part of a comprehensive case management program. Findings showed that having a home environmental assessment and case manager may decrease medical care use for children suffering from allergic rhinitis and asthma.[9]

HOME INTERVENTIONS—ENVIRONMENT AND EDUCATION

Barriers to obtaining proper asthma management in families of low income must be first identified to provide relief. Barriers to asthma management include the following: lack of allergy assessment and treatment, pessimistic parental beliefs regarding their ability to impact the disease, parental mental health problems, lack of health knowledge and inappropriate expectations for care, lack of access to a consistent health care professional, and competing household priorities.[10] Effective interventions include educating families and children to empower them to manage their disease.

Environmental conditions related to asthma morbidity were reviewed in a Michigan study evaluating the use of a program called Healthy Homes University (HHU) that was implemented for low-income families. The program assessed homes for asthma triggers and provided products and services to reduce exposures to triggers. Education was provided to families including identification of triggers and specific behaviors to reduce exposures. The study included 243 caregivers at baseline and at 6 months. HHU implemented several of the objectives from Healthy People 2010 into their educational program. HHU reduced levels of indoor allergen through home visits by providing asthma trigger reduction products to households and educated caregivers regarding how to decrease indoor allergens. HHU improved substandard housing though correction of physical housing problems including water leaks, electrical deficiencies, pest infestation, inoperable heating equipment, and peeling lead-based paint. HHU reduced the population's exposure to pesticides through education of households about integrated pest management techniques and provided them with traps, baits, food containers, and trash cans. Asthma symptoms were significantly reduced and acute care visits for asthma decreased by more than 47%.[11] A Canadian study enrolled 398 children and families into 2 groups to investigate the use of interactive education in a small group and the effect on asthma control by children and their families. The intervention group showed much improved asthma control, significantly fewer visits to the emergency room, and improvements in their quality-of-life scores. Education in a small group proved to be very effective in improving asthma management and decreasing acute episodes.[12]

The effectiveness of a low-cost approach to improve control of asthma symptoms in an urban population through lay educators was reviewed in 2008. The study concluded that low cost in-home education and environmental remediation improved outcomes for children with asthma. Lay educators were effective in delivering asthma-specific education, which resulted in improved asthma control.[13]

A pilot study of a home-based family intervention for low-income children with asthma was conducted in 2012. Low-income African American children have disproportionately higher rates of asthma morbidity and mortality. This study examined 43 families from an urban hospital and asthma camp, enrolling children aged 8 to 13 who had poorly controlled asthma. These children were randomized to a 4- to 6-session Home-Based Family Intervention or a single session of Enhanced Treatment As Usual. The Home-Based Family Intervention looked at family-selected goals targeting asthma management and stressors. Families were given an asthma action plan and dust mite covers. Children performed spirometry and demonstrated metered-dose inhaler/spacer technique at each home visit. Results suggest that home-based intervention addressing medical and psychosocial needs may prevent hospitalizations for children with poorly controlled asthma and parents/caregivers under stress.[14] Another important consideration when examining barriers is cultural sensitivity. The development of a program geared at the Latino children in urban areas provided improved asthma management. A 2008 study examined the experience of being an Asthma Amigo, a community-based educator who delivered asthma education to a Hispanic community using a train-the-trainer educational model. Focus groups evaluated participant experiences and program strengths and weaknesses. Findings suggested this program helped in highlighting asthma triggers and prevention in this population.[15]

A program called CALMA (an acronym of the Spanish for "Take Control, Empower Yourself, and Achieve Management of Asthma") was trialed in Puerto Rico. It provided a culturally adapted family-based intervention for decreasing asthma morbidity in poor Puerto Rican children aged 5 to 12 with persistent asthma. Puerto Rican children have the highest rates of asthma of any ethnic group and are more likely to die from asthma when compared with other children. When evaluating the educational intervention, Puerto Rican families had less asthma exacerbations and used fewer services after the CALMA program was implemented. Conclusions demonstrated that providing a culturally adapted program for families and tailoring the needs of low-income Puerto Rican families decreased asthma morbidity in the children.[16]

Parents frequently do not receive adequate information to help their children manage their asthma symptoms. Average clinic appointments last from 20 to 45 minutes with little time for in-depth discussion of asthma teaching. Different types of asthma education programs for parents were examined. A Web-based program, "My Child's Asthma," provides interactive tools for parents to become more engaged in learning about their child's disease. A 2011 study looked at 283 parents with children who had asthma. Surveys examined demographic and clinical characteristics, outcome expectations, and self-efficacy beliefs regarding asthma control for their child and attitudes about computers and the Internet. Results suggest it would be beneficial to find ways to increase engagement in a Web-based intervention for parents who are not yet engaging in recommended behaviors and/or those who report less positive outcome and efficacy expectations around asthma.[17]

PSYCHOSOCIAL/QUALITY OF LIFE

Asthma in the presence of other chronic medical illnesses is a concern for increased morbidity with asthma. Caregivers may have a positive impact on the health and well-being of children with medical and psychiatric comorbidities.[18] In a 2009 study examining the effect of routines on asthma management and rates of morbidity, outcomes for children with asthma and their parents were investigated. One hundred fifty children were enrolled and given quality-of-life scores comparing those with more versus those with less household routines, concluding that those with established routines may result in improved asthma morbidity outcomes.[19] In this systematic review, 16 studies measured quality-of-life issues in children or adolescents with asthma. The studies demonstrated an overall decrease of 0.8 symptom days in a 2-week period, or 21.0 fewer symptom days per year.[20] Allowing the child to participate in the clinic visit with parental coaching may be very helpful in solidifying the child's knowledge of their own asthma management plan. The goal for school-aged children is to change the dyadic interactions between the parent and provider into a triadic interaction, to include the child and thereby to improve their asthma management.[21] Shared decision-making in health care between the school-aged child and parents or medical professionals may also increase self-confidence and improve self-management skills.

ASTHMA IN THE SCHOOL
Absenteeism

Children with uncontrolled asthma are unable to perform at their best, and therefore, are at a disadvantage scholastically.[22] Identifying children with asthma and participating in their plan of care provide opportunities and challenges for the school system. School nurses play an important role in the care of asthmatic children in the creation and implementation of the care plan. However, many schools do not have school nurses on the premises and depend on office personnel to assist children with asthma management.[22,23] The School Health Policies and Programs Study of the Centers for Disease Control and Prevention assesses school health policies and programs at the state, district, school, and classroom levels. Their survey found that only 36% of schools have a full-time registered nurse or licensed practical nurse.[24] In some schools the school nurse is expected to maintain the attendance data and record keeping. Absence, extended absence, and repeated tardiness may occur because of asthma status. In a 2011 study by Mizan and coworkers, the mean days of absence in 86 students with asthma was 2.73 days compared with 1.89 days for 828 children without asthma. There was no difference in the number of days tardy. Students with asthma were more likely to be absent on Monday, Tuesday, and Friday than students without asthma.[22] Increased absenteeism may lead to decreased self-esteem and poor school performance. Subsequently, it may restrict future education and career opportunities.[4] The relationship between school absence, academic performance, and asthma status was examined in a predominantly African American urban school district. Children with absenteeism due to asthma symptoms did not test as well on standardized testing as those without asthma-related absenteeism.[23] Children with asthma are also more likely to be treated for mental health problems and demonstrate more negative social outcomes as well as decreased overall health and well-being.[25] Children with asthma who have parents with chronic disease show worsening health management and more absenteeism. It is important to understand how parents' health conditions influence children's health care and limit the child's participation in school and other activities.[26]

School-based Health Centers/Access to Care

The development of school-based health clinics (SBHC) may be the answer to providing improved asthma and general health care for the underserved. The National Association of School-based Health Centers has issued a policy statement identifying the implementation of SBHC to provide a medical home to provide primary care to this population.[27] The current health legislation provides for expansion of SBHC to provide primary care for children. The Patient Protection and Affordable Care Act (P.L.111–148), signed into law by President Obama in March 2012, provides language authorizing a federal SBHC grant program for operations, and an emergency appropriation that would provide $200 million for SBHC construction and equipment needs over 4 years. Provision of a funded federal program for SBHC will allow improved access to care for children and adolescents. Patient Protection and Affordable Care Act (Section 4101[a]) of the Affordable Care Act allows for SBHCs to access $200 million in competitive federal funds over the next 4 years. The grants are limited to facilities expenditures, such as the acquisition or improvement of land, construction costs, equipment, and similar expenditures. HR 1214 was passed in May 2011, by the House of Representatives, and provides for defunding of grants for SBHCs. Legislators are monitoring the pending of this law passing the senate and being signed by the President before it will go into effect.[27] SBHC currently provide onsite care by physicians or nurse practitioners in more than 1500 public schools in the United States. Revised National Institutes of Health, National Heart, Lung, and Blood Institute guidelines for the diagnosis and management of asthma provide evidence of the effectiveness of school-based programs to improve self-managed treatment of asthma among children.[24] The cost savings of implementing SBHC nationwide were reviewed. The costs considered not only the amount it would take to staff the SBHC, but also the cost savings of premature deaths, savings from absenteeism due to lost productivity for parents in the workplace, savings from decreased hospital costs, hospital costs at discharge for asthmatic school-aged children, medical costs for outpatient or physician office visits, decrease in emergency room use, actual cost of nursing salaries, actual emergency room use in acute asthma, and future earnings including fringe benefits and financial losses due to parent's need to stay home from work and provide care for the child at home. Medical savings alone did not offset the cost of implementing this program for asthma prevention. The reduction in asthma severity was estimated to save $260 million per year in emergency room and inpatient hospital costs.[28]

The Law

Liability for schools regarding asthma management and self-administration of medication may be of concern in many school districts. Because asthma attacks can occur without warning and require immediate emergency medication, children require access to their short-acting bronchodilators immediately. A delay in obtaining the medication may result in a required hospitalization or death. If a child needs to go to the nurse's office or principal to obtain the inhaler, this increases the risk for poor outcomes. Children with asthma should carry their rescue inhaler for facilitation of prompt administration. Several laws protect the right of children to carry emergency medications on their persons. These laws include the Individuals with Disabilities Education Act, Section 504 of the Rehabilitation Act of 1973, and Title III of the Americans with Disabilities Act.

The Individuals with Disabilities Education Act partly funds states to develop special education programs for children with disabilities. Children with asthma can be considered under the "other health impairment" section of the law, which would mandate that the school needs to meet the unique needs of the child and allow them to carry their inhaler. In the 504 plan of the Rehabilitation Act of 1973, discrimination is not allowed based on a disability. This plan defines individuals with a disability as someone with a "physical or mental impairment which substantially limits one or more major life activity and has a record of such impairment or is regarded as having such impairment."[29] By federal law, schools must make reasonable accommodations for children to carry their inhalers or have immediate access.

Last, Title III of the Americans with Disabilities Act provides public accommodations for people with disabilities in the private sector and for state and local entities that do not receive federal funding. Therefore, private schools would fall under this law and provide for nondiscrimination of students with disabilities in private schools.

Unfortunately, many school districts may be unaware of the laws and how they apply to children in school. It is necessary for the school nurse, and in some cases the parent, to serve as the child advocate to enlighten school districts of their legal responsibilities with regard to asthma management. School districts may need to adjust their policies to become updated with current laws allowing children to carry asthma medications. Some states have provided that, to comply with the federal law, state legislation identifies certain conditions must be met. For example, they require written authorization for parent or guardian for self-administration of asthma medication, a written statement from a licensed provider containing the student name, purpose, appropriate usage, dosage, time or times and under what circumstances the medication may be administered, and that the student has demonstrated the ability and understanding to self-administer the medication by passing an assessment by the school nurse who evaluates technique and level of understanding of the medication. In addition, the school district required parent acknowledgment in writing that they understand they will hold harmless the school, employees, agents, and school board from any injury resulting from self-administration of the medication.[29] In 2010 all 50 states agreed to allow the portability of asthma/allergy medication for children.[30] This agreement has allowed children to carry their rescue inhalers to class, lunch, and gym. Having a rescue inhaler available during known periods of possible asthma exacerbations improves access to care and decreases the incidence of asthma emergencies.

The school environment provides an excellent opportunity to screen for asthma in an effort to identify undiagnosed children and to deliver educational programs for children with asthma. Educating the teachers is extremely effective in decreasing the number of acute asthmatic episodes in children. Teachers may be the first to recognize early onset of a child who experiences respiratory distress/wheezing and requires short-acting bronchodilators per metered-dose inhaler with a spacer or even nebulized treatments in an effort to prevent an emergency room visit. In providing school-based asthma education, it is important to include the school personnel as well as children and families. The importance of providing an asthma-friendly school environment to provide improved asthma control was reviewed in 2008. Families need to be aware of school policies and procedures to navigate the school system better and to facilitate administration of medications while at school. Cicutto[31] suggests 8 goals to improve asthma management in school. The goals include the following:

1. Identify and track all students with asthma;
2. Assure immediate access to medications as prescribed;
3. Use an individualized asthma action plan for all students with asthma;
4. Encourage full participation in school-related activities, including physical activity;
5. Use standard emergency protocols for worsening asthma;
6. Educate all school personnel and students;
7. Identify and reduce common asthma triggers; and
8. Ensure communication and collaboration among school personnel, families, and health professionals/medical home, including discussion of asthma-related policies in school.

Immediate access to inhalers and an individualized asthma action plan give children the best possible opportunity to prevent acute exacerbations and to control them if they begin.[31]

Educational Programs in Schools

Multiple programs for schools have been studied to determine the best strategy for education in the school system. "Happy Air" is a school-based program for children and their families in primary grades with asthma. Children (n = 2765) and families were enrolled in the program that included diagnosis, clinical follow-up, education, self-management, and quality-of-life control aims to decrease the socioeconomic burden of asthma disease. Asthma management was significantly improved after the use of the program. An assessment to evaluate the need for educational programs was performed in 2010.[32] Findings showed that teachers' knowledge about asthma and asthma management is limited, especially among those whose students did not have active asthma. A more proactive approach to asthma management was recommended.[33] In the pilot testing, "Okay with Asthma," available at www.okay-with-asthma.org,[34] school-aged children aged 8 to 11 participated in an online asthma intervention program. This online asthma intervention program was originally developed for school nurses to use in health offices. The program was free and accessible to any school with Internet access. The self-guided program used a 20-minute animated story about a school-aged girl with asthma. It was used to convey asthma management strategies, including psychosocial strategies to adjust to asthma and the role of school personnel and peers in helping a child adjust to asthma. The efficacy of this program is not known, but could be replicated in larger samples over a longer period of time to learn the retention of asthma knowledge.[35] A review by Jones and colleagues looked at "How Asthma Friendly is Your School?" The questionnaire assessed 8 school health program components: health education, health services, physical education and activity, mental health and social services, nutrition services, healthy and safe school environment, faculty and staff health promotion, and family and community involvement. Administering this questionnaire highlighted the needs of the school system to provide additional programs for not only children and families but also all school ancillary personnel. Through the identification of deficiencies, improved educational programs can be implemented.[36]

Consulting Physician Role in Schools

Schools that have a consulting physician available provide improved asthma management and decrease absenteeism. It is hypothesized that parents have more confidence in the decisions of the school nurse when a consulting physician is in place.

In addition, school nurses have more self-confidence when they have the option of consulting with a physician regarding asthma treatment options. The 2009 study reviewing the implementation of a consulting physician in schools for children with asthma showed a decrease in absenteeism. The number of missed school days for students decreased from 8.9 to 7.5 after implementing the role of the consulting physician. The decreased absenteeism translates to increased reimbursement by school districts. More information is needed to examine the economic impact of implementing the consulting physician in school districts.[37]

SUMMARY

The incidence of pediatric asthma in the United States creates a huge financial burden to the economy as well as a negative impact on child health. The management of asthma in the home and school is positively impacted through improved education for children, their families, and all those who care for them. Identification and elimination of asthma triggers are helpful in reducing asthma exacerbations. The incidence of asthma is higher in African American and underserved populations. The implementation of effective asthma education improves the economic consequences for society and improves the health and future of children. Improved management of pediatric asthma leads to improved school performance and improved mental health and general well-being. The knowledge of the school nurse regarding federal and state laws is very helpful in providing improved asthma management for children. The use of an asthma action plan decreases the number of acute asthma exacerbations in children. It is the responsibility of the school nurse to educate school staff and ancillary personnel to assist in promoting child health and decreasing the health issues related to pediatric asthma.

REFERENCES

1. Stewart LJ. Pediatric asthma. Prim Care Clin Office Pract 2008;35:25–40.
2. CDC. National health Interview Survey (NHIS) data: 2008 lifetime and current asthma. Atlanta (GA): US Department of Health and Human Services, CDC; 2010. Available at: http://www.cdc.gov/asthma/nhis/08data.htm. Accessed August 6, 2012.
3. Barnett SB, Nurmagambetov TA. Costs of asthma in the United States: 2002-2008. J Allergy Clin Immunol 2011;127:145–52.
4. Crawford D. Understanding childhood asthma and the development of the respiratory tract. Nurs Child Young People 2011;23(7):25–34.
5. Centers for Disease Control and Prevention (CDC). Vital signs: asthma prevalence, disease characteristics, and self-management education. United States, 2001-2009. MMWR Morb Mortal Wkly Rep 2011;60:547–52.
6. Available at: http://www.healthypeople.gov/2020/topicsobjectives2020/objectiveslist.aspx?topicId=36. Accessed August 6, 2012.
7. National Institutes of Health, National Heart, Lung and Blood Institute (NHLBI). Guidelines for the diagnosis and management of asthma (EPR-3). Bethesda (MD): US Department of Health and Human Services, National institutes of health, National heart, Lung, and Blood Institute; 2007. Available at: http://www.nhlbi.nih.gov/guidelines/astha/asthgdln.pdf. Accessed August 8, 2012.
8. Breysse J, Wendt J, Dixon S, et al. Nurse case management and housing interventions reduce allergen exposures: the Milwaukee randomized controlled trial. Public Health Rep 2011;126(Suppl 1):89–99.

9. Barnes CS. Reduced clinic, emergency room, and hospital utilization after home environmental assessment and case management. Allergy Asthma Proc 2010; 31(4):317–23.
10. Davis D, Gordon M, Burns B. Educational interventions for childhood asthma: a review and integrative model for preschoolers from low-income families. Pediatr Nurs 2011;37(1):31–8.
11. Largo T, Borgialli M, Wisinski C, et al. Healthy Homes University: a home based environmental intervention and education program for families with pediatric asthma in Michigan. Public Health Rep 2011;126(Suppl 1):14–26.
12. Watson WT, Gillespie C, Thomas N, et al. Small group interactive education and the effect on asthma control by children and their families. CMAJ 2009;181(5): 257–63.
13. Bryant-Stephens T, Li Y. Outcomes of a home-based environmental remediation for urban children with asthma. J Natl Med Assoc 2008;100(3):306–16.
14. Celano MP. Home based family intervention for low income children with asthma a randomized controlled pilot study. J Fam Psychol 2012;26(2):171–8.
15. Lobar S. The experience of being an Asthma Amigo in a program to decrease asthma episodes in Hispanic children. J Pediatr Nurs 2008;23(5):364–71.
16. Canino G, Vila D, Normand S, et al. Reducing asthma health disparities in poor Puerto Rican children: the effectiveness of a culturally tailored family intervention. J Allergy Clin Immunol 2008;121(3):665–70.
17. Meischke H. Engagement in "My Child's Asthma" an interactive web-based pediatric asthma management intervention. Int J Med Inform 2011;80(11):765–74.
18. El Mallakh P, Howard PB, Inman SM. Medical and psychiatric comorbidities in children and adolescents: a guide to issues and treatment approaches. Nurs Clin North Am 2010;45(4):541–54.
19. Peterson-Sweeny K. The relationship of household routines to morbidity outcomes in childhood asthma. J Pediatr Nurs 2009;14(1):59–69.
20. Crocker D, Kinyota S, Dumitru G, et al. Effectiveness of home based, multi-trigger multicomponent interventions with an environmental focus for reducing asthma morbidity; a community guide systematic review. Am J Prev Med 2011;41(2 Suppl 1):S5–32.
21. Butz AM. Shared decision making in school age children with asthma. Pediatr Nurs 2007;33(2):111–6.
22. Mizan SS, Shendell DG, Rhoads GG. Absence extended absence, and repeat tardiness related to asthma status among elementary school children. J Asthma 2011;48(3):228–34.
23. Moonie S. The relationship between school absence, academic performance, and asthma status. J Sch Health 2008;78(3):140–8.
24. Bruzzese J, Evans D, Kattan M. School Based asthma programs. J Allergy Clin Immunol 2009;124:195–200.
25. Collins JE. Mental, emotional, and social problems among school children with asthma. J Asthma 2008;45(6):489–93.
26. Lipstein EA. School absenteeism, health status, and health care utilization among children with asthma: associations with parental chronic disease. Pediatrics 2009;123(1):360–6.
27. National Association of School Based Health Centers. Available at: http://www.nasbhc.org/site/c.ckLQKbOVLkK6E/b.7697107/apps/s/content.asp?ct=10884071. Accessed August 7, 2012.
28. Tai T, Bame S. Cost-benefit analysis of childhood asthma management through school based clinic programs. J Community Health 2011;36(2):253–60.

29. Putman-Casdorph H, Badzek L. Asthma and allergy medication self-administration by children in school: liability issues for the nurse. J Nurs Law 2011;14(1):32–6.
30. Allergy and Asthma Network Mothers of Asthmatics. Available at: http://www.aanma.org/advocacy/meds-at-school/. Accessed August 7, 2012.
31. Cicutto L. Supporting successful asthma management in schools: the role of the asthma care providers. J Allergy Clin Immunol 2009;124(2):390–3.
32. Chini L. Happy Air, a successful school based asthma educational and interventional program for primary school children. J Asthma 2011;48(4):419–26.
33. Bruzzese JM. Asthma knowledge and asthma management behavior in urban elementary school teachers. J Asthma 2010;47(2):185–91.
34. Okay with Asthma! Available at: www.okaywithasthma.org. Accessed August 7, 2012.
35. Wyatt RH, Hauenstein EJ. Pilot testing okay with asthma: an online asthma intervention for school-age children. J Sch Nurs 2008;24(3):145–50.
36. Jones SE, Wheeler LS, Smith AM, et al. Adherence to national Asthma Education and Prevention Program's "how asthma-friendly is your school?" recommendations. J Sch Nurs 2009;25(5):382–94.
37. Wilson K, Moonie S, Sterling D, et al. Examining the consulting physician model to enhance the school nurse role for children with asthma. J Sch Health 2009;79(1):1–7.

Difficult Childhood Asthma
Management and Future

Isabelle Tillie-Leblond, MD, PhD[a,b,*], Antoine Deschildre, MD[b,c],
Philippe Gosset, PhD[b], Jacques de Blic, MD[d]

KEYWORDS

- Asthma • Severe • Child • Difficult

KEY POINTS

- Severe childhood asthma, refractory to treatment, includes different phenotypes. Genetics mainly contribute to disease expression, progression, and response to treatment. The gene-environment interactions involving certain gene polymorphisms are probably essential for creating its severity.
- The quality of care and monitoring of children with severe asthma is as important as the prescription drug, and is also crucial for differentiating between severe asthma and difficult asthma, so expertise is required.
- Further studies (genetic and proteomic data), performed in well phenotyped children with severe asthma, should improve knowledge of the mechanisms involved in frequent exacerbations, persistent obstruction, sudden-onset severe asthma and help the pediatric pulmonologist to choose the appropriate monitoring and treatment of the phenotype.

This article originally appeared in Clinics in Chest Medicine, Volume 33, Issue 3, September 2012.
Conflict of interest: J.de B. has received grant research from GSK for immunohistopathologic analysis in severe asthma, honoraria for lectures and expert advice by CHIESI, GSK, MSD, and AstraZeneca. I.T.L. has received grant research from GSK for immunohistopathologic analysis in severe asthma, honoraria for lectures and expert advice by CHIESI, GSK, NOVARTIS, and AstraZeneca. A.D. has received honoraria for lectures and expert advises by NOVARTIS, GSK, and MSD.
[a] Pulmonary Department, University Hospital, Medical University of Lille, Hôpital Calmette, 1 Boulevard Leclercq, Lille Cedex 59037, France; [b] INSERM U 1019 Lung Infection and Innate Immunity, Université de Lille 2, Institut Pasteur, 1 rue du Professeur Calmette, BP 245, Lille Cedex 59019, France; [c] Unité de pneumopédiatrie, Centre de compétence des maladies respiratoires rares, Université Lille 2 et CHRU, Hôpital Jeanne de Flandre, Avenue Eugène Avinée, Lille 59037, France; [d] Service de pneumologie et allergologie pédiatriques, Centre de référence des maladies respiratoires rares, Hôpital Necker Enfants Malades, Assistance Publique des Hôpitaux de Paris; Université Paris Descartes, Paris 75015, France
* Corresponding author. Pulmonary Department, University Hospital, Medical University of Lille, Hôpital Calmette, 1 Boulevard Leclercq, 59037 Lille, Cedex, France.
E-mail address: i-tillie@chru-lille.fr

Severe asthma in children represents about 5% of asthmatics.[1] Diagnosis and management of severe asthma implies the definition of different entities, that is, difficult asthma and refractory severe asthma, but also the different phenotypes included in the term refractory severe asthma. A complete reevaluation by a physician expert in asthma is necessary, adapted for each child. Identification of mechanisms involved in different phenotypes in refractory severe asthma, may improve the therapeutic approach.

DEFINITION OF SEVERE CHILDHOOD ASTHMA

A wide variety of terms has been used by clinicians when referring to asthmatic children who have severe asthma: difficult-to-treat asthma, therapy-resistant asthma, difficult-to-control asthma, severe therapy-resistant asthma, severe refractory asthma and, more recently, problematic asthma.

The initial criteria for severe asthma in children were proposed in 1999 by the task force on difficult/therapy-resistant asthma.[2] A dose of beclomethasone or budesonide higher than 800 μg/d, or 400 μg/d of fluticasone was considered as reasonable threshold. In 2005, the American Thoracic Society (ATS) workshop reviewed by Wenzel[3] defined severe asthma in adults by the presence of one major criterion, namely, the need for high-dose inhaled corticosteroids or oral corticosteroids, and at least 2 of the following 7 minor criteria: (1) the need for a daily long-acting β2-agonist or leukotriene antagonist in addition to inhaled corticosteroids; (2) asthma symptoms requiring daily or near-daily use of a short-acting β2-agonist; (3) persistent airway obstruction, forced expiratory volume in 1 second (FEV_1) less than 80% predicted; (4) one or more emergency-care visits for asthma per year (5) 3 or more oral steroid "bursts" per year; (6) prompt deterioration with less than 25% reduction in oral or inhaled corticosteroid dose; (7) near-fatal asthma event in the past.[3]

More recently, in 2010, the Problematic Severe Asthma in Childhood Initiative Group has defined different categories of severe asthma.[4] Severe asthma should be considered in school-age children who, despite prescribed therapy with inhaled corticosteroid (ICS) (budesonide or equivalent 800 μg or more) with long-acting β-agonist (LABA) or leukotriene receptor antagonist, still have persistent chronic symptoms or exacerbations, or persistent airflow obstruction. Persistent chronic symptoms are defined if they occur most days (at least 3 times a week for ≥3 months) with poor quality of life. Acute exacerbations over the last year may require at least one admission to an intensive care unit, at least 2 hospital admissions, or at least 2 courses of oral steroids. Persistent airflow obstruction (following steroid trial) is defined by postbronchodilator FEV_1 less than 80% predicted value or Z score less than 1.96. The need for alternate-day or daily oral steroids, which is the last category, is extremely rare.

In preschool children, severe asthma should be considered when maximum treatment according to the recommended guidelines fails.

Severe asthma is a heterogeneous condition with different phenotypes:

- Persistence of symptoms or frequent exacerbations in a child with normal pulmonary function tests
- Persistence of symptoms or frequent exacerbations in a child associated with persistent airflow obstruction
- Persistent airflow obstruction in a child with few or no clinical symptoms

Severe or problematic asthma could also be split into 2 subcategories[5]:

- Difficult asthma, which should be reserved for asthma that remains uncontrolled because of persistent of poor compliance, aggravating factors, and comorbidities

- Severe refractory asthma, which should be reserved for children who are still uncontrolled despite optimum treatment of aggravating factors and comorbidities

Definition of severe asthma also implies 3 notions: (1) alternative diagnoses are excluded, (2) precipitating factors are correctly assessed, and (3) adherence to treatment is good.

DIAGNOSIS WORKUP EXPLORATIONS OF SEVERE ASTHMA IN CHILDREN

In a child referred for supposed severe asthma, explorations aim to confirm asthma, to detect precipitating factors and comorbidities, and to evaluate inflammation and airways remodeling,[5] constituting a main step in differentiating difficult from severe asthma.

Exclude Other Diagnoses to Differentiate Difficult Asthma from Severe Asthma

The first step is to arrive at the correct diagnosis.[5–7] **Box 1** summarizes the main alternative diagnoses. It should be noted that all these diseases may be associated with a true asthma.

The initial workup should include: inspiratory and expiratory chest radiographs; inspiratory and, if possible, expiratory low-dose high-resolution computed tomography (HRCT); nasal and exhaled nitric oxide; and, if sufficiently suspected: biopsy for primary ciliary dyskinesia, immunologic investigations with at least immunoglobulin (Ig)G, IgA, IgM measures, antibody response to vaccines, pHmetry, sweat test, and genotyping for cystic fibrosis. Vocal cord dysfunction, which is a possible comorbid condition in severe asthma, may induce inadequate overload treatment. Endoscopic visualization of an inappropriate adduction of the vocal cords during inspiration is the gold standard for the diagnosis.

Bronchoscopy may be part of this workup to exclude an anatomic or dynamic abnormality such as tracheal stenosis or tracheomalacia.

Not all of the workup is necessary for all children, and a focused approach based on history and physical examination is more appropriate.

Precipitating Factors and Comorbidities in Difficult-To-Treat Asthma

Inappropriate use of drug-delivery devices and poor adherence to medication are certainly the most frequent contributing factors for poor control of asthma.[8]

Precipitating factors include environmental tobacco smoke and ongoing allergen exposure. Data suggest that, as with active smoking, exposure to passive smoking leads to steroid resistance. Allergen exposure may induce both acute exacerbation and persistent airway inflammation. A complete allergic workup is necessary. Comorbid food allergy in asthma seems to reduce asthma control, whereas comorbid asthma in food allergy increases the risk of severe reactions and anaphylaxis.

The other main comorbidities associated with severe asthma in children are ear/nose/throat problems, mainly rhinitis and chronic rhinosinusitis, and gastroesophageal reflux. Complete examination, nasofibroscopy and sinus computed tomography (CT) scan, and esophageal pH testing may be necessary. In children, the impact of obesity on the severity and control of asthma is not evident, as in adults. However, obesity is associated with more severe acute asthma and also with a diminished response to ICSs.

Box 1
Alternative diagnoses of asthma in children

- Proximal airway obstruction
  - Inhaled foreign body
  - Tracheal or bronchial stenosis
  - Bronchopulmonary malformation
  - Benign or malignant tumor
  - Aortic arch abnormalities, pulmonary sling
  - Tracheomalacia, bronchomalacia
- Peripheral airway obstruction
  - Cystic fibrosis
  - Bronchopulmonary disease
  - Primary ciliary dyskinesia
  - Postinfectious (viral) obliterative bronchiolitis
- Recurrent aspirations
  - Tracheoesophageal fistula
  - Swallowing disorders
  - Gastroesophageal reflux
- Bronchiectasis
- Defect of host defense
- Chronic interstitial lung disease
- Extrinsic allergic alveolitis
- Eosinophilic lung
- Congenital heart disease (especially left to right shunt)
- Cardiac failure
- Vocal cord dysfunction
- Hyperventilation/panic attack

Evaluation of Inflammation and Remodeling by Indirect and Noninvasive Techniques in Severe Asthma

This step is certainly the most innovative part of the evaluation of severe asthma. For ethical and safety reasons, only few studies have been performed on children with asthma, and this is particularly true for studies involving bronchoscopy. In children, the use of invasive and direct techniques (ie, bronchoscopy, bronchoalveolar lavage [BAL], and biopsy) to clarify diagnosis and guide management is justified only in cases of refractory asthma (see later discussion). The development of noninvasive markers is necessary, given the ethical difficulties of conducting research in severe asthmatic children. These techniques include induced sputum, fractional exhaled nitric oxide (FE_{NO}), exhaled breath condensate, and HRCT scan.

Sputum induction is performed with hypertonic saline after pretreatment with a bronchodilator. The success rate is 60% to 90% and safety is good.[9–12] Normal sputum eosinophil percentage is assumed to be less than 3%.[11] In 38 children with difficult asthma, only one-third had abnormal sputum cytology, either eosinophils or neutrophils.[11,12]

To date, the best performing biomarker appears to be an inflammatory profile in sputum, but the practical difficulties of sputum induction, and technical variation in sputum analysis and processing limit the clinical application.

Extensive literature has been published on the value of FE_{NO} in asthmatic children. FE_{NO} is elevated in asthma, especially when eosinophilic inflammation is present. Recent ATS guidelines suggest that FE_{NO} may be useful for detecting eosinophilic airway inflammation, determining the likelihood of corticosteroid responsiveness, monitoring airway inflammation to determine the potential need for corticosteroids, and as a tool for nonadherence to corticosteroid.[13]

FE_{NO} and induced sputum have been used by Zacharasiewicz and colleagues[14] to predict the success or failure of reducing inhaled steroids in 40 children with stable asthma. Step-down was successful in all children who had no eosinophils in induced sputum, whereas increased FE_{NO} and elevated eosinophils were predictive of failed reduction.

Lex and colleagues[12] investigated the relationships between FE_{NO}, eosinophils in induced sputum, BAL, and bronchial subepithelium in a group of children with severe asthma. The investigators found significant correlations between eosinophils in the sputum and both BAL eosinophils and FE_{NO}, as well as between FE_{NO} and BAL eosinophils. However, they were not related to airway wall eosinophilia. Despite a good negative predictive value (89%), there was a poor positive predictive value (36%).

The measurement of FE_{NO} at different flows may allow partitioning of NO production to proximal and distal airways. In children with severe asthma, NO measurements were related to inflammation and several parameters of airway remodeling, suggesting that both subacute inflammation and remodeling influence NO output in refractory asthma.[15] At present, the clinical use of FE_{NO} routinely in severe asthma remains to be determined.

Condensate from exhaled breath (EBC) may reflect the composition of the airway lining fluid. EBC may be obtained in children even during exacerbation. However, no biomarkers have been validated for clinical use.[7]

HRCT is a noninvasive technique that may be valuable for quantifying airway remodeling in patients with severe asthma. It may also identify other diagnoses in asthma that are difficult to treat. In adults, evaluations of HRCT have shown that abnormalities of the airways, particularly the extent of bronchial wall thickening (BWT), correlate with lung functions, reticular basement membrane (RBM) thickness, and matrix metalloproteinase 9/tissue inhibitor metalloproteinase 1 production imbalance.[16,17]

In children with severe asthma, BWT was significantly higher than in control children.[18] Furthermore, bronchial thickening assessed by the BWT score on HRCT correlated with RBM thickening and NO production by the airway wall, but not with inflammatory markers determined by BAL or bronchial biopsy, or with pulmonary functions.[19]

The new generations of multislice CT scanners will allow higher definition and lower radiation exposure, and will probably give a better assessment of airway remodeling and efficacy of treatment in children with asthma. HRCT is not a routine procedure in children with severe asthma, and should be performed only if there is doubt as to the diagnosis. However, it could be incorporated in research protocols to determine correlation with airway structures.

In conclusion, the first steps in the exploration of severe asthma are to achieve the correct diagnosis (alternative or associated diagnosis) and to evaluate adherence to treatment, precipitating factors, and comorbidities. These first steps should be done systematically in all children presenting with difficult asthma.

The second level aims to evaluate the phenotype of severe asthma related to the clinical and/or functional features, and the patterns of airway inflammation and remodeling.

The techniques used, either direct and invasive or indirect and noninvasive, are not systematic but are reserved only for specialized units, whose staff are trained for techniques as well as analyses. Most of these techniques are still used for clinical or biological research.

When alternative diagnoses are excluded, comorbidities and environmental factors are evaluated, and adherence to treatment seems to have been obtained, difficult asthma is excluded. The diagnosis of severe childhood asthma refractory to treatment is probable.

PATHOPHYSIOLOGY OF SEVERE ASTHMA IN CHILDREN

Severe asthma in children displays heterogeneity and variability in its clinical and pathologic expression. Different phenotypes are described: persistent symptoms and/or frequent exacerbations, and/or persistent airway obstruction despite therapy, neutrophilic versus eosinophilic inflammation, and so forth. In addition, phenotypes can overlap and change over time. Although the pathophysiology is often detailed by concomitant and successive events, severe asthma results from many different pathways. The role of viral infection and allergen exposure is better known, but their implication and relationship with the severity is not well established.

Severe Asthma: An Early Determination

Cohort studies are in favor of an early onset of the severity. In cohort studies, severity was often defined by the appearance of an airway obstruction that persists in small and/or large airways. The greatest absolute loss of lung function seems to occur very early on in childhood.[20–22] In a cohort of children followed from birth until the age of 10 years, functional abnormalities associated with the risk of asthma existed in the first year of life.[23] Atopy plays a key role in the onset of asthma in children. Sensitization to perennial allergens developing in the first 3 years of life is associated with a loss of lung function at school age. This loss is increased with concomitant exposure to high levels of perennial allergens early on in life.[24] Cohort studies show that a combination of early sensitization and early lower respiratory tract infections (particularly human rhinovirus) in children is strongly associated with persistent asthma.[25–28] Holt and colleagues[29,30] suggest that the development of immune and inflammatory responses at the same time by these separate stimuli (allergen and virus) in the airways during a period of lung growth may perturb normal tissue-differentiation programs and result in disturbed respiratory function. Nevertheless, not all children exposed to these environmental factors develop a severe form of asthma. A combination of multiple environmental factors and genetic background (at risk or not) define the characteristics of the inflammatory and immune responses, with a particular important signature in resident cells such as epithelial cells. The nature of this host response is probably critical for the emergence of the disease and the development of a severe form of asthma. In children at risk of severe asthma, constitutional factors leading to an excessive remodeling process or persistent inflammation after rhinovirus infection, related to a defect in antioxidative response, an impaired phagocytosis function, or a deficiency in type I interferon (IFN) production, may play a role in the development of its severity.

Severe Asthma in Children and Cellular Infiltrate: Lack of Specificity

The presence of inflammatory cell infiltrate, mainly composed of eosinophils, neutrophils, and T lymphocytes, has been described in severe asthma in children, even if the role of resident cells (epithelial, fibroblasts, dendritic cells and macrophages) is central.

Most asthmatic children have eosinophilic airway inflammation.[31] Neutrophilia or a mixed cellularity is also often described.[11,32,33] BAL neutrophilia is a frequent pattern observed in preschool wheeze, whether or not associated with viral or bacterial infection.[34–36] The responsibility of exposure to passive smoking, infection, treatments, allergens, gastroesophageal reflux, endotoxins, and other environmental factors in influx of inflammatory cells is complex.[37] One hypothesis is that, in asthma, neutrophilic inflammation may precede eosinophilic inflammation.

In severe asthma in children, T-helper (Th)2-derived cytokines and eosinophils have been described.[31–33,38,39] Airway eosinophils may persist in difficult asthma in children, despite prednisolone therapy.[31] Noneosinophilic inflammation has also been reported.[11,40] In children, BAL neutrophilia may be correlated to the severity of asthma.[35,41] Persistence of bronchial eosinophilia does not mean uncontrolled asthma when mucosal eosinophilia persists in clinical remission of asthma.[42] The location of inflammatory infiltrate may be important. There are few data concerning the presence and the role of inflammatory cell microlocalization to structural cells (smooth muscle cells, glandular cells, airway nerves, and so forth) in severe childhood asthma. Mechanisms involved in their migration and their interactions with structural cells may play a role in bronchial hyperresponsiveness or the remodeling process, which could determine a factor of severity.[43] In severe asthma, eosinophils and neutrophils persist in bronchial biopsies, even under ICSs.[33] In severe asthma characterized by persistent airway obstruction, Th2 inflammation was associated with the presence of activated eosinophils and neutrophils in the epithelium in symptomatic children, whereas the inflammatory infiltrate was not found in paucisymptomatic asthmatic children.[33] This correlation does not exist with eosinophils and neutrophils in BAL or bronchial mucosa.[33] This study confirms that, as in adults, lumen and airway walls are different compartments.[12]

Balance of Th1/Th2?

Persistent airway obstruction was associated with a greater number of CD4$^+$ T cells in bronchial biopsies in difficult asthma under systemic corticosteroids, compared with controls in school-age children.[44]

After previous studies showed no difference in interleukin (IL-4), IL-5, and RANTES expression in bronchial biopsies between difficult asthma and controls in children,[44] Fitzpatrick and colleagues[32] recently described molecular phenotypes in children with severe asthma, based on cytokines, chemokines, BAL levels, and lysates from alveolar macrophages. In BAL, CXCL1, RANTES (CCL5), IL-12, IFN-γ, and IL-10 best characterized severe versus moderate asthma in children. In alveolar-macrophage lysate, a higher level of IL-6 was the strongest discriminator for severe asthma.[32] De Blic and colleagues[33] also showed an increase in Th1 cytokine levels in and paucisymptomatic (compared with symptomatic) children with severe asthma with persistent obstruction, whereas the IFN-γ/IL-4 balance was lower in symptomatic children. The high levels of IFN-γ in paucisymptomatic children suggest that this Th1 cytokine may modulate the local inflammatory response.[33] These studies clearly demonstrate that the classic Th1/Th2 pattern is not so constant in children with severe asthma.

Location of Inflammation

Bronchial or luminal, but also proximal or distal bronchial inflammation may also influence symptoms and severity. Involvement of distal airways in severe asthma in children is difficult to assess. BAL by definition evaluates a part of both compartments. Even if it has been performed,[45] there are some concerns about the practice of rigid bronchoscopy and transbronchial biopsies to evaluate respiratory symptoms routinely. Cohort studies with evaluation of lung function showed early distal impairment.[23,24]

IMMUNE RESPONSE: DO PREFERENTIAL PATHWAYS LEAD TO THE SEVERITY OF ASTHMA?
Environmental Factors: Virus and Allergen

Interaction of dendritic cells with allergens in the airway mucosa generates a Th2 cytokine response and, according to the genetic and environmental cofactors present, may lead to asthma induction.[46] Immune mechanisms involved in sensitization and allergic asthma have largely been developed. Recent developments provide new hypotheses concerning the immune response to respiratory viral infection in allergic asthmatics.[29,30,47]

Frequent exacerbations are associated with a phenotype of severe asthma, and repeated exacerbations are associated with an accelerated decline of lung function. The role of viral respiratory tract infections in severe asthma is probably essential, complex, and still widely debated. Virus produces wheezing episodes during the first 3 years of life in almost 50% of children.[48] In children at risk, rhinovirus infection is associated with a high risk of asthma.[49] The most recent hypothesis is that respiratory infection by rhinovirus, occurring in atopic asthmatic children (in a Th2 environment), is responsible for an enhanced FcεRI expression on dendritic cells. Thus, dendritic cells may produce proinflammatory mediators in response to allergens at challenge sites via nuclear factor κB–dependent mechanisms. Moreover, this may result in an enhanced capacity to capture the allergen (through its recognition by specific IgE) and to present the epitopes to specific allergen Th2 lymphocytes.[50] This process probably results in an enhanced activation of Th2 lymphocytes responsible for the production of Th2 cytokines IL-4, IL-5, and so forth. Their production may decrease or downregulate Th1 response to viral infection (IFN-γ) and increase airway inflammation. Signaling issued from the action of Th2 cytokines may enhance FcεRI expression on dendritic-cell precursors in bone marrow.[29,30] This concept needs to be confirmed, but represents an enticing reasoning. Genome-wide patterns of gene expression in sputum cells in children with asthma following an exacerbation showed that the activation of the Th1-like and IFN signaling pathways was decreased and was associated with airway obstruction.[47]

Virus-induced asthma/or wheezing episodes may also reveal a preexisting tendency toward asthma secondary to an impaired response to viral infection (decrease in type I IFN and viral clearance, increase in remodeling, and so forth).[27,51–53] There is a discrepancy in antiviral immune response in asthmatics compared with the healthy population. Increased risk of recurrent wheezing in the preschool and school-age years was associated with low concentrations of IFN-γ and IFN-λ (Th1 cytokine) in early life.[54–57] Respiratory viruses enter and replicate within airway epithelial cells. This step is the first toward initiating an innate and adaptive immune response. In reaction to rhinovirus, bronchial epithelial cells secrete proinflammatory cytokines and chemokines as well as an antiviral immune response.[58–60] Bronchial epithelial cells in asthmatics produced lower levels of type-I and type-III IFN (IFN-β and IFN-λ), which is associated with a higher level of rhinovirus replication.[53] Bullens and colleagues[61] showed that IFN-γ mRNA levels obtained from sputum cells correlated negatively with asthma symptoms in moderate to severe asthma, demonstrating a protective role for IFN-γ. The mechanisms behind deficient IFN-β and IFN-λ production in asthmatics remain unknown. It may result either from a polymorphism in its genes or their promoters, or from an excess of TGF-β secretion in asthmatic airways that mediates enhanced rhinovirus replication, potentially through its suppressive action on host type-I IFN responses.[62] Among mediators implicated in antiviral immunity, a recent study showed that IL-15 is reduced in BAL in asthmatics and in supernatants of macrophage stimulated by rhinovirus. This process may also play a role in virus-induced exacerbation in asthma.[63] In allergic mice, it has been shown that the immune response to respiratory viruses differs from that in control mice. Activation of pattern-recognition receptors such as Toll-like receptors (TLR)3 and TLR7/TLR8 as well as the RNA helicases are responsible for the innate response to respiratory viruses through the recognition of single-stranded and double-stranded RNA. The mobilization of these receptors is responsible for the antiviral response through the activation of an interferon regulatory factor (IRF)3/IRF7-dependent pathway. In asthmatic patients, an alteration of the expression and/or function of these receptors, and of the downstream signaling pathway, may be suspected.

The role of bacteria as superantigens, an exacerbating factor and risk factor of asthma, is also debated. Colonization with *Streptococcus pneumoniae*, *Haemophilus influenzae*, *Moraxella catarrhalis*, or *Staphylococcus aureus* is associated with an increased risk of recurrent wheezing and asthma before the age of 5 years.[64] The role of bacteria in the maintenance of a local inflammation and in the induction of a specific immune response to allergens remains a matter of debate. A recent discovery undermining the concept of sterility of the lower respiratory tract has been published.[65] Bronchial airways are not sterile; they contain bacterial flora, like the intestine, even if the number is much lower. Children with severe therapy-resistant asthma have different flora with more proteobacteria and fewer *Prevotella* species. This status could be related to the treatment, but could also be involved in the modulation of the local immune response to environmental factors. In germ-free mice, it has been shown that the presence of commensal bacteria is critical for ensuring control of allergic inflammation.[66] This effect may be related to a defect in the maturation of the immune system in the intestine, as demonstrated in mice. However, the role of the lung microbiome is still unknown, but may be involved in the maintenance of local inflammation and in the induction of a specific immune response to environmental factors.

One may hypothesize that rhinovirus induces severe asthma in predisposed children. A persistent obstructive pattern is a phenotype of severe asthma. In children with asthma, rhinovirus was detected in 45% by in situ hybridization on bronchial biopsies. Abnormal lung function was detected in 86% of rhinovirus-positive children and in 58% of rhinovirus-negative children. Persistence of the virus in the respiratory tract is associated with the severity of asthma, associated with persistent obstruction.[67] Resident cells, such as myofibroblasts, infected by rhinovirus in asthmatics, are associated with an enhanced viral replication and chemokine release involved in neutrophil recruitment.[62] In some predisposed children, local airway inflammation triggered by viral infection may alter lung growth and tissue differentiation, leading to alteration of lung function that persists for long time.[68] The immune (innate) response to rhinovirus or RSV differs between individuals, particularly between children at risk and not at risk of asthma. An aberrant innate immune response to repeated rhinovirus infections may facilitate airway remodeling and severe asthma via epithelial cell alterations, and enhance viral replication and persistence of bronchial inflammation.

Additional genetic factors that regulate the response to oxidative stress after viral infection or other environmental triggers also contribute to the quality of response.

Oxidative Stress and Genetic Factors in Severe Childhood Asthma

Excessive formation of reactive oxygen species and imbalance between pro-oxidant and antioxidant mediators are associated with severe asthma and reduced lung function. Systemic superoxide dismutase (SOD) deficiency was shown to correlate with airway obstruction.[69] The diminished systemic SOD activity associated with environmental tobacco-smoke exposure showed a specific oxidant mechanism by which tobacco-smoke exposure may affect patients with asthma.[70] SOD inhibition increased bronchial epithelial cell death through the cleavage/activation of caspases, and the oxidation and nitration of MnSOD, identified in the asthmatic airway, correlated with asthma severity.[71] These findings link oxidative stress to reduced SOD activity and downstream events that characterize asthma, including apoptosis and shedding of the airway epithelium. Glutathione is a powerful antioxidant. Fitzpatrick and colleagues[72] showed that in children with severe asthma associated with persistent airway obstruction, BAL fluid has more oxidized glutathione, compared with controls or children without airflow obstruction. This finding was associated in children with severe asthma with alveolar macrophage dysfunction (phagocytosis) after microbial stimulus. This macrophage dysfunction may compromise innate immune function and the clearance in pathogens.[73] The transcription nuclear factor (erythroid-derived 2)–like 2 (Nrf2) plays a main role in glutathione homeostasis and antioxidant defense. Children with severe asthma have a global disruption of thiol redox signaling and control in both the airway and systemic circulation that is associated with posttranslational modification of Nrf2.[74] Of note, Nrf2 deficiency in mice leads to the development of a severe form of asthma after allergen sensitization, a process associated with enhanced oxidative stress.[75] Increasing epithelial lining fluid glutathione level, that is, by Nrf2 reactivation, may reverse or limit the decrease in lung function in severe asthma in children.

Polymorphisms of the gene encoding for the glutathione transferase T1 and M1 is associated with the loss in lung function in utero when the pregnant woman is a tobacco smoker.[76] In early life, even in utero, the combination of tobacco smoke and a deficiency of antioxidants may lead, in children at risk, to more severe asthma with obstruction.

REMODELING IN SEVERE CHILDHOOD ASTHMA

The occurrence of remodeling is probably the consequence of interaction between both genetic (and epigenetic) and environmental factors. Decline in lung function may be a feature of airway remodeling, leading to a severe form of asthma and nonresponders to steroids, even if there are no studies on which to base conclusions. Many questions remain unanswered. What is the relationship between inflammation and remodeling? What is the impact of early anti-inflammatory treatment on prevention of remodeling? Does it occur in the early phase of the disease or later on? Does it respond to a specific trigger, or a combination of multiples?

Airway remodeling includes wall thickening, extracellular matrix deposition (including collagen), smooth muscle hyperplasia and hypertrophy, myofibroblast proliferation, mucus metaplasia, epithelial goblet-cell metaplasia and hyperplasia, subepithelial fibrosis, and thickening of the subepithelial reticular layer. The relative importance of each component is not clearly defined. Moreover, the nature of lung remodeling and of its evolution has not been extensively explored in children.

The concept explaining that airway remodeling in asthma is a process in response to long-term, unresolved airway inflammation, and that it may occur when asthma is not treated or controlled effectively, is widely discussed. Uncontrolled chronic bronchial inflammation is insufficient to explain the modification of bronchial structures.[77] Chronic inflammation may initiate tissue injury and repair, although remodeling may occur alongside inflammation.

Most studies in severe childhood asthma showed no correlation between RBM thickening and clinical characteristics or lung-function tests.[77–80] RBM thickening appears before the age of 3 years, as demonstrated in wheezy preschool children.[81] Children younger than 6 years with asthma ("confirmed wheeze" preschool children) had increased epithelial loss, RBM thickening, and eosinophilia compared with controls, showing that remodeling occurs early on in life,[81] but these modifications were not associated with the duration of symptoms, duration of asthma, and duration of treatment.[77,78] RBM is ultrastructurally similar to normal.[82] RBM thickening does not permit differentiation between moderate and severe asthma in children.[33,77,78] In severe asthma with an obstructive pattern, RBM thickening in children with persistent symptoms was similar to that seen in paucisymptomatic children.[33,78]

Even if this remodeling process may have a protective effect, smooth muscles encircling central and distal airways and muscular shortening produce constriction and shortening of the airways.[83] One hypothesis is that structural alterations can lead to fixed airway obstruction resistant to treatment, a feature of severe asthma,[84] which could contribute to loss of lung function. Airway smooth muscle is increased in severe asthma in children, correlated with an acute bronchodilation response to β2 agonists and inversely correlated with the FEV_1 value.[78,85] Hyperplasia and hypertrophy are important processes regulating increased smooth muscle mass in asthma.[86] Myofibroblasts display a phenotype intermediate between fibroblasts and smooth muscle cells, express a smooth muscle action, and have the ability to secrete matrix proteins and chemokines that prolong eosinophil survival.[87] Vitamin D seems to be an important immune-regulatory molecule. A recent study showed an inverse correlation between airway smooth muscle mass and 25(OH)D vitamin levels in severe therapy-resistant asthma,[88] and this was associated with a lower FEV_1 value. It is difficult to make conclusions because of the low number of patients included in this study[88] and the widespread vitamin D deficiency in the general population.

Vascular changes were demonstrated by the number of CD31-positive vascular structures in bronchial mucosa, significantly increased in severe childhood asthma with persistent obstruction, compared with those with normal function tests.[78] The CD31 expression was negatively correlated with FEV_1 and forced expiratory flow at 25% to 75% of vital capacity (FEF_{25-75}), and did not correlate with inflammatory infiltrates in bronchial mucosa.[78] Increased vessel numbers were confirmed to correlate with the severity of asthma in childhood asthma.[89] Increased vessel numbers, vasodilatation, and edema contribute to airway-wall thickening,[90] and also help cellular infiltration when endothelial cells express adhesion molecules in asthma.[91] Their expression (including intercellular adhesion molecule 1 and vascular cell adhesion molecule 1 [CD54 and CD104]) was controlled by both proinflammatory (TNF-α and IL-1β) and Th2 cytokines (IL-4, IL-13).

The role of epithelial cells and fibroblasts is essential in the pathogenesis of asthma (**Fig. 1**). The airway epithelium has a key role in the innate immunity. Epithelial cells interact with environmental agents and inflammatory mediators. In genetically susceptible children, impaired epithelial cells react to virus, allergen, and pollutant exposure, and may lead to an impaired repair response. An exaggerated remodeling response may lead to fixed airway obstruction associated with a more severe disease.[92] Factors responsible for bronchial remodeling are complex when inflammation does not always precede structural changes, as demonstrated in early life.[89,93,94] Comparing postmortem bronchial specimens from nonasthmatic with moderately to severely asthmatic

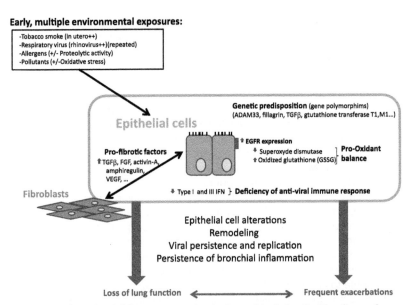

Fig. 1. Severe asthma in children: a central role for epithelial cells. The figure focuses on epithelial cell and its potential role in severe asthma. Early in life, bronchial epithelial cells are exposed to multiple environmental factors: tobacco smoke (in utero+++), respiratory virus (rhinovirus++, repeated episodes), allergens (+/− proteolytic activities), pollutants (+/− oxidatve stress). In asthma, EC have an increased expression of EGFR. Different gene polymorphisms seem to be associated with severe asthma (ADAM33, fillagrin, TGFβ, Gluta-thione transferase T1, M1...). Abnormal responses of EC to stress, in a predisposed genetic field, generate an excessive secretion of pro-fibrotic factors (TGFβ, FGF, Activin-A, VEGF, am-phiregulin that interact with fibroblats), a deficiency in anti-oxydant function and a defi-ciency in anti-viral immune response (a decrease in type I and III interferon that favors viral persistence and replication). This may lead to remodeling and enhanced and persistent bronchial inflammation and be an explanation for the frequent exacerbations, and the loss in lung function in refractory asthma in children.

children aged 5 to 15 years, Fedorov and colleagues[95] showed that the lamina retic-ularis was thicker in asthmatic biopsies, with increased deposition of collagen III, when eosinophils did not differ between groups. There was an upregulation of epidermal growth factor receptor (EGFR) expression in the bronchial epithelium, as demon-strated in adult asthma, with minimal evidence of increased proliferation.[95] This study showed that stressed epithelium exists without significant eosinophilic inflammation. Early treatment by inhaled steroids in children has a poor effect on the natural history of asthma, and eosinophils may persist under treatment in severely asthmatic chil-dren.[31,96,97] Activation of the epithelial-mesenchymal trophic unit early in life, even in utero, may support this hypothesis in the absence of recruited inflammatory cells. The first abnormality in asthma may be a disorder of repair relating to a dysregulation of EGFR-mediated repair, and the inflammation may be secondary to the abnormal tissue-repair processes.[98] Airway inflammation and remodeling could also have par-allel pathways. In children genetically predisposed to severe asthma, impaired im-mune response to environmental triggers associated with persistent inflammation of resident cells, particularly a damaged epithelium, could lead to severe asthma.[98] For example, enhanced surface expression and phosphorylation of EGFRs have been observed in severe childhood asthma, suggesting a key role played by epithelial injury in its severity. Proteases (included in some allergens such as dermatophagoides pteronyssimus) as well as tobacco smoke and pollutants generate reactive oxygen species and trigger the release of endogenous proteases. Proteases are implicated in damage to the airway epithelium. Impairment in antioxidant production, as demonstrated in severe asthmatic children,[72] associated with an enhanced surface expression and phosphorylation of EGFRs, may lead to a loss of integrity of the epithelium and be a factor in the severity of asthma in children.

Epithelial cells in reaction to stimuli are able to produce fibrogenic factors (growth factors) and inflammatory mediators. These factors may promote the transformation of fibroblasts in myofibroblasts. For example, TGF-β is produced and secreted by epithelial cells. TGF-β is involved in survival, proliferation, differentiation, and extracellular matrix regulation, and is particularly implicated in tissue repair and fibrosis.[99] Several genetic associations regarding the -509C>T polymorphism of TGF-β1 have been reported, and this polymorphism seems to contribute to the severity of asthma.[100] TGF-β2, a predominant isoform expressed in severe asthma, has an important role in regulating inflammation and remodeling in asthma, and may play a role in the development of childhood atopic asthma.[101,102] TGF-β2, as well as TGF-β1, is induced by IL-4 and IL-13 in epithelial cells.[101] Different polymorphisms of TGF-β2 are described.[101] Even if there are unrecognized differences in environmental exposure, particularly early on in childhood asthma, genetic factors, as illustrated by TGF-β polymorphisms, could affect the airway, the response to viral infection, and allergen or tobacco exposure, benefiting (or otherwise) excessive remodeling of the airway, the persistence of inflammation, and severity of asthma.

Another mediator that has been studied specifically in asthma is the ADAM33 (a disintegrin and metalloproteinase 33) polymorphism, implicated in airway caliber at the age of 3 and 5 years.[103]

Skin-barrier dysfunction is also being debated. Fillagrin gene variants are associated with a high risk of early-onset asthma, with a phenotype including acute severe asthma and recurrent wheeze but also with accelerated decline in lung function.[104–106] A recent cohort study conducted in Poland showed that fillagrin null variants were associated with the risk of atopic asthma (odds ratio [OR] 2.22, 95% confidence interval [CI] 1.24–3.96, $P = .006$),[107] revealing another potential factor of susceptibility to epithelial disease related to asthma.

There is a link between virus and remodeling. Rhinovirus infection of bronchial epithelial cells leads to upregulation of mediators implicated in airway remodeling: amphiregulin (a member of the EGF family), activin A (member of the TGF-β family), and vascular endothelial growth factor protein.[108] Fibroblasts have the ability to support rhinovirus replication and to promote inflammation through the secretion of IL-6 and IL-8.[109]

Remodeling in asthma may be initiated in early life, even in utero, and it can evolve in parallel with inflammatory infiltration. Some studies in children show that it may be associated with a phenotype of a persistent obstructive pattern (**Fig. 2**).

Many questions remain unresolved in identifying the determinant factor(s) of severity in childhood asthma. Even if the hypothesis of "ETMU" or the immune reaction occurring in response to a virus in allergic asthmatics related by Subrata and colleagues[30] are of great interest, only a few children will develop severe asthma. The role of triggers in early life, even in utero (allergen, protease, infection, tobacco smoke, pollutants, and so forth), particularly the combination of multiple environmental factors and the different modality of response related to genetic background (immune, antioxidant, repair process, epithelium junction, and so forth), probably act together to induce (or not) persistent inflammation and/or remodeling. Genetics mainly contribute to disease

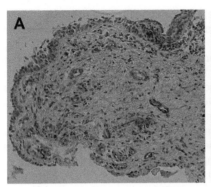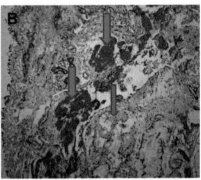

Fig. 2. (*A, B*) Diversity of airway remodeling in asthmatic children. Micrographs show indirect immunostaining (with fast *red*) obtained with antibody anti-alpha-smooth muscle actin mAb anti-SMA, clone asm-1 (Cymbus Biotech, Southampton, UK) on bronchial biopsies from children with severe asthma. In patient A (high magnification ×300), the airway epithelium is relatively untouched, and no hyperplasia of smooth muscle and mucous gland is detected. By contrast, in patient B (high magnification ×300) the airway epithelium is mainly desquamated, and a strong hyperplasia of mucous gland (*lower right*) and smooth muscle (in *red*) is observed. This appearance is associated with a different clinical profile, as reported in a previous article.[77]

expression, progression, and response to treatment, and the gene-environment interactions are probably essential in creating severity (**Figs. 1** and **2**).[110–112]

SEVERE ASTHMA PHENOTYPES IN CHILDREN

The definition of severe asthma does not take into account phenotypic characteristics and heterogeneity illustrated by some cross-sectional evaluation of cohorts of school-age children with severe asthma, and this may lead to suboptimal or inappropriate treatment. A predominance of males, atopy (86%), long duration of asthma (first symptoms: 1.25 years), and a large frequency of comorbidities (eg, food allergy: 24%; gastroesophageal reflux: 75%) was observed among 102 children with severe asthma, who presented with an obstructive pattern (FEV_1 67% ± 19.2%), a partial response to corticosteroid testing, and an eosinophilic and/or neutrophilic profile on BAL.[113] Fitzpatrick and colleagues[114] (SARP cohort) phenotyped 161 children with severe asthma (ATS criteria) according to their clinical features and inflammatory biomarkers (cluster analysis). Four clusters were identified, very different from those of adult severe asthma: late-onset symptomatic asthma with normal pulmonary function test and less atopy, early-onset atopic asthma with normal pulmonary function test, early-onset atopic asthma with greater comorbidity and mild airflow limitation, early-onset atopic asthma with advanced airflow limitation, and the greatest symptoms and use of medication. Asthma duration, number of controller medications, and baseline lung function, but not atopy were predictors of cluster assignment. Konradsen and colleagues[115] evaluated the features of 54 children with severe asthma according to GA2LEN Task Force guidelines, and compared them with age-matched peers with controlled persistent asthma. Children with severe asthma more frequently had parents with asthma, came from families of a lower socioeconomic status, were less active, had more comorbidities (rhinoconjunctivitis), and more lung-function abnormalities (lower FEV_1 and higher bronchial hyperresponsiveness). This study highlighted the difference between asthma that is difficult to treat with asthma-identified aggravating factors (39%) and therapy-resistant asthma (61%).[115] All these studies emphasize that definitions of asthma severity proposed by current guidelines do not reflect real life. A more specific approach is needed with the aim of assessing all the characteristics of severe asthma, including the history of respiratory symptoms since birth, exposures during pregnancy, comorbidity, and aggravating factors. The risk of impairment associated with the disorder, as well as the response to treatments, is also characterized by different possibilities.

Description of Severe Asthma Phenotypes in Children

Phenotypes based on allergic profile and comorbidities, clinical features (symptoms, exacerbations), lung function, or inflammation have been described in children with severe asthma. Children's phenotypes may not be stable with age-related profiles, and may also vary over time. Furthermore, there is a possible overlap between the features of the different phenotypes.

- *Allergy.* Allergic sensitization is a main feature of severe asthma in children.[113–116] Persistence of a severe atopic dermatitis has been related to filaggrin mutations, and is associated with a more severe asthma and accelerated decline of lung function.[106] Food allergy (peanut and tree-nuts) is overrepresented in children with severe asthma (24% of the Brompton series),[113] and is associated with the risk of life-threatening asthma.[117] Indeed, acute asthma is a feature of food anaphylaxis, needing inhaled β2 agonists and epinephrine injection.[118] Finally, a high IgE level and multisensitization are frequent in severe asthma. Some sensitizations (molds, cockroaches) may be overrepresented.[119] Severe asthma with fungal sensitization described in adults is very rare in childhood, according to anecdotal case reports.[120]
- *Brittle asthma phenotype.* Most information comes from adult studies, but this phenotype is also observed in pediatric patients.[121] Type 1 is characterized by prolonged chaotic swings of peak flow and type 2 by a single catastrophic decrease in peak flow in the context of good control.
- *Exacerbating phenotype.* Recurrent exacerbations requiring general corticosteroids and/or health care characterize severe asthma and are usually virally induced.[122] In the SARP cohort, median oral corticosteroid bursts and emergency-department visits for acute asthma exacerbations were significantly higher for the children with severe asthma than for those with moderate asthma, respectively 3 versus 1 and 3 versus 0.[114,116] Caroll and colleagues[123] describe a specific phenotype with isolated recurrent severe exacerbation requiring admission to the intensive care unit and sometimes assisted ventilation. This phenotype is also observed in preschool children, with personal or familial atopy.[124]
- *Pulmonary function abnormalities phenotype.* Pulmonary function abnormalities may be measured during early childhood and persist throughout the adult years.[125] Fixed obstruction with or without symptoms is also observed and may progress over time.[33,126] Decline in pulmonary function is also present in a subset of patients with mild to moderate asthma, as reported in 30% of the children in the CAMP study.[127] The clinical significance is not clear. However, these features may be associated with altered lung growth or specific airway remodeling, and possibly future asthma severity.

Inflammatory phenotypes also exist and are discussed in the pathophysiology section.[12,31,33,78,113,114,128] Cytology may be not sufficient, but the analysis of the nature of inflammation may improve the classification of severe asthma and the development of targeted treatments.

TREATMENT

The authors only consider the treatment of children uncontrolled under high-dose ICS (>400 µg/d fluticasone equivalent) and add-on therapies, long-acting β2-agonist (LABA) ± leukotriene receptor antagonist (LTRA), and an estimated correct medication adherence and inhaler technique. Allergic comorbidities, associated factors (gastroesophageal reflux, obesity, psychosocial condition), environment (allergens, tobacco, pollution) need also to be assessed and treated. Options can be divided into conventional treatments (ICS, oral corticosteroids [OCS], theophylline) with the new opportunity of biotherapy (omalizumab) and treatment not usually prescribed for asthma (macrolides, cytotoxics). Studies on daily lung-function monitoring or regular inflammation assessments have now been published. For all these options, pediatric data are lacking and the level of evidence for severe asthma in children remains poor. All these treatment strategies require the supervision of a specialist pediatric pulmonologist. Bush and colleagues[129] (PSACI group) recently published a review on the pharmacologic treatment of severe, therapy-resistant asthma.

Conventional Treatment

Inhaled corticosteroids

It is assumed that 80% to 90% of the ICS effect is obtained with 100 to 250 µg fluticasone equivalent in children with mild to moderate asthma.[130] However, poor glucocorticoid responsiveness or corticoresistance is a feature of severe asthma,[129,131] enhanced by some comorbidities (tobacco-smoke exposure, being overweight). A trial with a high dose of ICS, up to 2000 µg/d, may be prescribed for 3 to 6 months.[132] Thereafter, if benefits are observed the dose should gradually be tapered under regular monitoring. Budesonide nebulizations (1 mg × 2/d) may be considered, particularly for the youngest.[133] To target the distal airways and enhanced deposition, extrafine particle treatment (beclometasone HFA, ciclesonide) is another option.[134] ICS are usually associated with LABA therapy. Concerns about LABA's safety have recently been debated. On the basis of 20 systematic reviews and databases, Rodrigo and Castro-Rodríguez[135] concluded that concomitant use of LABA with ICS is not associated with these serious side effects.

Systemic corticosteroids

Until recently, OCS was the final conventional step in treatment recommendations.[136] There is no evidence about which protocol should be used. After a period (2–4 weeks) with 0.5 to 1 mg/kg/d of prednisolone equivalent, the daily dose should gradually be tapered (alternate dosing), according to clinical and functional monitoring, to the lowest efficient dose (best patient control). Adverse effects are common and should be monitored and prevented (height, blood pressure, glucose metabolism, cataract, and osteoporosis). The same warning should be given for patients with frequent OCS bursts for severe exacerbations. A trial of intramuscular triamcinolone given either as a single dose or as repeated monthly injections has also been tested, as a test for the potential steroid effect or as an alternative to OCS for children who have poor compliance or pulmonary inflammation that is resistant to OCS.[137] There is no randomized controlled study to evaluate whether this strategy has additional benefits, or risks, compared with OCS.

Omalizumab

The anti-IgE treatment (omalizumab) is a new, expensive option for children age 6 years and older with atopic allergic uncontrolled severe asthma and the appropriate level of IgE (upper limit: 1500 UI/mL). There are no tests to predict the response, and the total IgE level is often over the recommended limit in children with severe asthma. Pediatric controlled studies were conducted in moderate to severe asthma and showed a significant reduction in severe exacerbation rates, ICS dosage, and improvement in the control and quality of life.[138–140] Busse and colleagues[141] also observed the attenuation of spring and autumn peaks of exacerbation in children under omalizumab. Response to treatment has been observed, even if the total IgE level was greater than 1500 UI/mL (personal data, AD/French cohort). Meta-analysis by Rodrigo and colleagues[142] (8 studies, including 2 on children, 3429 patients) confirmed the significant impact on exacerbations during the stable phase of ICS treatment (relative risk [RR] = 0.57, 95% CI 0.48–0.66, P = .0001) as well as the tapered phase (RR = 0.55, 95% CI 0.47–0.64, P = .0001). Impact on lung function is more controversial, but should be studied in the long term, as should the impact on asthma progression. Omalizumab was safe and well tolerated in pediatric studies, up to 1 year.[142] However, adverse effects have been described, including anaphylaxis, and first injections should be performed under medical supervision.[143] Consequently, Omalizumab is now a valid option in children with uncontrolled asthma and/or frequent exacerbations under optimal inhaled treatment or oral steroids.

Other Treatments

- *Theophylline.* The conclusion of the meta-analysis by Seddon and colleagues[144] on xanthines in asthmatic children was that they may have a role as add-on therapy in severe asthma not controlled by ICS, but that further studies (not done) are needed to incorporate the risk-benefit ratio. Theophylline is now prescribed at low doses (blood level at 5–10 mol/L) for the immunomodulatory properties that have been described.[144]
- *Anti-infective treatments.* Therapeutic trials of macrolides are being prescribed in some patients with refractory asthma who fail to respond to standard therapy. Along with direct antimicrobial activity against gram-positive cocci and atypical pathogens, macrolides also have immune-modifying effects and effects on bronchial cells, and on cells of innate immunity.[145] Chronic infection with *Chlamydia* and *Mycoplasma pneumoniae* has been associated with severe asthma, as has nontuberculous mycobacteria.[146,147] However, no broad study confirms the role of macrolides in the treatment of severe asthma. Strunk and colleagues[148] were not able to demonstrate the role of azithromycin or montelukast as ICS-sparing agents in children with moderate to severe asthma controlled by medium ICS dose and LABA.
- *Cytotoxics.* These treatments have been tried in asthma that is resistant to conventional treatment or in asthma treated with OCS. Their side effects may outweigh the benefits and they need to be monitored.[149] Methotrexate and cyclosporine have been used with a small but significant effect in case series of children.[149,150] There are no pediatric data on azathioprine, anti–TNF-α, interferon-γ, or anti–IL-5 (mepolizumab).[151]

Monitoring Therapy

A few studies on lung-function telemonitoring in asthmatic patients have been published, mainly concerning the transmission of peak expiratory flow measures or the management program for asthma via the Internet.[152] A strategy based on daily home spirometry (FEV_1) with teletransmission to an expert medical center was applied in 50 children with severe uncontrolled asthma enrolled in a 12-month prospective study and randomized into 2 groups: treatment managed with daily home spirometry and medical feedback, and conventional treatment.[153] There was no significant difference in severe exacerbations, lung function (FEV_1, FEF_{25-75}), treatment outcome (daily ICS dose), or quality of life. These findings may highlight the weakness of the correlation between lung function and symptoms. The poor performance of this intensive management acts against telemonitoring with medical feedback, a position now supported by the latest ATS recommendations.[154]

Although asthma is an inflammatory disease, inflammation is not routinely assessed. FE_{NO} monitoring is easy, but was not more efficient than the conventional strategy in children with mild to moderate asthma (FE_{NO50}), and daily ICS dose may be higher.[155] Induced sputum cytology is another method of assessing bronchial inflammation. Fleming and colleagues[156] adopted this strategy in 55 children with severe asthma, randomized to either a conventional strategy or an inflammation strategy (first sputum eosinophilia and, if not obtained, FE_{NO}). Children were seen at 3-monthly intervals over a 1-year period. No improvement in the exacerbations rate or asthma control was observed. The investigators emphasize phenotypic variability (39% of children had at least one switch in phenotype over 1 year), the frequency of inflammation assessment, which is too low, and the use of FE_{NO} as a surrogate for sputum eosinophilia with the known nonconstant correlation between them. Development of biomarkers, which are easy to measure, is needed to optimize the choice of the treatment strategy according to the phenotype and to monitor the response to innovative therapy.

SUMMARY

Even if well defined, it is sometimes difficult to distinguish difficult from severe asthma in real life. When alternative diagnoses are excluded, comorbidities and environmental factors have been evaluated, and adherence to treatment seems to have been successful, difficult asthma is excluded. Severe asthma is probably determined early in life. Severe childhood asthma, refractory to treatment, includes different phenotypes. Genetics mainly contribute to disease expression, progression, and response to treatment. The gene-environment interactions involving certain gene polymorphisms are probably essential in creating its severity. An aberrant innate immune response to repeated rhinovirus infections may facilitate airway remodeling and severe asthma, via epithelial cell alterations, enhancing viral replication and persistence of bronchial inflammation. Additional genetic factors regulating the response to oxidative stress after viral infection or other environmental triggers also contribute to the quality of response. Different treatment strategies require the supervision of a specialist pediatric pulmonologist when the level of evidence remains poor. The quality of care and monitoring of children with severe asthma is as important as the prescription of drug. This factor is also crucial for differentiating between severe asthma and difficult asthma, and expertise is required. Further studies (genetic and proteomic data) performed in phenotypes of severe asthma in children should improve knowledge of the mechanisms involved in frequent exacerbations, persistent obstruction, and sudden-onset severe asthma, and help the pediatric pulmonologist to choose the appropriate monitoring and treatment for the phenotype.

REFERENCES

1. Lang A, Carlsen KH, Haaland G, et al. Severe asthma in childhood: assessed in 10 year olds in a birth cohort study. Allergy 2008;63:1054–60.
2. Chung KF, Godard P, Adelroth E, et al. Difficult/therapy-resistant asthma: the need for an integrated approach to define clinical phenotypes, evaluate risk factors, understand pathophysiology and find novel therapies. ERS Task Force on

Difficult/Therapy-Resistant Asthma. European Respiratory Society. Eur Respir J 1999;13:1198–208.

3. Wenzel S. Severe asthma in adults. Am J Respir Crit Care Med 2005;172:149–60.

4. Hedlin G, Bush A, Lødrup Carlsen K, et al. Problematic severe asthma in children, not one problem but many: a GA2LEN initiative. Eur Respir J 2010;36: 196–201.

5. Bel EH, Sousa A, Fleming L, et al. Unbiased Biomarkers for the Prediction of Respiratory Disease Outcome (U-BIOPRED) Consortium, Consensus Generation. Diagnosis and definition of severe refractory asthma: an international consensus statement from the Innovative Medicine Initiative (IMI). Thorax 2011;66:910–7.

6. Iliescu C, Tillie-Leblond I, Deschildre A, et al. Difficult asthma in children. Arch Pediatr 2002;9:1264–73.

7. Lødrup Carlsen KC, Hedlin G, Bush A, et al. PSACI (Problematic Severe Asthma in Childhood Initiative) group. Assessment of problematic severe asthma in children. Eur Respir J 2011;37:432–40.

8. de Groot EP, Duiverman EJ, Brand PL. Comorbidities of asthma during childhood: possibly important, yet poorly studied. Eur Respir J 2010;36:671–8.

9. Araújo L, Moreira A, Palmares C, et al. Induced sputum in children: success determinants, safety, and cell profiles. J Investig Allergol Clin Immunol 2011;21: 216–21.

10. Jones PD, Hankin R, Simpson J, et al. The tolerability, safety, and success of sputum induction and combined hypertonic saline challenge in children. Am J Respir Crit Care Med 2001;164:1146–9.

11. Lex C, Payne DN, Zacharasiewicz A, et al. Sputum induction in children with difficult asthma: safety, feasibility, and inflammatory cell pattern. Pediatr Pulmonol 2005;39:318–24.

12. Lex C, Ferreira F, Zacharasiewicz A, et al. Airway eosinophilia in children with severe asthma: predictive values of noninvasive tests. Am J Respir Crit Care Med 2006;174:1286–91.

13. Dweik RA, Boggs PB, Erzurum SC, et al. American Thoracic Society Committee on Interpretation of Exhaled Nitric Oxide Levels (FENO) for Clinical Applications. An official ATS clinical practice guideline: interpretation of exhaled nitric oxide levels (FENO) for clinical applications. Am J Respir Crit Care Med 2011; 184(5):602–15.

14. Zacharasiewicz A, Wilson N, Lex C, et al. Clinical use of noninvasive measurements of airway inflammation in steroid reduction in children. Am J Respir Crit Care Med 2005;171:1077–82.

15. Mahut B, Delclaux C, Tillie-Leblond I, et al. Both inflammation and remodeling influence nitric oxide output in children with refractory asthma. J Allergy Clin Immunol 2004;113:252–6.

16. Kasahara K, Shiba K, Ozawa T, et al. Correlation between the bronchial subepithelial layer and whole airway wall thickness in patients with asthma. Thorax 2002;57:242–6.

17. Vignola AM, Paganin F, Capieu L, et al. Airway remodelling assessed by sputum and high-resolution computed tomography in asthma and COPD. Eur Respir J 2004;24:910–7.

18. Marchac V, Emond S, Mamou-Mani T, et al. Thoracic CT in pediatric patients with difficult-to-treat asthma. AJR Am J Roentgenol 2002;179:1245–52.

19. de Blic J, Tillie-Leblond I, Emond S, et al. High-resolution computed tomography scan and airway remodeling in children with severe asthma. J Allergy Clin Immunol 2005;116:750–4.

20. Spahn JD, Covar R. Clinical assessment of asthma progression in children and adults. J Allergy Clin Immunol 2008;121:548–57.
21. Taussig LM, Wright AL, Holberg CJ, et al. Tucson Children's Respiratory Study: 1980 to present. J Allergy Clin Immunol 2003;111:661–75.
22. Borrego LM, Stocks J, Leiria-Pinto P, et al. Lung function and clinical risk factors for asthma in infants and young children with recurrent wheeze. Thorax 2009;64: 203–9.
23. Håland G, Carlsen KC, Sandvik L, et al. ORAACLE. Reduced lung function at birth and the risk of asthma at 10 years of age. N Engl J Med 2006;355:1682–9.
24. Illi S, von Mutius E, Lau S, et al, Multicentre Allergy Study (MAS) group. Perennial allergen sensitisation early in life and chronic asthma in children: a birth cohort study. Lancet 2006;368:763–70.
25. Oddy WH, de Klerk NH, Sly PD, et al. The effects of respiratory infections, atopy, and breastfeeding on childhood asthma. Eur Respir J 2002;19:899–905.
26. Holt PG, Rowe J, Kusel M, et al. Toward improved prediction of risk for atopy and asthma among preschoolers: a prospective cohort study. J Allergy Clin Immunol 2010;125:653–9.
27. Kusel MM, de Klerk NH, Kebadze T, et al. Early-life respiratory viral infections, atopic sensitization, and risk of subsequent development of persistent asthma. J Allergy Clin Immunol 2007;119:1105–10.
28. Lemanske RF Jr, Busse WW. Asthma: clinical expression and molecular mechanisms. J Allergy Clin Immunol 2010;125:S95–102.
29. Holt PG, Sly PD. Interaction between adaptive and innate immune pathways in the pathogenesis of atopic asthma: operation of a lung/bone marrow axis. Chest 2011;139:1165–71.
30. Subrata LS, Bizzintino J, Mamessier E, et al. Interactions between innate antiviral and atopic immunoinflammatory pathways precipitate and sustain asthma exacerbations in children. J Immunol 2009;183:2793–800.
31. Payne DN, Adcock IM, Wilson NM, et al. Relationship between exhaled nitric oxide and mucosal eosinophilic inflammation in children with difficult asthma, after treatment with oral prednisolone. Am J Respir Crit Care Med 2001;164: 1376–81.
32. Fitzpatrick AM, Higgins M, Holguin F, et al. National Institutes of Health/National Heart, Lung, and Blood Institute's Severe Asthma Research Program. The molecular phenotype of severe asthma in children. J Allergy Clin Immunol 2010; 125:851–7.
33. de Blic J, Tillie-Leblond I, Tonnel AB, et al. Difficult asthma in children: an analysis of airway inflammation. J Allergy Clin Immunol 2004;113:94–100.
34. Le Bourgeois M, Goncalves M, Le Clainche L, et al. Bronchoalveolar cells in children < 3 years old with severe recurrent wheezing. Chest 2002;122:791–7.
35. Marguet C, Jouen-Boedes F, Dean TP, et al. Bronchoalveolar cell profiles in children with asthma, infantile wheeze, chronic cough, or cystic fibrosis. Am J Respir Crit Care Med 1999;159:1533–40.
36. Stevenson EC, Turner G, Heaney LG, et al. Bronchoalveolar lavage findings suggest two different forms of childhood asthma. Clin Exp Allergy 1997;27: 1027–35.
37. Starosta V, Kitz R, Hartl D, et al. Bronchoalveolar pepsin, bile acids, oxidation, and inflammation in children with gastroesophageal reflux disease. Chest 2007;132:1557–64.
38. Moore WC, Bleecker ER, Curran-Everett D, et al, National Heart, Lung, Blood Institute's Severe Asthma Research Program. Characterization of the severe

asthma phenotype by the National Heart, Lung, and Blood Institute's Severe Asthma Research Program. J Allergy Clin Immunol 2007;119:405–13.

39. Miranda C, Busacker A, Balzar S, et al. Distinguishing severe asthma phenotypes: role of age at onset and eosinophilic inflammation. J Allergy Clin Immunol 2004;113:101–8.

40. Hauk PJ, Krawiec M, Murphy J, et al. Neutrophilic airway inflammation and association with bacterial lipopolysaccharide in children with asthma and wheezing. Pediatr Pulmonol 2008;43:916–23.

41. Just J, Fournier L, Momas I, et al. Clinical significance of bronchoalveolar eosinophils in childhood asthma. J Allergy Clin Immunol 2002;110:42–4.

42. Van den Toorn LM, Overbeek SE, de Jongste JC, et al. Airway inflammation is present during clinical remission of atopic asthma. Am J Respir Crit Care Med 2001;164:2107–13.

43. Siddiqui S, Hollins F, Saha S, et al. Inflammatory cell microlocalisation and airway dysfunction: cause and effect? Eur Respir J 2007;30:1043–56.

44. Payne DN, Qiu Y, Zhu J, et al. Airway inflammation in children with difficult asthma: relationships with airflow limitation and persistent symptoms. Thorax 2004;59:862–9.

45. Saglani S, Malmström K, Pelkonen AS, et al. Airway remodeling and inflammation in symptomatic infants with reversible airflow obstruction. Am J Respir Crit Care Med 2005;171:722–7.

46. Lambrecht BN, Hammad H. The role of dendritic and epithelial cells as master regulators of allergic airway inflammation. Lancet 2010;376:835–43.

47. Bosco A, Ehteshami S, Stern DA, et al. Decreased activation of inflammatory networks during acute asthma exacerbations is associated with chronic airflow obstruction. Mucosal Immunol 2010;3:399–409.

48. Stern DA, Morgan WJ, Halonen M, et al. Wheezing and bronchial hyperresponsiveness in early childhood as predictors of newly diagnosed asthma in early adulthood: a longitudinal birth-cohort study. Lancet 2008;372:1058–64.

49. Jackson DJ, Evans MD, Gangnon RE, et al. Evidence for a causal relationship between allergic sensitization and rhinovirus wheezing in early life. Am J Respir Crit Care Med 2012;185(3):281–5.

50. Maurer D, Fiebiger S, Ebner C, et al. Peripheral blood dendritic cells express Fc epsilon RI as a complex composed of Fc epsilon RI alpha- and Fc epsilon RI gamma-chains and can use this receptor for IgE-mediated allergen presentation. J Immunol 1996;157:607–16.

51. Singh AM, Moore PE, Gern JE, et al. Bronchiolitis to asthma: a review and call for studies of gene-virus interactions in asthma causation. Am J Respir Crit Care Med 2007;175:108–19.

52. Contoli M, Message SD, Laza-Stanca V, et al. Role of deficient type III interferon-lambda production in asthma exacerbations. Nat Med 2006;12:1023–6.

53. Wark PA, Johnston SL, Bucchieri F, et al. Asthmatic bronchial epithelial cells have a deficient innate immune response to infection with rhinovirus. J Exp Med 2005;201:937–47.

54. Message SD, Laza-Stanca V, Mallia P, et al. Rhinovirus-induced lower respiratory illness is increased in asthma and related to virus load and Th1/2 cytokine and IL-10 production. Proc Natl Acad Sci U S A 2008;105:13562–7.

55. Guerra S, Lohman IC, Halonen M, et al. Reduced interferon gamma production and soluble CD14 levels in early life predict recurrent wheezing by 1 year of age. Am J Respir Crit Care Med 2004;169:70–6.

56. Martinez FD. Viral infections and the development of asthma. Am J Respir Crit Care Med 1995;151:1644–7.
57. Tang ML, Kemp AS, Thorburn J, et al. Reduced interferon-gamma secretion in neonates and subsequent atopy. Lancet 1994;344:983–5.
58. Schroth MK, Grimm E, Frindt P, et al. Rhinovirus replication causes RANTES production in primary bronchial epithelial cells. Am J Respir Cell Mol Biol 1999;20: 1220–8.
59. Jackson DJ, Johnston SL. The role of viruses in acute exacerbations of asthma. J Allergy Clin Immunol 2010;125:1178–87.
60. Grünberg K, Sharon RF, Hiltermann TJ, et al. Experimental rhinovirus 16 infection increases intercellular adhesion molecule-1 expression in bronchial epithelium of asthmatics regardless of inhaled steroid treatment. Clin Exp Allergy 2000;30:1015–23.
61. Bullens DM, Decraene A, Dilissen E, et al. Type III IFN-lambda mRNA expression in sputum of adult and school-aged asthmatics. Clin Exp Allergy 2008; 38:1459–67.
62. Thomas BJ, Lindsay M, Dagher H, et al. Transforming growth factor-beta enhances rhinovirus infection by diminishing early innate responses. Am J Respir Cell Mol Biol 2009;41:339–47.
63. Laza-Stanca V, Message SD, Edwards MR, et al. The role of IL-15 deficiency in the pathogenesis of virus-induced asthma exacerbations. PLoS Pathog 2011;7: e1002114.
64. Bisgaard H, Hermansen MN, Buchvald F, et al. Childhood asthma after bacterial colonization of the airway in neonates. N Engl J Med 2007;357:1487–95.
65. Hilty M, Burke C, Pedro H, et al. Disordered microbial communities in asthmatic airways. PLoS One 2010;5:e8578.
66. Herbst T, Sichelstiel A, Schär C, et al. Dysregulation of allergic airway inflammation in the absence of microbial colonization. Am J Respir Crit Care Med 2011; 184:198–205.
67. Malmström K, Pitkäranta A, Carpen O, et al. Human rhinovirus in bronchial epithelium of infants with recurrent respiratory symptoms. J Allergy Clin Immunol 2006;118:591–6.
68. Holt PG, Upham JW, Sly PD. Contemporaneous maturation of immunologic and respiratory functions during early childhood: implications for development of asthma prevention strategies. J Allergy Clin Immunol 2005;116:16–24.
69. Comhair SA, Ricci KS, Arroliga M, et al. Correlation of systemic superoxide dismutase deficiency to airflow obstruction in asthma. Am J Respir Crit Care Med 2005;172:306–13.
70. Comhair SA, Gaston BM, Ricci KS, et al. Detrimental effects of environmental tobacco smoke in relation to asthma severity. PLoS One 2011;6:e18574.
71. Comhair SA, Xu W, Ghosh S, et al. Superoxide dismutase inactivation in pathophysiology of asthmatic airway remodeling and reactivity. Am J Pathol 2005;166: 663–74.
72. Fitzpatrick AM, Teague WG, Holguin F, et al. Airway glutathione homeostasis is altered in children with severe asthma: evidence for oxidant stress. J Allergy Clin Immunol 2009;123:146–52.
73. Fitzpatrick AM, Holguin F, Teague WG, et al. Alveolar macrophage phagocytosis is impaired in children with poorly controlled asthma. J Allergy Clin Immunol 2008;121:1372–8.
74. Fitzpatrick AM, Stephenson ST, Hadley GR, et al. Thiol redox disturbances in children with severe asthma are associated with posttranslational modification

of the transcription factor nuclear factor (erythroid-derived 2)-like 2. J Allergy Clin Immunol 2011;127:1604–11.

75. Rangasamy T, Guo J, Mitzner WA, et al. Disruption of Nrf2 enhances susceptibility to severe airway inflammation and asthma in mice. J Exp Med 2005;202: 47–59.

76. Gilliland FD, Gauderman WJ, Vora H, et al. Effects of glutathione-S-transferase M1, T1, and P1 on childhood lung function growth. Am J Respir Crit Care Med 2002;166:710–6.

77. Tillie-Leblond I, de Blic J, Jaubert F, et al. Airway remodeling is correlated with obstruction in children with severe asthma. Allergy 2008;63:533–41.

78. Payne DN, Rogers AV, Adelroth E, et al. Early thickening of the reticular basement membrane in children with difficult asthma. Am J Respir Crit Care Med 2003;167:78–82.

79. Barbato A, Turato G, Baraldo S, et al. Airway inflammation in childhood asthma. Am J Respir Crit Care Med 2003;168:798–803.

80. Kim ES, Kim SH, Kim KW, et al. Basement membrane thickening and clinical features of children with asthma. Allergy 2007;62:635–40.

81. Saglani S, Payne DN, Zhu J, et al. Early detection of airway wall remodeling and eosinophilic inflammation in preschool wheezers. Am J Respir Crit Care Med 2007;176:858–64.

82. Saglani S, Molyneux C, Gong H, et al. Ultrastructure of the reticular basement membrane in asthmatic adults, children and infants. Eur Respir J 2006;28:505–12.

83. Pascual RM, Peters SP. Airway remodeling contributes to the progressive loss of lung function in asthma: an overview. J Allergy Clin Immunol 2005;116:477–86.

84. Mauad T, Bel EH, Sterk PJ. Asthma therapy and airway remodeling. J Allergy Clin Immunol 2007;120:997–1009.

85. Regamey N, Ochs M, Hilliard TN, et al. Increased airway smooth muscle mass in children with asthma, cystic fibrosis, and non-cystic fibrosis bronchiectasis. Am J Respir Crit Care Med 2008;177:837–43.

86. Johnson PR, Roth M, Tamm M, et al. Airway smooth muscle cell proliferation is increased in asthma. Am J Respir Crit Care Med 2001;164:474–7.

87. Lazaar AL, Panettieri RA Jr. Airway smooth muscle as a regulator of immune responses and bronchomotor tone. Clin Chest Med 2006;27:53–69.

88. Gupta A, Sjoukes A, Richards D, et al. Relationship between serum vitamin D, disease severity, and airway remodeling in children with asthma. Am J Respir Crit Care Med 2011;184:1342–9.

89. Barbato A, Turato G, Baraldo S, et al. Epithelial damage and angiogenesis in the airways of children with asthma. Am J Respir Crit Care Med 2006;174:975–81.

90. Kanazawa H, Nomura S, Yoshikawa J. Role of microvascular permeability on physiologic differences in asthma and eosinophilic bronchitis. Am J Respir Crit Care Med 2004;169:1125–30.

91. Gosset P, Tillie-Leblond I, Janin A, et al. Expression of E-selectin, ICAM-1 and VCAM-1 on bronchial biopsies from allergic and non-allergic asthmatic patients. Int Arch Allergy Immunol 1995;106:69–77.

92. Holgate ST. The sentinel role of the airway epithelium in asthma pathogenesis. Immunol Rev 2011;242:205–19.

93. Baraldo S, Turato G, Bazzan E, et al. Noneosinophilic asthma in children: relation with airway remodelling. Eur Respir J 2011;38:575–83.

94. Malmström K, Pelkonen AS, Malmberg LP, et al. Lung function, airway remodelling and inflammation in symptomatic infants: outcome at 3 years. Thorax 2011; 66:157–62.

95. Fedorov IA, Wilson SJ, Davies DE, et al. Epithelial stress and structural remodelling in childhood asthma. Thorax 2005;60:389–94.

96. Guilbert TW, Morgan WJ, Zeiger RS, et al. Long-term inhaled corticosteroids in preschool children at high risk for asthma. N Engl J Med 2006;354:1985–97.

97. Murray CS, Woodcock A, Langley SJ, et al. IFWIN study team. Secondary prevention of asthma by the use of Inhaled Fluticasone propionate in Wheezy INfants (IFWIN): double-blind, randomised, controlled study. Lancet 2006;368: 754–62.

98. Holgate ST, Roberts G, Arshad HS, et al. The role of the airway epithelium and its interaction with environmental factors in asthma pathogenesis. Proc Am Thorac Soc 2009;6:655–9.

99. Blobe GC, Schiemann WP, Lodish HF. Role of transforming growth factor beta in human disease. N Engl J Med 2000;342:1350–8.

100. Pulleyn LJ, Newton R, Adcock IM, et al. TGFbeta1 allele association with asthma severity. Hum Genet 2001;109:623–7.

101. Hatsushika K, Hirota T, Harada M, et al. Transforming growth factor-beta(2) polymorphisms are associated with childhood atopic asthma. Clin Exp Allergy 2007; 37:1165–74.

102. Balzar S, Chu HW, Silkoff P, et al. Increased TGF-beta2 in severe asthma with eosinophilia. J Allergy Clin Immunol 2005;115:110–7.

103. Simpson A, Maniatis N, Jury F, et al. Polymorphisms in a disintegrin and metalloprotease 33 (ADAM33) predict impaired early-life lung function. Am J Respir Crit Care Med 2005;172:55–60.

104. Rodríguez E, Baurecht H, Herberich E, et al. Meta-analysis of filaggrin polymorphisms in eczema and asthma: robust risk factors in atopic disease. J Allergy Clin Immunol 2009;123:1361–70.

105. van den Oord RA, Sheikh A. Filaggrin gene defects and risk of developing allergic sensitisation and allergic disorders: systematic review and meta-analysis. BMJ 2009;339:b2433.

106. Marenholz I, Kerscher T, Bauerfeind A, et al. An interaction between filaggrin mutations and early food sensitization improves the prediction of childhood asthma. J Allergy Clin Immunol 2009;123:911–6.

107. Ponińska J, Samoliński B, Tomaszewska A, et al. Filaggrin gene defects are independent risk factors for atopic asthma in a Polish population: a study in ECAP cohort. PLoS One 2011;6:e16933.

108. Leigh R, Oyelusi W, Wiehler S, et al. Human rhinovirus infection enhances airway epithelial cell production of growth factors involved in airway remodeling. J Allergy Clin Immunol 2008;121:1238–45.

109. Bedke N, Haitchi HM, Xatzipsalti M, et al. Contribution of bronchial fibroblasts to the antiviral response in asthma. J Immunol 2009;182:3660–7.

110. Ober C, Hoffjan S. Asthma genetics 2006: the long and winding road to gene discovery. Genes Immun 2006;7:95–100.

111. Yang IA, Holloway JW. Asthma: advancing gene-environment studies. Clin Exp Allergy 2007;37:1264–6.

112. von Mutius E. Genes and the environment: two readings of their interaction. J Allergy Clin Immunol 2008;122:99–100.

113. Bossley CJ, Saglani S, Kavanagh C, et al. Corticosteroid responsiveness and clinical characteristics in childhood difficult asthma. Eur Respir J 2009;34: 1052–9.

114. Fitzpatrick AM, Teague WG, Meyers DA, et al, National Institutes of Health/ National Heart, Lung, and Blood Institute Severe Asthma Research Program.

Heterogeneity of severe asthma in childhood: confirmation by cluster analysis of children in the National Institutes of Health/National Heart, Lung, and Blood Institute Severe Asthma Research Program. J Allergy Clin Immunol 2011;127: 382–9.

115. Konradsen JR, Nordlund B, Lidegran M, et al, Swedish Network of Pediatric Allergists, Severe Asthma Network. Problematic severe asthma: a proposed approach to identifying children who are severely resistant to therapy. Pediatr Allergy Immunol 2011;22:9–18.

116. Fitzpatrick AM, Gaston BM, Erzurum SC, et al. National Institutes of Health/National Heart, Lung, and Blood Institute Severe Asthma Research Program. Features of severe asthma in school-age children: Atopy and increased exhaled nitric oxide. J Allergy Clin Immunol 2006;118:1218–25.

117. Roberts G, Patel N, Levi-Schaffer F, et al. Food allergy as a risk factor for life-threatening asthma in childhood: a case-controlled study. J Allergy Clin Immunol 2003;112:168–74.

118. Sampson HA, Muñoz-Furlong A, Campbell RL, et al. Second symposium on the definition and management of anaphylaxis: summary report—Second National Institute of Allergy and Infectious Disease/Food Allergy and Anaphylaxis Network symposium. J Allergy Clin Immunol 2006;117:391–7.

119. O'Driscoll BR, Hopkinson LC, Denning DW. Mold sensitization is common amongst patients with severe asthma requiring multiple hospital admissions. BMC Pulm Med 2005;5:4.

120. Vicencio AG, Muzumdar H, Tsirilakis K, et al. Severe asthma with fungal sensitization in a child: response to itraconazole therapy. Pediatrics 2010;125:e1255–8.

121. Ayres JG, Jyothish D, Ninan T. Brittle asthma. Paediatr Respir Rev 2004;5:40–4.

122. Dougherty RH, Fahy JV. Acute exacerbations of asthma: epidemiology, biology and the exacerbation-prone phenotype. Clin Exp Allergy 2009;39:193–202.

123. Carroll CL, Schramm CM, Zucker AR. Severe exacerbations in children with mild asthma: characterizing a pediatric phenotype. J Asthma 2008;45:513–7.

124. Bacharier LB, Phillips BR, Bloomberg GR, et al, Childhood Asthma Research and Education Network, National Heart, Lung, and Blood Institute. Severe intermittent wheezing in preschool children: a distinct phenotype. J Allergy Clin Immunol 2007;119:604–10.

125. Phelan PD, Robertson CF, Olinsky A. The Melbourne Asthma Study: 1964-1999. J Allergy Clin Immunol 2002;109:189–94.

126. Fitzpatrick AM, Teague WG, National Institutes of Health/National Heart, Lung, and Blood Institute's Severe Asthma Research Program. Progressive airflow limitation is a feature of children with severe asthma. J Allergy Clin Immunol 2011; 127:282–4.

127. Covar RA, Spahn JD, Murphy JR, et al, Childhood Asthma Management Program Research Group. Progression of asthma measured by lung function in the childhood asthma management program. Am J Respir Crit Care Med 2004;170: 234–41.

128. He XY, Simpson JL, Wang F. Inflammatory phenotypes in stable and acute childhood asthma. Paediatr Respir Rev 2011;12:165–9.

129. Bush A, Pedersen S, Hedlin G, et al, PSACI (Problematic Severe Asthma in Childhood Initiative) group. Pharmacological treatment of severe, therapy-resistant asthma in children: what can we learn from where? Eur Respir J 2011;38:947–58.

130. Holt S, Suder A, Weatherall M, et al. Dose-response relation of inhaled fluticasone propionate in adolescents and adults with asthma: meta-analysis. BMJ 2001;323:253–6.

131. Lex C, Payne DN, Zacharasiewicz A, et al. Is a two-week trial of oral predniso-lone predictive of target lung function in pediatric asthma? Pediatr Pulmonol 2005;39:521–7.

132. Adams NP, Bestall JC, Jones P, et al. Fluticasone at different doses for chronic asthma in adults and children. Cochrane Database Syst Rev 2008; 4:CD003534.

133. de Blic J, Delacourt C, Le Bourgeois M, et al. Efficacy of nebulized budesonide in treatment of severe infantile asthma: a double-blind study. J Allergy Clin Im-munol 1996;98:14–20.

134. Cohen J, Postma DS, Douma WR, et al. Particle size matters: diagnostics and treatment of small airways involvement in asthma. Eur Respir J 2011;37:532–40.

135. Rodrigo GJ, Castro-Rodríguez JA. Safety of long-acting {beta} agonists for the treatment of asthma: clearing the air. Thorax 2012;67(4):342–9.

136. Global Strategy for Asthma Management and Prevention, Global Initiative for Asthma (GINA) 2011. Available at: http://www.ginasthma.org/. Accessed May 26, 2012.

137. Panickar JR, Kenia P, Silverman M, et al. Intramuscular triamcinolone for difficult asthma. Pediatr Pulmonol 2005;39:421–5.

138. Milgrom H, Berger W, Nayak A, et al. Treatment of childhood asthma with anti-immunoglobulin E antibody (omalizumab). Pediatrics 2001;108:e36.

139. Lanier B, Bridges T, Kulus M, et al. Omalizumab for the treatment of exacerba-tions in children with inadequately controlled allergic (IgE-mediated) asthma. J Allergy Clin Immunol 2009;124:1210–6.

140. Lemanske RF Jr, Nayak A, McAlary M, et al. Omalizumab improves asthma-related quality of life in children with allergic asthma. Pediatrics 2002;110:e55.

141. Busse WW, Morgan WJ, Gergen PJ, et al. Randomized trial of omalizumab (anti-IgE) for asthma in inner-city children. N Engl J Med 2011;364:1005–15.

142. Rodrigo GJ, Neffen H, Castro-Rodriguez JA. Efficacy and safety of subcutane-ous omalizumab vs placebo as add-on therapy to corticosteroids for children and adults with asthma: a systematic review. Chest 2011;139:28–35.

143. Cox L, Platts-Mills TA, Finegold I, et al, American Academy of Allergy, Asthma & Immunology; American College of Allergy, Asthma and Immunology. American Academy of Allergy, Asthma & Immunology/American College of Allergy, Asthma and Immunology Joint Task Force Report on omalizumab-associated anaphylaxis. J Allergy Clin Immunol 2007;120:1373–7.

144. Seddon P, Bara A, Ducharme FM, et al. Oral xanthines as maintenance treat-ment for asthma in children. Cochrane Database Syst Rev 2006;1:CD002885.

145. Rottier BL, Duiverman EJ. Anti-inflammatory drug therapy in asthma. Paediatr Respir Rev 2009;10:214–9.

146. Metz G, Kraft M. Effects of atypical infections with Mycoplasma and Chlamydia on asthma. Immunol Allergy Clin North Am 2010;30:575–85.

147. Patel KK, Vicencio AG, Du Z, et al. Infectious *Chlamydia pneumoniae* is associ-ated with elevated interleukin-8 and airway neutrophilia in children with refrac-tory asthma. Pediatr Infect Dis J 2010;29:1093–8.

148. Strunk RC, Bacharier LB, Phillips BR, et al, CARE Network. Azithromycin or mon-telukast as inhaled corticosteroid-sparing agents in moderate-to-severe child-hood asthma study. J Allergy Clin Immunol 2008;122:1138–44.

149. Evans DJ, Cullinan P, Geddes DM. Cyclosporin as an oral corticosteroid sparing agent in stable asthma. Cochrane Database Syst Rev 2001;2:CD002993.

150. Davies H, Olson L, Gibson P. Methotrexate as a steroid sparing agent for asthma in adults. Cochrane Database Syst Rev 2000;2:CD000391.

151. Firszt R, Kraft M. Pharmacotherapy of severe asthma. Curr Opin Pharmacol 2010;10:266–71.
152. Rasmussen LM, Phanareth K, Nolte H, et al. Internet-based monitoring of asthma: a long-term, randomized clinical study of 300 asthmatic subjects. J Allergy Clin Immunol 2005;115:1137–42.
153. Deschildre A, Béghin L, Salleron J, et al. Home telemonitoring (FEV1) in children with severe asthma does not reduce exacerbations. Eur Respir J 2012;39(2): 290–6.
154. Reddel HK, Taylor DR, Bateman ED, et al, American Thoracic Society/European Respiratory Society Task Force on Asthma Control and Exacerbations. An official American Thoracic Society/European Respiratory Society statement: asthma control and exacerbations: standardizing endpoints for clinical asthma trials and clinical practice. Am J Respir Crit Care Med 2009;180:59–99.
155. Petsky HL, Cates CJ, Lasseron TJ, et al. A systematic review and meta-analysis: tailoring asthma treatment on eosinophilic markers (exhaled nitric oxide or sputum eosinophils). Thorax 2012;67:199–208.
156. Fleming L, Wilson N, Regamey N, et al. Use of sputum eosinophil counts to guide management in children with severe asthma. Thorax 2012;67:193–8.

Challenges in Providing Preventive Care To Inner-City Children with Asthma

Arlene M. Butz, ScD, MSN[a,b],*, Joan Kub, PhD, MSN[b],
Melissa H. Bellin, PhD, LCSW[c], Kevin D. Frick, PhD[d]

KEYWORDS

- Asthma • Inner city • Preventive care

KEY POINTS

- Major challenges to preventive asthma care are encountered by inner-city children and include family and patient attitudes and beliefs, lack of access to quality medical care, and psychosocial and environmental factors.
- Pediatric nurses can affect these challenges by identifying parental attitudes and beliefs about asthma medications, parental depression and stress, and environmental exposures. Remediation of these challenges may require referral to community resources such as an asthma specialist, community mental health clinics, and smoking-cessation clinics.
- Alternative or supplemental health care sites such as school-based asthma programs, community or mobile health care clinics, or disease case management programs may enhance access to preventive care for high-risk inner-city children.

INTRODUCTION

Asthma affects 7.1 million children in the United States and is the number 1 cause of pediatric emergency department (ED) visits.[1–3] Although the scientific understanding of the pathophysiology of asthma and the quality of asthma therapies have significantly improved over the past 30 years, asthma morbidity remains high and preventive care low for inner-city children. Low-income, African American children have a 4.1-times higher rate of ED visits and a death rate 7.6 times higher than rates of non-Hispanic white children,[4] although minority low-income children are the least

This article originally appeared in Nursing Clinics of North America, Volume 48, Issue 2, June 2013.
[a] Department of Pediatrics, The Johns Hopkins University School of Medicine, 200 North Wolfe Street, Baltimore, MD 21287, USA; [b] Department of Community Health, School of Nursing, Johns Hopkins University, 525 North Wolfe street, Baltimore, MD 21287, USA; [c] School of Social Work, The University of Maryland at Baltimore, 525 West Redwood Street, Baltimore, MD 21201, USA; [d] Department of Health Policy and Management, The Johns Hopkins University Bloomberg School of Public Health, 615 North Wolfes Street, Baltimore, MD 21205, USA
* Corresponding author. Division of General Pediatrics, Johns Hopkins University School of Medicine, 200 North Wolfe Street Room 2051, Baltimore, MD 21287.
E-mail address: abutz@jhmi.edu

likely to receive adequate guideline-based therapy.[5–7] Furthermore, Hispanic and black children have higher rates of inadequate health care insurance in comparison with white children.[8] This disparity in asthma morbidity among inner-city children often results from inadequacies of the health care delivery system[8] as well as from individual factors regarding the patient, caregiver, and health care provider.

Preventive asthma care among inner-city children is challenging because of a variety of factors including health care system/organizational and provider characteristics, patient and family attitudes and beliefs, and psychosocial and environmental factors. These factors affect a child's opportunity to receive preventive care for asthma and, if missed, can result in increased asthma morbidity and health care costs (**Fig. 1**). Specific health care system/organizational challenges are lack of access to quality medical care, including long wait times and unavailability of health care appointments, lack of transportation to clinic sites, and lack of access to specialty asthma care. Especially challenging to preventive care for inner-city children with asthma is nonadherence to national asthma guidelines by health care providers. Self-reported rates of adherence of primary care providers to national asthma guidelines are low,[9–11] and may lead to misclassification of asthma severity and control for the child owing to unfamiliarity with guidelines. This misclassification of severity may contribute to the underuse of anti-inflammatory medications consistently reported in inner-city children.[12–15] Family and patient attitudes and beliefs about asthma care, psychosocial factors including caregiver depression and life stress,[16–19] and environmental factors found in the child's home and neighborhood are other major challenges to preventive asthma care in inner-city children. This article purposely focuses on 4 major challenges to providing preventive care (family and patient attitudes and beliefs, lack of access to quality medical care, psychosocial factors, and environmental factors) based on prior evidence and the authors' own observation of these challenges in research with inner-city children with asthma over the past decade. Pediatric nurses are in contact with children with asthma and their families in a variety of settings including schools, community health, primary care, EDs, and inpatient units. The goal of this article is to describe the aforementioned challenges, address cost issues related to preventive care, and provide recommendations for pediatric nurses across settings.

CHALLENGES TO PREVENTIVE ASTHMA CARE
Caregiver/Family Attitudes and Beliefs About Asthma Care

Common caregiver/family attitudes and beliefs about asthma preventive care are (1) lack of appreciation for preventive asthma medication and follow-up care when a child with asthma is asymptomatic, and (2) distrust and worry about side effects of medications.[5,20,21] The evidence from several studies indicates that even when appropriate preventive asthma medications are prescribed, only 30% to 50% of children with asthma who require daily preventive medications receive adequate doses anti-inflammatory medications.[13,14,22] The most common contributor to nonadherence to daily preventive medication use in children with asthma is misunderstanding by both caregiver and child of the role of daily anti-inflammatory medications in treating asthma. For instance, caregivers may believe that the child's asthma is not severe enough to require daily medication, noted in many nonadherent adult patients with asthma[21] and consistent with caregiver reports of high symptom days but low use of daily preventive medications by their children.[6,14,23] Moreover, administration of daily preventive medications is complex, with complicated regimens and delivery systems. Accurate use of metered dose inhalers (MDIs), dry powder inhalers, and nebulizers requires cooperation and coordination from the child. The use of spacers

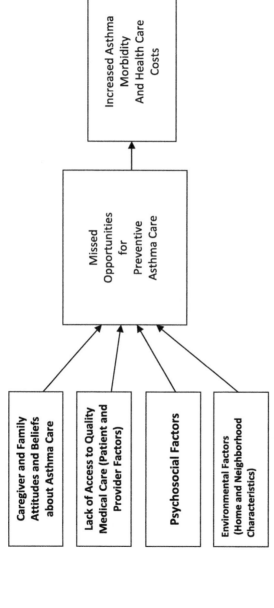

Fig. 1. Challenges to preventive care for inner-city children with asthma.

with MDIs significantly enhances aerosolized medication deposition into the lung instead of the mouth or pharynx, and is recommended for use by all children and adolescents who are prescribed MDI-administered asthma medications.

Parental worry about medication dependence and reduced effectiveness of long-term use of asthma medications has been reported.[14,21] In the authors' current study of 300 inner-city children aged 3 to 10 years with persistent asthma and frequent ED visits for asthma, nearly one-third of parents reported that they were very worried about the side effects of their child's asthma medications (**Table 1**). This level of parental worry is most likely related to concerns of potential long-term effects, misperception of the type of steroid medication (nonanabolic steroid), and the perceived risk of dependence.[25]

Child age appears to be associated with adherence to preventive care appointments because of the competing demands of school and work. In the authors' behavioral intervention study of children with persistent asthma, younger children were significantly more likely to attend a primary care follow-up visit for asthma than older children, most likely because competing school or work obligations of older children impeded attending an appointment with the primary care physician during daytime hours.[26] Alternatively, caregivers may be more concerned about asthma symptoms and acute exacerbations in younger children who are less able to communicate their asthma symptoms or unable to communicate their symptoms as clearly as older children. Furthermore, because older children may self-manage their asthma, parental awareness of symptoms may be decreased.

Guideline-based asthma treatment is based on accurate recognition and reporting of symptoms by the family, and appropriate classification of severity by the health care provider. A critical premise of effective asthma self-management is the caregiver's and/or child's ability to communicate the symptom level to the health care provider and have the provider accurately assign a severity level that indicates treatment guidelines. Communication about asthma severity may be impaired by poor symptom perception on the part of the child or parent,[27,28] or inappropriate symptom labeling by the parent or health care provider. For example, mislabeling cough as nonasthma may result in misdiagnosis and inadequate treatment of asthma. Perceptions of asthma symptoms by parents and children are multidimensional and include nonspecific symptoms such as fatigue, malaise, and fear.[29] Miscommunication about symptom frequency and severity between parents and providers may result in an inaccurate assessment of severity, leading to an inappropriate medication regimen and uncontrolled asthma.[13]

Recommendations to improve understanding of caregiver/family attitudes and beliefs about asthma care

- Identify and discuss parental attitudes, beliefs, and worries about medications, including potential side effects and dependence on asthma medications.
- Teach parents and school-age children specific and nonspecific symptoms of asthma, and identify descriptors of child symptoms for parents and teachers to use.
- Monitor younger and newly diagnosed children with asthma more frequently through the evolving ability of the parent and child to recognize asthma symptoms.[27,30]

Lack of Access to Quality Medical Care: Patient and Health Care Provider Factors

Common health care system/organizational barriers to preventive care encountered by inner-city children with asthma include lack of available primary care appointments, long wait times or inconvenient times for scheduled appointments,[31,32] lack of endorsement by the child's primary care provider for the need to follow up after ED visits,[33,34] lack of transportation, lack of affordable child care, fear of losing one's job through attending multiple medical appointments, and lack of referral to specialty care for treatment when indicated.[23]

Several behavioral interventions targeting system/organizational barriers have shown modest improvement in providing preventive asthma care; these include school-based screening, health care provider prompting for guideline-based care, and parent Web-based feedback interventions.[35–39] Successful physician feedback interventions for asthma include providing feedback on specific asthma health information to the child's primary care provider regarding the child's symptom frequency and frequency of ED visits,[15] and information sent by providers regarding their patients' adherence to inhaled corticosteroid (ICS) use as compared with prescribed doses.[38] Although case management, another successful organizational intervention for high-risk children, is usually reimbursable, it is not standard practice in all health care settings. Moreover, case management is often inadequately structured to have any significant impact on inner-city children with complex social problems such as family mental health issues[18] or poor-quality housing.

Alternative health care delivery models, such as school-based and mobile health vans, have shown potential in tackling system/organizational barriers to preventive care for inner-city children with asthma. One promising intervention is an asthma therapy program consisting of monitoring asthma control and administering daily preventive medications, which is delivered in public schools.[39] Based on the research team's prior successful model using directly observed therapy (DOT) of preventive medications to children with persistent asthma by school health staff,[39] the asthma therapy intervention was improved by the addition of a Web-based communication between an asthma care coordinator, the child's health care provider, and the school. The intervention is integrated within school and community systems, and pilot data indicate that the majority of children received preventive medications during school hours.[40]

Use of mobile health vans is increasing in popularity as a way to improve access to care for a variety of medical and dental diseases.[41,42] The mobile clinics are predominantly used at schools that offer the advantages of providing multiple sites for care, eliminating transportation issues and resulting in a decrease in missed appointments.[42] The Breathmobile program, a mobile health clinic providing specialty asthma care, is an innovative solution to help increase access to specialty care for underserved children with asthma.[43] Children attending the Baltimore Breathmobile had a significant reduction in symptom-free days, urgent care visits, and improved controller medication use, and has proved to be an effective model of health care delivery for underserved children.[41]

Nonadherence by health care providers to national asthma guidelines is another significant challenge to preventive care for inner-city children with asthma. More than a decade ago, national asthma guidelines were published by the National Heart, Lung, and Blood Institute (NHLBI) National Asthma Education and Prevention Program (NAEPP) in an attempt to standardize and improve the quality of asthma care and to disseminate best practices for asthma management.[44] However, provision of preventive asthma medication is strikingly low in minority inner-city children,[5] with rates of anti-inflammatory medication use of between 40% and 60% for inner-city children with persistent asthma.[9,45] Less than half (44%) receive a written asthma action plan, only half (51%) receive advice regarding environmental control,[7] and only 23% to 24% of these children are seen by an asthma specialist.[23,46] Despite most pediatricians (88%) indicating awareness and access to the guidelines, there is a wide gap

Table 1
Baseline characteristics of inner-city children with persistent asthma enrolled in pediatric asthma alert intervention (N = 300)

Characteristic	Number (%)
Child's age	
Mean (SD)	5.65 (2.2)
Race/Ethnicity	
African American	286 (95.4)
Hispanic/Latino	3 (1.0)
White	4 (1.3)
Other	7 (2.3)
Health insurance type	
Medicaid	275 (91.7)
Private	24 (8.0)
Self-pay	1 (0.3)
Caregiver Characteristics	
Caregiver age	
Mean (SD)	31.5 (7.0)
Marital status	
Single	210 (70.0)
Married	56 (18.7)
Other	34 (11.3)
Center for Epidemiologic Studies Depression Scale (n = 298)	
≥16 (Clinical cutoff for depressive symptoms)	102 (34.2)
Caregiver Daily Life Stress	
Mean (SD) (Range: 0 = No stress and 10 = high stress)	6.33 (2.9)
Caregiver Asthma Life Stress	
Mean (SD) (Range: 0 = No stress and 10 = high stress)	5.16 (3.7)
Child Health Characteristics	
Symptom days past 2 wk	
0–3	98 (32.7)
4 or more (not controlled)	202 (67.3)
Symptom nights (n = 299)	
0–2	101 (33.8)
3 or more (not controlled)	198 (66.2)
Number of ED visits for asthma past 6 mo	
None	13 (4.4)
1–2	157 (52.3)
3 or more	130 (43.3)
Routine preventive asthma care visits past 6 mo	
None	29 (9.7)
1	75 (25.0)
2	76 (25.3)
3 or more	120 (40.0)
Seen by asthma specialist last 2 y	
Yes	58 (19.3)
Asthma Action Plan in the home	
Yes	103 (34.3)
Uses a spacer for inhaled medications	
Yes	276 (92.0)
Uses a peak flow meter in home	
Yes	73 (24.3)

(continued on next page)

Table 1 (continued)	
Characteristic	**Number (%)**
Uses home remedies for asthma (n = 296)	
Yes	100 (33.8)
Worried or concerned about child's asthma medications and side effects[a] (n = 299)	
Very, very worried or very worried	92 (30.8)
Fairly or somewhat or a little worried	65 (21.7)
Hardly or not worried	142 (47.5)
Smoker in the home	
Yes	177 (59.0)
Cockroaches in the home	
Yes	84 (28.0)
Mice in the home	
Yes	137 (45.7)
Violence exposure (seeing violence in the neighborhood)	69 (23.0)

[a] Item from Pediatric Asthma Caregivers Quality of Life Questionnaire.[24]

between preventive care of children with asthma and the NAEPP guidelines, with low rates of adherence by primary care providers.[9–11] Rates of 39% to 53% have been reported for specific guideline components: 53% for prescribing corticosteroids and 39% for complying with instructions for daily peak flowmeter use.[47,48] Several reasons for physician nonadherence to the NAEPP guidelines include time and staff limitations for delivery of recommendations, low reimbursement for visits that provide patient education and medication monitoring, low self-efficacy among clinicians for correctly dosing anti-inflammatory medications and teaching peak flowmeter use,[49] lack of time for education specific to guideline components that involve intensive teaching and counseling,[48] low self-efficacy about counseling for smoking cessation, and clinical inertia or the failure to change therapy when the disease is uncontrolled.[50] Other reasons for nonadherence to guidelines are based in part on provider beliefs, including lack of agreement with safety of long-term corticosteroid use (concerns of cushingoid effects, osteoporosis, growth stunting, cataract development),[47] underestimation by clinicians of children's asthma severity,[13,51] difficulty convincing parents to administer ICSs when they are concerned about side effects,[47] and language barriers in families with English as a second language who may be unable to understand proper medication dosage and administration. In summary, most pediatric providers are aware of the national asthma guidelines and have access to a copy of the guidelines, yet adherence to specific guideline components remains low.

Recommendations to improve access to quality medical care

- Provide alternative health care sites for inner-city children with asthma through school-based asthma programs and community or mobile health care clinics when available.
- Enroll patients into comprehensive disease-management or case-management programs that provide transportation, appointment reminders, and electronic communication with the patient's health care provider to improve the quality of care and monitor asthma status on a regular basis.
- Encourage endorsement of national asthma guidelines by local pediatric professional organizations (American Academy of Pediatrics, National Association of

Pediatric Nurse Practitioners and Nurses, and National Association of School Health Nurses) to improve pediatric health care provider awareness and encourage more use of national asthma guidelines.[9,47,48]

- Provide practical workshops for health care providers, parents, and children to provide hands-on experience with asthma devices, medications, and smoking-cessation counseling.

Psychosocial Factors

Several psychosocial factors are also known to create barriers to preventive care for children with asthma. In particular, caregiver psychological symptoms and life stress related to residence in low-income, inner-city communities negatively influence decisions about asthma self-management and increase asthma morbidity through treatment nonadherence and unnecessary use of health care.[52–56] Both caregiver anxiety and depressive symptoms are associated with poor asthma outcomes,[57,58] but research with inner-city populations increasingly suggests that caregiver depression is a particularly strong predictor of child asthma attacks,[59] ED visits,[60] and hospitalizations.[61] Even when the child's asthma severity is taken into account, caregivers with high levels of depressive symptoms are 30% more likely to report an ED visit by their child than those with low symptomatology.[62]

It is well established that successful asthma self-management requires the caregiver to possess both skill competencies and focused attention to carefully assess and monitor the child's symptoms, administer the correct dosage of preventive medication and stepped-up therapy when needed, and be cognizant of environmental hazards such as mold, rodent infestation, and dust.[44,63] However, depressive symptoms may reduce the caregiver's capacity for the quick and critical thinking that is essential to proper decision making regarding asthma management and health care utilization.[64,65] The clouded judgment may in turn result in avoidable ED and urgent care visits.

Life stress associated with inner-city residence similarly creates barriers to preventive care by disrupting asthma self-management activities.[66] Intimate partner violence (IPV), one example of life stress, is related to poorer health outcomes. The relationship between IPV and asthma in children was examined using the Behavioral Risk Factor Surveillance System survey conducted in 10 US states/territories. Women who experienced IPV at any point in their lifetime were significantly more likely to report that their children ever had or currently have asthma, compared with women who had never experienced IPV.[67]

Both acute (eg, exposure to violence) and chronic (eg, housing instability, poverty) stressors divert attention away from monitoring the child's symptoms and administering controlling medicine.[68] Simply stated, inner-city, low-income caregivers mobilize sparse resources to support "the family's daily survival and future stability".[69(p706)] Adverse social conditions create a barrier to preventive care when a caregiver's physical, financial, and psychological resources are consumed in their efforts to ensure the safety and well-being of the family unit, leaving little time or energy for proper asthma self-management. In summary, symptoms of caregiver depression and life stress may erode the caregiver's ability to perform asthma self-management behaviors as prescribed by the NHLBI, leading to increased asthma morbidity, health care use, and cost.

Recommendations to improve psychosocial challenges

- Provide regular screening of caregiver depression in clinical encounters with child asthma, with referrals to community mental health treatment providers for follow-up care.

- Provide screening for IPV during child asthma encounters, and make appropriate referrals to mental health treatment and community resources to address IPV.
- Caregivers of inner-city minority children with asthma may benefit from counseling strategies to help them cope with contemporary life stressors associated with poverty.[70]

Environmental Factors: Home and Neighborhood Characteristics

Physical and psychosocial aspects of the environment, in both the home and neighborhood, play a significant role in pediatric asthma morbidity. Children in rural environments are at lower risk of asthma compared with children in urban environments.[71] In inner-city environments air pollution is one significant factor, and the home serves as another primary source of allergen and irritant exposures for children, contributing to an increased sensitization to allergens.[72] Allergen sensitivity and exposure are associated with increased asthma morbidity, particularly in sensitized individuals with asthma.[73] The factors associated with this increased sensitization are often related to poverty and poor housing conditions in inner cities, and low-income children are more frequently exposed to environmental triggers,[74] including high levels of indoor allergens,[75] in comparison with children who are not poor. Substandard housing conditions result in exposure to high cockroach and mouse allergen levels,[76] dust mites, and mold related to water and roof leaks. Increased moisture in the home not only augments mold growth but provides a rich environment for dust-mite proliferation. A recent study that pooled allergen, housing conditions, and other data from 9 asthma studies found that high levels of cockroach allergen were associated with cracks or holes in walls, high dust-mite allergen levels with mold odors, and mouse allergen levels with signs of rodents.[77] Furthermore, water leaks and below-average housekeeping was associated with high levels of cockroach allergen. Increased moisture in the home not only augments mold growth but provides a rich environment for dust-mite proliferation. Without pest management, these infestations result in high allergen load in the home, resulting in an increased risk of asthma exacerbation. These high indoor exposures are supported by observations in the authors' current cohort of 300 inner-city children with asthma who reported high levels of rodent and cockroach exposure (mice: 46%; cockroach infestation: 28%) (see **Table 1**).

Other indoor exposures include nitrogen dioxide associated with the use of gas stoves, and exposure to second-hand smoke (SHS). Both indoor exposure to nitrogen dioxide and SHS are associated with negative respiratory effects in asthma.[78] In a recent study of 469 families of children with asthma in a large city, gas stoves were present in 88% of the homes and the median level of indoor nitrogen dioxide was high.[78] This higher level of nitrogen dioxide was related to lower peak flow levels among the children during the colder months.[78] Another prevalent indoor exposure for children is SHS. Of note, between 40% and 67% of inner-city children with asthma reside in a dwelling with at least 1 smoker,[74] which has important implications for children living in substandard housing with poor ventilation. Objective evidence of SHS exposure in a large study of children with asthma reported that the median level of cotinine/creatinine, a biomarker for SHS exposure, was 42.4 ng/mg in children living in homes with a smoker, compared with 18.0 ng/mg in children not residing with a smoker.[78] The authors' data confirm the high prevalence of SHS exposure in inner-city children with asthma, with more than half (59%) of the children residing with a smoker in their home (see **Table 1**).

Besides the physical home environment, psychosocial aspects of neighborhoods and communities influence asthma morbidity. Even though some communities may share low SHS and environmental exposures, such as poor housing or high outdoor pollution, they may not share excess asthma morbidity.[68,79–81] This paradox has resulted in studies examining the role of psychosocial factors within neighborhoods to help explain these differences. For example, researchers have found that individual perceptions of stressors related to living in high-risk neighborhoods and actual community-level indicators are also significantly related to asthma morbidity. Community-level stressors include poverty, unemployment or underemployment, limited social capital, and high exposure to crime and violence.[81] Exposure to community violence is one specific factor related to asthma morbidity. Caretakers of children with asthma and who were exposed to community violence reported more lost sleep and symptom days among their children.[82] In a recent longitudinal study of children with asthma younger than 10 years and residing in Chicago, community violence was also associated with increased asthma risk, although it did not fully explain asthma risk when controlling for individual-level and other neighborhood-level factors.[83]

On the other hand, protective factors at the community level have been described. Cagney and colleagues,[79] for example, studied the paradox of foreign-born Latinos having a respiratory health advantage if they lived in an enclave of other foreign-born Latinos. The explanation for this protective advantage was described as the sense of cohesiveness or collective efficacy present in the community. This level of trust and attachment within a community may be protective for families who feel a sense of cohesiveness and know they can rely on neighbors for assistance if their child has asthma symptoms.[68]

Recommendations to improve physical and neighborhood factors

- Assist families to identify specific allergen triggers for their child, including awareness of both indoor and outdoor allergens and air-pollutant exposures. Provide individualized and comprehensive education about simple household preventive measures such as use of mousetraps, cockroach bait, and repair of water leaks to avoid mold exposure.
- Provide smoking-cessation resources to families with a smoker in the home. National Quitline 1-800-Quit Now.
- Families living in substandard housing may benefit from referral and counseling strategies to help them seek alternative living conditions.
- Assess for exposure to violence; referral to stress-reduction program or to programs that provide counseling to those exposed to violence.
- Promote social cohesion in communities and build social capital (ie, connections within and between social networks) to create better living conditions to improve health.

Cost of Challenges to Providing Preventive Care to Inner-City Children with Asthma

Costs create challenges, with respect to asthma generally and preventive care specifically, in several ways. First, asthma is costly for families. A recent report indicated that the mean out-of-pocket costs for medication related to asthma was $151 for children younger than 5 years and just slightly higher ($154) for children ages 5 to 18.[84] Another study, this time focusing on families of children with asthma in which an adult is employed, found that children having asthma was associated with higher employee costs (health care, prescriptions, sick leave, and short-term disability), and the children's health care ($862) and prescription ($534) spending.[85] With a 20% copayment (common in many insurance policies), the combination of health care and prescriptions for children would result in approximately $280 of additional out-of-pocket costs per year for the family.

A key in interpreting these results is to recognize that these costs are not a small amount for families in difficult economic situations and that asthma in general (and uncontrolled asthma specifically) is associated with poverty.[1] The resources required for routine asthma care compete with other uses of familial resources, including child care for other children and a variety of costs to help improve the environment. For

Table 2
Summary of recommendations by challenge

Challenge	Recommendations
Caregiver and family attitudes and beliefs about asthma care	Identify and discuss parental attitudes, beliefs, and worries about medications Teach parents and school-age children specific and nonspecific symptoms of asthma, and identify child-symptom descriptors for parents and teachers to understand Monitor younger and newly diagnosed children with asthma more frequently, owing to evolving ability to recognize asthma symptoms
Lack of access to quality medical care	Provide alternative health care sites such as school-based asthma programs, community or mobile health care clinics when available Enroll patients into comprehensive disease-management or case-management programs Encourage endorsement of guidelines by local pediatric professional organizations (American Academy of Pediatrics, National Association of Pediatric Nurse Practitioners and Nurses, and National Association of School Health Nurses) to improve pediatric health care provider awareness and use of national asthma guidelines Provide practical workshops to provide hands-on experience with asthma devices, medications, smoking-cessation counseling, and models of asthma care
Psychosocial factors	Regular screening of caregiver depression in child asthma clinical encounters, with referrals to community mental health treatment providers for follow-up care Caregivers of inner-city minority children with asthma may benefit from counseling strategies to help them cope with contemporary life stressors associated with poverty
Environmental factors	Assist families to identify specific allergen triggers for their child. Provide individualized and comprehensive education about simple household preventive measures such as use of mousetraps, cockroach bait, and repair of water leaks to avoid mold exposure Provide smoking-cessation resources to families with smokers in the home. National Quitline 1-800-Quit Now. Families living in substandard housing may benefit from referral and counseling strategies to help them seek alternative living conditions Assess for exposure to violence; referral to stress-reduction program or to programs that provide counseling to those exposed to violence Promote social cohesion in communities and build social capital (ie, connections within and between social networks) to create better living conditions to improve health

example, extermination for mice and cockroaches, air cleaners in the child's bedroom, and mattress covers for dust-mite prevention are all nonnegligible expenses and are usually not covered by insurance. These preventive activities may be given even lower priority than preventive medications, as the impact is apparent only in the longer term, and individuals with limited financial resources tend to focus on the use of resources with the most immediate outcomes.

SUMMARY AND IMPLICATIONS

Preventive asthma care for inner-city children is challenging because of multiple health care system/organizational, caregiver and family, health care provider, psychosocial, and environmental factors that negatively affect preventive care (**Table 2**). Several recommendations to help minimize the barriers to preventive asthma care are suggested for pediatric nurses who care for these high-risk children across multiple settings. To enhance asthma self-management and reduce barriers to preventive care, clinical work with this population must extend beyond screening for traditional environmental risk factors (eg, allergens and irritants) to also include comprehensive assessment of caregiver attitudes and beliefs, caregiver stressors, and targeted referrals for modifiable psychosocial stressors that influence caregiver behaviors. Furthermore, pediatric health care providers can monitor the level of stress, anxiety, or depression, and recommend either management strategies or links to services that might help patients and caregivers to manage these stressors. Because exposure to allergens and irritants plays a significant role in asthma morbidity, families may need assistance with identification of specific allergen triggers and awareness of indoor and outdoor exposures, and their effects on children with asthma. Effective remediation of allergen and pollutant exposure involves individualized and comprehensive family education about household preventive measures such as use of mousetraps and cockroach bait, and repair of water leaks to avoid mold exposure. Lastly, endorsement of national guidelines by local pediatric professional organizations to improve awareness in pediatric health care providers is recommended, along with the use of national asthma guidelines.

REFERENCES

1. Akinbami LJ, Moorman JE, Bailey C, et al. Trends in asthma prevalence, health care use and mortality in the United States, 2001-2010. NCHS Data Brief 2012; 94:1–7.
2. Akinbami LJ, Moorman JE, Garbe PL, et al. Status of childhood asthma in the United States, 1980-2007. Pediatrics 2009;123(S3):S131–45.
3. Akinbami L. The state of childhood asthma, United States, 1980-2005. Centers for Disease Control and Prevention National Center for Health Statistics. Adv Data 2006 Dec 12;(381):1–24.
4. Akinbami LJ, Moorman JE, Liu X. Asthma prevalence, health care use and mortality: United States, 2005-2009. Natl Health Stat Report 2011;12(32):1–14.
5. Diaz T, Sturm T, Matte T, et al. Medication use among children with asthma in East Harlem. Pediatrics 2000;105(6):1188–93.
6. Ortega AN, Gergen PJ, Paltiel AD, et al. Impact of site of care, race, and Hispanic ethnicity on medication use for childhood asthma. Pediatrics 2002; 109(1):E1.
7. Centers for Disease Control and Prevention (CDC). Vital signs: asthma prevalence, disease characteristics, and self-management education—United States, 2001-2009. MMWR Morb Mortal Wkly Rep 2011;60(17):547–52.

8. Bethell CD, Kogan MD, Strickland BB, et al. A National and State profile of leading health problems and heath care quality for US children: key insurance disparities and across-state variations. Academic Pediatrics 2011;11(Suppl 3): S22–33.

9. Finkelstein JA, Lozano P, Shulruff R, et al. Self-reported physician practices for children with asthma: are national guidelines followed? Pediatrics 2000; 106(Suppl 4):886–96.

10. Crain EF, Weiss KB, Fagan MJ. Pediatric asthma care in US emergency departments. Current practice in the context of the National Institutes of Health Guidelines. Arch Pediatr Adolesc Med 1995;149:893–901.

11. Wisnivesky JP, Lorenzo J, Lyn-cook R, et al. Barriers to adherence to asthma management guidelines among inner-city primary care providers. Ann Allergy Asthma Immunol 2008;101:264–70.

12. Van den Berg NJ, Hagmolen W, Nagelkerke AF, et al. What general practitioners and paediatricians think about their patients' asthma. Patient Educ Couns 2005; 59:182–95.

13. Halterman JS, Yoos HL, Kaczorowski JM, et al. Providers underestimate symptom severity among urban children with asthma. Archives of Pediatric and Adolescent Medicine 2002;156:141–6.

14. Butz AM, Tsoukleris M, Donithan M, et al. Patterns of inhaled anti-inflammatory medication use in young underserved children with asthma. Pediatrics 2006; 118:2504–13.

15. Kattan M, Crain EF, Steinbach S, et al. A randomized clinical trial of clinician feedback to improve quality of care for inner-city children with asthma. Pediatrics 2006;117:e1095–103.

16. Gregor MA, Wheeler JR, Stanley RM, et al, Great Lakes Emergency Medical Services for Children Research Network. Caregiver adherence to follow-up after an emergency department visit for common pediatric illnesses: impact on future ED use. Med Care 2009;47(3):326–33.

17. Brousseau D, Dansereau L, Linakis J, et al. Pediatric emergency department utilization within a statewide Medicaid managed care system. Academic Emergency Medicine 2002;9:296–9.

18. Otsuki M, Eakin M, Arceneaux LL, et al. Prospective relationship between maternal depressive symptoms and asthma morbidity among inner-city African American Children. J Pediatr Psychology 2010;35(7):758–67.

19. Turyk ME, Hernandez E, Wright RJ, et al. Stressful life events and asthma in adolescents. Pediatr Allergy Immunol 2008;19(3):255–63.

20. Conn KM, Halterman JS, Fisher SG, et al. Parental beliefs about medications and medication adherence among urban children with asthma. Ambulatory Pediatrics 2005;5:306–10.

21. Bender BG, Bender SE. Patient-identified barriers to asthma treatment adherence: response to interviews, focus groups and questionnaires. Immunol Allergy Clin N Am 2005;25:107–30.

22. Halterman JS, McConnochie KM, Conn KM, et al. A randomized trial of primary care provider prompting to enhance preventive asthma therapy. Arch Pediatr Adolesc Med 2005;159(5):422–7.

23. Flores G, Snowden-Bridon C, Torres S, et al. Urban minority children with asthma: substantial morbidity, compromised quality and access to specialists, and the importance of poverty and specialty care. J Asthma 2009;46:392–8.

24. Juniper EF, Guyatt GH, Feeny DH, et al. Measuring quality of life in the parents and children with asthma. Qual Life Res 1996;5(1):27–34.

25. Horne R, Weinman J. Self-regulation and self-management in asthma: exploring the role of illness perceptions and treatment beliefs in explaining non-adherence to preventer medication. Psychology and Health 2002;17(1):17–32.

26. Butz AM, Halterman JS, Bellin M, et al. Factors associated with caregiver completion of a behavioral intervention for primary care providers and caregivers of urban children with asthma. J Asthma 2012;49(9):977–88. http://dx.doi.org/10.3109/02770903.2012.721435.

27. Yoos HL, Kitzman H, McMullen A, et al. Symptom perception in childhood asthma: how accurate are children and their parents? Journal of Asthma 2003;40:27–39.

28. Fritz GK, Yeung A, Wamboldt MZ, et al. Conceptual and methodological issues in quantifying perceptual accuracy in childhood asthma. J Pediatr Psychol 1996;21:153–73.

29. Yoos HL, Kitzman H, McMullen A, et al. The language of breathlessness: do families and health care providers speak the same language when describing asthma symptoms? J Pediatr Health Care 2005;19:197–205.

30. Diette GB, Skinner EA, Markson LE, et al. Consistency of care with national guidelines for children with asthma in managed care. J Pediatrics 2001;138:59–64.

31. Zorc JJ, Scarfone RJ, Li Y. Predictors of primary care follow-up after a pediatric emergency visits for asthma. J Asthma 2005;42:571–6.

32. Armstrong HE, Ishiki D, Heiman J, et al. Service utilization by black and white clientele in an urban community mental health center. Revised assessment of an old problem. Community Mental Health Journal 1984;20:269–81.

33. Smith SR, Highstein GR, Jaffe DM, et al. Parental impressions of the benefits (pros) and barriers (cons) of follow-up care after an acute emergency department visit for children with asthma. Pediatrics 2002;110:323–30.

34. Smith SR, Jaffe DM, Fisher EB, et al. Improving follow-up for children with asthma after an acute emergency department visit. J Pediatr 2004;145:772–7.

35. Baren JM, Boudreaux ED, Brenner BE, et al. Randomized controlled trial of emergency department interventions to improve primary care follow-up for patients with acute asthma. Chest 2006;129:257–65.

36. Teach SJ, Crain EF, Quint DM, et al. Improved asthma outcomes in a high-morbidity pediatric population. Arch Pediatr Adolesc Med 2006;160:535–41.

37. Meischke H, Lozano P, Zhou C, et al. Engagement in "My Child's Asthma", an incentive web-based pediatric asthma management intervention. Int J Medical Informatics 2011;80(11):765–74.

38. Onyirimba F, Apter A, Reisine S, et al. Direct clinician-to-patient feedback discussion of inhaled steroid use: its effect on adherence. Ann Allergy Asthma Immunol 2003;90:411–5.

39. Halterman JS, Szilagyi P, Fisher S, et al. A randomized controlled trial to improve care for urban children with asthma: results of the School-Based Asthma Therapy trial. Arch Pediatr Adolesc Med 2011;165:262–8.

40. Halterman JS, Sauer J, Fagnano M, et al. Working toward a sustainable system of asthma care: development of the school-based preventive asthma care technology (SB-PACT) Trial. J Asthma 2012;49(4):395–400.

41. Bollinger ME, Morphew T, Mullins CD. The Breathmobile program: a good investment for underserved children with asthma. Ann Allergy Asthma Immunol 2010;105:274–81.

42. Douglas JM. Mobile dental vans: planning considerations and productivity. J Public Health Dentistry 2005;65(2):110–3.

43. Jones CA, Clement LT, Hanley-Lopez J, et al. The Breathmobile Program: structure, implementation and evolution of a large-scale, urban, pediatric asthma disease management program. Dis Manag 2005;8:205–22.
44. U.S. Department of Health and Human Services (USDHHS). The National Asthma Education and Prevention Program. Expert Panel Report 3 (EPR3): Guidelines for the diagnosis and management of asthma. NIH Publication No. 07-4051, August 2007.
45. Celano MP, Linzer JF, Demi A, et al. Treatment adherence among low-income, African American children with persistent asthma. J Asthma 2010;47:317–22.
46. Butz AM, Walker J, Land CL, et al. Improving asthma communication in high-risk children. J Asthma 2007;44:739–45.
47. Cabana MD, Ebel BE, Cooper-Patrick L, et al. Barriers pediatricians face when using asthma practice guidelines. Arch Pediatr Adolesc Med 2000;154:685–93.
48. Cabana MD, Rand CS, Becher OJ, et al. Reasons for pediatrician nonadherence to asthma guidelines. Arch Pediatr Adolesc Med 2001;155:1057–62.
49. Cabana MD, Flores G. The role of clinical practice guidelines in enhancing quality and reducing racial/ethnic disparities in pediatrics. Paediatric Respiratory Reviews 2002;3:52–8.
50. Phillips LS, Branch WT Jr, Cook CB. Clinical inertia. Ann Intern Med 2001;135:825–34.
51. Revicki D, Weiss KB. Clinical assessment of asthma symptom control: review of current assessment instruments. J Asthma 2006;43:481–7.
52. Wolf JM, Miller GE, Chen E. Parent psychological states predict changes in inflammatory markers in children with asthma and healthy children. Brain Behav Immun 2008;22:433–41.
53. Mangan JM, Wittich AR, Gerald LB. The potential for reducing asthma disparities through improved family and social function and modified health behaviors. Chest 2007;132:789S–801S.
54. Shalowitz MU, Mijanovich T, Berry CA, et al. Context matters: a community-based study of maternal mental health, life stressors, social support, and children's asthma. Pediatrics 2006;117:e940–8.
55. Strunk RC, Ford JG, Taggart V. Reducing disparities in asthma care: priorities for research—National Heart, Lung, and Blood Institute Workshop Report. J Allergy Clin Immunol 2002;109:229–37.
56. Szabo A, Mezei G, Kovari E, et al. Depressive symptoms amongst asthmatic children's caregivers. Pediatr Allergy Immunol 2010;21:e667–73.
57. Brown SE, Gan V, Jeffress J, et al. Psychiatric symptomatology and disorders in caregivers of children with asthma. Pediatrics 2006;118:e1715–20.
58. Silver EJ, Warman KL, Stein RE. The relationship of caretaker anxiety to children's asthma morbidity and acute care utilization. J Asthma 2005;42:379–83.
59. Feldman JM, Perez EA, Canino G, et al. The role of caregiver major depression in the relationship between anxiety disorders and asthma attacks in Island Puerto Rican youth and young adults. J Nerv Ment Dis 2011;119:313–8.
60. Lange NE, Bunyavanich S, Silberg JL, et al. Parental psychosocial stress and asthma morbidity in Puerto Rican twins. J Allergy Clin Immunol 2010;127:734–40.
61. Flynn HA, Davis M, Marcus SM, et al. Rates of maternal depression in pediatric emergency department and relationship to child service utilization. Gen Hosp Psychiatry 2004;26:316–22.
62. Bartlett SJ, Kolodner K, Butz AM, et al. Maternal depressive symptoms and emergency department use among inner-city children with asthma. Arch Pediatr Adolesc Med 2001;155:347–53.

63. Martinez KG, Perez EA, Ramirez R, et al. The role of caregivers' depressive symptoms and asthma beliefs on asthma outcomes among low-income Puerto Rican children. J Asthma 2009;46:136–41.

64. Bartlett S, Krishnan J, Riekert K, et al. Maternal depressive symptoms and adherence to therapy in inner-city children with asthma. Pediatr 2004;113:229–37.

65. DiMatteo MR, Lepper HS, Croghan TW. Depression is a risk factor for noncompliance with medical treatment. Arch Intern Med 2000;160:2101–7.

66. Quinn K, Kaufman JS, Siddiqi A, et al. Stress and the city: housing stressors are associated with respiratory health among low socioeconomic status Chicago children. J Urban Health 2010;87:688–702.

67. Breiding MJ, Ziembroski JS. The relationship between intimate partner violence and children's asthma in 10 US states/territories. Pediatr Allergy Immunol 2011; 22(1 Pt 2):e95–100.

68. Quinn K, Kaufman JS, Siddiqi A, et al. Parent perceptions of neighborhood stressors are associated with general health and child respiratory health among low-income urban families. J Asthma 2010;47:281–9.

69. Yinusa-Nyahkoon LS, Cohn ES, Cortes DE, et al. Ecological barriers and social forces in childhood asthma management: examining routines of African American families living in the inner city. J Asthma 2010;47:701–10.

70. Bellin MH, Kub J, Frick K, et al. Stress and quality of life in caregivers of inner-city minority children with poorly controlled asthma. J Pediatric Health Care 2013;27(2).

71. Priftis KN, Mantzouranis EC, Antrhacopoulos MB. Asthma symptoms and airway narrowing in children growing up in an urban versus rural environment. J Asthma 2009;46:244–51.

72. Eggleston PA. The environment and asthma in US inner cities. Chest 2007; 132(Suppl 5):782S–8S.

73. Sheehan WJ, Sheehan MD, Rangsithienchal PA, et al. Pest and allergen exposure and abatement in inner-city asthma: a Work Group Report of the American Academy of Allergy, Asthma & Immunology Indoor Allergy/Air Pollution Committee. J Allergy Clin Immunol 2010;125:575–81.

74. Gruchalla RS, Pongracic J, Plaut M, et al. Inner-city Asthma Study: relationship among sensitivity, allergen exposure, and asthma morbidity. J Allergy Clin Immunol 2005;115(3):478–85.

75. National Research Council "Front Matter". Clearing the air: asthma and indoor air exposures. Washington, DC: National Academy Press; 2000.

76. Krieger J, Jacobs DE, Ashley PJ, et al. Housing interventions and control of asthma-related indoor biologic agents: a review of evidence. J Public Health Management Practice 2010;16(5):S11–20.

77. Wilson J, Dixon SL, Breysse P, et al. Housing and allergens: a pooled analysis of nine US cities. Environ Research 2010;110:189–98.

78. Kattan M, Gergen PJ, Eggleston P. Health effects of indoor nitrogen dioxide and passive smoking on urban asthmatic children. J Allergy Clin Immunol 2007; 120(3):618–24.

79. Cagney KA, Browning CR, Wallace DM. The Latino paradox in neighborhood context: the case of asthma and other respiratory conditions. Am J Public Health 2007;97:919–25.

80. Sandel M, Wright RJ. When home is where the stress is: expanding the dimensions of housing that influence asthma morbidity. Arch Dis Child 2006;91:942–8.

81. Wright RJ, Subramanian SV. Advancing a multilevel framework for epidemiologic research on asthma disparities. Chest 2007;132(Suppl 5):757S–69S.

82. Wright RJ, Mitchell H, Visness CM, et al. Community violence and asthma morbidity: the inner-city asthma study. Am J Public Health 2004;94(4):625–32.
83. Sternthal MJ, Jun HJ, Earls F, et al. Community violence and urban childhood asthma: a multilevel analysis. Eur Respir J 2010;36(6):1400–9.
84. Karaca-Mandic P, Jena AB, Joyce GF, et al. Out-of-pocket medication costs and use of medications and health care services among children with asthma. JAMA 2012;307(12):1284–91.
85. Kleinman NL, Brook RA, Ramachandran S. An employer perspective on annual employee and dependent costs for pediatric asthma. Ann Allergy Asthma and Immunol 2009;103:114–20.

Pediatric Obesity and Asthma Quality of Life

Barbara Velsor-Friedrich, PhD, RN[a],*,
Lisa K. Militello, MSN, MPH, CPNP[b], Joanne Kouba[c],
Patrick R. Harrison, BS, MA[d], Amy Manion, PhD, RN, PNP[e],
Rita Doumit, PhD, RN[f]

KEYWORDS

- Asthma • Obesity • Youth • Quality of life

KEY POINTS

- The literature to date highlights existing gaps and provides several outlets for future research.
- The comorbid prevalence of obesity and asthma in youth is clearly an area requiring additional research.
- It is evident that health disparities exist for both asthma and obesity, especially in both Hispanic and African American youth.
- It is suggested that for these at-risk populations, weight-management and weight-reduction education should be included in every health-related visit.
- In addition, because of the negative effect of asthma and obesity on quality of life, tools such as the Pediatric Asthma Quality of Life Questionnaire should be used at every asthma evaluation visit and quality-of-life issues discussed, and incorporated into the asthma treatment plan.

BACKGROUND AND SIGNIFICANCE

Adult Obesity

The phenomenon of unhealthy weight status in the United States has captured the attention of health professionals and the public alike. Dramatic increases in body

This article originally appeared in Nursing Clinics of North America, Volume 48, Issue 2, June 2013.
[a] Niehoff School of Nursing, Loyola University Chicago, Granada Center Room 355B, 1032 West Loyola Avenue, Chicago, IL 60626, USA; [b] College of Nursing, Arizona State University, 500 North 3rd Street, Phoenix, AZ 85004-0698, USA; [c] Niehoff School of Nursing, Loyola University Chicago, 2160 South First Avenue, Maywood, IL 60153, USA; [d] Department of Psychology, Loyola University Chicago, 1032 West Loyola Avenue, Coffee Hall, Chicago, IL 60626, USA; [e] College of Nursing, 600 South Paulina Avenue Suite 440, Amour Academic Center, Chicago, IL 60612, USA; [f] University of Lebanon Beirut Campus
* Corresponding author.
E-mail address: bvelsor@luc.edu

mass index (BMI; weight in kilograms divided by height in meters squared, ie, kg/m^2) have been reported through public health surveillance programs such as the National Health and Nutrition Examination Survey (NHANES) starting in the 1970s to the 1990s for both adults and youth, making obesity and overweight common conditions in the United States. According to the most recent NHANES reports, using data from 2009 to 2010, age-adjusted obesity prevalence for adults is 35.7% and overweight prevalence for this group is 33.1%. In other words, 68.8% of adults in the United States have a BMI greater than is considered healthy.[1]

The burden of high BMI is not equally distributed among all segments of the adult population. Analysis of NHANES trends from 1999 to 2010 suggests that significant increases in obesity prevalence have occurred for white, non-Hispanic black, and Mexican American men, and non-Hispanic black and Mexican American women.[1]

Obesity in Youth

The obesity phenomenon in youth parallels that of adults in the United States. Childhood obesity has tripled in the last 4 decades. Current estimates are that 16.9% of youth between 2 and 19 years of age are obese (BMI ≥95th percentile for age) and 14.9% are overweight (BMI between the 85th and 94th percentile for age), which results in a total of 31.8% of youth in the United States meeting criteria for unhealthy weight.[2] As a child's age increases, so does their likelihood of being overweight or obese, as shown in **Table 1**. Preschool children aged 2 to 5 years have lower odds (0.58 for males; 0.62 for females) of obesity compared with adolescents aged 12 to 19 years.[2] Similar to disparities in adults, the burden of excess weight is more prevalent in black and Hispanic youth, and in both genders, as shown in **Table 1**. For youth combined between 2 and 19 years old, males have a significantly higher prevalence of obesity (18.6%) than females (15%)[2]; this holds true for white but not Hispanic or non-Hispanic black youth.

Youth Obesity and Asthma

The prevalence of both asthma and obesity has increased dramatically over the last several decades, which has led to an increase in the number of studies examining the relationship between these 2 variables.[3,4] However, despite the increased interest in these comorbidities, much of the research in this area has focused on adults.[3,5–7]

A study examining the prevalence of obesity among adults, using data from the NHANES I, II, and III, showed that adults with asthma are far more likely to be obese than adults without asthma.[3] In a retrospective study of 143 adult individuals aged 18 to 88 years, the prevalence of obesity increased along with increasing asthma severity in adults.[5] Furthermore, the results showed that females with asthma were

Table 1
Prevalence of high body mass index (BMI; ≥85th percentile) in United States youth: both genders combined for selected groups

BMI ≥85th Percentile	2–19 Years Old	2–5 Years Old	6–11 Years Old	12–19 Years Old
All racial/ethnic groups	31.8	26.7	32.6	33.6
Non-Hispanic white	27.9	23.8	27.6	30.0
Mexican American	39.4	33.3	39	43.4
Non-Hispanic black	39.1	41.8	42.7	41.2

Data from Ogden CL, Carroll MD, Kit BK, et al. Prevalence of obesity and trends in body mass index among US children and adolescents, 1999–2010. JAMA 2012;307(5):483–90.

significantly more overweight than males, with a mean BMI of 35.9 versus 32.14 ($P =$ .01). These findings suggest that obesity may be a potentially modifiable risk factor for asthma.[5]

The relationship between asthma and high BMI has also been examined in youth. Much of this research has focused on low-income urban and minority populations, owing to the higher prevalence of asthma and obesity in these groups. In a sample (N = 171) of predominantly Hispanic (78%) youth, 45.9% of those with asthma were overweight or obese compared with 30.2% of those without asthma who were overweight or obese ($P =$ .04).[8] It was unclear whether exercise-induced asthma symptoms resulted in exercise avoidance and obesity, or if obesity exacerbated asthma symptoms with exercise. Belamarich and colleagues[9] examined inner-city children with asthma and determined that there was a higher incidence of obesity in Latino study subjects. In addition, obese children with asthma used more asthma medications, wheezed more, and had a greater proportion of unscheduled visits to the emergency department (ED).

A cross-sectional study using data from the 1988 to 1994 NHANES documented that 2 of the highest-risk groups for developing asthma were children older than 10 years with a BMI greater than or equal to the 85th percentile, and children with a parental history of asthma who were 10 years or younger and of African American ethnicity.[10] A subsequent study of NHANES data between 1999 and 2006 included 16,074 youth between the ages of 2 and 19 years.[11] The odds of asthma for those categorized as overweight and obese were 1.32 and 1.68, respectively, after adjustment for age, survey period, race/ethnicity, gender, and other social factors. Overweight and obesity were also associated with a higher likelihood for an asthma attack, visits to the ED, wheezing episodes, missed school, or ambulatory care visit in the last year. Limitations of studies based on NHANES data are the cross-sectional study design and the self-reporting of asthma.

A large cross-sectional study examined relationships between current asthma diagnosis, weight status, and race/ethnicity using information from 681,122 electronic medical records of youth in the Kaiser Permanente health system between 2007 and 2009.[12] The prevalence of current physician-diagnosed asthma with current medication use was 10.9%. Black youth were more likely to have asthma than non-Hispanic white youth (odds ratio = 1.93). When asthma diagnosis was examined for various weight categories, a dose-response relationship was noted, with increasing odds of asthma for those who were classified as overweight, obese, or extremely obese reported as 1.22, 1.37, and 1.68, respectively ($P<.001$ for trend).

When the data were further stratified by race/ethnicity and weight status, differences were noted. The dose-response relationship between weight status and risk of asthma was most pronounced in the Native American/Alaskan population, with odds of asthma for the extremely obese being 3.65 times that of asthma for normal-weight Native Americans/Alaskan youth. However, because of the small sample size (n = 610), statistical significance was not established. This dose-response relationship was statistically significant for the white sample, with odds of 1.3, 1.47, and 1.93 for those who were overweight, obese, and extremely obese in comparison with normal weight. This relationship was also identified in black youth, although with smaller and narrower odds. Also interesting was that the odds for asthma with increasing weight status was less in Hispanic youth with high BMI than in white youth with high BMI, though still higher than in normal-weight Hispanic youth. Researchers also found that those with extreme obesity were 18% more likely to use oral corticosteroids ($P<.001$), and 9% more likely to use inhaled corticosteroids ($P<.001$) than normal-weight youth. Extremely obese youth with asthma made 274 more ambulatory care visits per 1000 youth (*P*<.001) and 23 more ED visits (*P*<.001) than normal-weight youth with asthma. Strengths of this study included physician-diagnosed asthma and the large sample.

International studies report similar findings. A study conducted in Taiwan examined the relationship between asthma, lung function, and BMI in more than 15,000 school-aged children. The prevalence of asthma increased as BMI increased in both males and females.[13] A similar result was found in a study conducted in Nova Scotia, Canada, which examined 3804 students 10 to 11 years of age. Controlling for socioeconomic factors, there was a linear association between BMI and asthma, with a 6% increase in prevalence per unit increase of BMI.[14]

The consistency of the studies noted offer promising support of the correlation between high BMI and asthma. However, many used a cross-sectional design aiding in hypothesis generation but not adding to insights about causation.

The systematic review of Noal and colleagues[15] provides insights into the temporal relationship between BMI and asthma and the causal path. Ten longitudinal studies examined the relationship between weight status in early childhood and the development of asthma in adolescence. With one exception, all studies reported sample sizes greater than 1000. The majority (8 of 10) of the studies reported a positive association between overweight or obesity in early childhood and the development of asthma in adolescence. For example, Mannino and colleagues[16] followed 4393 asthma-free children for up to 14 years. Analysis of the data showed that boys with a BMI at or greater than the 85th percentile at age 2 to 3 years and boys with a BMI consistently at or above the 85th percentile were at higher risk for subsequent asthma development. Three of the studies reported in the systematic review by Noal and colleagues[15] reported higher risk for females, 3 studies reported higher risk for males, and 2 reported that the relationship was independent of gender. Although this review provides support for the causative role of high BMI in asthma incidence because of its longitudinal study design, the mechanisms for this relationship are still unclear. Proposed hypotheses have included a mechanical effect of obesity on respiratory function, the role of obesity in fueling inflammatory responses leading to asthma and/or obesity-induced immune changes that trigger genetic or hormonal pathways for asthma. Environmental factors that promote obesity, such as sedentary lifestyle, diet, and low birth weight, may also promote asthma development.[15] Clearly the rising incidence of asthma and obesity, and their combined impact on youth's quality of life (QOL), requires additional investigation.

REVIEW OF THE LITERATURE
Pediatric Asthma Quality of Life

The need to address QOL issues in chronically ill youth has become a priority in the United States.[17] There are several reasons for examining QOL in adolescents with asthma as a unique group distinct from young children and adults. Adolescence is a period of emergence of independent thinking and behavior which, along with various stressors, such as peer pressure, may affect the interpretation of asthma symptoms and adherence to prescribed asthma therapy.[18–20] This concept was supported in a study by Bruzzese and colleagues,[20] which found that early adolescents' asthma self-management was suboptimal. Although they perceive themselves to have greater responsibility for managing their asthma, early adolescents did less to care for their asthma, suggesting they may be given responsibility for asthma care prematurely.

Clinicians and researchers routinely use QOL as an indicator of successful management of asthma in youth. Measures of QOL are thought to indicate how much an adolescent's illness interferes with daily life and how well the teenager is adapting to his or her illness across several areas of functioning such as social, emotional, and physical.

A systematic review by Everhart and Fiese[21] found that asthma severity was a correlate of QOL in youth with asthma. Youth whose asthma symptoms were not well managed were more likely to experience an impaired level of QOL. Everhart and Fiese[21] concluded that researchers and health care providers basing clinical outcomes on QOL assessments should consider asthma severity in their evaluations.

These findings were supported by another study conducted with 533 Dutch adolescents. Symptom severity affected overall and positive QOL, both directly and indirectly, via coping. The lifestyle restricted by coping strategies and worrying about asthma were associated with poorer overall QOL. The use of the coping strategies-restricted lifestyle, positive reappraisal, and information seeking was related to increased scores on the positive QOL domain, whereas hiding asthma was related to lower scores on the positive QOL domain.[22]

Burkhart and colleagues[18] explored the predictors of QOL among adolescents from the United States and Iceland. Statistically significant predictors of higher asthma QOL were a better rating of overall health ($P<.01$), not having had a severe asthma attack in the last 6 months ($P<.01$), and lower depressive symptoms ($P<.01$). The researchers concluded that interventions designed to decrease depression and prevent asthma exacerbations might improve QOL for adolescents with asthma. In line with this study, Mohangoo and colleagues[23] evaluated health-related QOL (HRQOL) in adolescents with wheezing attacks using self-reported data, and determined independent associations between wheezing attacks and QOL. The presence of at least 4 wheezing attacks during the past year was associated with relevant deficits in QOL.

Another study conducted by Schmier and colleagues[24] evaluated asthma-related activity limitations and productivity losses among children and adolescents (age 4–18 years). Both HRQOL and productivity were significantly lower in patients with inadequately controlled asthma when compared with those with controlled asthma. Inadequately controlled asthma had a significant impact on asthma-specific HRQOL, school productivity and attendance, and work productivity of children and their caregivers.

Bruzzese and colleagues[25] tested the efficacy of an 8-week school-based intervention (Asthma Self-Management for Adolescents, ASMA) on 345 primarily Latino (46%) and African American (31%) high school students (mean age 15.1 years, 70% female) reporting an asthma diagnosis, symptoms of moderate to severe persistent asthma, and use of asthma medication in the last 12 months. Primary outcomes were asthma self-management, symptom frequency, and QOL; secondary outcomes were asthma medical management, school absences, days with activity limitations, and urgent health care use. Participants reported significant increases in confidently managing their asthma; use of controller medication and written treatment plans; fewer night awakenings, days with activity limitation, and school absences due to asthma; improved QOL; and fewer acute care visits, ED visits, and hospitalizations.

The feasibility of a motivational interviewing–based asthma self-management program (5 home visits) was developed and assessed in 37 African American adolescents with asthma (age 10–15 years). The teens had recently been seen in an inner-city ED for asthma symptoms and were prescribed an asthma controller medication.[26,27] Although there were no pre-post differences in adolescent-reported medication adherence, participants did report increased motivation and readiness to adhere to treatment. Teens and their caregivers reported statistically significant increases in their asthma QOL. The findings from this pilot study suggest that motivational interviewing is a feasible and promising approach for increasing medication adherence among inner-city adolescents with asthma, and is worthy of further evaluation in a randomized trial.

Pediatric Asthma, Obesity, and QOL

Although asthma severity has been shown to negatively affect QOL, there has been limited research conducted on the effects of both obesity and asthma on QOL despite the increasing prevalence of both diseases. The few studies that have explored QOL, asthma, and obesity in adults have demonstrated mixed results. A study of 382 adults with asthma discovered that the patients with higher BMIs reported lower QOL scores regardless of asthma severity.[25] Grammer and colleagues[28] studied 352 adults with asthma, 191 of whom were obese. Using the Asthma Quality of Life Questionnaire (AQLQ), results showed that obesity directly correlated with decreased QOL and increased health care utilization as demonstrated by ED/urgent care encounters. A second study using the AQLQ examined more than 900 patients, both adults and children, and found similar results in the adult group; obesity significantly correlated with decreased QOL. However, the researchers found no correlation between AQLQ scores and obesity in the children studied. There was no increase in health care use for either the obese adults or children.[29]

Researchers in Germany compared QOL in children with obesity, asthma/atopic dermatitis, or both, using the German KINDL QOL questionnaire. Among the 3 groups, the results showed lower QOL scores in children with obesity, which improved following obesity treatment.[30]

In another international study, Blandon and colleagues[31] examined 100 obese, overweight, and normal-weight children in Mexico with intermittent or mild persistent asthma. There were significant differences in QOL in the obese asthmatic group ($P<.000$). A third study conducted in the Netherlands by van Gent and colleagues,[32] using the Pediatric Asthma Quality of Life Questionnaire, found children with both asthma and obesity had lower (25%) QOL scores than children with either asthma alone (14%) or obesity alone (1%).

From the review of the literature, there appears to be a relationship between asthma and obesity. However, the exact nature of this relationship has yet to be fully determined.[33] Given the rising prevalence of obesity and asthma, additional studies regarding asthma, obesity, and QOL are warranted in order to better understand the interaction between the two comorbidities. In addition, the mechanism behind the link between asthma and obesity needs to be further investigated. The knowledge gained from further studies will aid in the development of more effective treatments and prevention programs for both asthma and obesity.

School-Based Asthma Education Programs

Coffman and colleagues[34] conducted a systematic review of the literature on school-based asthma education programs for youth aged 4 to 17 years with a clinical diagnosis of asthma or symptoms consistent with asthma. Synthesizing across studies was difficult because the characteristics of interventions and target populations varied widely, as did the outcomes assessed. Most studies that compared asthma education with usual care found that school-based asthma education programs improved knowledge of asthma, self-efficacy, and self-management behaviors. Fewer studies reported favorable effects on QOL, symptom days, symptom nights, and school absences.

More recently other supportive interventions, such as cognitive behavior modification strategies, have been found to be successful in treating children and adolescents with chronic illnesses. Interventions that use behavioral strategies are more effective in supporting change than are solely knowledge-based interventions.[35–37] Coping skills training (CST) is based on social cognitive theory, and stresses the use of adaptive coping methods and problem-solving skills. The goal of CST is to teach children and adolescents personal and social coping skills that can assist them in dealing with potential stressors they encounter in their daily lives and the stress reactions that may result from these situations.[38] The use of such skills can increase a teen's sense of competence and self-efficacy in dealing with a wide range of daily demands and health issues. In the youth population, CST has resulted in decreasing substance abuse,[39] increased social skills and reduction of aggressive behaviors,[40] and a decrease in negative responses to stressors.[41] It has also been used successfully in children with chronic illnesses such as cancer and diabetes[42–44] and in minority youth with diabetes.[45,46]

STUDY BY THE AUTHOR
Purpose

The purpose of this study is to report on the specific effects of childhood obesity and asthma on self-reported asthma QOL, coping, and control of asthma health outcomes in low-income African American teens with asthma. A randomized controlled trial (n = 137) was conducted to evaluate the efficacy of a school-based asthma education/management program on asthma-related QOL and other psychosocial and health outcomes in urban African American teens with asthma. The intervention components and results of the study have been reported in detail elsewhere.[47] In brief, the TEAM program (Teen Education and Asthma Management) is composed of 3 elements: (1) asthma education; (2) CST; and (3) nurse practitioner re-enforcement visits.

Methods

Students were recruited from 5 African American dominant urban high schools. Approximately 94% of students and their families received public assistance. Student assent and parent/guardian assent was obtained. Randomization occurred by school because individual randomization within schools could lead to contamination. Students in both the treatment and control groups attended 2 asthma education sessions (group format), 3 educational re-enforcement sessions (group sessions), and an individual clinic visit with the TEAM nurse practitioner at baseline and at the end of program.

Students in the intervention group participated in CST. Five CST sessions were offered once a week during the extended homeroom period for 45 minutes. A makeup session was offered at the end of the fifth session. The following skills were taught: (1) social problem solving; (2) effective communication; (3) managing stress; (4) conflict resolution; and (5) cognitive restructuring (guided self-dialogue). At each session a skill was taught and then students were asked to role-play the skill within an asthma-based scenario. Each week the previous skill was reviewed and the new skills were taught in the same manner. Data were collected at baseline and at 2, 6, and 12 months.

Measures
The Parent Questionnaire was completed by the student's parent/guardian and supplies information regarding demographics and the adolescent's current and prior asthma health status.

The Pediatric Asthma Quality of Life Questionnaire[48] is a 23-item, 7-point Likert-scale instrument that assesses both physiologic and emotional functional impairments experienced by children and adolescents. There are 3 subscales: symptoms experienced (10 items), activity limitation (5 items), and emotional functional (8 items). Total scale α values ranged from 0.93 to 0.94 across all time periods.

Coping was measured using the Kid Cope,[49,50] a 17-item inventory designed to assess 10 cognitive and behavioral strategies used by adolescents. These strategies include distraction, social withdrawal, cognitive restructuring, self-criticism, blaming others, problem-solving, emotional regulation, wishful thinking, social support, and resignation. Total scale α values ranged from 0.73 to 0.86 across time periods.

Control of Asthma Health Outcomes was operationally defined as according to the National Asthma Education and Prevention Program guidelines.[51] For this study, well-controlled was defined as meeting all of the following criteria: mean peak flow reading in the green zone, asthma symptom frequency less than 2 days a week, asthma symptom frequency less than 2 nights per month, and the use of asthma rescue medicine less than 2 days per week.

Overweight and obesity were operationally defined per the Centers for Disease Control criterion and plotted on age-appropriate and gender-appropriate growth charts. If a student had a BMI greater than or equal to 85% to 94% the diagnosis of overweight was made, and if their BMI was equal to or greater than 95% the diagnosis of obesity was made.[52]

Data analysis

Using correlation and regression analyses, relations among study variables were examined. Correlational analyses were used to examine the bivariate relations among intent to treat approach, a series of mixed-model analyses of variance examined the interaction between BMI and obesity and asthma QOL. Regression analyses were used to determine which variables predicted significant variability in asthma QOL. Finally, a series of t-tests were conducted to determine whether those who were overweight or obese had significantly worse outcomes than those who were of normal weight. Two-sided test were used and a P value of less than .05 was considered significant.

Results

At baseline, self-reported asthma QOL scores indicated a moderate level of impairment for all students, with only 53% of students determined to be in control of their asthma. Correlational results indicated that BMI was negatively associated with asthma QOL at baseline ($r = -0.16$), 2 months ($r = -0.10$), 6 months ($r = -0.09$), and 12 months ($r = -0.24$), although this relationship was only significant at 12 months ($P<.01$). These findings suggest that increased BMI is negatively associated with self-reported asthma QOL.

To further explore the nature of the relation between BMI and asthma QOL, t-tests were conducted to determine whether those who were overweight or obese had significantly worse asthma QOL relative to those who were of normal weight. Results indicated that those who were overweight or obese at baseline had marginally significantly lower asthma QOL (mean = 4.65, standard deviation [SD] = 1.11) compared with those who were normal weight (mean = 4.97, SD = 0.83), $t(121) = 1.78$, $P = .07$. Furthermore, at 12 months, those who were overweight or obese reported higher levels of negative coping (mean = 1.42, SD = 0.63) compared with those who were of normal weight (mean = 1.20, SD = 0.52), $t(121) = 2.06$, $P = .04$. In addition, those who were not in control of their asthma reported lower asthma QOL (mean = 4.67, SD = 1.10), $t(132) = 2.51$, $P = .01$. There were no significant differences between those who were overweight or obese and those who were normal at any other time point.

To examine the role of BMI in determining asthma QOL relative to other important predictors, a series of regression equations tested the relative importance of BMI in asthma QOL. Results indicated that when including symptom frequency, asthma classification (intermittent, mild, moderate, severe), asthma knowledge, asthma self-efficacy, and asthma self-care levels, BMI remained the strongest predictor of asthma QOL ($\beta = -0.28$, $P = .002$) along with asthma knowledge ($\beta = 0.28$, $P = .003$). These findings suggest that even when controlling for the influence of symptom frequency and asthma classification, BMI remains a most important factor in determining self-reported QOL among teens with asthma.

To determine whether BMI and obesity inhibits the effectiveness of an asthma treatment program (TEAM), an additional series or regression models were used to test the moderating role of BMI and obesity. Contrary to hypotheses, results indicated that when controlling for baseline levels of asthma QOL, neither BMI nor obesity had a significant moderating effect on the effectiveness of an asthma treatment program at 6 months ($\beta = -0.07$, $P = .82$; $\beta = 0.03$, $P = .86$, respectively). Similarly, when controlling for baseline levels of asthma QOL, neither BMI nor obesity had a significant moderating effect on the effectiveness of an asthma treatment program on asthma QOL at 12 months ($\beta = -0.05$, $P = .73$; $\beta = 0.03$, $P = .91$, respectively). These findings suggest that although BMI and obesity are important predictors of asthma-related QOL in their own right, they did not influence the effectiveness of the asthma treatment program in this study.

Discussion and Clinical Implications

Although the results showed that overweight and obesity did not change the effectiveness of the asthma treatment program, the impact obesity plays on QOL should not be ignored.

These findings support previous literature suggesting that overweight/obese adolescents experience poorer physical health than their nonoverweight peers. In a sample of 923 adolescents, Wake and colleagues[53] found that obesity was associated with a lower QOL. However, special needs related to asthma only slightly rose with increased BMI, and not to the point of significance. It was found that many adverse health and psychological effects of childhood obesity could be reversed if the obesity were treated before adolescence. However, specific health problems that would prompt a reduction in the BMI of adolescence were not reported. Although the strength of the random sampling method, parallel adolescent self-reports and parent proxy reporting, and large sample size add weight to the study findings, the study was limited by potential bias owing to attrition and a higher rate of obese participants lost.

In another study, Burkhart and colleagues[18] found that gender was statistically significantly associated with QOL in a sample of 30 adolescents with asthma. Males had a higher QOL compared with females ($P = .003$), and QOL scores were poorer with the experience of an asthma attack in the past 6 months. Asthma severity did not correlate with asthma QOL. However, the majority of the participants reported their asthma as mild (57%) and more than half said their activity was occasionally limited by asthma (56%). This study lends interesting insights into the predictors of QOL in adolescents with asthma; however, the weight of the contribution is limited by the small sample size, exploratory nature, and cross-sectional design.

The literature to date does highlight existing gaps and provides several outlets for future research. The comorbid prevalence of obesity and asthma in youth is clearly an area requiring to be understood. It is evident that health disparities exist for both asthma and obesity, especially in both Hispanic and African American youth. It is suggested that for these at-risk populations, weight-management and weight-reduction education should be included in every health-related visit. In addition, because of the negative effect of asthma and obesity on QOL, tools such as the Pediatric AQLQ should be used at every asthma evaluation visit, and QOL issues discussed as well as being incorporated into the asthma treatment plan.

REFERENCES

1. Flegal KM, Carroll MD, Kit BK, et al. Prevalence of obesity and trends in the distribution of body mass index among US adults, 1999-2010. JAMA 2012;307(5): 491–7.
2. Ogden CL, Carroll MD, Kit BK, et al. Prevalence of obesity and trends in body mass index among US children and adolescents, 1999-2010. JAMA 2012; 307(5):483–90.
3. Ford ES, Mannino DM. Time trends in obesity among adults with asthma in the United States: findings from three national surveys. J Asthma 2005;42(2): 91–5.
4. Chen AY, Kim SE, Houtrow AJ, et al. Prevalence of obesity among children with chronic conditions. Obesity 2009;17(6):1–4.
5. Akerman MJ, Calacanis CM, Madsen MK. Relationship between asthma severity and obesity. J Asthma 2004;41(5):521–6.
6. Luder E, Ehrlich RI, Lou WY, et al. Body mass index and the risk of asthma in adults. Respir Med 2004;98(1):29–37.
7. Spivak H, Hewitt MF, Onn A, et al. Weight loss and improvement of obesity-related illness in 500 U.S. patients following laparoscopic adjustable gastric banding. Am J Surg 2005;189(1):27–32.
8. Gennuso J, Epstein LH, Paluch RA, et al. The relationship between asthma and obesity in urban minority children and adolescents. Arch Pediatr Adolesc Med 1998;152:1197–2000.
9. Belamarich PF, Luder E, Kattan M, et al. Do obese inner-city children with asthma have more symptoms than nonobese children with asthma? Pediatrics 2000; 106(6):1436–41.
10. Rodriguez MA, Winkleby MA, Ahn D, et al. Identification of population subgroups of children and adolescents with high asthma prevalence: findings from the Third National Health and Nutrition Examination Survey. Arch Pediatr Adolesc Med 2005;156(3):269–75.
11. Visness CM, London SJ, Daniels JL, et al. Association of childhood obesity with atopic and non-atopic asthma: results from the National Health and Nutrition Examination Survey 1999-2006. J Asthma 2010;47:822–9.
12. Black MH, Smith N, Porter AH, et al. Higher prevalence of obesity among children with asthma. Obesity 2012;20:1041–7.
13. Chu YT, Chen WY, Wang TN, et al. Extreme BMI predicts higher asthma prevalence and is associated with lung function impairment in school-aged children. Pediatr Pulmonol 2009;44(5):472–9.
14. Sithole F, Douwes J, Burstyn I, et al. Body mass index and childhood asthma: a linear association? J Asthma 2008;45(6):473–7.
15. Noal RB, Menezes AMB, Macedo EC, et al. Childhood body mass index and risk of asthma in adolescence: a systematic review. Obes Rev 2011;12:93–104.
16. Mannino DM, Mott J, Ferdinands J, et al. Boys with high body masses have an increased risk of developing asthma: findings from the National Longitudinal Survey of Youth (NLSY). Int J Obes 2006;30:6–13.
17. Centers for Disease Control and DC. Healthy People. 2020. Available at: www.cdc.gov/nchs/healthy-people.htm. Accessed July 20, 2012.

18. Burkhart P, Svavardottir EK, Rayens MK, et al. Adolescents with asthma: predictors of quality of life. J Adv Nurs 2009;64(4):860–6.
19. Velsor-Friedrich B, Vlasses F, Moberley J, et al. Talking with teens about asthma management. J Sch Nurs 2004;20(3):140–8.
20. Bruzzese JM, Stepney C, Fiorino EK, et al. Asthma self-management is suboptimal in urban Hispanic and African American/black early adolescents with uncontrolled persistent asthma. J Asthma 2011;183:998–1006.
21. Everhart RS, Fiese BH. Asthma severity and child quality of life in pediatric asthma: a systematic review. Patient Educ Couns 2008;75:162–8.
22. Van De Ven MO, Engels RC, Sawyer SM, et al. The role of coping strategies in quality of life adolescents with asthma. Qual Life Res 2007;16:625–34.
23. Mohangoo AD, deKoning HJ, Mangunkusumg RT, et al. Health-related quality of life in adolescents with wheezing attacks. J Adolesc Health 2007;41(5): 464–71.
24. Schmier JK, Manjunath R, Halpern MT, et al. The impact of inadequately controlled asthma in urban children on quality of life and productivity. Ann Allergy Asthma Immunol 2007;98(3):245–51.
25. Bruzzese JM, Sheares BJ, Vincent JE, et al. Effects of a school-based intervention for urban adolescents with asthma. Am J Respir Crit Care Med 2011;49(1): 90–7.
26. Riekert KA, Borrelli B, Bilderback A, et al. The development of a motivational interviewing intervention to promote medication adherence among inner-city, African American adolescents with asthma. Patient Educ Couns 2011;82(1): 117–22.
27. Lavoie KL, Bacon SL, Labrecque M, et al. Higher BMI is associated with worse asthma control and quality of life but not asthma severity. Respir Med 2006; 100:648–57.
28. Grammer LC, Weiss KB, Pedicano JB, et al. Obesity and asthma morbidity in a community-based adult cohort in a large urban area: The Chicago Initiative to Raise Asthma Health Equity (CHIRAH). J Asthma 2010;47:491–5.
29. Peters JI, McKinney JM, Smith B, et al. Impact of obesity in asthma: evidence from a large prospective disease management study. Ann Allergy Asthma Immunol 2011;106:30–5.
30. Ravens-Sieberer U, Redegeld M, Bullinger M. Quality of life after in-patient rehabilitation in children with obesity. Int J Obes Relat Metab Disord 2001;25(S1): S63–5.
31. Blandon VV, del Rio Navarro B, Berber Eslava A, et al. Quality of life in pediatric patients with asthma with or without obesity: a pilot study. Allergol Immunopathol (Madr) 2004;32(5):259–64.
32. van Gent R, van der Ent CK, Rovers MM, et al. Excessive body weight is associated with additional loss of quality of life in children with asthma. J Allergy Clin Immunol 2007;119:591–6.
33. Michelson PH, Williams LW, Benjamin DK, et al. Obesity, inflammation, and asthma severity in childhood: data from the National Health and Nutrition Examination Survey 2001-2004. Ann Allergy Asthma Immunol 2009;103(5):381–5.
34. Coffman JM, Cabana MD, Yelin EH. Do school-based asthma education programs improve self-management and health outcomes? Pediatrics 2009;124: 729–42, 729.
35. Cristensin H, Griffins K, Korten A. Web-based cognitive behavior therapy: analysis of site usage and changes in depression and anxiety scores. J Med Internet Res 2002;4(1):e3.

36. Wright J. Cognitive behavior therapy. Basic principles and recent advances. Focus: The Journal of Lifelong Learning in Psychiatry American Psychology Association 2006;4(2):173–8.

37. Glick B. Cognitive behavioral interventions for at-risk youth. Kingston (NJ): Civic Research Institute; 2006.

38. Forman S. Coping skills for children and adolescents. San Francisco (CA): Josey-Bass; 1993.

39. Forman S, Linney J, Brondion M. Effects of coping-skills training on adolescents at risk for substance abuse. Psychol Addict Behav 1990;4:67–76.

40. Prinz R, Blechman E, Dumas J. An evaluation of peer coping-skills training for childhood aggression. Clin Child Fam Psychol Rev 1994;23:193–203.

41. Elias MJ, Gara M, Ubriaco M, et al. Impact of a preventive social problem solving intervention children's coping with middle-school stressors. Am J Community Psychol 1986;14:259–75.

42. Grey M, Boland E, Davidson M, et al. Coping skills training for youths with diabetes on intensive therapy. Appl Nurs Res 1999;12:3–12.

43. Grey M, Whittemore R, Jaser S, et al. Efforts of coping skills training in school-age children with type 1 diabetes. Res Nurs Health 2009;32:405–18.

44. Varni JW, Katz ER, Colegrove R, et al. The impact of social skills training on the adjustment of children with newly diagnosed cancer. J Pediatr Psychol 1993;18:751–67.

45. Jefferson V, Jaser S, Lindemann E, et al. Coping skills training in a telephone health coaching program for youth at risk for type 2 diabetes. J Pediatr Health Care 2011;25:153–61.

46. Grey M, Berry D, Davidson M, et al. Preliminary testing of a program to prevent type 2 diabetes among high-risk youth. J Sch Health 2004;74:10–5.

47. Velsor-Friedrich B, Militello L, Richards M, et al. Effects of coping skills training in low-income urban African-American adolescents with asthma. J Asthma 2011;49(4):372–9.

48. Junniper E, Guyatt G, Feeny D, et al. Measuring quality of life in children with asthma. Qual Life Res 1996;5:35–46.

49. Spirito A, Star L, Willimas C. Development of a brief coping checklist for use with pediatric populations. J Pediatr Psychol 1988;13:555–74.

50. Spirito A, Stark L, Kanpp L. Stress and coping in child health. In: Wallander JL, Walker CE, editors. The assessment of coping in chronically ill children: implications for clinical practice. New York: Guilford Press; 1992. p. 327–44.

51. National Asthma Education and Prevention Program. Expert Panel report. Guidelines for the diagnosis and management of asthma update on selected topics. 2007. Available at: http://www.nhlbi.nih.gov/guidelines/asthma/asthgdln.pdf. Accessed July 20, 2012.

52. Centers for Disease Control and Prevention (CDC). About BMI for children and teens. Available at: http://www.cdc.gov/healthyweight/assessing/bmi/childrens_bmi/about_childrens_bmi.html. Accessed May 27, 2012.

53. Wake M, Canterford L, Patton GC, et al. Comorbidities of overweight/obesity experienced in adolescence: longitudinal study. Arch Dis Child 2010;95:162–8.

Asthma Action Plans and Self-Management

Beyond the Traffic Light

Anna L. Edwards, NP-C, MSN

KEYWORDS

- Asthma action plan • Self-management • Health literacy • Outcomes • Measures
- Interventions

KEY POINTS

- Use of asthma action plans may be more effective in populations with a high use of services.
- Asthma outcome measures are variable but primarily focus on use.
- Asthma interventions should be appropriate for the population and/or the individual.

INTRODUCTION

Large health care organizations and health plans support care practices that incorporate self-management and action planning for the benefit of the patient and the potential savings in high-cost service use (emergency room/inpatient hospitalization). Smaller organizations and private practices are also incentivized as the health care industry emphasizes quality outcomes and financially compensates practitioners for meeting or exceeding quality benchmarks. Pay-for-performance is an example of a program that is "designed to offer financial incentives to physicians and other health care providers to meet defined quality, efficiency, or other targets," such as increasing the number of patients with asthma who are taking controller medications.[1]

Improving the care and management of chronic conditions, such as asthma, is a vital area of focus for individuals, providers, payers, and health systems. Because time and resources are limited in the care environment, it is important to identify what interventions are evidence-based, effective, and most plausible to implement. Clinicians and support staff must invest time in providing interventions that yield the best result and are appropriate for the population. Interventions that make practical sense may be

This article originally appeared in Nursing Clinics of North America, Volume 48, Issue 1, March 2013.

Disclosure: The author has disclosed that she does not have any relationship with a commercial company that has a direct financial interest in the subject matter or materials discussed in the article or with a company making a competing product.

400 West Leadora Avenue, Glendora, CA 91741, USA

E-mail address: anedwards@dhs.lacounty.gov

difficult to implement in busy practice settings with multilevel challenges (ie, different individual patient educational needs).

ACTION PLANS

Action plans provide a guide for patients and families to self-manage chronic conditions, such as heart failure or asthma. Written action plans consist of 2 components: an algorithm consisting of clinical scenarios indicating the need to adjust medications or seek emergent medical care, and detailed information on the medication adjustment according to the clinical scenario.[2]

Asthma action plan templates are readily available through public and private professional medical organizations, and the use of these tools is supported by third-party payers. The National Asthma Education Prevention Program (NAEPP) Expert Panel Report 3 (EPR-3) recommends that every person diagnosed with asthma should have a written asthma action plan.[3] However, according to the National Health Interview Surveys (NHIS) information, one-third of all children and adults diagnosed with asthma here reported having a written asthma action plan.[4] Why is this the case? Some factors may include the length of time it takes to work on an action plan with a patient, or the complexity of the action plan tool may be a deterrent. The process of educating the patient may be time-consuming. With little or stretched staffing resources, extra time is a precious commodity. Perhaps providers lack the confidence that patients can follow an action plan.

Asthma action plans are used as a tool to support self-management of the condition. These plans provide concrete indicators for changes in health status with the steps/actions to make improvements. In asthma action plans, indicators of change in respiratory status are measured using peak flow meter performance figures (percentage ranges of personal best) or defined symptoms (eg, cough, shortness of breath).

However, asthma action plans are not necessarily the most appropriate tool for all patients with asthma. Lefevre and colleagues[2] suggest that perhaps the most appropriate population to develop an action plan is the high users of services. Although written asthma action plans may be appropriate for some patients, this intervention involves a significant time investment on the clinician's part and a level of confidence that patients understand how to use the plan. The use of a written asthma action plan alone does not demonstrate a significant improvement in several outcome measures, such as health care resource use, despite the wide support for use.[2]

Review of the current literature relating written asthma action plans to specific outcome measures provides relevant information on what intervention is most appropriate for patients. The literature examines the effect of asthma intervention variables on key outcome measures (**Box 1**).

Research and meta-analytic review identifies promising interventions or combinations of interventions that positively influence key asthma outcome measures. The remainder of this article highlights the following interventions derived from the literature: self-management education and asthma education that considers the patient's health literacy level.

SELF-MANAGEMENT EDUCATION

The area of self-management is a growing and widely recognized health promotion skill, particularly in chronic disease management. The skills needed for effective self-management must be cultivated and developed on both the provider and patient sides. The provider must learn to focus the care plan around what the patient views as their most important problem (collaboration), which is a shift from the ingrained

---

Box 1
Effect of asthma intervention variables on key outcome measures

Common asthma outcome measures in the literature

- Health care utilization (emergency room/hospitalization)
- Quality of life
- Medication adherence
- Frequency of rescue inhaler use
- Symptom control
- Missed work/school
- Functional status

Variables influencing the outcome measures

- Written action plan
- Peak flow meter use
- Asthma education
- Provider review
- Health literacy
- Self-management education

---

medical model wherein the plan of care is designed around the medical facts and available treatments. The patient side of self-management is learning problem-solving skills that can be applied to their personal health care issues.[5] Asthma-specific self-management education, such as trigger avoidance, medication use, and recognition of asthma control indicators, becomes more meaningful when patients are empowered with the skills to problem solve and have the support from their health care provider or team. A systematic review of research studies on educational and behavioral interventions for asthma suggests that a combined approach that includes self-management and regular communication between the patient and provider or clinical team have the "greatest effect on most outcomes."[6] The confidence that accompanies self-management education and skills can be the basis for complimentary interventions or tools, such as using written action plans or symptom recognition to make the decision to self-adjust medications.[7]

The Cochrane Collaboration's review of multiple study results on adult patients with asthma and the effects of self-management education and regular provider review versus usual care[8] on multiple outcome measures reinforces practitioner–patient skills and effort in asthma care interventions. Regularly scheduled practitioner follow-up for asthma care and monitoring of self-management behaviors yielded decreased use of acute services and improvement in asthma symptoms (nocturnal) and perceived quality of life.

HEALTH LITERACY–BASED ASTHMA EDUCATION

Patient-centered/focused care is a major health care focus in today's times. Developing a patient-centered clinical practice involves changes to access and new approaches to care delivery, such as taking into consideration the patient's health beliefs and understanding of health and illness.[9] Patient understanding, and therefore their ability to grasp information or important skills such as self-management education about their condition, depends on their health literacy. Health literacy is defined in

Healthy People 2010 as "The degree to which individuals have the capacity to obtain, process, and understand basic health information and services needed to make appropriate health decisions."[10] The level of health literacy is not, however, measured in the number of years of formal education or reading level.

Studies focused on asthma health literacy levels have shown relationships between low health literacy levels and increased asthma severity, functional level, perceived quality of life, and higher resource use.[11] Additionally, depressive symptoms may be higher in individuals with low health literacy according to Mancuso and Rincon's[11] review of related research studies.

For a patient to learn skills such as self-management, the level of health literacy should be evaluated and an individualized approach to improving the level should be designed. Where does a practitioner begin with this task? A resource such as the Office of Disease Prevention and Health Promotion offers information on health literacy basics and supporting research that is helpful for the interested practitioner. A starting point is to evaluate patients with chronic conditions, such as asthma, about their understanding of the condition and treatment. Tailoring an individualized education plan can pave the way for future self-management development skills, which has been shown to have a positive effect on multiple outcome measures.[12] Increasing practitioner awareness of support options, such as a health plan or community programs, is another important step in improving the supporting health literacy in the clinic practice.

DISCUSSION

A need exists for future studies to isolate the intervention variables and replicate the studies across populations to generalize the result findings. Self-management programs show a positive impact on chronic condition care, such as asthma. However, wide variations in program approaches make best practices difficult to isolate in the available literature. It would be valuable for future studies to test specific aspects of asthma self-management education relative to health literacy levels.

REFERENCES

1. Agency for Healthcare Research and Quality Web site. Available at: http://www.ahrq.gov/qual/pay4per.htm. Accessed July 30, 2012.
2. Lefevre F, Piper MP, Weiss K, et al. Do written action plans improve patient outcomes in asthma? An evidence-based analysis. J Fam Pract 2002;51(10): 842–8.
3. National Institutes of Health, National Heart, Lung, Blood Institute (NHLBI). Guidelines for the diagnosis and management of asthma (EPR-3). Available at: http://www.nhlbi.nih.gov/guidelines/astha/asthgdln.pdf. Accessed August 8, 2012.
4. Centers for Disease Control and Prevention (CDC) website. Available at: http://www.cdc.gov/mmwr/preview/mmwrhtml/mm6017a4.htm?s_cid=mm6017a4_w. Accessed July 23, 2012.
5. Bodenheimer T, Lorig K, Holman H, et al. Patient self-management of chronic disease in primary care. JAMA 2002;288(19):2469–75.
6. Clark NM, Griffiths C, Keteyian SR, et al. Educational and behavioral interventions for asthma: who achieves which outcomes? A systematic review. J Asthma Allergy 2010;3:187–97.
7. Powell H, Gibson PG. Options for self-management education for adults with asthma. Cochrane Database Syst Rev 2002;(1):CD004107.

8. Gibson PG, Powell H, Wilson A, et al. Self-management education and regular practitioner review for adults with asthma. Cochrane Database Syst Rev 2003;(1):CD001117.

9. Bergeson SC, Dean JD. A systems approach to patient-centered care. JAMA 2006;296(23):2848–51.

10. National Network of Libraries of Medicine. Available at: http://nnlm.gov/outreach/consumer/hlthlit.html. Accessed July 23, 2012.

11. Mancuso CA, Rincon M. Impact of health literacy on longitudinal asthma outcomes. J Gen Intern Med 2006;21:813–7.

12. Janson SL, McGrath KW, Covington JK, et al. Individualized asthma self-management improves medication adherence and markers of asthma control. J Allergy Clin Immunol 2009;123(4):840–6.

Work-Exacerbated Asthma

Anthony M. Szema, MD[a,b,*]

KEYWORDS

- Work-exacerbated asthma • Allergy • Occupational exposures • Chemical irritants
- Work-related asthma

KEY POINTS

- A spectrum of workplace exposures can result in work-exacerbated asthma (WEA), including exposures to chemical, smoke, paints, solvents, cleaning agents, allergens, cold temperature, and exercise.
- Patients with WEA are more symptomatic, use more health care resources and have a lower quality of life than those with asthma exacerbations unrelated to work.
- Materials safety data sheets (MSDSs) may identify agents that may exacerbate asthma in the workplace.
- The NIOSH Pocket Guide to Chemical Hazards may help identify potential triggers of WEA.
- The Americans with Disabilities Act mandates that employers adjust for reasonable accommodations for disabilities, including asthma.

GENERAL PRINCIPLES

A spectrum of workplace exposures can result in work-exacerbated asthma (WEA). These exposures include chemical irritants, paints, solvents,[1] and cleaning agents.[2–4] Additional potentially hazardous exposures include dust, indoor and outdoor aeroallergens (sources include molds, cats, trees, grasses, weeds), cold temperature, emotional stress, and exercise.[5]

Patients with WEA are more symptomatic, use more health care resources, and report a lower quality of life compared with those who have asthma exacerbations unrelated to work. Patients with WEA resemble patients with occupational asthma (OA) with respect to asthma severity; medication requirements; and socioeconomic factors, including unemployment and loss of income from work.[6–8]

This article originally appeared in Clinics in Chest Medicine, Volume 33, Issue 4, December 2012.
Disclosure: Dr Szema's research is funded by Merck (through the Naussau Health Care Foundation), Garnett McKeen Laboratory, and The New York State Center for Biotechnology.
a Department of Medicine, Allergy Section, Veterans Affairs Medical Center, Northport, NY 11768, USA; b Department of Medicine, Stony Brook University School of Medicine, Stony Brook, NY 11794-8161, USA
* Department of Medicine, Stony Brook University School of Medicine, Stony Brook, NY 11794-8161.
E-mail address: anthony.szema@stonybrookmedicine.edu

Clinics Collections 2 (2014) 339–348
http://dx.doi.org/10.1016/j.ccol.2014.09.019
2352-7986/14/$ – see front matter Published by Elsevier Inc.

Evidence-based reports regarding the prevention of WEA and its natural history are limited, although common management strategies include (1) avoidance of common triggers (ie, primary prevention), (2) diagnosing early in the course of the disease by assessing the temporal relationship between asthma exacerbations and work (ie, secondary prevention), and (3) eliminating exposures once the diagnosis is confirmed (ie, tertiary prevention). Eliminating the source of the exposure is important. Examples of such interventions include installing pigeon guards on windowsills to prevent bird-dropping contamination of indoor air, improved heating ventilation and air conditioning (HVAC) filtration systems, and using high-efficiency particulate air filters to remove airborne particles. Depending on the work setting, respirators may be beneficial. However, the World Trade Center disaster showed that in a setting where job duties require intense physical exertion, workers may remove their masks in response to a sensation of suffocation while working.[9,10] In other settings, personal respiratory protection may be practical and well accepted (eg, respirators for spray painters).[11–13]

Materials safety data sheets (MSDSs) may identify agents that exacerbate asthma in the workplace. MSDSs may be incomplete or inaccurate and, therefore, should be viewed as just one tool for exploring potentially relevant workplace exposures. The *NIOSH Pocket Guide to Chemical Hazards* and Web-based searches are additional sources for identifying the potential respiratory effects of agents encountered in the workplace.

The Americans with Disabilities Act mandates that employers adjust for reasonable accommodations for disabilities, including asthma.[14] Although a complete review of the legal obligations of employers for promoting workplace safety is beyond the purview of this article, it merits emphasis that a diagnosis of WEA has vocational and socioeconomic consequences in addition to medical implications.

More research is needed to understand dose-response relationships, to identify causal agents in complex environments, and to model these situations. For example, some soldiers in Iraq and Afghanistan who have developed respiratory complaints have been exposed to burning trash, improvised explosive devices, indoor and outdoor aeroallergens, and dust storms.[15–18] Another complex setting is exposure to multiple cleaning agents in the context of domestic chores and janitorial services.[4,19] In these complex exposure settings, it is difficult to establish clear causal relationships between a specific airborne exposure and respiratory health effects, including asthma. These types of complex exposures are difficult and perhaps impossible to study in an experimental model.

CASE DEFINITION OF WEA

In 2011, the American Thoracic Society Ad Hoc Committee on Work-Exacerbated Asthma published the following case definition of WEA:

1. Worker has pre-existing or concurrent asthma. Pre-existing asthma is defined as asthma that was present before the worker entered the worksite of interest, or asthma predated changes in exposures at an existing job due to the introduction of new processes or materials, which trigger asthma. Concurrent asthma or co-incident asthma is defined as asthma with onset while employed in a worksite of interest, but not due to exposures in that worksite.
2. Temporally-related asthma exacerbations at work, with exacerbations based on self-reports of symptoms or medication use at work, or based on peak expiratory flow rates.
3. Conditions exist at work that can exacerbate asthma.
4. OA (asthma caused by work) is unlikely.[20]

PREVALENCE OF WEA

The prevalence of asthma varies depending on the population studied. In one study, 23% of adult patients with asthma in a health maintenance organization (HMO) had WEA.[6] Another study showed 14% of members in an HMO with self-reported peak expiratory flow rates had WEA.[21] In the European Community Respiratory Health Survey, 4% of workers had WEA; this was associated with low schooling and socio-economic status.[22] In an analysis of 12 published reports, the prevalence of WEA ranged from 13% (in an analysis that included all adults with asthma) to 58% (in an analysis of working adults with asthma) with a median of 21%.[20]

JOBS ASSOCIATED WITH WEA

Jobs with exposures associated with WEA include those with secondhand tobacco smoke exposure (eg, hospitality workers), dust exposure, HVAC maintenance professionals, poultry workers, and firefighters (although asthma is an exclusion criterion for hiring in some jurisdictions).[23–25] Other occupations at an increased risk for WEA include medical technicians (exposed to latex or larger proteins, such as psyllium dispensed by nurses), farmers, welders, cleaners, bleachers, bakers, spray painters, cabinetmakers, and carpenters.[26,27]

A spectrum of organic and inorganic exposures can cause exacerbations of asthma, including work with animals (animal dander); work near incinerators producing high concentrations of ambient airborne pollutants (**Fig. 1**); pollen, natural disasters, such as active volcanoes; mold related to water accumulation (**Fig. 2**); tobacco smoke; and hairdressers' aerosolized products.[28–35]

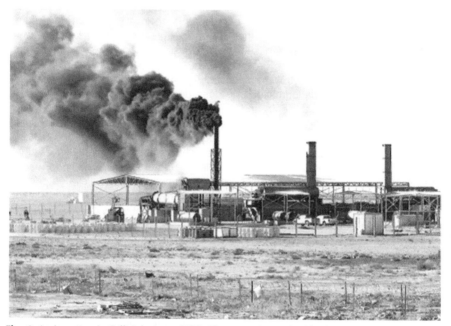

Fig. 1. Incinerator in Fallujah, Iraq, 2008. Photograph used with permission from a soldier who wishes to remain anonymous. This incinerator is a source of particulate matter air pollution, which can exacerbate a soldier's asthma.

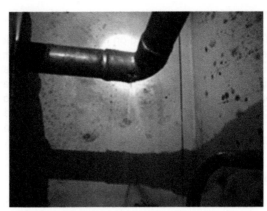

Fig. 2. Black mold (*Epicoccum* by culture) on wall of furnace room after water pipe burst from a water heater.

Ragweed and particulate matter air pollution may trigger asthma among workers who work outdoors, such as landscapers, even in those not allergically sensitized.[36] **Table 1** shows high-risk occupations for WEA. Many cases of WEA may be attributed to irritant exposure. Among these are ethanol, paints, solvents, calcium oxide, acids, ammonia, cigarette smoke, glutaraldehyde (eg, technicians who clean endoscopes), and welders exposed to fumes.

In an analysis of 5600 health care providers, 3650 replied to a questionnaire about their occupation, asthma diagnosis, variability of asthma symptoms at and away from work, and exposure to individual cleaning substances. WEA was defined as a categorical variable with 4 mutually exclusive categories: work-related asthma symptoms (WRAS), WEA, OA, and none. Multivariable logistic regression analysis was used to evaluate the association between self-reported use of cleaning substances and asthma outcomes among health care providers. Prevalence of WRAS, WEA, and OA were 3.3%, 1.1%, and 0.8%, respectively. Women had higher prevalence estimates than men. The odds increased in a dose-dependent manner for exposure in the longest job to cleaning agents and disinfectants, respectively. For exposure in any job, the odds of WRAS were significantly elevated for both factor 1 exposures (bleach, cleaners/abrasives, toilet cleaners, detergents, and ammonia) and factor 2 exposures (glutaraldehyde/ortho-phtaldehyde, chloramines, and ethylene oxide). Risk for WEA was observed for exposure to bleach, factor 2, and formalin/formaldehyde. Exposure to chloramines was associated with nearly fivefold elevated odds of OA. These investigators determined that health care providers are at risk of developing work-related asthma (WRA) from exposure to cleaning substances.[19]

Another study examined the frequency of claims for OA and WEA allowed by the compensation board in Ontario, Canada for which industry was coded as *health care* between 1998 and 2002. Five claims were allowed for sensitizer OA, 2 for natural rubber latex (NRL), and 3 for glutaraldehyde/photographic chemicals. The 2 NRL cases occurred in nurses who had worked for more than 10 years before the date of the accident. There were 115 allowed claims for WEA; health care was the most frequent industry for WEA. Compared with the rest of the province, claims in health care made up a significantly greater proportion of WEA claims (17.8%) than OA (5.1%) (odds ratio, 4.1). The WEA claims rate was 2.1 times greater than that in the rest of the workforce. WEA claims occurred in many jobs (eg, clerk) other than classic

Table 1
High-risk occupations for work-exacerbated asthma

Occupation	Things that can Cause or Worsen Asthma
Autobody workers	Acrylate in resins, glues, sealants, adhesives
Animal handlers, veterinarians, animal researchers, farmers	Dander, hair, scales, fur, saliva, and body wastes
Bakers, grain workers, farmers	Cereal grains, flour, amylase, enzymes, tobacco
Carpet makers	Gums
Dental hygienists	Latex gloves, material for filings, impressions, disinfectants
Forestry workers, carpenters, sawmill workers, cabinetmakers, woodworkers	Wood dust
Firefighters	Smoke
Hairdressers	Bleach, dye
Health care professionals	Latex gloves, formaldehyde, glutaraldehyde, antibiotics, detergent enzymes
Janitors, cleaning staff	Disinfectants, detergent enzymes, mixtures of chemicals (eg, mixing bleach and ammonia), fragrances
Jewelry, alloy, and catalyst makers	Platinum
Landscapers, gardeners, other outdoor workers	Cold air, humidity, mold, pollens, smog pollution, exercise
Manicurists	Acrylate in artificial nails
Office workers	Mold, fungus, dust
Pharmaceutical workers	Antibiotics, psyllium, enzymes
Printing industry	Gum arabic, reactive dyes, acrylates
Seafood processors who work with lobster, crab, shrimp, clam, oyster, scallop, squid, mussel, whelk, sea urchins, sea cucumber	Proteins in the shellfish
Shellac handlers	Amines
Teachers	Viral or other kinds of lung infections, mold, dust
Waiters, bar staff	Secondhand smoke
Welders, refiners, metal platers	Metals, nickel sulfate, solder fluxes
Spray painters, autobody shop painters, insulation installers, plastics, foam, and foundry industry workers	Diisocyanates (chemicals found in polyurethane products like flexible and rigid foams); molded parts; coatings, such as paints and varnishes; building insulation materials
Textile workers	Dyes
Users of plastics, epoxy resins	Chemicals, such as anhydrides

From The Canadian Lung Association (www.lung.ca/diseases-maladies/asthma-asthme/work-travail/who-qui_e.php); with permission.

health care jobs, such as nurses, and were associated with a variety of agents: construction dust, secondhand smoke, paint fumes. These investigators concluded that WEA occurs frequently in this professional sector. Those affected and attributed agents include many not typically expected in health care.[37]

WEA shares many features with asthma unrelated to work and with OA, but important differences exist. At an HMO in Massachusetts, patients with WEA were more likely to be men and to be affected by asthma symptoms on more days during the past week than other adults with asthma. Nevertheless, the 2 types of patients with asthma were similar in age, race/ethnicity, education, annual income level, cigarette smoking, severity of asthma, and number of treatments for acute asthma attacks and number of workdays missed because of asthma in the previous year.[6] Patients with WEA from the workers' compensation system in Washington were more likely to be women than patients with OA. In this analysis, the median age of workers with WEA and OA was similar. The patients with WEA were less likely than their counterparts with OA to have received treatment from a specialist or to have completed pulmonary function and allergy tests.[38,39]

In Quebec, WEA often led to workers leaving their jobs after diagnosis. WRA can have an adverse impact on patients' working life and income. Spirometry, methacholine challenge results, sputum cell counts, and symptom frequency were compared between when patients were diagnosed and at follow-up. The patients with OA and WEA were similar, with improvement in respiratory symptoms and little change in other clinical features by follow-up. In another study comparing 115 patients with WEA with 82 patients with OA, atopy was more common among the patients with OA (87%) than the patients with WEA (74%). The 2 types of WRA were similar in other clinical and functional features, except for differences in specific inhalation challenge findings that were used to delineate OA from WEA.[40]

WORK-RELATED RHINITIS AND WEA

Some patients are affected by both work-related rhinitis and WEA. Work-related rhinitis includes work-exacerbated rhinitis and occupational rhinoconjunctivitis. Implicated substances leading to occupational rhinitis include (1) high-molecular-weight proteins and (2) low-molecular-weight chemicals. The diagnosis of work-related rhinitis is established based on occupational history and documentation of immunoglobulin E (IgE)–mediated sensitization to the causative agent, if possible. The treatment of occupational rhinoconjunctivitis includes elimination or reduction of exposure to causative agents combined with pharmacotherapy, which is similar to other causes of rhinitis. Allergen immunotherapy is one option.[41]

In one study, 105 out of 363 patients with clinical WEA who demonstrated nonspecific bronchial hyperresponsiveness to histamine, but a negative response to a specific inhalation challenge with the suspected occupational agents, were considered as having WEA. Their characteristics were compared with those of 172 patients with OA ascertained by a positive response to a specific inhalation challenge. A high proportion of patients with WEA (83%) and OA (90%) reported at least one nasal symptom at work. Symptoms of (1) sneezing/itching or (2) rhinorrhea were more frequent in patients with OA (78% for sneezing/itching and 70% for rhinorrhea) than in those with WEA (61% for sneezing/itching and 57% for rhinorrhea), whereas postnasal discharge was more common in WEA (30%) than in OA (18%). Nasal symptoms were less severe in WEA (median [25th–75th percentiles] global severity score: 4 [2–6]) as compared with OA (median global severity score: 5 [4–7]). Nasal symptoms preceded less frequently those of asthma in patients with WEA (17%) than in patients with OA (43%). Nasal symptoms are highly prevalent in patients with WEA, although their clinical pattern differs from that found in OA.[42]

PREVENTION AND MANAGEMENT

Early in the course of disease, identification and mitigation of triggers is crucial. Reviewing MSDSs may help in addition to reviewing processes at work. Environmental controls including ensuring adequate ventilation and air filtration, and the use of personal respirators, are cornerstones of prevention. Medical surveillance may identify early cases of WEA. Work rotation, and even worker's compensation policies may influence the motivation of workers to seek treatment. The American with Disabilities Act

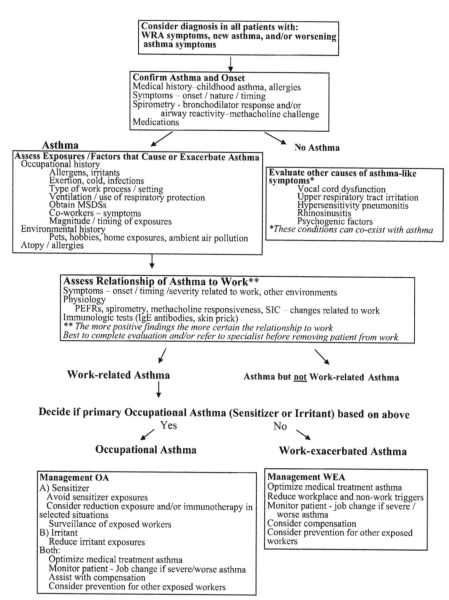

Fig. 3. Summary flow chart of clinical evaluation and management of WRA. PEFRs, peak expiratory flow rate; SIC, Specific Inhalational Challenge; WRA, Work Related Asthma. (*From* Tarlo SM, Balmes J, Balkissoon R, et al. Diagnosis and management of work-related asthma: American College of Chest Physicians Consensus Statement. Chest 2008;134:1S–41S; with permission.)

mandates that employers make reasonable accommodations for individuals with disabilities such as asthma.

The Ontario Work-Related Asthma Surveillance System: Physician Reporting (OWRAS) Network was established in 2007 to estimate the prevalence of WRA in Ontario and to test the feasibility of collecting data for cases of WRA from physicians voluntarily. More than 300 respirologists, occupational medicine physicians, allergists, and primary care providers in Ontario were invited to participate in monthly reporting of WRA cases by telephone, postal service, or e-mail. Since 2007, 49 physicians have registered with the OWRAS Network and, to date, have reported 34 cases of OA and 49 cases of WEA. Highly reactive chemicals were the most frequently reported suspected causative agent of the 108 suspected exposures reported. Despite the challenge of enlisting a representative sample of physicians in Ontario willing to report, the OWRAS Network has shown that it is feasible to implement a voluntary reporting system for WRA; however, its long-term sustainability is unknown.[43]

Reducing exposure to relevant workplace triggers (ie, prevention) is a cornerstone to disease management. Medication management is similar to that of asthma unrelated to work. A summary flow chart (**Fig. 3**) reviews the American College of Chest Physicians' recommendations for clinical evaluation and management of WEA.

SUMMARY AND FUTURE RESEARCH

WEA is defined as preexisting asthma exacerbated by conditions at work, making it different from OA, which is caused by work. Jobs associated with WEA may entail exposure to secondhand smoke, dust, and cleaning agents, especially in health care and office workers. Work-related rhinitis and conjunctivitis may be concurrent. Prevention and management principles are based on identifying triggers, removing exposure, cleaning the work environment, and medications. Future research is needed to help understand dose-response relationships and causal agents in complex environments.

ACKNOWLEDGMENTS

The author would like to acknowledge medical student Edward Forsyth for his assistance.

REFERENCES

1. Kurt E, Demir AU, Cadirci O, et al. Occupational exposures as risk factors for asthma and allergic diseases in a Turkish population. Int Arch Occup Environ Health 2011;84:45–52.
2. Omland O, Hjort C, Pedersen OF, et al. New-onset asthma and the effect of environment and occupation among farming and nonfarming rural subjects. J Allergy Clin Immunol 2011;128:761–5.
3. Lieberman JA, Sicherer SH. The diagnosis of food allergy. Am J Rhinol Allergy 2010;24:439–43.
4. Quirce S, Barranco P. Cleaning agents and asthma. J Investig Allergol Clin Immunol 2010;20:542–50 [quiz: 542–50].
5. Henneberger PK. Work-exacerbated asthma. Curr Opin Allergy Clin Immunol 2007;7:146–51.
6. Henneberger PK, Derk SJ, Sama SR, et al. The frequency of workplace exacerbation among health maintenance organisation members with asthma. Occup Environ Med 2006;63:551–7.

7. Larbanois A, Jamart J, Delwiche JP, et al. Socioeconomic outcome of subjects experiencing asthma symptoms at work. Eur Respir J 2002;19:1107–13.
8. Henneberger PK, Hoffman CD, Magid DJ, et al. Work-related exacerbation of asthma. Int J Occup Environ Health 2002;8:291–6.
9. Antao VC, Pallos LL, Shim YK, et al. Respiratory protective equipment, mask use, and respiratory outcomes among World Trade Center rescue and recovery workers. Am J Ind Med 2011;54:897–905.
10. Wheeler K, McKelvey W, Thorpe L, et al. Asthma diagnosed after 11 September 2001 among rescue and recovery workers: findings from the World Trade Center Health Registry. Environ Health Perspect 2007;115:1584–90.
11. Liu Y, Stowe MH, Bello D, et al. Respiratory protection from isocyanate exposure in the autobody repair and refinishing industry. J Occup Environ Hyg 2006;3:234–49.
12. Sparer J, Stowe MH, Bello D, et al. Isocyanate exposures in autobody shop work: the SPRAY study. J Occup Environ Hyg 2004;1:570–81.
13. Cullen MR, Redlich CA, Beckett WS, et al. Feasibility study of respiratory questionnaire and peak flow recordings in autobody shop workers exposed to isocyanate-containing spray paint: observations and limitations. Occup Med (Lond) 1996;46:197–204.
14. Portman C. Determining a qualifying disability under the ADA: case study–mild asthma and indoor air quality. AAOHN J 1994;42:230–5.
15. Szema AM, Schmidt MP, Lanzirotti A, et al. Titanium and iron in lung of a soldier with nonspecific interstitial pneumonitis and bronchiolitis after returning from Iraq. J Occup Environ Med 2012;54:1–2.
16. Szema AM, Salihi W, Savary K, et al. Respiratory symptoms necessitating spirometry among soldiers with Iraq/Afghanistan war lung injury. J Occup Environ Med 2011;53:961–5.
17. Szema AM, Peters MC, Weissinger KM, et al. New-onset asthma among soldiers serving in Iraq and Afghanistan. Allergy Asthma Proc 2010;31:67–71.
18. King MS, Eisenberg R, Newman JH, et al. Constrictive bronchiolitis in soldiers returning from Iraq and Afghanistan. N Engl J Med 2011;365:222–30.
19. Arif AA, Delclos GL. Association between cleaning-related chemicals and work-related asthma and asthma symptoms among healthcare professionals. Occup Environ Med 2012;69:35–40.
20. Henneberger PK, Redlich CA, Callahan DB, et al. An official American Thoracic Society statement: work-exacerbated asthma. Am J Respir Crit Care Med 2011;184:368–78.
21. Bolen AR, Henneberger PK, Liang X, et al. The validation of work-related self-reported asthma exacerbation. Occup Environ Med 2007;64:343–8.
22. Caldeira RD, Bettiol H, Barbieri MA, et al. Prevalence and risk factors for work related asthma in young adults. Occup Environ Med 2006;63:694–9.
23. Szema AM, Khedkar M, Maloney PF, et al. Clinical deterioration in pediatric asthmatic patients after September 11, 2001. J Allergy Clin Immunol 2004;113:420–6.
24. Landrigan PJ, Lioy PJ, Thurston G, et al. Health and environmental consequences of the world trade center disaster. Environ Health Perspect 2004;112:731–9.
25. Endres M, Kullmann L, Simon G, et al. Rehabilitation of hemiplegic leg amputees. Orv Hetil 1987;128:2741–3 [in Hungarian].
26. Blanc PD, Ellbjar S, Janson C, et al. Asthma-related work disability in Sweden. The impact of workplace exposures. Am J Respir Crit Care Med 1999;160:2028–33.

27. Bernedo N, Garcia M, Gastaminza G, et al. Allergy to laxative compound (Plantago ovata seed) among health care professionals. J Investig Allergol Clin Immunol 2008;18:181–9.
28. Erwin EA, Woodfolk JA, Custis N, et al. Animal danders. Immunol Allergy Clin North Am 2003;23:469–81.
29. Terzano C, Di Stefano F, Conti V, et al. Air pollution ultrafine particles: toxicity beyond the lung. Eur Rev Med Pharmacol Sci 2010;14:809–21.
30. van der Walt A, Lopata AL, Nieuwenhuizen NE, et al. Work-related allergy and asthma in spice mill workers - the impact of processing dried spices on IgE reactivity patterns. Int Arch Allergy Immunol 2010;152:271–8.
31. Carlsen HK, Gislason T, Benediktsdottir B, et al. A survey of early health effects of the Eyjafjallajokull 2010 eruption in Iceland: a population-based study. BMJ Open 2012;2:e000343.
32. Dahlman-Hoglund A, Renstrom A, Larsson PH, et al. Salmon allergen exposure, occupational asthma, and respiratory symptoms among salmon processing workers. Am J Ind Med 2012;55:624–30.
33. Jarvholm B, Reuterwall C, Bystedt J. Mortality attributable to occupational exposure in Sweden. Scand J Work Environ Health 2012;3284 [Epub ahead of print].
34. Remen T, Acouetey DS, Paris C, et al. Diet, occupational exposure and early asthma incidence among bakers, pastry makers and hairdressers. BMC Public Health 2012;12:387.
35. Bernstein RS, Sorenson WG, Garabrant D, et al. Exposures to respirable, airborne Penicillium from a contaminated ventilation system: clinical, environmental and epidemiological aspects. Am Ind Hyg Assoc J 1983;44:161–9.
36. Wiszniewska M, Palczynski C, Krawczyk-Szulc P, et al. Occupational allergy to Limonium sinuatum: a case report. Int J Occup Med Environ Health 2011;24:304–7.
37. Liss GM, Buyantseva L, Luce CE, et al. Work-related asthma in health care in Ontario. Am J Ind Med 2011;54:278–84.
38. Anderson NJ, Reeb-Whitaker CK, Bonauto DK, et al. Work-related asthma in Washington State. J Asthma 2011;48:773–82.
39. Curwick CC, Bonauto DK, Adams DA. Use of objective testing in the diagnosis of work-related asthma by physician specialty. Ann Allergy Asthma Immunol 2006;97:546–50.
40. Singh T, Bello B, Jeebhay MF. Risk factors associated with asthma phenotypes in dental healthcare workers. Am J Ind Med 2012 Apr 2. [Epub ahead of print].
41. Sublett JW, Bernstein DI. Occupational rhinitis. Immunol Allergy Clin North Am 2011;31:787–96, vii.
42. Vandenplas O, Van Brussel P, D'Alpaos V, et al. Rhinitis in subjects with work-exacerbated asthma. Respir Med 2010;104:497–503.
43. To T, Tarlo SM, McLimont S, et al. Feasibility of a provincial voluntary reporting system for work-related asthma in Ontario. Can Respir J 2011;18:275–7.

Treating According to Asthma Control: Does it Work in Real Life?

Helen K. Reddel, MB, BS, PhD, FRACP

KEYWORDS

- Asthma control • Guidelines • Exacerbations • Primary health care • Drug therapy
- Adults

KEY POINTS

- Control-based asthma management, adjusting the patient's treatment upward or downward according to simple measures of control, has been incorporated in asthma guidelines for many years.
- This article reviews the evidence for its utility in adults, describes its strengths and limitations in real life, and proposes areas for further research, particularly about incorporation of future risk and identification of patients for whom phenotype-guided treatment would be effective and efficient.
- The strengths of control-based management include its simplicity and feasibility for primary care, and its limitations include the nonspecific nature of asthma symptoms, the complex role of β_2-agonist use, barriers to stepping down treatment, and the underlying assumptions about asthma pathophysiology and treatment responses.

WHAT IS CONTROL-BASED MANAGEMENT?

The concept of adjusting asthma treatment according to the patient's \ level of asthma control has been embedded in asthma guidelines for so long that it is easy to forget that this approach is somewhat unusual in other areas of clinical practice. With many chronic diseases, patient assessment and treatment is guided by disease severity, an intrinsic feature usually manifest at the initial presentation and correlated with the underlying pathologic condition. However, for asthma, information about

This article originally appeared in Clinics in Chest Medicine, Volume 33, Issue 3, September 2012.

Disclosure of interests: H.K.R. is Chair of the Science Committee of the Global Initiative for Asthma (GINA) and a member of the Steering Committee for the 2012 update of the *Australian Asthma Management Handbook*. She has participated in asthma advisory boards for AstraZeneca, GlaxoSmithKline, and Novartis; has received unrestricted research funding from AstraZeneca and GlaxoSmithKline; is a member of a data monitoring committee for AstraZeneca, GlaxoSmithKline, Merck, and Novartis; and has given continuing medical education presentations at symposia funded by AstraZeneca, GlaxoSmithKline, and Novartis.

Clinical Management Group, Woolcock Institute of Medical Research, PO Box M77, Missenden Road Post Office, New South Wales 2050, Australia

E-mail address: hkr@med.usyd.edu.au

airway pathology was not (and is still not) generally available to clinicians, so the initial concept of asthma severity was based on the patient's clinical features at presentation (ie, symptoms, reliever use, and airflow limitation).[1,2] Early studies had shown that

- Symptoms and airflow limitation could be temporarily relieved by the use of short-acting β_2-agonist medications (SABA).
- More sustained control of symptoms required longer-term treatment with inhaled corticosteroids (ICS).[3]
- Patients with more severe asthma at baseline, already using ICS or oral corticosteroids, generally responded to higher ICS doses[4,5] or the addition of long-acting β_2-agonist (LABA).[6]
- Once symptoms and airflow limitation were well controlled (ie, occurring only a couple of times a week), the ICS dose could be reduced to minimize the potential for side effects.[7]

These principles, initially empiric and consensus based but later formalized with extensive randomized controlled trials and meta-analyses, still largely form the basis for current clinical practice recommendations, including from the Global Initiative for Asthma (GINA),[8] the National Heart Lung and Blood Institute's Expert Panel 3 Report,[9] and the British Thoracic Society/Scottish Intercollegiate Guidelines Network (BTS/SIGN).[10] The current recommended treatment steps for adults are:

- As-needed SABA
- Low-dose ICS
- Low-dose ICS/LABA
- Moderate-high dose ICS/LABA
- Add-on prednisone or other agents.

At each level, the guidelines also provide options for alternative medications to allow for patient preference, side effects, and cost.

From the start, the concept of control-based management also included:

- Short-term management of worsening asthma, with patients adjusting their medications according to a written asthma action plan based on worsening symptoms or lung function and returning to pre-exacerbation treatment levels once asthma was controlled
- Management of asthma within a framework of a good patient-doctor relationship, self-management education, and regular review.

Although evidence-based medicine places a high value on systematic reviews of good-quality randomized controlled trials, it is now recognized that:

- Only a small minority of community patients would have satisfied the entry criteria for the major studies on which asthma guidelines are based.[11]
- Substantial heterogeneity occurs in responses to ICS and other medications, with patients with similar clinical characteristics at baseline having widely differing responses to treatment.[12–14]
- Treatment strategies may have different effects on clinical measures of control and on exacerbations.[15]
- Finally, with sputum induction and bronchial biopsies more readily available, it was found that variation in treatment response could be at least partly attributed to heterogeneity in the underlying inflammatory processes.[16,17]

As a result, asthma, rather than being considered as a single disease, is gaining recognition as a syndromic descriptor for a group of conditions with similar clinical manifestations but different pathophysiologic mechanisms and responses to treatment,[18,19] as occurred with arthritis.

The assessment of asthma was recently reviewed to develop standardized definitions and criteria for asthma control, severity, and exacerbations for use in clinical trials and clinical practice.[20,21] The diversity of underlying pathophysiological phenotypes was emphasized; the assessment of asthma control was expanded from current clinical features, such as symptoms, airway obstruction, and impaired activity, to also include the assessment of patient's risks of adverse events, such as exacerbations, accelerated lung function decline, and side effects. These two components were named *current clinical control* and *future risk*.[20] Future risk was incorporated in recognition that symptoms were a superficial marker of asthma control in that they could be suppressed by LABA monotherapy while exacerbations remained uncontrolled, and that there were other predictors of future risk, such as smoking, low lung function, and airway eosinophilia, which were independent of the level of symptoms.[20]

The present article reviews the evidence for the utility of control-based asthma management in adults, describes the strengths and limitations of this approach in real life, and proposes areas for further research to improve its utility and to identify patients and populations for whom control-based management is appropriate.

EVIDENCE ABOUT CONTROL-BASED MANAGEMENT IN REAL LIFE

The first clinical practice guidelines for asthma were published in Australia in 1989.[2] They recommended the adjustment of treatment based on lung function and "severity", which was similar to the present assessment of asthma "control". A similar approach was taken in Canada the following year, with both countries undertaking intensive dissemination activities.[22] At the time, evidence-based medicine was in its infancy, so the guidelines were largely consensus based, and there were no formal studies comparing control-based management with the previous more ad hoc approach.

Assessing the impact of the control-based strategy in real life is difficult because it was intended to be part of a package of asthma care and education and to include both stepping up and stepping down. By contrast, most research evidence comes from closely monitored randomized controlled trials with a single-step treatment change at randomization. Planning clinical trials to examine medication adjustment strategies is challenging because the cumulative effect of algorithmic interventions can magnify any design flaws.[23]

Pre-Post Studies in Real Life

- Ecological evidence for the impact of control-based management may be suggested by the dramatic decrease in asthma mortality in countries, such as Australia and Canada, in the 20 years after the publication of their asthma guidelines despite increasing asthma prevalence.[24,25]
- In 1994, Finland adopted a comprehensive 10-year asthma-management program incorporating systematic implementation strategies, which achieved remarkable national penetration across all levels of health care. Again, hospitalizations and deaths caused by asthma were halved despite and increase in asthma prevalence, and there was a decrease in asthma-related costs.[26]
- In 1998 to 2000, the International Union Against Tuberculosis and Lung Disease (IUATLD) conducted asthma-management studies in 9 countries, using a control-based algorithm customized for developing countries. Over 1 year of follow-up, the proportion of patients with poorly controlled asthma decreased from 43% to 16%.[27]

However, evidence that the control-based approach to asthma management has not been (sufficiently) successful in real life comes from the many cross-sectional studies that have shown that a high proportion of patients, even in countries with well-established guidelines and ready access to controller medications, still experience frequent symptoms and interference with daily activities and many still require urgent health care for asthma.[28] From administrative datasets, too, comes evidence that prescribing and/or dispensing of controller medications are inconsistent with control-based guidelines. For example, according to control-based management, most patients should be started on low-dose ICS, and most should achieve good asthma control when this is taken regularly. However, in Australia, most ICS is dispensed as moderate/high potency ICS/LABA and only 9% of ICS recipients aged 15 to 34 years have dispensing rates consistent with daily use.[24] In a US claims database, patients with mild persistent asthma were more often initiated on more expensive treatments than on the low-dose ICS recommended by guidelines.[29]

Control-Based Management Versus Usual Care in Real Life

Because control-based management has been recommended by clinical practice guidelines for more than 20 years, the outcomes of studies that compare guidelines-based management with usual care reflect the extent to which guidelines have been adopted in clinical practice as well as the effectiveness of the control-driven regimen itself. For example, a cohort analysis from a large managed care organization showed that patients with uncontrolled asthma (n = 7177) had better asthma control, as indicated by reduced reliever use, if their treatment was stepped up in accordance with guidelines than those with no step-up; however there was no significant difference between groups in exacerbation rates.[30]

In several intervention studies, practical tools have increased the implementation of a control-based approach, with improved outcomes compared with usual care. For example:

- In Spain, a GINA-based management system with computerized decision support led to improved quality of life and reduced health care utilization and was cost-effective, compared with usual care.[31]
- In a US managed care organization with existing control-based processes for managing asthma, protocolized implementation of stepped-care guidelines by trained care managers, using customized worksheets and educational tools, led to significant improvements in medication adherence, asthma control and asthma-related quality of life, and a significant reduction in health care utilization compared with usual care within the same organisation.[32] Medication adherence was even higher when care managers used a shared decision-making process for medication choices,[32] emphasizing the importance of patient-clinician communication in the implementation of control-based management.

Control-Based Management Versus Inflammation-Guided Management

It might be expected that treatment guided by biomarkers which reflect the nature of underlying airway inflammation would improve overall outcomes. Studies comparing control-based management with inflammation-guided management are dealt with in detail by Nair and colleagues elsewhere in this issue, but the key issues for clinical practice are summarized below.

Sputum-guided management

The pivotal studies of sputum-guided treatment showed a halving of severe exacerbations and similar levels of current asthma control compared with control-based treatment.[33] However, the results are not directly applicable to real-life clinical practice because the studies involved very selected populations and research sites. Patients with moderate-severe asthma were recruited through specialist chest clinics with existing research expertise in sputum cell counting, and who were generally excluded if they were thought to have adherence problems or comorbidities, were current smokers, or had a significant smoking history. There was some variation between these studies in the details of the sputum-based and control-based algorithms, and there was a delay of 1 to 7 days between the patient visit and the treatment decision.

Now that the evidence for the efficacy of sputum-guided treatment has been established in these rigorously conducted studies, further research is needed to investigate its feasibility, cost-effectiveness, and acceptability to patients and clinicians within more general secondary care. In post hoc analysis of one study,[34] the advantages of sputum-guided treatment were seen in patients with discordant symptoms and eosinophilic inflammation, with lower ICS doses achieved in those with high symptoms but low inflammation, and fewer severe exacerbations in those with few symptoms but marked sputum eosinophilia.[35]

Fractional concentration of exhaled nitric oxide–guided treatment

There has been considerable interest in the use of the fractional concentration of exhaled nitric oxide (FeNO) as a more feasible surrogate marker of eosinophilic airway inflammation. However, the overall results of studies comparing FeNO-guided treatment with control-based treatment in children and adults have not been as convincing as for sputum-guided treatment, with meta-analysis failing to show an overall benefit either in clinical control or exacerbation rates.[36] Wide variation was seen between studies in the selection of patients and the design of the FeNO and control algorithms, including in the extent to which the control algorithm reflected guideline recommendations.

Gibson[23] recently highlighted several methodological issues that likely contributed to the lack of difference between the FeNO-based and control-based algorithms in these studies. These issues included the narrow range of patient ICS doses at entry, the use of 1 rather than 2 FeNO cut points, and the low probability that the selected algorithms within most of the studies would result in different treatment decisions. The implementation of these methodological principles in a subsequent algorithm study of pregnant women with asthma led to striking reductions in exacerbation rates, and lower ICS doses, with FeNO-guided compared with a control-based algorithm, although the latter differed in several respects from current guidelines, although the latter differed in several respects from current recommendations.[37] Given the ease of measurement of FeNO and the rapidity with which results are obtained, further studies are awaited with interest.

As with sputum-guided treatment, it will be important to identify the patients and settings in which FeNO-guided management gives better outcomes than control-based management.

STRENGTHS OF CONTROL-BASED MANAGEMENT IN REAL LIFE

The major strengths of control-based management for real-life application are its simplicity, feasibility, and patient-centered approach.

The control-based strategy for medication adjustment is feasible for use in primary and secondary care:

- It can be implemented across broad populations, including in developing countries,[26,27,38] because it involves only a few simple questions about clinical features and the patient's risk factors for longer-term adverse outcomes.

- The measurement of forced expiratory volume in the first second of expiration (FEV_1) or peak flow is a component of the assessment of asthma control when available and is readily accessible (although currently underutilized) in primary care.
- Medication decisions can be made immediately during consultations without the need for specialized equipment, personnel, or processing.

Because a patient's individual experience of asthma is largely driven by their symptoms,[39] the concept of adjusting treatments based on symptoms can emphasize that the approach is patient-centered. Several studies have shown that patients taking maintenance controller treatment already adjust their usage in response to symptoms, although the reported level of use is less than that needed for good asthma control.[40,41]

LIMITATIONS OF CONTROL-BASED MANAGEMENT IN REAL LIFE

Despite, or perhaps because of, its simplicity, control-based management has some important limitations in real life. These limitations may not be sufficient to influence group mean results in a research study but are relevant to the management of individual patients in clinical practice.

Incorrect Diagnosis of Asthma

Integral to the concept of control-based management is the assumption that the diagnosis of asthma has been confirmed, because symptoms not caused by bronchoconstriction or airway inflammation are unlikely to respond to conventional asthma pharmacotherapy. However, studies of community-based populations in Sweden,[42,43] the Netherlands,[44] and Canada[45] report that objective evidence of asthma cannot be found in 24% to 34% of patients with a reported diagnosis of asthma.

High rates of overdiagnosis may be partly attributable to the success of previous public and medical awareness campaigns, encouraging clinicians to think of asthma for patients with respiratory symptoms[22,46]; however, the situation is worsened by barriers to use of spirometry in primary care.[47,48] Only 43% of Canadian patients with a new diagnosis of asthma had undergone spirometric testing in the 3.5 years around the time of diagnosis.[49]

Correct diagnosis of asthma is crucial because, in patients with respiratory symptoms, control-based management would otherwise promote a progressive increase in medication, with patients eventually likely labeled as having severe refractory asthma.

Heterogeneity in Inflammatory Profile

The stepwise treatment options recommended in current guidelines were based on the assumption from group mean data that asthma is usually characterized by eosinophilic inflammation, which in turn causes airway hyperresponsiveness, thence bronchoconstriction, and symptoms, and that an ICS-based strategy would be most effective. Alternative medication options are offered at each step but their selection is described as depending on patient preference, side effects, or cost. Although each medication change is regarded as a therapeutic trial, failure to respond usually prompts a step-up to the next level rather than trial of one of the other medication options at the same level.

However, as described previously, one of the most striking advances in asthma in recent years has been in the growing awareness of heterogeneity in the relationship between symptoms and eosinophilic airway inflammation, and in the existence of other inflammatory phenotypes with different response profiles to ICS. As yet, inflammometry (inflammation-guided treatment) is only available in specialized centers.

Reliance on Symptoms

Asthma symptoms are nonspecific

Even once the diagnosis of asthma has been confirmed, it cannot be assumed that all subsequent respiratory symptoms are also caused by asthma. It is important in clinical practice to consider the possibility that new respiratory symptoms may be caused by a comorbidity, such as sinusitis, deconditioning, obesity, or vocal cord dysfunction, before stepping up the patient's asthma treatment. In the past, patients were considered to be mislabeling asthma symptoms if lung function was not reduced at the time,[50] but, with reduced reliance on the assessment of lung function in clinical practice, clinicians now have fewer tools for distinguishing asthma from nonasthma symptoms.

Symptom perception is variable

Substantial variation is seen between patients in their ability to perceive airflow limitation and, hence, in their level of symptoms. Contributing factors include age, baseline lung function, airway hyperresponsiveness, and airway inflammation.[51,52] The ability to identify bronchoconstriction improves with improved asthma control.[51]

The extent of symptoms experienced for a given level of lung function may also vary according to the patient's level of physical activity. Patients with a sedentary lifestyle are unlikely to experience exercise-induced bronchoconstriction and may not experience day-to-day symptoms until moderate to severe airflow limitation is present.

The no-symptoms-no-asthma belief

Core to the concept of control-based management is that patients who respond to treatment with ICS should continue to take them every day even if they have no symptoms, because the treatment is for control rather than for a cure. Patients may perceive this to be inconsistent with the use of symptoms to guide treatment. The no-symptoms-no-asthma belief, in which asthma is perceived and managed by patients as an acute episodic condition rather than a chronic disease, is associated with worse asthma control and greater need for prednisone courses.[53]

Subjective measures of control may respond to placebo treatment

The importance of monitoring both subjective and objective measures of asthma control has been highlighted by recent studies that have shown significant effects of placebo or sham interventions on symptoms in patients with mild asthma, without significant effects on lung function.[54,55]

β_2-Agonist Use as a Measure of Asthma Control

Factors affecting usage of β_2-agonist

The frequency of reliever use is likely to be affected by the patient's level of physical activity, by doses taken before exercise, by psychological dependence, and by the use of LABA. As expected, β_2-agonist use typically decreases after the addition of LABA to maintenance ICS treatment; however, cessation of LABA does not necessarily lead to an increase in SABA use,[56,57] suggesting a contribution of tachyphylaxis or habitual use of SABA, which may impact the assessment of asthma control in these patients.

Adverse effects of excess β_2-agonist

Guidelines recommend that rapid-acting β_2-agonist should be used as needed for relief of symptoms and bronchoconstriction, including acute severe asthma. Less well known, particularly in primary care, is that the regular or frequent use of SABA is associated with increased symptoms, bronchial reactivity, airway inflammation, and risk of exacerbations compared with placebo or twice-daily LABA.[58] One of the most difficult aspects of the assessment of asthma control in clinical practice is to identify when β_2-agonist use, rather than being an *indicator* of poor asthma control, is *contributing* to poor asthma control. Clinical pointers may include the long-term use of high SABA dosages (eg, albuterol 8+ puffs per day or daily use of nebulizer); well-preserved lung function despite very frequent symptoms and β_2-agonist use; and a lack of improvement in lung function with the administration of extra SABA (although this can also be seen during viral exacerbations[59]). Improved asthma control has been seen in around one-third of patients when strategies are implemented to reduce β_2-agonist exposure.[60,61]

Instability of Control Measures in Poorly Controlled Asthma

Patients with untreated asthma demonstrate substantial variability in measures of asthma control from week to week. For example, in a 12-week study in which patients at baseline had daily symptoms consistent with uncontrolled asthma, those who received as-needed SABA alone had symptoms and reliever use consistent with well-controlled asthma in 18% and 30% of the study weeks, respectively.[62] The need for preventer treatment may, therefore, be underestimated if it is based on the short-term assessment of asthma control. However, after patients commence regular preventer treatment, week-to-week variability in control measures is substantially reduced.[63]

Patient Understanding of Control

Many studies have reported that patients overestimate their level of asthma control, based on the discordance between patient-reported asthma control and the guidelines-based assessment of control.[28] However, this is more likely to indicate that patients attribute a different meaning to control, such as self-control or the ease with which they can relieve their symptoms with SABA, compared with the medical usage of the term.[20,64] Similar differences are seen in the medical and lay usage of the term shock.

Patient-reported level of control is included in the Asthma Control Test (ACT).[65] It has been suggested that the discordance between responses to this item and the 4 clinical items might serve as a red flag to identify patients who would benefit from further education about their disease[65]; however, the impact that this might have on subsequent ACT scores has not been evaluated.

Barriers to Stepping Down Asthma Treatment

Control-based management is predicated on regular review by the clinician, with stepwise increases in treatment when asthma control is worse and stepwise decreases when symptoms improve. However, in a review of more than 2000 visits by 397 patients in a community population over 2 years, 85% of medication changes were a step-up and only 13% were a step-down. A contributory factor is that patients often fail to attend for scheduled follow-ups or review visits; in the same study, there were 2.3 times as many visits for acute asthma problems as for asthma evaluations or follow-up.[66]

Despite evidence that step-down can be performed safely once asthma is well controlled,[67] clinicians seem to be reluctant to reduce even high-intensity treatment,[68] presumably because of the potential for destabilizing patients. Both the patient's and the physician's personality may contribute to overtreatment in asthma.[69] In addition, there are few barriers for the physician to maintaining high doses, given the low side-effect profile of ICS. This factor contrasts with conditions, such as diabetes or hypertension, whereby overtreatment can have serious adverse effects. Nevertheless, patient-reported side effects increase with increasing ICS dose[70] and are associated with lower medication adherence.[71]

Other Factors Contributing to Poor Asthma Control

Teaching materials about asthma guidelines often focus on the key table or figure that summarizes the recommended stepwise changes in medications and doses that should be followed in response to worsening asthma control. This approach omits some of the most important components of asthma management, which are usually emphasized in the accompanying text, particularly the need to establish a patient-doctor partnership and to assess common factors, such as adherence and inhaler technique, before considering a step-up in asthma medication.[72]

Poor inhaler technique

Poor technique with respiratory devices is so common that, for practical purposes, inhaler technique should be considered to be incorrect until proven otherwise. Poor technique, regardless of inhaler type, is associated with poor asthma control and an increased risk of hospitalization, emergency department visits, and need for systemic corticosteroids.[73] Sadly, most health professionals are also unable to demonstrate correct inhaler technique,[74] showing errors similar to those demonstrated by patients.[75] Increasing the prescribed dose of an inhaled medication is unlikely to be effective if patients are unable to use the relevant inhaler correctly.

Poor adherence

Poor adherence, likewise, is so common in asthma that it is to be considered almost the norm. Although there is evidence that patients self-reporting less-than-perfect adherence can be believed,[71,76] clinicians have difficulty in identifying patients who, through embarrassment or fear, deliberately conceal poor adherence.[77]

HOW CAN CONTROL-BASED MANAGEMENT BE IMPROVED?
Improve the Diagnosis of Asthma

Improving the diagnosis of asthma should reduce the number of patients who seem to fail control-based management, but this is not a simple task. There is no gold standard for the diagnosis of asthma and, like most other chronic diseases, it does not seem to be dichotomous, with the most typical features of symptoms and variable lung function existing on a continuum.[78] Wheezing, shortness of breath, cough, and chest tightness may occur with many other conditions. Strategies that may assist with asthma diagnosis are:

- A useful tool provided by the BTS/SIGN guidelines is a list of simple features that increase or decrease the probability that patients with respiratory symptoms have asthma.[10]
- Increasing the availability of good-quality spirometry in primary care is essential for improving the quality of diagnosis[79]; this may include providing online diagnostic and technical support, or centralized spirometry services.

Improve Implementation of Control-Based Management

Provide access to basic medications
Most of the benefit of ICS is obtained at low daily doses,[80,81] but these medications are not currently available widely in all countries. The Asthma Drug Facility of the IUATLD provides generic ICS at low cost to developing countries in conjunction with simple documentation of process measures and clinical outcomes.[82]

Reinforce existing components of control-based management

Simple tools, such as Asthma Control Questionnaire (ACQ)[83] and ACT, can standardize the assessment of asthma control from visit to visit; they can be completed on paper in the waiting room, online,[84,85] or by telephone.[86] For an individual patient, a change in ACT score of 3 is regarded as clinically important.[87]

Guidelines emphasize the importance of confirming that symptoms are caused by asthma and that inhaler technique and adherence are satisfactory before considering a step-up in treatment but these basic steps are often overlooked. The dissemination of simple tools may help. For example:

- Inhaler technique assessment and training takes an average of only 2.5 minutes and is effective in improving asthma control.[88,89]
- Brief questionnaires can screen for poor adherence,[71,90] and shared decision-making can improve adherence.[32]
- Automated text messaging can reduce no-shows with follow-up visits.[91]

Tools for integrating future risk assessment

In recent years, GINA reports[8] have emphasized that clinicians should not rely only on the assessment of the patient's current control status but should also consider their future risk.[20] Because this concept is unfamiliar, it may be helpful to develop simple tools for primary care to assist clinicians in identifying patients who report few symptoms but who should have their treatment stepped up and patients with frequent symptoms who should have further investigations or whose treatment should be reduced or modified. For example:

- Patients with asthma who continue to smoke may be considered for treatment with higher ICS doses[92] or a leukotriene receptor antagonist.[93]
- Patients with frequent β_2-agonist use may benefit from breathing exercises[94] or transfer to an alternative bronchodilator.[60]

Improve the Control Algorithm

More frequent control-based adjustments

Current control-based guidelines recommend that maintenance treatment should be reviewed at intervals of approximately 1 to 3 months. More frequent adjustment of inhaled controller medication may possibly lead to improved outcomes and may be better matched to patient preferences.[40] This concept is supported by 2 approaches to patient-driven control-based management that have been evaluated in recent years.

- The first approach is the prescription of ICS and rapid-acting LABA both as a low-dose maintenance treatment, which is adjusted at intervals by the clinician according to asthma control in the conventional manner, and as reliever medication, which is adjusted by patients in response to asthma symptoms. This regimen is incorporated into asthma guidelines as one option for patients whose asthma is inadequately controlled on step 2 therapy (low-dose ICS). Compared with conventional maintenance therapy, this strategy with low-dose budesonide/formoterol leads to similar or better levels of current asthma control, together with reduced exacerbation rates or lower ICS doses.[95,96] The reduction in exacerbation rates relative to overall ICS dose, including during reported colds,[97] may be related to more frequent adjustments of ICS/LABA dose.
- The second approach is again driven by patients, this time using weekly ACQ.[83] Van der Meer and colleagues[98] showed that asthma education with an internet-based algorithm for monthly patient-driven adjustment of controller medication,

led to improved asthma control and lung function and similar exacerbation rates compared with usual care.

Clarify the role of spirometry

Some, but not all, control assessment tools include the assessment of lung function.

- Lung function is 1 of 5 criteria in the GINA[8] and National Asthma Education and Prevention Program Expert Panel Report 3 (EPR3)[9] control classifications (GINA: FEV_1 [or peak expiratory flow]: $\geq$80% or <80% predicted or best; EPR3: >80%, 60%–80%, and <60% predicted or best).
- In the ACQ,[83] prebronchodilator FEV_1 is equally weighted with 6 symptom-related components. At a population level, the inclusion of FEV_1 in ACQ does not add significantly to the assessment of asthma control.[99]

Spirometry correlates poorly with symptom-based measures of asthma control,[100] so it may be more useful in asthma monitoring as an independent measure both for identifying patients at risk of exacerbations[101] and, when discordant with symptoms, by alerting the clinician to the possibility of alternative diagnoses.

Research to Improve Control-Based Management

Research is essential to improve the quality of asthma care. Further research will provide opportunities to improve asthma outcomes, particularly in primary care where most asthma is managed and where effective, efficient, and low-cost treatment is an important goal.

Carry out pragmatic research in community-based populations

Clinical practice guidelines for asthma are based largely on regulatory studies, with rigorous inclusion/exclusion criteria and a closely monitored environment. However, the generalizability of these studies is limited because a median of only 4% (range 0%–36%) of community patients with doctor-diagnosed asthma and variable airflow limitation would meet the eligibility criteria for major clinical asthma trials.[11] To clarify the role of control-based management, further research is needed in broad community-based populations. Pragmatic study designs can also markedly improve generalizability without sacrificing quality.[102]

Investigate cut points for control-based management

The schemas for control-based management were developed from consensus, and further research is needed to clarify the most appropriate control cut points for changing treatment[103] because repeated application of any guideline or algorithm with inappropriate cut points will magnify problems regardless of the treatment approach.[23] At present, a step-up is considered if asthma is "Partly Controlled" (GINA,[8]) or "Not Well Controlled" (EPR3,[9]); but in a retrospective analysis, the average ACQ score for patients with Partly Controlled asthma was 0.75,[104] a level at which most physicians would not increase asthma treatment.[105]

Analyze responder variation

In the past, the analysis of clinical trial results was often limited to group mean responses and these formed the basis for treatment guidelines on the assumption that they would be relevant to most patients. However, this approach often concealed substantial heterogeneity in individual responses.[12] Progress can be made through analysis of variation in response in asthma studies using simple baseline characteristics, such as age, gender, lung function, atopy, and smoking status, as well as more specialized biomarkers.[14]

For research about responder analysis to be reliable, it should be planned prospectively, and standardized measures should be recorded for all patients at baseline.[21] Utility for primary care is improved by examining the predictive ability of simple and deep phenotyping and in broad rather than highly selected populations.

Identify patients for whom control-based management is not appropriate

The identification of phenotypic clusters of patients with different treatment responses is one of the most exciting areas of asthma research at present because it provides the potential for better customization of asthma management and greater efficiency in the use of health resources. Although several randomized controlled trials have demonstrated better outcomes, a lower risk of side effects, or lower costs with phenotype-guided treatment compared with control-guided treatment, even the most enthusiastic supporters do not expect that this approach will be appropriate or necessary for all patients and all health care settings. For example, sputum-guided treatment was most effective in patients for whom symptoms were not a reliable indicator of eosinophilic inflammation; such discordance was found in about 60% of patients with treatment-resistant asthma recruited from secondary care but only about 15% of patients recruited from primary care.[35] Similar analysis is needed with other large databases to identify patients for whom control-based treatment would be appropriate and those for whom referral for phenotype-guided treatment would be more effective and efficient. Recently-published guidelines suggest that FeNO may be particularly useful in managing patients with respiratory symptoms due to comorbidities such as anxiety.[106]

Develop practical tools for patient-centered implementation of asthma care

As already reported, asthma outcomes have improved substantially compared with usual care when control-based management is actively implemented in clinical practice. This finding suggests that, in parallel with the research described previously, more work is needed to improve the dissemination and implementation of asthma guidelines within primary care.

Clinicians are more likely to adopt guidelines when the recommendations are clearly presented and explained, when they are integrated into existing practice routines and software, and when system barriers are addressed.[107,108] Patients are more likely to be adherent with the resulting treatment recommendations when they understand the reasons for treatment and are involved in the decision-making process.[32]

SUMMARY

In summary, control-based management (ie, adjusting the patient's asthma treatment upwards or downwards according to simple measures of control) has been incorporated in asthma guidelines, in concept if not in name, for the past 20 years. As a result, it is difficult to obtain evidence about its effectiveness in real life. However, when this approach has been actively disseminated and implemented, asthma outcomes have improved at a population level in both developed and developing countries. The advantages of this approach include its simplicity and feasibility for implementation. Its limitations include the lack of specificity of asthma symptoms; the complex role of β_2-agonist use; barriers to stepping down treatment; and the underlying assumption that, in most patients, symptoms will be concordant with eosinophilic airway inflammation and, therefore, responsive to ICS. Potential improvements include increasing the frequency of dose adjustment and use of Internet or telephone-based support. More research is needed in community-based populations to identify the patients for whom control-based management is appropriate and those for whom phenotype-guided treatment will lead to more effective and efficient treatment. The broadening of the definition of asthma control in recent years to include an assessment of future risk, independent of the patient's level of symptoms, provides a mechanism for incorporating feasible elements of phenotype-guided treatment into control-based asthma management.

ACKNOWLEDGMENTS

The contribution of D. Robin Taylor to the discussion of these concepts is appreciated.

REFERENCES

1. National Asthma Education Program. Expert panel report on diagnosis and management of asthma. Washington, DC: National Institutes of Health. NIH Publication No. 92–2113a; 1992.
2. Woolcock A, Rubinfeld AR, Seale JP, et al. Thoracic Society of Australia and New Zealand. Asthma management plan, 1989. Med J Aust 1989;151(11–12): 650–3.
3. Juniper EF, Kline PA, Vanzieleghem MA, et al. Effect of long-term treatment with an inhaled corticosteroid (budesonide) on airway hyperresponsiveness and clinical asthma in nonsteroid-dependent asthmatics. Am Rev Respir Dis 1990; 142:832–6.
4. Toogood JH, Lefcoe NM, Haines DS, et al. A graded dose assessment of the efficacy of beclomethasone dipropionate aerosol for severe chronic asthma. J Allergy Clin Immunol 1977;59(4):298–308.
5. Busse WW, Chervinsky P, Condemi J, et al. Budesonide delivered by Turbuhaler® is effective in a dose-dependent fashion when used in the treatment of adult patients with chronic asthma [Erratum appears in J Allergy Clin Immunol 1998;102:511]. J Allergy Clin Immunol 1998;101:457–63.
6. Fitzpatrick MF, Mackay T, Driver H, et al. Salmeterol in nocturnal asthma: a double blind, placebo controlled trial of a long acting inhaled beta 2 agonist. BMJ 1990; 301(6765):1365–8.
7. Juniper EF, Kline PA, Vanzieleghem MA, et al. Reduction of budesonide after a year of increased use: a randomized controlled trial to evaluate whether improvements in airway responsiveness and clinical asthma are maintained. J Allergy Clin Immunol 1991;87:483–9.
8. Global Initiative for Asthma. Global strategy for asthma management and prevention. 2011. Available at: www.ginasthma.com. Accessed July 1, 2012.
9. National Heart Lung and Blood Institute National Asthma Education and Prevention Program. Expert panel report 3: guidelines for the diagnosis and management of asthma. 2007. Available at: http://www.nhlbi.nih.gov/guidelines/asthma/asthgdln.htm. Accessed July 1, 2012.
10. British Thoracic Society, Scottish Intercollegiate Guidelines Network. British guideline on the management of asthma. 2011. Available at: http://www.brit-thoracic.org.uk/guidelines/asthma-guidelines.aspx. Accessed December 1, 2011.
11. Travers J, Marsh S, Williams M, et al. External validity of randomised controlled trials in asthma: to whom do the results of the trials apply? Thorax 2007;62(3): 219–23.
12. Malmstrom K, Rodriguez-Gomez G, Guerra J, et al. Oral montelukast, inhaled beclomethasone, and placebo for chronic asthma. A randomized, controlled trial. Montelukast/beclomethasone study group. Ann Intern Med 1999;130(6):487–95.

13. Szefler SJ, Martin RJ, King TS, et al. Significant variability in response to inhaled corticosteroids for persistent asthma. J Allergy Clin Immunol 2002;109(3): 410–8.
14. Szefler SJ, Martin RJ. Lessons learned from variation in response to therapy in clinical trials. J Allergy Clin Immunol 2010;125(2):285–92.
15. Gibson PG, Powell H, Ducharme FM. Differential effects of maintenance long-acting beta-agonist and inhaled corticosteroid on asthma control and asthma exacerbations. J Allergy Clin Immunol 2007;119(2):344–50.
16. Pavord ID, Brightling CE, Woltmann G, et al. Non-eosinophilic corticosteroid unresponsive asthma. Lancet 1999;353(9171):2213–4.
17. Berry M, Morgan A, Shaw DE, et al. Pathological features and inhaled cortico-steroid response of eosinophilic and non-eosinophilic asthma. Thorax 2007; 62(12):1043–9.
18. Bel EH. Clinical phenotypes of asthma. Curr Opin Pulm Med 2004;10(1):44–50.
19. Wenzel SE. Asthma: defining of the persistent adult phenotypes. Lancet 2006; 368(9537):804–13.
20. Taylor DR, Bateman ED, Boulet LP, et al. A new perspective on concepts of asthma severity and control. Eur Respir J 2008;32:545–54.
21. Reddel HK, Taylor DR, Bateman ED, et al. An official American Thoracic Society/European Respiratory Society statement: asthma control and exacerbations: standardizing endpoints for clinical asthma trials and clinical practice. Am J Respir Crit Care Med 2009;180(1):59–99.
22. Bauman A, Antic R, Rubinfeld A, et al. "Could it be asthma?": the impact of a mass media campaign aimed at raising awareness about asthma in Australia. Health Educ Res 1993;8(4):581–7.
23. Gibson PG. Using fractional exhaled nitric oxide to guide asthma therapy: design and methodological issues for ASthma TReatment ALgorithm studies. Clin Exp Allergy 2009;39(4):478–90.
24. Australian Centre for Asthma Monitoring. Asthma in Australia 2011. Australian Institute of Health and Welfare, Canberra; 2011. Available at: www.asthmamonitoring. org. Accessed July 1, 2012.
25. Public Health Agency of Canada. Life and breath: respiratory disease in Canada. 2007. Available at: http://www.phac-aspc.gc.ca/publicat/2007/lbrdc-vsmrc/pdf/PHAC-Respiratory-WEB-eng.pdf. Accessed December 1, 2011.
26. Haahtela T, Tuomisto LE, Pietinalho A, et al. A 10 year asthma programme in Finland: major change for the better. Thorax 2006;61(8):663–70.
27. Ait-Khaled N, Enarson DA, Bencharif N, et al. Treatment outcome of asthma after one year follow-up in health centres of several developing countries. Int J Tuberc Lung Dis 2006;10(8):911–6.
28. Rabe KF, Adachi M, Lai CK, et al. Worldwide severity and control of asthma in children and adults: the global asthma insights and reality surveys. J Allergy Clin Immunol 2004;114(1):40–7.
29. Colice GL, Yu AP, Ivanova JI, et al. Costs and resource use of mild persistent asthma patients initiated on controller therapy. J Asthma 2008;45(4):293–9.
30. Zeiger RS, Schatz M, Li Q, et al. Step-up care improves impairment in uncontrolled asthma: an administrative data study. Am J Manag Care 2010;16(12): 897–906.
31. Plaza V, Cobos A, Ignacio-Garcia JM, et al. Cost-effectiveness of an intervention based on the Global INitiative for Asthma (GINA) recommendations using a computerized clinical decision support system: a physicians randomized trial. Med Clin (Barc) 2005;124(6):201–6 [in Spanish].

32. Wilson SR, Strub P, Buist AS, et al. Shared treatment decision making improves adherence and outcomes in poorly controlled asthma. Am J Respir Crit Care Med 2010;181(6):566–77.
33. Petsky HL, Kynaston JA, Turner C, et al. Tailored interventions based on sputum eosinophils versus clinical symptoms for asthma in children and adults. Cochrane Database Syst Rev 2007;2:CD005603.
34. Green RH, Brightling CE, McKenna S, et al. Asthma exacerbations and sputum eosinophil counts: a randomised controlled trial. Lancet 2002;360(9347): 1715–21.
35. Haldar P, Pavord ID, Shaw DE, et al. Cluster analysis and clinical asthma phenotypes. Am J Respir Crit Care Med 2008;178(3):218–24.
36. Petsky HL, Cates CJ, Li A, et al. Tailored interventions based on exhaled nitric oxide versus clinical symptoms for asthma in children and adults. Cochrane Database Syst Rev 2009;4:CD006340.
37. Powell H, Murphy VE, Taylor DR, et al. Management of asthma in pregnancy guided by measurement of fraction of exhaled nitric oxide: a double-blind, randomised controlled trial. Lancet 2011;378(9795):983–90.
38. Guarnaccia S, Lombardi A, Gaffurini A, et al. Application and implementation of the GINA asthma guidelines by specialist and primary care physicians: a longitudinal follow-up study on 264 children. Prim Care Respir J 2007;16(6):357–62.
39. Osman LM, McKenzie L, Cairns J, et al. Patient weighting of importance of asthma symptoms. Thorax 2001;56(2):138–42.
40. Partridge MR, van der Molen T, Myrseth SE, et al. Attitudes and actions of asthma patients on regular maintenance therapy: the INSPIRE study. BMC Pulm Med 2006;6:13.
41. Ulrik C, Backer V, Soes-Petersen U, et al. The patient's perspective: adherence or non-adherence to asthma controller therapy? J Asthma 2006;43(9):701–4.
42. Marklund B, Tunsäter A, Bengtsson C. How often is the diagnosis bronchial asthma correct? Fam Pract 1999;16(2):112–6.
43. Montnémery P, Hansson L, Lanke J, et al. Accuracy of a first diagnosis of asthma in primary health care. Fam Pract 2002;19(4):365–8.
44. Lucas AE, Smeenk FW, Smeele IJ, et al. Overtreatment with inhaled corticosteroids and diagnostic problems in primary care patients, an exploratory study. Fam Pract 2008;25(2):86–91.
45. Aaron SD, Vandemheen KL, Boulet LP, et al. Overdiagnosis of asthma in obese and nonobese adults. Can Med Assoc J 2008;179(11):1121–31.
46. Carman PG, Landau LI. Increased paediatric admissions with asthma in Western Australia–a problem of diagnosis? Med J Aust 1990;152(1):23–6.
47. O'Dowd LC, Fife D, Tenhave T, et al. Attitudes of physicians toward objective measures of airway function in asthma. Am J Med 2003;114(5):391–6.
48. Dennis SM, Zwar NA, Marks GB. Diagnosing asthma in adults in primary care: a qualitative study of Australian GPs' experiences. Prim Care Respir J 2010;19(1):52–6.
49. Gershon AS, Victor JC, Guan J, et al. Pulmonary function testing in the diagnosis of asthma: a population study. Chest 2012;141(5). 1190-0–6.
50. Dirks JF, Schraa JC, Robinson SK. Patient mislabeling of symptoms: implications for patient-physician communication and medical outcome. Int J Psychiatry Med 1982;12(1):15–27.
51. Salome CM, Reddel HK, Ware SI, et al. Effect of budesonide on the perception of induced airway narrowing in subjects with asthma. Am J Respir Crit Care Med 2002;165(1):15–21.

52. Rosi E, Stendardi L, Binazzi B, et al. Perception of airway obstruction and airway inflammation in asthma: a review. Lung 2006;184(5):251–8.

53. Halm EA, Mora P, Leventhal H. No symptoms, no asthma: the acute episodic disease belief is associated with poor self-management among inner-city adults with persistent asthma. Chest 2006;129(3):573–80.

54. Wise RA, Bartlett SJ, Brown ED, et al. Randomized trial of the effect of drug presentation on asthma outcomes: the American Lung Association Asthma Clinical Research Centers. J Allergy Clin Immunol 2009;124(3):436–44.

55. Wechsler ME, Kelley JM, Boyd IO, et al. Active albuterol or placebo, sham acupuncture, or no intervention in asthma. N Engl J Med 2011;365(2):119–26.

56. Godard P, Greillier P, Pigearias B, et al. Maintaining asthma control in persistent asthma: comparison of three strategies in a 6-month double-blind randomised study. Respir Med 2008;102(8):1124–31.

57. Reddel HK, Gibson PG, Peters MJ, et al. Down-titration from high-dose combination therapy in asthma: removal of long-acting β_2-agonist. Respir Med 2010; 104(8):1110–20.

58. Taylor DR. The beta-agonist saga and its clinical relevance: on and on it goes. Am J Respir Crit Care Med 2009;179(11):976–8.

59. Reddel H, Ware S, Marks G, et al. Differences between asthma exacerbations and poor asthma control [Erratum in Lancet 1999;353:758]. Lancet 1999; 353(9150):364–9.

60. Taylor DR, Hannah D. Management of beta-agonist overuse: why and how? J Allergy Clin Immunol 2008;122(4):836–8.

61. Taylor DR, Sears MR, Cockcroft DW. The beta-agonist controversy. Med Clin North Am 1996;80(4):719–48.

62. Calhoun WJ, Sutton LB, Emmett A, et al. Asthma variability in patients previously treated with beta2-agonists alone. J Allergy Clin Immunol 2003;112(6):1088–94.

63. Bateman ED, Bousquet J, Busse WW, et al. Stability of asthma control with regular treatment: an analysis of the Gaining Optimal Asthma controL (GOAL) study. Allergy 2008;63(7):932–8.

64. Aroni R, Goeman D, Stewart K, et al. Enhancing validity: what counts as an asthma attack? J Asthma 2004;41(7):729–37.

65. Nathan RA, Sorkness CA, Kosinski M, et al. Development of the Asthma Control Test: a survey for assessing asthma control. J Allergy Clin Immunol 2004;113(1): 59–65.

66. Yawn BP, Wollan PC, Bertram SL, et al. Asthma treatment in a population-based cohort: putting step-up and step-down treatment changes in context. Mayo Clin Proc 2007;82(4):414–21.

67. Hawkins G, McMahon AD, Twaddle S, et al. Stepping down inhaled corticosteroids in asthma: randomised controlled trial. BMJ 2003;326(7399):1115.

68. Diette GB, Patino CM, Merriman B, et al. Patient factors that physicians use to assign asthma treatment. Arch Intern Med 2007;167(13):1360–6.

69. Dirks JF, Horton DJ, Kinsman RA, et al. Patient and physician characteristics influencing medical decisions in asthma. J Asthma Res 1978;15(4):171–8.

70. Foster JM, van Sonderen E, Lee AJ, et al. A self-rating scale for patient-perceived side effects of inhaled corticosteroids. Respir Res 2006;7:131.

71. Foster JM, Smith L, Bosnic-Anticevich SZ, et al. Identifying patient-specific beliefs and behaviours for conversations about adherence in asthma. Intern Med J 2011;42(6):e136–44.

72. Hancox RJ, Souëf PL, Anderson GP, et al. Asthma - time to confront some inconvenient truths. Respirology 2010;15(2):194–201.

73. Melani AS, Bonavia M, Cilenti V, et al. Inhaler mishandling remains common in real life and is associated with reduced disease control. Respir Med 2011; 105(6):930–8.
74. Guidry GG, Brown WD, Stogner SW, et al. Incorrect use of metered dose inhalers by medical personnel. Chest 1992;101(1):31–3.
75. Basheti IA, Qunaibi E, Bosnic-Anticevich SZ, et al. Investigation of errors in accuhaler and turbuhaler technique by asthma patients and pharmacists from Jordan and Australia. Respir Care 2011;56(12):1916–23.
76. Rand CS, Nides M, Cowles MK, et al. Long-term metered-dose inhaler adherence in a clinical trial. Am J Respir Crit Care Med 1995;152:580–8.
77. Simmons MS, Nides MA, Rand CS, et al. Unpredictability of deception in compliance with physician-prescribed bronchodilator inhaler use in a clinical trial. Chest 2000;118(2):290–5.
78. Marks GB. Identifying asthma in population studies: from single entity to a multi-component approach. Eur Respir J 2005;26(1):3–5.
79. Levy ML, Quanjer PH, Booker R, et al. Diagnostic spirometry in primary care: proposed standards for general practice compliant with American Thoracic Society and European Respiratory Society recommendations: a General Practice Airways Group (GPIAG) document, in association with the Association for Respiratory Technology & Physiology (ARTP) and Education for Health. Prim Care Respir J 2009;18(3):130–47.
80. Powell H, Gibson PG. Inhaled corticosteroid doses in asthma: an evidence-based approach. Med J Aust 2003;178(5):223–5.
81. Suissa S, Ernst P, Benayoun S, et al. Low-dose inhaled corticosteroids and the prevention of death from asthma. N Engl J Med 2000;343(5):332–6.
82. International Union Against Tuberculosis and Lung Disease. Asthma Drug Facility. Available at: http://www.globaladf.org/. Accessed December 1, 2011.
83. Juniper EF, O'Byrne PM, Guyatt GH, et al. Development and validation of a questionnaire to measure asthma control. Eur Respir J 1999;14:902–7.
84. Peters SP, Jones CA, Haselkorn T, et al. Real-world Evaluation of Asthma Control and Treatment (REACT): findings from a national Web-based survey. J Allergy Clin Immunol 2007;119(6):1454–61.
85. Juniper EF, Langlands JM, Juniper BA. Patients may respond differently to paper and electronic versions of the same questionnaires. Respir Med 2009; 103(6):932–4.
86. Kosinski M, Kite A, Yang M, et al. Comparability of the Asthma Control Test telephone interview administration format with self-administered mail-out mail-back format. Curr Med Res Opin 2009;25(3):717–27.
87. Schatz M, Kosinski M, Yarlas AS, et al. The minimally important difference of the Asthma Control Test. J Allergy Clin Immunol 2009;124(4):719–23.e711.
88. Basheti IA, Reddel HK, Armour CL, et al. Improved asthma outcomes with a simple inhaler technique intervention by community pharmacists. J Allergy Clin Immunol 2007;119(6):1537–8.
89. Basheti IA, Armour CL, Bosnic-Anticevich SZ, et al. Evaluation of a novel educational strategy, including inhaler-based reminder labels, to improve asthma inhaler technique. Patient Educ Couns 2008;72(1):26–33.
90. Morisky DE, Green LW, Levine DM. Concurrent and predictive validity of a self-reported measure of medication adherence. Med Care 1986;24(1): 67–74.
91. Downer SR, Meara JG, Da Costa AC, et al. SMS text messaging improves outpatient attendance. Aust Health Rev 2006;30(3):389–96.

92. Tomlinson JE, McMahon AD, Chaudhuri R, et al. Efficacy of low and high dose inhaled corticosteroid in smokers versus non-smokers with mild asthma. Thorax 2005;60(4):282–7.

93. Lazarus SC, Chinchilli VM, Rollings NJ, et al. Smoking affects response to inhaled corticosteroids or leukotriene receptor antagonists in asthma. Am J Respir Crit Care Med 2007;175(8):783–90.

94. Slader CA, Reddel HK, Spencer LM, et al. Double-blind randomised controlled trial of two different breathing techniques in the management of asthma. Thorax 2006;61:651–6.

95. Demoly P, Louis R, Soes-Petersen U, et al. Budesonide/formoterol maintenance and reliever therapy versus conventional best practice. Respir Med 2009; 103(11):1623–32.

96. Bateman ED, Reddel HK, Eriksson G, et al. Overall asthma control: the relationship between current control and future risk. J Allergy Clin Immunol 2010;125(3): 600–8.

97. Reddel HK, Jenkins C, Quirce S, et al. Effect of different asthma treatments on risk of cold-related exacerbations. Eur Respir J 2011;38:584–93.

98. van der Meer V, Bakker MJ, van den Hout WB, et al. Internet-based self-management plus education compared with usual care in asthma: a randomized trial. Ann Intern Med 2009;151(2):110–20.

99. Juniper EF, O'Byrne PM, Roberts JN. Measuring asthma control in group studies: do we need airway calibre and rescue beta2-agonist use? Respir Med 2001;95(5):319–23.

100. Schatz M, Sorkness CA, Li JT, et al. Asthma Control Test: reliability, validity, and responsiveness in patients not previously followed by asthma specialists. J Allergy Clin Immunol 2006;117(3):549–56.

101. Osborne ML, Pedula KL, O'Hollaren M, et al. Assessing future need for acute care in adult asthmatics: the profile of asthma risk study: a prospective health maintenance organization-based study. Chest 2007;132(4):1151–61.

102. Zwarenstein M, Treweek S, Gagnier JJ, et al. Improving the reporting of pragmatic trials: an extension of the CONSORT statement. BMJ 2008;337:a2390.

103. O'Byrne PM, Reddel HK, Colice GL. A pro-con debate: does the current stepwise approach to asthma pharmacotherapy encourage over-treatment? Respirology 2010;15(4):596–602.

104. O'Byrne PM, Reddel HK, Eriksson G, et al. Measuring asthma control: a comparison of three classification systems. Eur Respir J 2010;36:269–76.

105. Juniper EF, Bousquet J, Abetz L, et al. Identifying 'well-controlled' and 'not well-controlled' asthma using the Asthma Control Questionnaire. Respir Med 2006; 100(4):616–21.

106. Dweik RA, Boggs PB, Erzurum SC, et al. American Thoracic Society Committee on Interpretation of Exhaled Nitric Oxide Levels for Clinical A: An official ATS clinical practice guideline: interpretation of exhaled nitric oxide levels (FENO) for clinical applications. Am J Respir Crit Care Med 2011;184:602–15.

107. Grol R, Dalhuijsen J, Thomas S, et al. Attributes of clinical guidelines that influence use of guidelines in general practice: observational study. BMJ 1998;317: 858–61.

108. Grol RP, Bosch MC, Hulscher ME, et al. Planning and studying improvement in patient care: the use of theoretical perspectives. Milbank Q 2007;85(1):93–138.

Occupational Asthma
New Deleterious Agents at the Workplace

Catherine Lemiere, MD, MSc[a],*, Jacques Ameille, MD[b],
Piera Boschetto, MD, PhD[c], Manon Labrecque, MD, MSc[a],
Jacques-André Pralong, MD, MSc[d]

KEYWORDS

- Occupational asthma • Irritant-induced asthma • RADS • Occupational agents
- High-molecular-weight agents • Low-molecular-weight agents • Irritant agents

KEY POINTS

- This article summarizes the main new categories of occupational agents responsible for causing occupational asthma, with and without a latency period reported in the last 10 years.
- This article also reports examples of occupational agents for which the fabrication processing or use have influenced the outcome of occupational asthma.

INTRODUCTION

Occupational asthma (OA) refers to de novo asthma or the recurrence of previously quiescent asthma (ie, asthma as a child or in the distant past that has been in remission) induced by either sensitization to a specific substance, which is termed sensitizer-induced OA, or by exposure to an inhaled irritant at work, which is termed irritant-induced OA.

More than 400 distinct agents have been documented as causing OA.[1,2] The agents responsible for OA are classically divided according to their molecular weight. High-molecular-weight (HMW) agents (>10 kDa[3]) include proteins and microorganisms of

This article originally appeared in Clinics in Chest Medicine, Volume 33, Issue 3, September 2012.

Disclosures: Catherine Lemière, Jacques Ameille, Piera Boschetto, Manon Labrecque, and Jacques-André Pralong do not have any conflict of interest in relation to this article.

[a] Chest Department, Sacré-Coeur Hospital, Montreal, 5400 Gouin Ouest, Montreal, Quebec H4J 1C5, Canada; [b] AP-HP, Unité de pathologie professionnelle, Hôpital Raymond Poincaré, Université de Versailles, 104 Boulevard Raymond Poincaré, Garches 92380, France; [c] Department of Clinical and Experimental Medicine, University of Ferrara, Via Fossato di Mortara, 64B, Ferrara 44100, Italy; [d] Research Center, Sacre-Coeur Hospital, Montreal, Université de Montréal, 5400 Gouin Ouest, Montreal, Quebec H4J 1C5, Canada

* Corresponding author. Hôpital du Sacré-Coeur de Montréal, 5400 Gouin Ouest, Montreal, Quebec H4J 1C5, Canada.

E-mail address: catherine.lemiere@umontreal.ca

http://dx.doi.org/10.1016/j.ccol.2014.09.021
2352-7986/14/$ – see front matter

animal and vegetable origins. Low-molecular-weight (LMW) agents include wood dust, drugs, metals, and other chemicals. The list of agents that cause OA is constantly growing[4] (www.asthme.cssst.qc.ca). The causes of irritant-induced asthma (IIA; OA without a latency period) are also steadily increasing.[5] Ammonia, chlorine, and sulfur dioxide are the most frequent causes of IIA.

Many agents, especially LMW agents can have both sensitizing and irritant properties. For example, isocyanates can induce OA by an immunologic mechanism but, at higher concentrations, they have been reported to induce irritant-induced asthma.[6]

Publications continue to report new causes of OA. This article reviews the new causes of sensitizer-induced OA and IIA reported in the last 10 years. It describes how interventions such as surveillance programs or changes in the fabrication process can influence the incidence of OA.

ALLERGIC OA
Newly Identified HMW Agents

HMW agents encountered at the workplace are natural proteins, derived from animal or plant sources that induce classic immunoglobulin (Ig) E–mediated sensitization after months or years of exposure.[4] HMW agents act as complete antigens and cause an allergic or immunologic asthma by producing specific IgE antibodies. Some newly recognized HMW agents that induce OA are discussed in this article.

Laboratory animals
Small animals represent a frequent cause of OA in laboratory technicians and veterinarians. Proteins excreted in urine, especially those produced by male rats, are the most potent source of sensitization.[7] A new gerbil allergen (*Meriones unguiculatus*) of 23 kDa has been identified in the gerbil urine, epithelium, hair, and airborne samples. Partial characterization of this allergen suggests that it could be a lipocalin.[8] Inhalation of bovine serum albumin (BSA) powder, commonly used in research laboratories, has been shown to cause OA and rhinitis in a laboratory worker in whom an IgE-mediated response was shown.[9] The patient had a high serum-specific IgE level to BSA, and a 66-kDa IgE-binding component was detected within the BSA extract on immunoblot analysis. During a bronchial provocation test with a BSA solution, the patient experienced severe systemic reactions, including eye itching, conjunctivitis, rhinorrhea, nasal obstructions, sneezing, shortness of breath, and bronchospasm, with a 30% decrease in forced expiratory volume in 1 second (FEV$_1$), 52% of predicted, and decreased blood pressure.

Allergens derived from flour, cereal, and vegetable matter
Cereals and flour are the oldest and most commonly identified causes of OA.[1,4] Purified wheat proteins either in natural or recombinant forms have been implicated in the pathogenesis of baker's asthma. The thaumatinlike protein and lipid transfer protein 2G were identified to be newly identified allergens associated with baker's asthma in a group of 20 patients with baker's rhinitis, asthma, or both who had positive skin-prick test reactions and specific IgE antibodies to wheat flour.[10] The recombinant wheat lipid transfer protein (Tri a 14) has also recently been recognized as a potential novel tool for the diagnosis of baker's asthma.[11] The possibility of discriminating baker's asthma, wheat-induced food allergy, and grass pollen allergy was investigated by serologic tests based on microarrayed recombinant wheat seed and grass pollen allergens.[12] Recombinant wheat flour allergens, specifically recognized by patients suffering from baker's asthma, but not from patients with food allergy to wheat or pollen allergy, were identified.

The first known case of an IgE-mediated OA to malt has been reported in a machine operator in a malt manufacturing plant.[13] Pirson and colleagues[14] described a case of a patient employed in a factory producing inulin from chicory who developed rhinoconjunctivitis and asthma to the dust of dry chicory roots. A specific inhalation challenge (SIC) with dry chicory was performed and an acute rhinoconjunctivitis and an immediate asthmatic response was seen. This case documents occupational rhinoconjunctivitis and asthma caused by IgE sensitization to inhaled chicory allergens, including one identified for the first time as a 17-kDa Bet v 1 homologous protein.

In addition, the first case of IgE-mediated occupational allergy (rhinitis and asthma) to marigold flour has been reported.[15] Marigold flour has been largely used by the food additive industry as poultry feed colorant. The sensitization was confirmed by a skin-prick test, a nasal challenge test, and specific IgE determination.

Food and fishing industry

Various foods, food additives, and contaminants have been associated with OA.[16] In the commercial fishing industry, crustaceans are the main source of sensitization, followed by mollusks and fin fish.[17] Patients who are allergic to fish can suffer asthma attacks when they breathe airborne particles from fish. Rosado and colleagues[18] described the first case of OA caused by handling and exposure to aerosolized octopus allergens in a seafood processing worker. Immunoblotting revealed IgE-binding bands of 43 and 32 kDa that likely correspond with tropomyosin (38–40 kDa) as the culprit allergen. Three workers experienced symptoms of rhinoconjunctivitis and bronchial asthma while classifying fish by size at the same fish farm.[19] Although they could eat turbot, they were sensitized to this fish probably by inhalation. Parvalbumin was identified as the causal allergen in 1 of the cases. Simultaneous type I and type IV allergic reactions (asthma and contact dermatitis) caused by occupational contact with fish parasitized by *Anisakis simplex* have been reported.[20] *A simplex* is a nematode that is a parasite of several marine organisms during its life cycle. It is known as an accidental gastrointestinal parasite in subjects who had ingested raw fish, but it has also been suggested to be the cause of allergic reactions in subjects who frequently eat or manipulate parasitized fish.

Pests and arthropods

Molds have been identified as causal agents of OA in workers exposed to coffee grounds (*Chrysonilia sitophila* [asexual state of *Neurospora sitophila*])[21,22] as well as in a pork butcher worker (dry sausage mold, *Penicillium nalgiovensis*[23]). The case of an electric power company engineer who suffered from OA caused by caddis flies (Phryganeiae) has been reported and proved by using an extract of these insects in a SIC.[24] In addition, Skousgaard and colleagues[25] pointed out that *Amblyseius californicus*, a beneficial predatory mite present in microbiological pesticides, was able to induce IgE sensitization and OA among greenhouse workers. The different agents are summarized in **Table 1**.

Key Points

- HMW act through an IgE-dependent mechanism to induce OA.
- The identification of proteins responsible for the sensitization can help to improve diagnosis and management of OA.

Table 1
Newly identified HMW agents

Agents	Allergen	Workplace	Diagnosis Tests	Symptoms	Reference
Laboratory animals					
M unguiculatus (gerbil allergen)	23 kDa protein, lipocalin?	Biologist, laboratory animals	SPT, nasal challenge and SIC	Rhinoconjunctivitis asthma	7
BSA	BSA, 66 kDa binding protein	Research laboratory	SIC	Rhinitis, asthma	8
Flour, cereals					
Flour	Thaumatinlike protein; lipid transfer protein 2G	Baker	SPT, specific IgE	Rhinitis, asthma	9
Malt	—	Malt manufacturing plant	SPT, SIC	Rhinitis, asthma, alveolitis	12
Chicory	17 kDa Bet v 1 homologous protein	Factory producing inulin from chicory	SPT, specific IgE SIC	Rhinoconjunctivitis asthma	13
Marigold flour	—	Food additive industry	SPT nasal challenge	Rhinitis, asthma	14
Food and fishing industry					
Octopus	Tropomyosin (38–40 kDa)	Seafood processing industry	SPT, specific IgE SIC	Rhinitis, asthma	17
Turbot	Parvalbumin	Fish farm	SPT, specific IgE, Serial PEF monitoring	Rhinoconjunctivitis, asthma	18
A simplex	—	Fish industry	SPT, specific IgE	Dyspnea and contact dermatitis	19
Pests and arthropods					
C sitophila (mold)	—	Coffee dispenser operators	Mycologic analysis, SPT serial PEF monitoring, specific IgE	Asthma	21
P nalgiovensis (mold)	—	Pork butcher industry	SPT; favorable outcome after removal from exposure	Asthma	22
Phryganeiae (caddis flies)	—	Electric power company engineer	SPT; SIC	Rhinoconjunctivitis, asthma	23
A californicus (mite)	—	Greenhouse workers	Specific IgE, SIC	Cutaneous rash, rhinoconjunctivitis, asthma	24

Abbreviations: PEF, peak expiratory flow; SPT, skin-prick tests.

Newly Identified LMW Agents

Given the high number of new chemicals produced each year, many workers are exposed to LMW agents (<10 kDa). They include drugs, wood dusts, metals, chemicals, and biocides. The literature reported 42 new LMW agents causing OA for the period 2000 to 2011, including 12 drugs, 11 wood species, 4 metals, 10 chemicals, and 5 biocides/fungicides.

Drugs

Antibiotics, and especially penicillin-derived antibiotics, have long been known to induce OA.[26] During recent years, several new antibiotics or their precursors have been reported as causes of OA. Choi and colleagues[27] reported the case of a man working in a pharmaceutical company and exposed to vancomycin powder. The diagnosis of OA was based on history and peak expiratory flow (PEF) monitoring. The postulated mechanism to explain OA was a direct histamine-releasing effect. Gomez-Olles and colleagues[28] reported a case of colistin-induced OA and rhinitis presenting an immediate asthmatic reaction during the SIC. A type I hypersensitivity reaction was associated with OA in workers exposed to thiamphenicol, 7-aminocephalosporanic acid (7-ACSA; an intermediate metabolite of the synthesis of ceftriaxone), and cefteram.[29–31] Two workers exposed to 7-ACSA developed an immediate asthmatic reaction but no reaction was noted when they were exposed to ceftriaxone.[29] A case of OA caused by 7-amino-3-thiomethyl-3-cephalosporanic acid confirmed by an immediate asthmatic reaction during the SIC has also been reported.[32]

Several other drug categories have been reported to cause OA. An antineoplastic drug, mitoxantrone, induced OA and rhinitis in a nurse, which was confirmed by the occurrence of a late asthmatic reaction during SIC.[33] Two cases of OA have been reported among anesthetic staff workers using sevoflurane and isoflurane,[34] 1 confirmed by a late asthmatic reaction during the SIC and the second by a positive methacholine challenge, an equivocal SIC for isoflurane, and a 14% decrease in FEV_1 after indirect exposure to sevoflurane. Klusackova and colleagues[35] reported 3 cases of OA caused by exposure to lasamide (a precursor of the diuretic furosemide) in a pharmaceutical plant; all 3 experienced an immediate asthmatic reaction during the SIC. Sastre and colleagues[36] reported a case of OA caused by 5-aminosalicylic acid (used to treat inflammatory bowel disease) with a late asthmatic reaction during the SIC. OA has been showed in a worker employed in a pharmaceutical company and exposed to aescin, the compound inducing an atypical asthmatic reaction during the SIC.[37] Drought and colleagues[38] reported 2 cases of OA caused by thiamine in cereal manufacture, the diagnosis being confirmed by late asthmatic reactions during the SIC.

Wood dusts

Most wood species reported as occupational sensitizers during the past years are exotic woods from Africa, Asia, or South America.[39–48] It is difficult to estimate the number of woodworkers exposed to such species worldwide. A recent meta-analysis of 19 studies estimated that the relative risk of developing OA in workers exposed to wood dust was 1.53 (95% confidence interval [CI] 1.25–1.87).[49] During the past 11 years, 11 new species have been reported to induce OA.[39–48] Except for sapele, the diagnosis has been confirmed by SIC showing immediate (n = 5), late (n = 3), and dual (n = 3) reactions. Specific IgE antibodies were positive for 4 wood species (cedro arana, angelim pedra, antiaris, and sapele),[39,41–43] confirming a type I allergic reaction, even if the nature of the chemical compound responsible for OA remains unknown. Specific IgG have been found in a worker exposed to falcate,[47] postulating the presence of another immune mechanism.

Metals

Metal salts are known to be respiratory sensitizers.[50] Most of them belong to the transition series. In the first series of transition metals, chromium, cobalt, and nickel are all known to induce OA.[51–53] Manganese belongs to the same series and has been reported to induce OA in a welder working in a train factory.[54] The diagnosis has been confirmed by an immediate asthmatic reaction during SIC. Iron also belongs to the first series of transition metals. Munoz and colleagues[55] reported 3 cases of OA induced by iron welding fumes. Air analysis during the SIC found a high number of metals and gases, many of them known to be respiratory irritants (such as O_3, NO_2, NO, and CO). Even if none of these components exceeded the threshold limit value in the laboratory, it is possible that they participated in the mechanism of OA. Sputum cell count analysis showed an increase in neutrophils.

In the second series of transition metals, palladium has been reported to cause OA.[56] In the same series, Merget and colleagues[57] reported a case of OA and rhinitis induced by rhodium salt and confirmed by an immediate asthmatic reaction during the SIC.

Apart from the metal salts, alloys are also known to induce OA. Hannu and colleagues[58] reported the case of a welder exposed to stellite, an alloy made of cobalt (60%), chromium (30%), tungsten, and carbon. A positive SIC confirmed the diagnosis of OA when the worker was exposed to stellite fumes but not when he was exposed to cobalt or chromium solutions. Therefore, it seems that the alloy was responsible of OA and not the individual metals, even if cobalt and chromium are known to induce OA.

Biocides and fungicides

Several biocides have been described as causes of OA. For example, glutaraldehyde[59] and chlorhexidine[60] are disinfectants frequently used in hospitals and known to be respiratory sensitizers. Two new agents used by hospital staff in endoscopic units have been reported as causes of OA, namely a peracetic acid–hydrogen peroxide mixture and orthophthalaldehyde.[61,62] Chlorine-releasing agents are another type of disinfectant commonly used in swimming pools. The role of theses agents was recently evoked in the pathogenesis of asthma in swimmers and children[63–65] but, to date, no study has produced a definite conclusion. Thickett and colleagues[66] reported the cases of 2 lifeguards and a swimming pool instructor (working in separate indoor swimming pools) who developed OA, confirmed by either SIC to nitrogen trichloride (belonging to the chloramine family) in 2 workers or by a positive poolside challenge test. Draper and colleagues[67] published 2 cases of OA in workers employed in fungicides manufacturing. They were exposed to fluazinam and chlorothalonil respectively and SIC induced late asthmatic reactions.

Various chemicals

Many different chemicals are able to induce OA. Various chemicals responsible for OA that have been identified in the last 10 years are summarized in **Table 2**.[68–77]

Key Points

- Forty-two new LMW agents have been identified in the last 10 years as causing OA.
- An effort should be made to identify agents responsible for OA to facilitate an effective prevention program.

Table 2
Newly identified LMW agents

Agents	Workplace	Diagnosis	Symptoms	Reference
Drugs				
Cefteram	Pharmaceutical company	SPT, specific IgE, SIC	Asthma	30
Colistin	Pharmaceutical company	SIC	Rhinitis, asthma	28
Vancomycin	Pharmaceutical company	PEF, histamine release test	Rhinitis, asthma	27
Lasamide and precursors	Pharmaceutical company	SIC	Rhinitis, asthma	35
Sevoflurane and isoflurane	Hospital, anesthetic staff	PEF, SIC	Rhinitis, asthma	34
Thiamphenicol	Pharmaceutical company	SPT, specific IgE, SIC	Rhinitis, asthma	31
Aescin	Pharmaceutical company	PEF, SIC	Rhinitis, asthma	37
Thiamine	Cereal manufacture	PEF, SIC	Asthma	38
7-ACSA	Pharmaceutical company	SPT, specific IgE, SIC	Rhinitis, asthma	29
7-TACA	Pharmaceutical company	SIC	Rhinitis, asthma	32
Mitoxantrone	Hospital, oncology staff	SIC	Rhinitis, asthma	33
5-ASA	Pharmaceutical company	SIC	Asthma	36
Wood Dusts				
Chengal	Carpentry	PEF, SIC	Rhinitis, asthma	44
Tali	Carpentry	PEF, SIC	Rhinitis, asthma	44
Jatoba	Carpentry	PEF, SIC	Rhinitis, asthma	46
Falcata	Wood furniture plant	Specific IgG, SIC	Asthma	47
Cedroarana	Carpentry	SPT, specific IgE, SIC	Rhinitis, asthma	42
Bethabara	Railway platform	SIC	Asthma	48
Angelim pedra	Carpentry	SPT, specific IgE, SIC	Rhinitis, asthma	39
Ipe	Wood work	SPT, SIC	Asthma	40
Antiaris	Door manufacture	SPT, specific IgE, SIC	Rhinitis, asthma	43
African cherry	Carpentry	SIC	Asthma	45
Sapele	Carpentry	Specific IgE, history	Rhinitis, asthma, dermatitis	41
Metals				
Rhodium	Electroplating plant	SPT, SIC	Rhinitis, asthma	57
Iron (fumes)	Welding	PEF, SIC	Asthma	55
Manganese	Welding	PEF, SIC	Asthma	54

(continued on next page)

Table 2
(continued)

Agents	Workplace	Diagnosis	Symptoms	Reference
Stellite	Machine manufacture	PEF, SIC	Asthma	58
Biocides and Fungicides				
PA-HP	Endoscopic unit	PEF, SIC	Rhinitis, asthma	61
Nitrogen trichloride	Swimming pool	PEF, SIC	Asthma	66
Orthophthalaldehyde	Endoscopic unit	History	Asthma, dermatitis	62
Fluazinam	Fungicides manufacture	PEF, SIC	Asthma	67
Chlorothalonil	Fungicide manufacture	PEF, SIC	Asthma	67
Various Chemicals				
Sodium disulfite	Lobster fishing	PEF, SIC	Asthma	74
Adipic acid flux	Soldering	PEF, SIC	Asthma	68
Dodecanedioic acid gel flux	Electronics company	PEF, SIC	Rhinitis, asthma	69
Tetramethrin	Insect extermination firm	SIC	Asthma	72
Uronium salts	Peptide synthesis laboratory	SPT, SIC	Rhinitis, asthma	71
Eugenol	Hairdressing salon	SIC	Rhinitis, asthma, dermatitis	75
3-Amino-5-mercapto-1,2,4-triazole	Production of herbicides	PEF	Rhinitis, asthma	70
Artificial flavor	Popcorn popping company	History	Asthma	73
Chlorendic anhydride	Mechanic work	SPT, specific IgE, PEF	Asthma, dermatitis	77
Reactive dye Synozol Red-K 3BS	Textile industry	Specific IgE, SIC	Rhinitis, asthma	76

Abbreviations: 7-ACSA, 7-aminocephalosporanic acid; 5-ASA, 5-aminosalicylic acid; PA-HP, peracetic acid-hydrogen peroxide; PEF, peak expiratory flow; SPT, skin prick tests; 7-TACA, 7-amino-3-thiomethyl-3-cephalosporanic acid.

New Processing or New Utilization of Known Sensitizers

Many new agents responsible for OA are reported annually. However, some agents have been known to cause OA for a long time but their use or processing have changed with time, inducing an increase or decrease in the number of OA cases associated with their exposure.

Latex

Evidence that natural rubber latex (NRL) was acting as an aeroallergen causing OA was first published in 1990.[78,79] During the late 1990s, latex became widely used, especially in health care settings because of the extensive use of gloves or other medical devices. This wide use of NRL has been associated with a large increase in positive NRL skin-prick tests among exposed working groups,[80–82] especially in health care settings. The number of annual new cases increased in Belgium from 1 in 1982 to 20 in 1998.[83] This increase was also reported in other countries such as Canada[84] or Germany.[85] Policies were established in the health care system for replacing powdered latex gloves (associated with a high level of airborne latex allergen) with nonpowdered gloves.[83–85] Furthermore, the protein and allergen content of NRL gloves declined in the mid to late 1990s.[86] These changes resulted in a substantial decrease in the number of cases of OA to latex[83–85,87] in the last decade. Although latex remains a potential sensitizer for causing OA, the numbers of cases seen in clinical practice have markedly decreased.

Enzymes

Proteolytic enzymes were introduced the mid-1960s in washing powder for increasing their cleaning efficacy.[88] The enzymes were proteases produced from the growth of *Bacillus subtilis*, termed subtilisins. As a results of their wide use, many reports of OA and sensitization caused by subtilisin exposure occurred.[89] Their use in a powered form was discontinued but these enzymes were reintroduced in encapsulated form. The capsulated form of the enzyme was not associated with a recurrence of OA and allergy cases. However, subtilisin started to be used in the health care setting for cleaning and/or disinfection of medical instruments. A first case report of OA caused by subtilisin in a health care worker was published in 1996.[90] More recently, 2 cases of OA and 4 other cases of possible OA or rhinitis associated with the use of detergent enzymes for cleaning medical instruments were reported in health care settings.[91] The use of enzymes as cleaning agents should be monitored and considered as a potential cause of OA or allergy.

Isocyanates

Isocyanates have been the leading cause of OA caused by LMW agents for many years. There have been efforts to lower and monitor the threshold of exposures to isocyanates in the occupational environment and to improve protective measures for workers, such as efficient respirators. Efficient surveillance programs have been implemented.[92] Although isocyanates remain one of the most frequent LMW agents causing OA, there has been a decrease of the number of OA cases caused by isocyanates compared with the late 1980s. In Ontario, there has been a substantial decrease in the number of cases of OA caused by isocyanates in the late 1990s,[93] which is likely to be caused by the implementation of surveillance programs.

Key Point

- The change in the fabrication processing of occupational agents or the implementation of effective surveillance programs can influence and improve the outcome of OA.

IIA

IIA encompasses a spectrum of clinical presentations. The most typical form is represented by reactive airways dysfunction syndrome (RADS),[94] which refers to a type of OA without latency and immunologic sensitization, occurring after a single massive irritant exposure, causing severe airway injury and resulting in persistent airway inflammation and nonspecific bronchial hyperresponsiveness (NSBH). Comprehensive lists of agents associated with RADS have been published.[95] The 7 most frequently reported agents for work-related RADS were, in decreasing order: cleaning materials; chemicals not otherwise specified (NOS); chlorine; solvents NOS; acids, bases, oxidizers NOS, smoke NOS; and diesel exhaust.[96]

In many cases, onset of asthma is not sudden and follows repeated low-dose exposure to 1 or more bronchial irritants. Various names have been proposed for this phenotype of IIA: low-dose RADS,[97] not-so-sudden IIA,[98] and low-intensity chronic exposure dysfunction syndrome (LICEDS).[2,95] The role of repeated exposure to occupational irritants in the pathogenesis of new-onset asthma has been shown or suggested by several epidemiologic studies or case reports.[95] These publications particularly concern workers exposed to chlorine gas in pulp mills and paper mills; meat wrappers; workers exposed to formaldehyde; aluminum smelters exposed to pot fume emissions containing gaseous fluorides, hydrofluoric acid, and sulfur dioxide (potroom asthma); or workers exposed to machining fluids.

More recently, the hypothesis of asthma induced by recurrent episodes of irritant gas exposure has been supported by an epidemiologic study showing that the incidence of adult-onset, physician-diagnosed asthma among sulfite mill workers reporting SO_2 gassing was 6.2 per 1000 person years, compared with 1.9 per 1000 person years among subjects not exposed to SO_2 and any gassing (hazard ratio 4.0, 95% CI 2.1–7.7).[99] However, the pathophysiologic mechanisms leading to IIA seem to be different from OA. For example, a single exposure to those irritants at low concentration does not induce an acute asthmatic reaction.

In the last 10 years, the most important findings concerning IIA and its causal agents have come from studies that described the health problems observed in rescue and recovery workers following the terrorist attack on the World Trade Center (WTC), and from additional data on OA in cleaners.

The WTC Tragedy and the Onset of IIA

It has been estimated that more than 50,000 people worked on the rescue and recovery effort that followed destruction of the WTC on September 11, 2001, including first responders such as firefighters, police officers, and paramedics but also operating engineers, iron workers, railway tunnel workers, telecommunication workers, and sanitation workers. WTC rescue and recovery workers were exposed to a complex mix of airborne contaminants. Collapse of the towers pulverized building materials and created a dense cloud of dust that was found to consist predominantly of coarse particles and contained cement, glass fibers, asbestos, lead, polycyclic aromatic hydrocarbons, polychlorinated biphenyls, and polychlorinated furans and dioxins.[100] The WTC dust was highly alkaline (pH 9.0–11.0) and consequently irritant. Despite most particles being greater than 10 μm in diameter, the dust burden on day 1 was so high that a substantial number of particles in the respirable range was present and inhaled into the small airways, as shown by induced sputum analysis in firefighters exposed to WTC dust.[10,101] Prezant and colleagues[102] investigated the incidence of severe cough and NSBH in firefighters in the first 6 months after the WTC collapse, according to the level of exposure to WTC dust. Severe cough, defined as persistent cough that developed after exposure to the site, and accompanied by respiratory symptoms severe enough to require medical leave for at least 4 weeks, named WTC cough, occurred in 128 of 1636 (8%) firefighters who arrived at the scene during the collapse, on the morning of September 11, 2001 (high level of exposure); 187 of 6958 (3%) firefighters with moderate level of exposure (arrival after the collapse but within the first 2 days); and 17 of 1320 (1%) firefighters with a low level of exposure (arrival between days 3 and 7). A provocative concentration of methacholine inducing a 20% fall in FEV1 which is less than 16 mg/mL was found in 47 (24%) of 196 firefighters with WTC cough who performed a methacholine challenge test. The time of arrival at the WTC site predicted the presence of NSBH and the incidence of WTC cough. NSBH was found in about one-quarter of the firefighters with a high level of exposure, whether or not they had WTC cough. One month after the WTC tragedy, the prevalence of NSBH was much higher in the exposed firefighters (24.6%) compared with a control group of firefighters who were absent from the WTC site for at least the first 2 weeks (3.6%).[103]

There is evidence that RADS may be an outcome of injury by inorganic particulates.[104] Two recently published longitudinal studies have shown high cumulative incidence of asthma in subjects exposed to WTC dust.[105,106] The prolonged increased incidence of asthma after the WTC collapse is in accordance with clinician observations that the onset of asthma symptoms in many cases was slow, without a complete clinical expression until several months after leaving the WTC site.[18]

Cleaning Activities and IIA

Cleaners represent a significant proportion of workers in all industrialized countries, with diverse jobs ranging from domestic cleaning to cleaning offices, plants, and kitchens. Professional cleaners have emerged, in the last 10 years, as one of the high-risk groups for work-related asthma in industrialized nations.[95,107] The main airway irritants in cleaning products are bleach (sodium hypochlorite), hydrochloric acid, and alkaline agents (ammonia and sodium hydroxide), which are commonly mixed together.[108] Recent studies have suggested that respiratory irritants probably play a key role in the increased risk of asthma among cleaners.[109,110]

Key Points

- Exposure to inorganic particulates can induce various forms of occupational IIA (RADS and LICEDS).
- In cleaners, RADS seems to be predominantly related to inappropriate mixtures of bleach with either hydrochloric acid or ammonia, leading to the release of large amounts of chlorine gas or chloramines, respectively.
- Cleaning workers may also have an increased risk of new-onset asthma caused by prolonged low-to-moderate exposure to respiratory irritants.

SUMMARY

Many occupational agents can potentially cause OA through different pathophysiologic mechanisms. The list of those agents is constantly growing. The causal agent of OA should be identified because effective interventions can be implemented in the workplace. As shown with the examples of latex or isocyanates, appropriate changes in the fabrication process, or effective measures of prevention, can substantially decrease the incidence of OA.

REFERENCES

1. Malo J, Chan-Yeung M. Agents causing occupational asthma with key references. In: Bernstein IL, Chan-Yeung M, Malo JL, et al, editors. Asthma in the workplace. New York: Taylor & Francis; 2006. p. 825–66.
2. Tarlo SM, Balmes J, Balkissoon R, et al. Diagnosis and management of work-related asthma: American College Of Chest Physicians Consensus Statement. Chest 2008;134(Suppl 3):1S–41S.

3. Dykewicz MS. Occupational asthma: current concepts in pathogenesis, diagnosis, and management. J Allergy Clin Immunol 2009;123(3):519–28 [quiz: 29–30].

4. Malo JL, Chan-Yeung M. Agents causing occupational asthma. J Allergy Clin Immunol 2009;123(3):545–50.

5. Lemière C, Malo J, Gautrin D. Nonsensitizing causes of occupational asthma. Med Clin North Am 1996;80:749–74.

6. Leroyer C, Perfetti L, Cartier A, et al. Can reactive airways dysfunction syndrome (RADS) transform into occupational asthma due to "sensitisation" to isocyanates? Thorax 1998;53:152–3.

7. Smith AM, Bernstein D. Occupational allergens. Clin Allergy Immunol 2008;21: 261–71.

8. de las Heras M, Cuesta-Herranz J, Cases B, et al. Occupational asthma caused by gerbil: purification and partial characterization of a new gerbil allergen. Ann Allergy Asthma Immunol 2010;104(6):540–2.

9. Choi GS, Kim JH, Lee HN, et al. Occupational asthma caused by inhalation of bovine serum albumin powder. Allergy Asthma Immunol Res 2009;1(1):45–7.

10. Lehto M, Airaksinen L, Puustinen A, et al. Thaumatin-like protein and baker's respiratory allergy. Ann Allergy Asthma Immunol 2010;104(2):139–46.

11. Palacin A, Varela J, Quirce S, et al. Recombinant lipid transfer protein Tri a 14: a novel heat and proteolytic resistant tool for the diagnosis of baker's asthma. Clin Exp Allergy 2009;39(8):1267–76.

12. Constantin C, Quirce S, Poorafshar M, et al. Micro-arrayed wheat seed and grass pollen allergens for component-resolved diagnosis. Allergy 2009;64(7): 1030–7.

13. Miedinger D, Malo JL, Cartier A, et al. Malt can cause both occupational asthma and allergic alveolitis. Allergy 2009;64(8):1228–9.

14. Pirson F, Detry B, Pilette C. Occupational rhinoconjunctivitis and asthma caused by chicory and oral allergy syndrome associated with bet v 1-related protein. J Investig Allergol Clin Immunol 2009;19(4):306–10.

15. Lluch-Perez M, Garcia-Rodriguez RM, Malet A, et al. Occupational allergy caused by marigold (*Tagetes erecta*) flour inhalation. Allergy 2009;64(7): 1100–1.

16. Cartier A. The role of inhalant food allergens in occupational asthma. Curr Allergy Asthma Rep 2010;10(5):349–56.

17. Lucas D, Lucas R, Boniface K, et al. Occupational asthma in the commercial fishing industry: a case series and review of the literature. Int Marit Health 2010;61(1):13–6.

18. Rosado A, Tejedor MA, Benito C, et al. Occupational asthma caused by octopus particles. Allergy 2009;64(7):1101–2.

19. Perez Carral C, Martin-Lazaro J, Ledesma A, et al. Occupational asthma caused by turbot allergy in 3 fish-farm workers. J Investig Allergol Clin Immunol 2010; 20(4):349–51.

20. Barbuzza O, Guarneri F, Galtieri G, et al. Protein contact dermatitis and allergic asthma caused by *Anisakis simplex*. Contact Dermatitis 2009;60(4):239–40.

21. Heffler E, Nebiolo F, Pizzimenti S, et al. Occupational asthma caused by *Neurospora sitophila* sensitization in a coffee dispenser service operator. Ann Allergy Asthma Immunol 2009;102(2):168–9.

22. Francuz B, Yera H, Geraut L, et al. Occupational asthma induced by *Chrysonilia sitophila* in a worker exposed to coffee grounds. Clin Vaccine Immunol 2010; 17(10):1645–6.

23. Talleu C, Delourme J, Dumas C, et al. Allergic asthma due to sausage mould. Rev Mal Respir 2009;26(5):557–9 [in French].
24. Miedinger D, Cartier A, Lehrer SB, et al. Occupational asthma to caddis flies (Phryganeiae). Occup Environ Med 2010;67(7):503.
25. Skousgaard SG, Thisling T, Bindslev-Jensen C, et al. Occupational asthma caused by the predatory beneficial mites *Amblyseius californicus* and *Amblyseius cucumeris*. Occup Environ Med 2010;67(4):287.
26. Diaz Angulo S, Szram J, Welch J, et al. Occupational asthma in antibiotic manufacturing workers: case reports and systematic review. J Allergy (Cairo) 2011;2011:365683.
27. Choi GS, Sung JM, Lee JW, et al. A case of occupational asthma caused by inhalation of vancomycin powder. Allergy 2009;64(9):1391–2.
28. Gomez-Olles S, Madrid-San Martin F, Cruz MJ, et al. Occupational asthma due to colistin in a pharmaceutical worker. Chest 2010;137(5):1200–2.
29. Park HS, Kim KU, Lee YM, et al. Occupational asthma and IgE sensitization to 7-aminocephalosporanic acid. J Allergy Clin Immunol 2004;113(4):785–7.
30. Suh YJ, Lee YM, Choi JH, et al. Heterogeneity of IgE response to cefteram pivoxil was noted in 2 patients with cefteram-induced occupational asthma. J Allergy Clin Immunol 2003;112(1):209–10.
31. Ye YM, Kim HM, Suh CH, et al. Three cases of occupational asthma induced by thiamphenicol: detection of serum-specific IgE. Allergy 2006; 61(3):394–5.
32. Pala G, Pignatti P, Perfetti L, et al. Occupational asthma and rhinitis induced by a cephalosporin intermediate product: description of a case. Allergy 2009; 64(9):1390–1.
33. Walusiak J, Wittczak T, Ruta U, et al. Occupational asthma due to mitoxantrone. Allergy 2002;57(5):461.
34. Vellore AD, Drought VJ, Sherwood-Jones D, et al. Occupational asthma and allergy to sevoflurane and isoflurane in anaesthetic staff. Allergy 2006;61(12): 1485–6.
35. Klusackova P, Lebedova J, Pelclova D, et al. Occupational asthma and rhinitis in workers from a lasamide production line. Scand J Work Environ Health 2007; 33(1):74–8.
36. Sastre J, Garcia del Potro M, Aguado E, et al. Occupational asthma due to 5-aminosalicylic acid. Occup Environ Med 2010;67(11):798–9.
37. Munoz X, Culebras M, Cruz MJ, et al. Occupational asthma related to aescin inhalation. Ann Allergy Asthma Immunol 2006;96(3):494–6.
38. Drought VJ, Francis HC, Mc LNR, et al. Occupational asthma induced by thiamine in a vitamin supplement for breakfast cereals. Allergy 2005;60(9): 1213–4.
39. Alday E, Gomez M, Ojeda P, et al. IgE-mediated asthma associated with a unique allergen from *Angelim pedra* (*Hymenolobium petraeum*) wood. J Allergy Clin Immunol 2005;115(3):634–6.
40. Algranti E, Mendonca EM, Ali SA, et al. Occupational asthma caused by Ipe (*Tabebuia* spp) dust. J Investig Allergol Clin Immunol 2005;15(1):81–3.
41. Alvarez-Cuesta C, Gala Ortiz G, Rodriguez Diaz E, et al. Occupational asthma and IgE-mediated contact dermatitis from sapele wood. Contact Dermatitis 2004;51(2):88–98.
42. Eire MA, Pineda F, Losada SV, et al. Occupational rhinitis and asthma due to cedroarana (*Cedrelinga catenaeformis* Ducke) wood dust allergy. J Investig Allergol Clin Immunol 2006;16(6):385–7.

43. Higuero NC, Zabala BB, Villamuza YG, et al. Occupational asthma caused by IgE-mediated reactivity to *Antiaris* wood dust. J Allergy Clin Immunol 2001; 107(3):554–6.
44. Lee LT, Tan KL. Occupational asthma due to exposure to chengal wood dust. Occup Med (Lond) 2009;59(5):357–9.
45. Obata H, Dittrick M, Chan H, et al. Occupational asthma due to exposure to African cherry (Makore) wood dust. Intern Med 2000;39(11):947–9.
46. Quirce S, Parra A, Anton E, et al. Occupational asthma caused by tali and jatoba wood dusts. J Allergy Clin Immunol 2004;113(2):361–3.
47. Tomioka K, Kumagai S, Kameda M, et al. A case of occupational asthma induced by falcata wood (*Albizia falcataria*). J Occup Health 2006;48(5):392–5.
48. Yacoub MR, Lemiere C, Labrecque M, et al. Occupational asthma due to bethabara wood dust. Allergy 2005;60(12):1544–5.
49. Perez-Rios M, Ruano-Ravina A, Etminan M, et al. A meta-analysis on wood dust exposure and risk of asthma. Allergy 2010;65(4):467–73.
50. Malo JL. Occupational rhinitis and asthma due to metal salts. Allergy 2005; 60(2):138–9.
51. Gheysens B, Auwerx J, Van den Eeckhout A, et al. Cobalt-induced bronchial asthma in diamond polishers. Chest 1985;88(5):740–4.
52. Malo JL, Cartier A, Doepner M, et al. Occupational asthma caused by nickel sulfate. J Allergy Clin Immunol 1982;69(1 Pt 1):55–9.
53. Novey HS, Habib M, Wells ID. Asthma and IgE antibodies induced by chromium and nickel salts. J Allergy Clin Immunol 1983;72(4):407–12.
54. Wittczak T, Dudek W, Krakowiak A, et al. Occupational asthma due to manganese exposure: a case report. Int J Occup Med Environ Health 2008;21(1):81–3.
55. Munoz X, Cruz MJ, Freixa A, et al. Occupational asthma caused by metal arc welding of iron. Respiration 2009;78(4):455–9.
56. Daenen M, Rogiers P, Van de Walle C, et al. Occupational asthma caused by palladium. Eur Respir J 1999;13(1):213–6.
57. Merget R, Sander I, van Kampen V, et al. Occupational immediate-type asthma and rhinitis due to rhodium salts. Am J Ind Med 2010;53(1):42–6.
58. Hannu T, Piipari R, Tuppurainen M, et al. Occupational asthma due to welding fumes from stellite. J Occup Environ Med 2007;49(5):473–4.
59. Corrado OJ, Osman J, Davies RJ. Asthma and rhinitis after exposure to glutaraldehyde in endoscopy units. Hum Toxicol 1986;5(5):325–8.
60. Waclawski ER, McAlpine LG, Thomson NC. Occupational asthma in nurses caused by chlorhexidine and alcohol aerosols. BMJ 1989;298(6678):929–30.
61. Cristofari-Marquand E, Kacel M, Milhe F, et al. Asthma caused by peracetic acid-hydrogen peroxide mixture. J Occup Health 2007;49(2):155–8.
62. Fujita H, Ogawa M, Endo Y. A case of occupational bronchial asthma and contact dermatitis caused by ortho-phthalaldehyde exposure in a medical worker. J Occup Health 2006;48(6):413–6.
63. Bernard A, Nickmilder M, Voisin C. Outdoor swimming pools and the risks of asthma and allergies during adolescence. Eur Respir J 2008;32(4):979–88.
64. Bernard A, Nickmilder M, Voisin C, et al. Impact of chlorinated swimming pool attendance on the respiratory health of adolescents. Pediatrics 2009;124(4): 1110–8.
65. Goodman M, Hays S. Asthma and swimming: a meta-analysis. J Asthma 2008; 45(8):639–47.
66. Thickett KM, McCoach JS, Gerber JM, et al. Occupational asthma caused by chloramines in indoor swimming-pool air. Eur Respir J 2002;19(5):827–32.

67. Draper A, Cullinan P, Campbell C, et al. Occupational asthma from fungicides fluazinam and chlorothalonil. Occup Environ Med 2003;60(1):76–7.
68. Moore VC, Burge PS. Occupational asthma to solder wire containing an adipic acid flux. Eur Respir J 2010;36(4):962–3.
69. Moore VC, Manney S, Vellore AD, et al. Occupational asthma to gel flux containing dodecanedioic acid. Allergy 2009;64(7):1099–100.
70. Hnizdo E, Sylvain D, Lewis DM, et al. New-onset asthma associated with exposure to 3-amino-5-mercapto-1,2,4-triazole. J Occup Environ Med 2004;46(12):1246–52.
71. Vandenplas O, Hereng MP, Heymans J, et al. Respiratory and skin hypersensitivity reactions caused by a peptide coupling reagent. Occup Environ Med 2008;65(10):715–6.
72. Vandenplas O, Delwiche JP, Auverdin J, et al. Asthma to tetramethrin. Allergy 2000;55(4):417–8.
73. Sahakian N, Kullman G, Lynch D, et al. Asthma arising in flavoring-exposed food production workers. Int J Occup Med Environ Health 2008;21(2):173–7.
74. Madsen J, Sherson D, Kjoller H, et al. Occupational asthma caused by sodium disulphite in Norwegian lobster fishing. Occup Environ Med 2004;61(10):873–4.
75. Quirce S, Fernandez-Nieto M, del Pozo V, et al. Occupational asthma and rhinitis caused by eugenol in a hairdresser. Allergy 2008;63(1):137–8.
76. Jin HJ, Kim JH, Kim JE, et al. Occupational asthma induced by the reactive dye Synozol Red-K 3BS. Allergy Asthma Immunol Res 2011;3(3):212–4.
77. Keskinen H, Pfaffli P, Pelttari M, et al. Chlorendic anhydride allergy. Allergy 2000;55(1):98–9.
78. Baur X, Jager D. Airborne antigens from latex gloves. Lancet 1990;335(8694):912.
79. Lagier F, Badier M, Charpin D, et al. Latex as aeroallergen. Lancet 1990;2:516–7.
80. Lagier F, Vervloet D, Lhermet I, et al. Prevalence of latex allergy in operating room nurses. J Allergy Clin Immunol 1992;90:319–22.
81. Liss G, Sussman G, Deal K, et al. Latex allergy: epidemiological study of 1351 hospital workers. Occup Environ Med 1997;54:335–42.
82. Vandenplas O. Occupational asthma caused by natural rubber latex. Eur Respir J 1995;8:1957–65.
83. Vandenplas O, Larbanois A, Vanassche F, et al. Latex-induced occupational asthma: time trend in incidence and relationship with hospital glove policies. Allergy 2009;64(3):415–20.
84. Liss G, Tarlo S. Natural rubber latex-related occupational asthma: association with interventions and glove changes over time. Am J Ind Med 2001;40:347–53.
85. Latza U, Haamann F, Baur X. Effectiveness of a nationwide interdisciplinary preventive programme for latex allergy. Int Arch Occup Environ Health 2005;78:394–402.
86. Sussman G, Liss G, Deal K, et al. Incidence of latex sensitization among latex glove users. J Allergy Clin Immunol 1998;101:171–8.
87. Turjanmaa K, Kanto M, Kautiainen H, et al. Long-term outcome of 160 adult patients with natural rubber latex allergy. J Allergy Clin Immunol 2002;110(Suppl 2):S70–4.
88. Hole A, Draper A, Jolliffe G, et al. Occupational asthma caused by bacillary amylase used in the detergent industry. Occup Environ Med 2000;57:840–2.
89. Pepys J, Longbottom J, Hargreave F, et al. Allergic reactions of the lungs to enzymes of *Bacillus subtilis*. Lancet 1969;1:1811–4.

90. Lemière C, Cartier A, Dolovich J, et al. Isolated late asthmatic reaction after exposure to a high-molecular-weight occupational agent, subtilisin. Chest 1996;110:823–4.

91. Adisesh A, Murphy E, Barber CM, et al. Occupational asthma and rhinitis due to detergent enzymes in healthcare. Occup Med (Lond) 2011;61(5):364–9.

92. Labrecque M, Malo JL, Alaoui KM, et al. Medical surveillance programme for diisocyanate exposure. Occup Environ Med 2011;68(4):302–7.

93. Buyantseva LV, Liss GM, Ribeiro M, et al. Reduction in diisocyanate and non-diisocyanate sensitizer-induced occupational asthma in Ontario. J Occup Environ Med 2011;53(4):420–6.

94. Brooks S, Weiss M, Bernstein I. Reactive airways dysfunction syndrome (RADS). Persistent asthma syndrome after high level irritant exposures. Chest 1985;88:376–84.

95. Gautrin D, Bernstein I, Brooks S, et al. Reactive airways dysfunction syndrome and irritant-induced asthma. In: Bernstein IL, Chan-Yeung M, Malo JL, et al, editors. Asthma in the workplace. 3rd edition. New York: Taylor & Francis; 2006. p. 579–627.

96. Henneberger P, Derk S, Davis L, et al. Work-related reactive airways dysfunction syndrome cases from surveillance in selected US States. J Occup Environ Med 2003;45:360–8.

97. Kipen H, Blume R, Hutt D. Occupational and environmental Medicine Clinic. Low-dose reactive airways dysfunction syndrome. J Occup Med 1994;36:1133–7.

98. Brooks S, Hammad Y, Richards I, et al. The spectrum of irritant-induced asthma. Chest 1998;113:42–9.

99. Andersson E, Knutsson A, Hagberg S, et al. Incidence of asthma among workers exposed to sulphur dioxide and other irritant gases. Eur Respir J 2006;27:720–5.

100. Landrigan PJ, Lioy PJ, Thurston G, et al. Health and environmental consequences of the World Trade Center disaster. Environ Health Perspect 2004;112(6):731–9.

101. Fireman EM, Lerman Y, Ganor E, et al. Induced sputum assessment in New York City firefighters exposed to World Trade Center dust. Environ Health Perspect 2004;112(15):1564–9.

102. Prezant D, Weiden M, Banauch G, et al. Cough and bronchial responsiveness in firefighters at the World Trade Center site. N Engl J Med 2002;347:806–15.

103. Banauch G, Alleyne D, Sanchez R, et al. Persistent hyperreactivity and reactive airway dysfunction syndrome in firefighters at the World Trade Center. Am J Respir Crit Care Med 2003;168:54–62.

104. Nemery B. Reactive fallout of World Trade Center dust. Am J Respir Crit Care Med 2003;168(1):2–3.

105. Brackbill RM, Hadler JL, DiGrande L, et al. Asthma and posttraumatic stress symptoms 5 to 6 years following exposure to the World Trade Center terrorist attack. JAMA 2009;302(5):502–16.

106. Wisnivesky JP, Teitelbaum SL, Todd AC, et al. Persistence of multiple illnesses in World Trade Center rescue and recovery workers: a cohort study. Lancet 2011;378(9794):888–97.

107. Jaakkola J, Jaakkola M. Professional cleaning and asthma. Curr Opin Allergy Clin Immunol 2006;6:85–90.

108. Quirce S, Barranco P. Cleaning agents and asthma. J Investig Allergol Clin Immunol 2010;20(7):542–50 [quiz: 2p following 50].

109. Medina-Ramon M, Zock J, Kogevinas M, et al. Asthma, chronic bronchitis, and exposure to irritant agents in occupational domestic cleaning: a nested case-control study. Occup Environ Med 2005;62:598–606.
110. Vizcaya D, Mirabelli MC, Anto JM, et al. A workforce-based study of occupational exposures and asthma symptoms in cleaning workers. Occup Environ Med 2011;68(12):914–9.

Asthma and Obesity
The Dose Effect

Amy Manion, PhD, RN, PNP[a,b],*

KEYWORDS

- Asthma • Obesity • Dose effect

KEY POINTS

- Asthma is one of the most common chronic illnesses in the world, affecting an estimated 300 million people.
- Globally, the prevalence of asthma has continued to spread as economic improvements in developing countries create a population trend toward urbanization and adoption of a western lifestyle.
- Research supports an association between obesity and asthma.

As the populations of the world have evolved from a mainly rural, mainly agrarian society, to a more urban and industrial society, the challenges facing modern medicine have also evolved. What were once the mainstays of concern, infectious diseases, such as polio, tuberculosis, and typhoid, have now been replaced with an equally fatal, if not more insidious problem. As the new millennium begins, the high rate of mortality from infectious diseases has been replaced with chronic illnesses, such as heart disease, diabetes, and asthma.

ASTHMA

Asthma is one of the most common chronic illnesses in the world, affecting an estimated 300 million people.[1] Over the period 1980 through 1996, there was a dramatic increase in the prevalence of asthma among all ages, genders, and racial groups, especially in more urbanized nations such as the United States.[2] Currently, 24.6 million people living in the United States have been diagnosed with asthma.[3] Globally, the prevalence of asthma has continued to spread as economic improvements in

This article originally appeared in Nursing Clinics of North America, Volume 48, Issue 1, March 2013.
Funding Sources: Nil.
Conflict of Interest: Nil.
[a] Northwestern Children's Practice, Chicago, IL, USA; [b] College of Nursing, Rush University, 600 South Paulina Street, Chicago, IL 60612, USA
* Armour Academic Center, College of Nursing, Rush University, 600 South Paulina Street, 1080, Chicago, IL 60612.
E-mail address: Amy_manion@rush.edu

developing countries create a population trend toward urbanization and adoption of a western lifestyle.[4,5] Based on this urbanization trend, it has been predicted that by 2025 an additional 100 million people will be diagnosed with asthma, increasing the global impact to 400 million.[1]

There is no cure for asthma. However, it can be controlled and managed with proper treatment. The general goals of asthma therapy consist of preventing chronic asthma symptoms and exacerbations, maintaining normal levels of activity, having normal or near-normal lung function, and having minimal side effects, while receiving optimal medication management.[6] Standard treatment of asthma consists of bronchodilators to relieve airway constriction, inhaled or oral corticosteroids to control inflammation, and avoidance of asthma triggers, such as smoke and other environmental irritants.[6]

Recently, combination therapy, consisting of an inhaled long-acting β_2-agonist along with an inhaled corticosteroid, has become the center of therapy for patients with moderate or severe persistent asthma.[7] In addition, leukotriene modifiers, which can prevent bronchoconstriction at a cellular level, are being used as add-on therapy.[7]

Despite the advances in therapeutic options, the economic burden of treating asthma in the United States has been expanding at an alarming rate because of the ever-increasing number of individuals diagnosed with the disease. In 1990, total costs due to asthma were estimated to be $6.2 billion.[8] By 1998, the cost of asthma had almost doubled to $11.3 billion, with direct costs accounting for $7.5 billion and indirect costs amounting to $3.8 billion.[9] Currently, the economic burden of asthma in the United States is staggering, with direct health care costs estimated at over $50 billion and indirect costs at $5.9 billion annually.[10]

Although asthma affects people of all ages, it disproportionately affects more children than adults, especially minority and poor children.[11,12] Currently, in the United States, over 10 million children and adolescents have been diagnosed with asthma, making it the leading chronic childhood illness.[13] Since 1999, children 5 to 17 years of age have demonstrated the highest prevalence rates with 109.3 per 1000 diagnosed with asthma, compared with 76.8 per 1000 in those over 18 years of age.[10] In 2009, the Centers for Disease Control and Prevention in the United States reported asthma prevalence ratios to be higher in children with approximately 1 in 12 for adults having asthma compared with 1 in 10 children.[14] The higher prevalence of asthma among children is not restricted to the United States; it is evident worldwide, especially in other industrial countries, such as the United Kingdom, where 1 in 7 children have been diagnosed with asthma compared with 1 in 25 adults.[15]

Furthermore, besides economic and age-related disparities, significant racial inequalities exist as well, especially in the more industrialized countries with the highest numbers of asthma prevalence. For example, in the United States, the asthma rate of prevalence is 43% higher for non-Hispanic blacks compared with non-Hispanic whites.[10] Even among children, these differences are evident. An analysis using results from the National Health Interview Survey 1997 to 2003 found that rate of asthma prevalence was consistently greater among non-Hispanic black children (15.7%) compared with non-Hispanic white children (11.5%) across all levels of income.[12] In addition, non-Hispanic black children are 3.6 times more likely to use the emergency department for asthma-related issues than non-Hispanic white children.[16] Multiple asthma-related emergency department visits are considered risk factors for fatal asthma, which is reflected in the rates of asthma mortality seen among minority groups, especially African Americans.[17] In 2006, non-Hispanic blacks had a rate of asthma mortality over 200% higher than non-Hispanic whites.[18] Furthermore, from 2003 to 2005, the Centers for Disease Control and Prevention reported that African American children had a rate of asthma mortality 7 times higher than non-Hispanic white children.[19] The World Health Organization has estimated the global rate of mortality from asthma to be 250,000 people annually.[20]

OBESITY

The high global prevalence of asthma and its continued drain on medical resources make it a major cause for concern. Nevertheless, another disturbing trend in health care use has revealed itself in the past decade as millions of American waistlines have grown to uncomfortable and unhealthy sizes. The prevalence of obesity in the United States is increasing at an alarming rate. Body mass index (BMI), defined as the weight in kilograms divided by the square of the height in meters, is commonly used to classify overweight and obesity among adults.[21] In adults, a BMI between 25 and 29.9 is defined as overweight, and a BMI of 30 or higher is considered obese. For children, overweight is defined as a BMI between the 85th and 94th percentile for age and gender, and obese is defined at a BMI at or above the 95th percentile for age and gender.[21]

According to data from the 2005 to 2006 National Health and Nutrition Examination Survey (NHANES), more than one-third of adults, or over 72 million people, are obese.[22] The incidence of obesity is increasing not only in the United States but also globally. Worldwide there are more than 1.5 billion overweight adults, with at least 500 million clinically obese adults.[23] The World Health Organization has predicted that by 2015, approximately 2.3 billion adults will be overweight and over 700 million will be obese.[24]

The worldwide increase in the prevalence of obesity is especially concerning because of the multitude of health problems associated with obesity. Obese and overweight adults are at greater risk of cardiovascular disease, hypertension, stroke, type 2 diabetes, and certain forms of cancer, such as breast, pancreas, kidney, thyroid, and esophagus.[25] Approximately 85% of people with diabetes are type 2, and of these, 90% are overweight or obese.[23]

The true economic impact associated with the rise in obesity prevalence is difficult to determine due to the number of obesity-related conditions. The direct obesity-related medical costs in the United States have been estimated at $51.6 billion, whereas the indirect costs have been estimated at $47.6 billion.[26]

The increase in the prevalence of obesity in adults has been accompanied by a similar increase in the prevalence of obesity in children.[27] Furthermore, there is a strong cyclical relationship between adult and childhood obesity. For example, parental obesity more than doubles the risk of adult obesity in both obese and nonobese children.[28,29] If both parents are lean, a healthy child has a 14% chance of becoming overweight; however, if both parents are obese, the risk jumps to 80%.[30]

In the United States, the number of overweight children has doubled and the number of overweight adolescents has tripled over the last 2 decades.[31] The results from the 2003 to 2006 NHANES study showed an estimated 17% of children ages 6 to 11 years are overweight, which represents more than a 60% increase from the overweight estimates of 11% obtained from the 1988 to 1994 NHANES.[21]

The increasing prevalence of childhood overweight is not restricted to the United States alone. An estimated 22 million children under the age of 5 are considered overweight worldwide.[24] Childhood overweight is becoming prevalent even in the developing world; for example, in Thailand, the prevalence of overweight in children 5 to 12 years of age increased from 12.2% to 15.6% in just 2 years.[23]

Similar to asthma, racial and ethnic disparities exist with obesity prevalence as well. In the United States, non-Hispanic blacks have a 51% higher rate of obesity, and

Hispanics have a 21% higher rate of obesity compared with non-Hispanic whites.[32] Similar to adults, NHANES data have shown the prevalence of obesity and overweight combined to be higher in non-Hispanic black children (35.4%) compared with non-Hispanic white children (28.2%).[33] The NHANES data found Mexican American boys ages 6 to 11 to have the highest combined obesity and overweight prevalence (43.9%).[33]

ASTHMA AND OBESITY

The increase in prevalence of both asthma and obesity has led to several studies examining the possible relationship between these 2 variables. Much of the research in this area has focused on the adult population. A study examining the trends in obesity among adults, using data from the NHANES I (1971–1975), II (1976–1980), and III (1988–1994), found that BMI increased universally among adults with asthma and those without; however, the prevalence of obesity rose more in the asthma group (21.3-32.8%) compared with the nonasthma group (14.6-22.8%).[34] A retrospective study of 143 individuals ages 18 to 88 found that the prevalence of obesity increased along with increasing asthma severity.[35]

The relationship between asthma and obesity demonstrated in studies conducted with adults has also been replicated in the pediatric population. A cross-sectional study using data from the Third National Health and Nutrition Examination Survey 1988 to 1994 showed that 2 of the highest risk groups for developing asthma were children over the age of 10 with a BMI greater than or equal to the 85th percentile (overweight and obese category) and children with a parental history of asthma who were 10 years or younger and of African American ethnicity.[36] A study conducted in the United Kingdom found that obesity among children 4 to 11 years of age was associated with asthma regardless of ethnicity, especially among girls.[37] Findings from the National Longitudinal Survey of Youth, which followed more than 4000 asthma-free children for 14 years, discovered a BMI at or greater than the 85th percentile at age 2 to 3 years was a risk factor for subsequent asthma development in boys.[38]

DOSE EFFECT

Research seems to support a relationship between obesity and asthma. Obesity has proven to be a risk factor for asthma in both adults and children.[39,40] There is a growing body of evidence to support a dose effect for asthma severity with obesity; however, a causal relationship has not been proven.

The evidence of a dose effect between obesity and asthma symptoms and severity is most strongly supported by the results from research conducted with patients who have experienced weight loss. In a study of 500 morbidly obese patients who underwent laparoscopic adjustable gastric banding surgery, greater than 80% of the patients who had asthma symptoms before surgery reported resolution or improvement in their symptoms.[41] A systematic review of studies examining asthma and weight loss found there was reversibility of at least 1 asthma outcome irrespective of whether weight loss was a result of surgical or medical intervention.[42] A meta-analysis of prospective studies involving obesity and asthma risk found asthma incidence increased by 50% in overweight and obese individuals regardless of gender, demonstrating a dose-dependent relationship between obesity and asthma.[43]

The dose effect relationship between obesity and asthma has also been researched in children. A study examining non-Hispanic black and Hispanic children age 2 to 18 years with asthma found the prevalence of overweight to be higher in children with moderate to severe asthma symptoms compared with the control group.[44] A more recent study found obese children with asthma used more asthma medications, wheezed more, and had a higher number of unscheduled emergency department visits than the nonobese children with asthma.[45] A large cross-sectional study of more than 400,000 adolescents found a significantly higher likelihood of asthma diagnosis occurring at higher BMI percentiles regardless of gender and race/ethnicity, indicating a positive dose response relationship between increasing BMI and asthma risk.[46]

Internationally, the dose effect relationship between obesity and asthma has also been documented. A large Norwegian study of more than 135,000 men and women found a 10% increase in asthma prevalence per unit of increase in BMI in men and a 7% increase in prevalence per unit increase in BMI in women.[47] A study in Taiwan of greater than 15,000 school-aged children found the prevalence of asthma increased as BMI elevated and high BMI coincided with low FEV_1/FCV scores on lung function testing, which is associated with lung impairment.[48] A similar result was found in a study conducted in Nova Scotia, Canada, that examined over 3000 students 10 to 11 years of age and found a linear association between BMI and asthma with a 6% increase in prevalence per unit increase of BMI.[49]

The exact mechanism creating the dose effect seen between obesity and asthma still needs further investigation. One theory proposed, which supports the less common view that asthma causes obesity, is that individuals with asthma restrict their levels of activity for fear of inducing an asthma exacerbation, which then leads to a more sedentary lifestyle and an increased risk of obesity.[37] Although many individuals with asthma might avoid vigorous physical activity and thus put on weight, this would seem, at best, an incomplete explanation for asthma causing obesity.[50]

The reverse association, that obesity causes asthma, and is the driving force behind the dose effect seen between these diseases has the most support. Proposed theories include mechanical, dietary, genetic, and hormonal.[46,51] One main theory that has generated the most discussion is the role pro-inflammatory cytokines such as leptin play in the process because adipose tissue is known as a primary source of these systemic immunomodulating agents and could be contributing to the chronic inflammation seen in asthma, creating more symptoms of the disease.[46,52] Cytokines are already believed to play a role in exercise-induced asthma, which could lead to proposals to add similar obesity-induced asthma nomenclature to the list of asthma categories.[53]

IMPLICATIONS

Whether the relationship between obesity and asthma is direct or indirect has yet to be determined. Nevertheless, the affects of obesity on asthma are evident and need to be incorporated into the management of the disease. Because prevention is the key to combating the steady rise in obesity, weight management should be addressed at each health care visit regardless of the individual's weight. For those individuals who are overweight or obese, nutritional counseling should be provided and a follow-up plan for weight loss should be developed. The positive effects of weight loss on asthma symptoms should be shared with patients to provide motivation and encouragement. Only by making weight management a priority in the treatment of asthma can the rising prevalence of both diseases be hindered and global health improved.

REFERENCES

1. Global Initiative for Asthma (GINA). The Global Strategy for Asthma Management and Prevention. 2011. Available at: http://www.Ginasthma.org/. Accessed June 15, 2012.

2. Akinbami LJ, Moorman JE, Garbe PL, et al. Status of childhood asthma in the United States, 1980–2007. Pediatrics 2009;123(Suppl 3):S131–45.

3. Centers for Disease Control and Prevention (CDC). Vital signs: asthma prevalence, disease characteristics, and self-management education: United States, 2001-2009. MMWR Morb Mortal Wkly Rep 2011;60(17):547–52 [0149-2195].

4. Bai J, Zhao J, Shen K, et al. Current trends of the prevalence of childhood asthma in three Chinese cities: a multicenter epidemiological survey. Biomed Environ Sci 2010;23:453–7.

5. Ait-Khaled N, Enarson DA, Bissell K, et al. Access to inhaled corticosteroids is key to improving quality of care for asthma in developing countries. Allergy 2007;62:230–6.

6. National Asthma Education and Prevention Program. Expert panel report 3: Guidelines for the diagnosis and management of asthma (No. NIH publication no. 07-4051). Bethesda (MD): National Heart Lung and Blood Institute; 2007.

7. Arellano FM, Arana A, Wentworth CE, et al. Prescription patterns for asthma medications in children and adolescents with health care insurance in the United States. Pediatr Allergy Immunol 2011;22:469–76.

8. Weiss KB, Sullivan SD. The health economics of asthma and rhinitis. Assessing the economic impact. J Allergy Clin Immunol 2001;107:3–8.

9. National Heart Lung and Blood Institute. Data fact sheet: asthma statistics. 1999. Available at: http://www.nhlbi.nih.gov/health/prof/lung/asthma/asthstat. pdf. Accessed March 3, 2006.

10. American Lung Association. Trends in morbidity and mortality. 2011. Available at: www.lung.org/finding-cures/our-research/trend-reports/asthma-trend-report. pdf. Accessed August 5, 2012.

11. Flores G, The Committee on Pediatric Research. Technical report- Racial and ethnic disparities in the health and health care of children. Pediatrics 2010; 125(4):e979–1021.

12. McDaniel M, Paxson C, Waldfogel J. Racial disparities in childhood asthma in the United States: Evidence from the National Health Interview Survey, 1997 to 2003. Pediatrics 2006;117(5):868–77.

13. Bloom B, Cohen RA, Freeman G. Summary health statistics for U.S. children: National health interview survey, 2010. Vital Health Stat 10 2010;(250):1–89.

14. CDC. 2011 Asthma in the U.S., Vital Signs. 2011. Available at: http://www.cdc. gov/VitalSigns/Asthma/. Accessed August 5, 2012.

15. Braman SS. The global burden of asthma. Chest 2006;130(1):4S–12S.

16. U.S. Department of Health and Human Services, Agency for Healthcare Research and Quality, National Healthcare Quality and Disparities Reports. 2011. Available at: www.ahrq.gov/qual/qrdr11/6_maternalchildhealth/T6_4_14_ 1_1.htm. Accessed June 19, 2012.

17. Carroll CL, Uygungil B, Zucker AR, et al. Identifying an at-risk population of children with recurrent near-fatal asthma exacerbations. J Asthma 2010;47:460–4.

18. CDC. Asthma prevalence, health care use and mortality: United States, 2003-2005. 2006. Available at: http://www.cdc.gov/nchs. Accessed August 15, 2009.

19. Akinbami LJ. The state of childhood asthma, United States, 1980-2005, Advance data from vital health statistics; no. 381. Hyattsville (MD): National Center for Health Statistics; 2006.

20. World Health Organization. Global surveillance, prevention and control of chronic respiratory diseases: a comprehensive approach. Geneva, Switzerland: World Health Organization; 2007.

21. CDC. Overweight and obesity. 2012. Available at: http://www.cdc.gov/obesity/adult/defining.html. Accessed June 19, 2012.
22. Ogden CL, Carroll MD, McDowell MA, et al. Obesity among adults in the United States- no change since 2003-2004. Hyattsville (MD): National Center for Health Statistics; 2007.
23. World Health Organization. Obesity and overweight. 2011. Available at: http://www.who.int/mediacentre/factsheets/fs311/en/index.html. Accessed July 6, 2012.
24. World Health Organization. WHO: global database on body mass index. 2012. Available at: http://www.who.int/bmi/index.jsp. Accessed July 6, 2012.
25. Kopelman P. Health risks associated with overweight and obesity. Obes Rev 2007;8(Suppl 1):13-7.
26. Li Z, Bowerman S, Heber D. Health ramifications of the obesity epidemic. Surg Clin North Am 2005;85(4):681-701.
27. Maffeis C, Tato L. Long-term effects of childhood obesity on morbidity and morality. Horm Res 2001;55(Suppl 1):42-5.
28. Krebs NF, Jacobson MS, American Academy of Pediatrics Committee on Nutrition. Prevention of pediatric overweight and obesity. Pediatrics 2003;112(2):424-30.
29. Whitaker RC, Wright JA, Pepe MS, et al. Predicting obesity in young adulthood from childhood and parental obesity. N Engl J Med 1997;337(13):869-73.
30. Hagarty MA, Schmidt C, Bernaix L, et al. Adolescent obesity: Current trends in identification and management. J Am Acad Nurse Pract 2004;16(11):481-9.
31. U.S. Preventative Services Task Force. Screening and interventions for overweight in children and adolescents: recommendation statement. Pediatrics 2005;116(1):205-9.
32. CDC. Differences in prevalence of obesity among black, white, and hispanic adults-United States, 2006-2008. MMWR Morb Mortal Wkly Rep 2009;58(27):740-4.
33. Wang Y, Beydoun MA. The obesity epidemic in the United States—Gender, age socioeconomic, racial/ethnic, and geographic characteristics: A systemic review and meta-regression analysis. Epidemiol Rev 2007;29:6-28.
34. Ford ES, Mannino DM. Time trends in obesity among adults with asthma in the United States: findings from three national surveys. J Asthma 2005; 42(2):91-5.
35. Akerman MJ, Calacanis CM, Madsen MK. Relationship between asthma severity and obesity. J Asthma 2004;41(5):521-6.
36. Rodriguez MA, Winkleby MA, Ahn D, et al. Identification of population subgroups of children and adolescents with high asthma prevalence: findings from the Third National Health and Nutrition Examination Survey. Arch Pediatr Adolesc Med 2002;156(3):269-75.
37. Figueroa-Munoz JI, Chinn S, Rona RJ. Association between obesity and asthma in 4-11 year old children in the U.K. Thorax 2001;56:133-7.
38. Mannino DM, Mott J, Ferdinands JM, et al. Boys with high body masses have an increased risk of developing asthma: findings from the National Longitudinal Survey of Youth (NLSY). Int J Obes 2006;30(1):6-13.
39. Guerra S, Sherrill DL, Bobadilla A, et al. The relation of body mass index to asthma, chronic bronchitis, and emphysema. Chest 2002;122:1256-63.
40. Hjellvik V, Tverdal A, Furu K. Body mass index as predictor for asthma: a cohort study of 118, 723 males and females. Eur Respir J 2010;35(6):1235-42.

41. Spivak H, Hewitt MF, Onn A, et al. Weight loss and improvement of obesity-related illness in 500 U.S. patients following laparoscopic adjustable gastric banding procedure. Am J Surg 2005;189(1):27–32.
42. Eneli IU, Skybo T, Camargo CA Jr. Weight loss and asthma: a systematic review. Thorax 2008;63:671–6.
43. Beuther DA, Sutherland ER. Overweight, obesity, and incident of asthma. Am J Respir Crit Care Med 2007;175:661–6.
44. Luder E, Melnik TA, DiMaio M. Association of being overweight with greater asthma symptoms in inner city black and Hispanic children. J Pediatr 1998; 132(4):699–703.
45. Belamarich PF, Luder E, Kattan M, et al. Do obese inner-city children with asthma have more symptoms than nonobese children with asthma? Pediatrics 2000;106(6):1436–41.
46. Davis A, Lipsett M, Milet M, et al. An association between asthma and BMI in adolescents: results from the California Healthy Kids survey. J Asthma 2007; 44:873–9.
47. Nystad W, Meyer HE, Nafstad P, et al. Body mass index in relation to adult asthma among 135,000 Norwegian men and women. Am J Epidemiol 2004; 160:969–76.
48. Chiu YT, Chen WY, Wang TN, et al. Extreme BMI predicts higher asthma prevalence and is associated with lung function impairment in school-aged children. Pediatr Pulmonol 2009;44:472–9.
49. Sithole F, Douwes J, Burstyn I, et al. Body mass index and childhood asthma: a linear association? J Asthma 2008;45:473–7.
50. Shaneen SO. Obesity and asthma: cause for concern? Clin Exp Allergy 1999; 29(3):291–3.
51. Chin S. Obesity and asthma: evidence for and against a causal relation. J Asthma 2003;40(1):1–16.
52. Silva P, Mello M, Cheik N, et al. The role of pro-inflammatory and anti-inflammatory adipokines on exercise-induced bronchospasm in obese adolescents undergoing treatment. Respir Care 2012;57(4):572–82.
53. Hallstrand TS, Moody MW, Aitken ML, et al. Airway immunopathology of asthma with exercise-induced bronchoconstriction. J Allergy Clin Immunol 2005;116(3): 586–93.

Why Otolaryngologists and Asthma Are a Good Match
The Allergic Rhinitis-Asthma Connection

Rachel Georgopoulos, MD, John H. Krouse, MD, PhD,
Elina Toskala, MD, PhD*

KEYWORDS

• Asthma • Rhinitis • Allergy • Immunology

KEY POINTS

- In the unified airway model, the nose and the paranasal sinuses through the respiratory bronchi are considered as components of 1 functional unit.
- Rhinitis and asthma are linked epidemiologically and pathophysiologically.
- Rhinitis is not only associated with but is a risk factor for the development of asthma.
- Atopy/allergy and disease severity are important factors affecting the association between rhinitis and asthma.
- Hygiene hypothesis suggests that a lack of microbial exposures as a child may result in modification of immunity toward T helper 2 (Th_2) skewing and the increased risk for asthma and other atopic diseases.
- Proper management of allergic rhinitis can concomitantly allow better asthma control.
- In evaluating and treating patients with rhinitis, the diagnosis of asthma should be considered.
- It is important that physicians managing rhinitis/rhinosinusitis become familiar with the diagnosis and management of asthma.

INTRODUCTION

Although rhinitis and asthma are frequently comorbid conditions, physicians managing patients with rhinitis and or rhinosinusitis have traditionally not taken part in the diagnosis or management of asthma. Rhinitis, sinusitis, and asthma are linked both epidemiologically and pathophysiologically and thus the nose through the paranasal sinuses to the distal bronchioles should not be thought of as separate entities but rather constituents of 1 functional unit. This unit is referred to as the unified airway

This article originally appeared in Otolaryngologic Clinics of North America, Volume 47, Issue 1, February 2014.

Department of Otolaryngology, Temple University Health System, 3509 North Broad Street, Philadelphia, PA 19140-4105, USA

* Corresponding author.

E-mail address: elina.toskala@tuhs.temple.edu

Clinics Collections 2 (2014) 393–404

http://dx.doi.org/10.1016/j.ccol.2014.09.023

Abbreviations	
AR	Allergic rhinitis
BHR	Bronchial hyperresponsiveness
CGRP	Calcitonin gene-related peptide
ICS	Inhaled corticosteroids
LABA	Long-acting β2-agonists
RSV	Respiratory syncytial virus
SABAs	Short-acting bronchodilators

model.[1–3] Rhinitis is not only associated with but is a risk factor for the development of asthma.[4–11] Although both allergic and nonallergic forms of rhinitis are associated with asthma, the association between asthma and allergic rhinitis (AR) is even stronger.[4,11] The use of allergen-directed immunotherapy in young children with allergic rhinitis has been shown to prevent the development of asthma in later life.[12–14] Irritants and allergens presented at one portion of the airway have distal effects. It is thought that the upper and lower airways communicate through a complex interaction of inflammatory mediators and the autonomic system. Furthermore, disease severities in rhinitis and asthma often parallel each other.[4,15] Adequate treatment of allergic rhinitis can allow better asthma control and, in some situations, may even prevent the development of asthma.[16–20] With the substantial evidence to support the link between upper and lower airway disease it is imperative that physicians who manage patients with rhinitis and sinusitis become familiar with the diagnosis and management of asthma.

AR AND ASTHMA DEFINED

AR is defined as a symptomatic immunoglobulin E (IgE)–mediated inflammation of the nasal mucosa.[9] Symptoms of rhinitis are reversible and include nasal congestion/obstruction, rhinorrhea, sneezing, pruritus, postnasal drip, chronic cough, throat clearing, and conjunctivitis.[9,21] Rhinitis is categorized, based on duration of symptoms and by the disease's impact on quality of life, as intermittent or persistent mild or moderate to severe (**Table 1**).[9]

Asthma is a chronic inflammatory disorder of the airways that results in reversible airway obstruction and bronchial hyperresponsiveness (BHR) to a variety of stimuli. Inflammatory mediators and mainly mast cells, eosinophils, T lymphocytes, neutrophils, and epithelial cells are known to play an important role in this process. In advanced cases, airway remodeling can occur, with irreversible injury to the pulmonary mucosa. The airway inflammation and subsequent airway obstruction experienced by these individuals can result in symptoms of wheezing, breathlessness, chest tightness, and coughing.[22,23]

Although the focus of asthma pathophysiology was once on the hyperresponsiveness of the airways, it is now known that inflammation is the driving mechanism, with the increased bronchial reactivity being caused by this inflammatory state. This concept is important to understanding the pathophysiology and treatment of asthmatics.

EPIDEMIOLOGY
Asthma-Rhinitis Link

AR and asthma affect about 30% and 7% to 8% of people respectively.[6,24,25] Between 75% and 80% of atopic and nonatopic individuals with asthma have rhinitis.[9] Between 10% and 40% of individuals with rhinitis have asthma.[26] Not only are rhinitis and

Table 1 Classification of allergic rhinitis	
Intermittent	Symptoms present for: • Less than 4 d/wk • Or for less than 4 wk/y
Persistent	Symptoms present for: • More than 4 d/wk • Or for more than 4 wk/y
Mild	Patient does not experience: • Sleep disturbance • Impairment of daily activities, leisure, and/or sport • Impairment of school or work • Troublesome symptoms
Moderate to severe	Patient experiences 1 or more of the following: • Sleep disturbance • Impairment of daily activities, leisure, and/or sport • Impairment of school or work • Troublesome symptoms

Adapted from Bousquet J, Van Cauwenberge P, Khaltaev N, ARIA Workshop Group, World Health Organization. Allergic rhinitis and its impact on asthma. J Allergy Clin Immunol 2001;108(5):147–336; with permission.

asthma associated but rhinitis is a risk factor for the development of asthma. Twenty percent of individuals with rhinitis go on to develop asthma later in life. Studies suggest that individuals with rhinitis have a 3-fold increased risk for the development of asthma.[4,5,7] Rhinitis often precedes the development of asthma.

This association is influenced by a variety of factors. The development of atopy in early childhood, before 6 years of age, is an important risk factor for the development of BHR in late childhood.[27] However, although early sensitization to inhalant allergens is a known risk factor for the development of atopic disease later in life, only about 25% of individuals sensitized to one or more inhalant allergen go on to develop asthma.[28] Among individuals with AR and atopy the type of protein to which the individual is sensitized correlates with differing propensities for development of asthma. Individuals sensitized to perennial allergens have a significantly higher likelihood for developing asthma than individuals sensitized to seasonal allergens.[11,29] In a study by Linneberg and colleagues,[11] compared with their nonallergic counterparts, individuals sensitized to pollen, a seasonal allergen, had a 10-fold increased risk for developing asthma, whereas those who were sensitized to dust mite, a perennial allergen, had a 50-fold increased risk for developing asthma.

Genetics

In addition, there seems to be a genetic predilection to the development of these diseases. In a study in northern Sweden, a family history of atopic rhinitis and atopic asthma increased the risk of developing those conditions up to 6-fold and 4-fold respectively.[30]

Geography

Significant geographic variability exists in reference to the prevalence of allergic respiratory diseases. Dahl and colleagues[31] performed a study looking at the prevalence of patient-reported allergic respiratory disorders in 10 European countries. Spain had a significantly lower prevalence and Italy a significantly higher prevalence of allergic respiratory disorder compared with other European countries: 11.7% and 33.6%, respectively (**Table 2**).[31]

Table 2
Prevalence of allergic respiratory disorder in 10 European countries

Country	Prevalence (%)[a]
Italy	33.6
Norway	26.8
Sweden	26.8
United Kingdom	26.2
Finland	26.0
The Netherlands	24.2
Germany	23.5
Denmark	20.6
Austria	15.9
Spain	11.7

[a] Nationally balanced prevalence % weighted against size of national population.
Adapted from Dahl R, Andersen PS, Chivato T, et al. National prevalence of respiratory allergic disorders. Respir Med 2004;98(5):398–403; with permission.

Disease Severity

Disease severity also has an important influence on this association. Individuals with severe, persistent forms of rhinitis are more likely to have symptomatic asthma than individuals with intermittent forms of rhinitis.[4,15] Patients with asthma and severe rhinitis experience a higher rate of nighttime awakenings and increased absences from work than asthmatics with less severe rhinitis.[15]

Environmental Factors Beyond Allergens

In addition to allergens, there are a variety of environmental factors that have been implicated in the development of asthma. As an example, there is a known association between respiratory symptoms such as dyspnea on exertion, breathlessness, and cough with air pollution.[32] Furthermore, exposure to moisture damage at work or at home and other causes of occupational rhinitis are well-studied risk factors.[33–35] The risk of asthma has been shown to be as high as 7 times that of controls among farmers with occupational rhinitis.[34] Although further studies need to be performed, reduced exposure to known occupational triggers for rhinitis is important not only for symptom management but also for the potential prevention of occupational asthma. Furthermore, tobacco smoke, drugs such as aspirin, obesity, and viral infections such as respiratory syncytial virus are known risk factors for the development of asthma.[36–40]

Allergens and/or irritants cause local inflammation in the nasal mucosa that leads to an increased ability for inhaled irritants to get to the distal bronchioles by disrupting the filtering capabilities of the nose, which results in the inhalation of unfiltered irritants into the distal airways and subsequently pulmonary symptoms. However, even in the absence of a local response, allergens/irritants presented to an isolated portion of the respiratory system exert distal effects.

PATHOPHYSIOLOGY

Two mechanisms have been proposed to explain the communication between the nasal and bronchial mucosa:

1. Inflammatory crosstalk in which local irritation leads to upregulation of a variety of inflammatory mediators at a distal site within the respiratory tract[41–43]

2. Neurogenic reflexes, in which neuronal stimulation in the nose can result in the release of cholinergic neurotransmitters and subsequent contraction of the bronchial smooth muscle[44,45]

Inflammatory Response

A series of studies were performed by Braunstahl and colleagues[41–43] in which antigen placed in the nose resulted in upregulation of inflammatory mediators at the distal bronchi, and inoculation of an antigen into the bronchi using a bronchoscope resulted in upregulation of inflammatory mediators in the nose. The upregulation of inflammatory mediators at a site distal to inoculation suggests an inflammatory crosstalk between the upper and lower airway systems. Bronchoconstriction results from the interaction between resident inflammatory cells, such as mast cells and alveolar macrophages, with upregulated inflammatory mediators such as eosinophils, lymphocytes, neutrophils, and basophils. Mediators such as histamine, leukotrienes, prostaglandin D_2, and platelet-activating factor, are subsequently released and act on bronchial smooth muscle to cause muscle contraction.[22,46]

Autonomic Response

Either by direct activation of the vagus nerve or via secondary activation of the parasympathetic system, neuroregulatory mechanisms act at the level of the bronchial smooth muscle to result in bronchoconstriction. Neuromediators such as substance P and calcitonin gene-related peptide, affect the release of histamine and bradykinin. These mediators work at the vascular epithelium to cause an unrestricted passage of proteins and fluid. In addition, cholinergic neurotransmitters cause contraction of the bronchial smooth muscle.[46–50] Moreover, mucus plugging from excessive mucus production further contributes to airflow obstruction.[46]

Histopathology

The nose, paranasal sinuses, trachea, and primary and secondary bronchi are all lined by a pseudostratified ciliated columnar epithelium.[1] The inflammatory cell profile in the nasal mucosa of patients with AR is similar to that seen in the bronchial mucosa of patients with atopic asthma, with both having an increased infiltration of mainly eosinophils, as well as a variety of other cytokines.[51,52]

Unlike the lower respiratory tract, the nasal passages have an extensive vascular system with subepithelial capillaries, arteries, and venous and cavernous sinusoids.[9] Vessel engorgement results in symptomatic nasal obstruction, which is one of the characteristic features of rhinitis. In contrast, the trachea through the respiratory bronchi is lined by smooth muscle. It is the contraction of this smooth muscle system either through the inflammatory or neuroregulatory mechanisms discussed earlier that causes the acute, reversible airway obstruction that is the pathognomonic feature of asthma.

T helper 2 (Th_2) cells are responsible for allergic inflammation. Interleukin (IL)-4, IL-5, and IL-13, along with other inflammatory mediators and chemokines, result in the transendothelial migration and activation of eosinophils.[46,53–56] In addition, endothelial adhesion proteins intercellular adhesion molecule-1 and vascular cell adhesion molecule-1 assist in the migration of neutrophils, lymphocytes, and eosinophils from the intravascular space into the airway. Mast cell degranulation and histamine release lead to the production of leukotrienes. Eosinophils present in the inflamed tissue causes the release of toxic basic proteins, which leads to epithelial damage and airflow obstruction.[46] This processes results in the characteristic histologic features of mucosal edema, submucosal gland and bronchial smooth muscle hypertrophy, mucus hypersecretion, and basement membrane thickening and fibrosis seen in asthma.[46,57–59]

Chronic inflammation in asthmatics can result in airway remodeling. Remodeling is a process in which tissue injury and subsequent repair leads to mucosal edema, submucosal gland and bronchial smooth muscle hypertrophy, mucus gland and goblet cell hyperplasia, angiogenesis, collagen deposition, basement membrane thickening, and subepithelial fibrosis in the lamina reticularis.[46,57–59] Although similar finding are seen in patients with chronic rhinosinusitis, remodeling has not been well shown in patients with allergic rhinitis. Further, the reticular basement membrane thickening is not as pronounced in nasal epithelium in rhinitis as it is in the bronchial epithelium in patients with asthma.[60]

ASTHMA AND ATOPY

There are 2 categories of T lymphocytes, Th_1 and Th_2, with atopic patients having a skewed predilection for the Th_2 phenotype.[61–63] Th_2 cells lead to the production of IgE antibodies and the upregulation of eosinophils, and various interleukins such as IL-4, IL-5, and IL-13.[18,46,54–56,61] This process is sustained by cytokines such as IL-4 that work through positive feedback mechanisms to perpetuate the Th_2 pathway and downregulate Th_1 cells.[62]

Many theories have been proposed to explain the increased prevalence of asthma, particularly in the pediatric population. One theory is referred to as the hygiene hypothesis. In this model, the increased predilection for the Th_2 cytokine response is attributed to a decreased microbial exposure in the postnatal period.[61] Microbial exposure early in life is a known stimulus for normal Th_1 maturation.[64] With improvements in management and prevention of infection through advancements in antibiotics, vaccination, and various public health measures, there has been a decreased microbial stimulus for the Th_1 phenotype. This theory has been supported by multiple studies. Children with increased exposure to infection early in life have fewer symptoms of BHR.[65] In addition, it has been shown that atopy is less prevalent among children raised in large families and or on farms.

DIAGNOSIS

The work-up and evaluation of patients with rhinitis and or asthma should include a thorough assessment of both the upper and lower airways. In light of the significant association with allergy, it is important to inquire about presence of atopic disease; seasonality of symptoms; known triggers; or locations, such as work, in which symptoms worsen; and family history of atopic disease. In addition, it is important to ask whether allergy or pulmonary function testing has been performed and whether the patient has been or is on inhaled, topical, or oral medications for upper or lower airway disease. Along with asking about nasal symptoms such as nasal congestion/obstruction, hyposmia/anosmia, sneezing, postnasal drip, throat clearing, and chronic cough, it is important to ask about symptoms of shortness of breath with exercise, prolonged cough after viral infections, and nighttime cough. However, patients with cough-variant asthma may not present with the classic asthma symptoms such as wheezing.

Physical examination in these patients should include a thorough head and neck examination with particular attention to signs of atopy. Some examples include darkening of the skin beneath the eyes, referred to as allergic shiners, fine lines of the eyelids, referred to as Dennie lines, and a horizontal crease across the lower bridge of the nose referred to as the allergic salute.[66] Conjunctival erythema may also be appreciated. Rhinoscopy is a valuable tool in the evaluation of patients with AR and or asthma. Rigid or flexible endoscopy is preferred but in their absence an otoscope can be placed in the nares. Attention should be paid to the appearance of the nasal mucosa. In cases of AR the nasal mucosa is often boggy and pale, whereas in cases of nonallergic rhinitis the mucosa is often erythematous and inflamed. The quality of nasal secretion, position of the nasal septum, and/or the presence of polyps should also be noted. Examination of the oropharynx in patients with AR may reveal irregularities of the posterior pharynx, referred to as cobblestoning, which is often seen in patients with atopy. Otoscopic examination may reveal signs of effusion. The skin should be examined for signs of eczema and/or dermatitis, which can be present in atopic patients. In addition, a pulmonary examination should be performed. Auscultation may reveal prolonged forced exhalation and expiratory wheezes. Percussion of the lungs may reveal hyper-resonant breath sounds as a result of air trapping.[1]

A diagnosis of asthma is based on the presence of a variety of symptoms with episodic and at least partially reversible airway obstruction.[22] Although symptoms of breathlessness, cough, recurrent wheezing, and/or chest tightness are common in asthma, they are not diagnostic. Objective measures of pulmonary function can help delineate asthma from a variety of other pulmonary disorders including restrictive airway diseases, other obstructive pulmonary diseases, vocal fold dysfunction, and central airway obstruction. There are a variety of tests used to assess pulmonary function, including lung volumes, spirometry, flow volume loops, diffusion capacity, and body plethysmography.[1]

In patients with allergic rhinitis, allergy testing with either skin prick test or allergen-specific IgE (radioallergosorbent testing [RAST]) should be performed. Although test results take longer with RAST, it is useful in patients with dermographism, dermatitis, and in cases in which antihistamines cannot be discontinued.[67]

TREATMENT

In patients with known IgE-mediated sensitization, avoidance of sensitized allergens has been shown to improve rhinitis and asthma control and is therefore recommended in all atopic patients.[68]

Treatment of rhinitis has been shown to improve asthma control.[16,17,53,69,70] Intranasal corticosteroids are often used as first-line agents in the management of AR. Not only have intranasal corticosteroids been found to be efficacious in the management of moderate to severe rhinitis they have also been shown to reduce BHR and improve asthma symptoms.[16,17]

At present, there are 2 classes of medications used in the management of asthmatics, referred to as controller and reliever medications.[71]

- Controller medications such as corticosteroids and immunomodulators are used to treat the underlying inflammatory process in an attempt to prevent adverse outcomes.
- Reliever or rescue medications, including short-acting bronchodilators and inhaled anticholinergics, are used to treat the acute symptoms of bronchoconstriction including dyspnea, wheezing, and cough.

Inhaled corticosteroids (ICSs) are the first-line controller therapy used in the treatment of asthma.[22] Not only has ICS been shown to decrease airway inflammation and BHR but it has also been shown to improve nasal symptoms and pulmonary function scores, reduce the frequency and severity of asthma exacerbations, and reduce asthma-related mortality.[71] Long-acting β2-agonists (LABA) are used in combination with ICSs for long-term control and prevention in moderate or severe persistent asthma.

LABAs are not used as a monotherapy because they do not have efficacy as an antiinflammatory agent and are associated with increased risk of asthma-related deaths.[69]

The use of both intranasal and inhaled steroids has been shown to reduce the number of emergency department visits, as well as the number of asthma-related work absences and asthma-related episodes of nighttime awakening.[16]

Systemic corticosteroids have been efficacious in the management of both rhinitis and asthma but, as a result of their side effect profile, systemic corticosteroid therapy is only used in severe refractory cases.

Immunomodulators such as omalizumab, a monoclonal anti-IgE antibody, has shown efficacy in both the treatment of asthma and allergic rhinitis but its use is limited because of significantly high costs.[22,72,73]

AR often precedes the development of asthma, and therefore early and aggressive management of AR should be used in order to potentially prevent the development of asthma in later life. Immunotherapy to sensitized allergens in patients with AR has shown promising results in terms of reduced symptoms, reduced need for medication, and potential prevention of asthma.[12]

SUMMARY

Consideration of the unified airway model when managing patients with rhinitis and or asthma allows a more comprehensive care plan and therefore improved patient outcomes. Asthma is clearly linked to rhinitis both epidemiologically and biologically, and this association is even stronger in individuals with atopy. Rhinitis is not only associated with but is a risk factor for the development of asthma.[4–10] As a result, physicians managing rhinitis may be the first health care providers able to identify early signs of asthma. Management of rhinitis has been shown to improve asthma control. Early and aggressive treatment of allergic rhinitis may prevent the development of asthma. In patients with allergic rhinitis that is not sufficiently controlled by allergy medication, allergen-directed immunotherapy should be considered.

REFERENCES

1. Krouse JH, Brown RW, Fineman SM, et al. Asthma and the unified airway. Otolaryngol Head Neck Surg 2007;136(5):S75–106.
2. Krouse JH. Allergy and chronic rhinosinusitis. Otolaryngol Clin North Am 2005; 38:1257–66.
3. Krouse JH. The unified airway–conceptual framework. Otolaryngol Clin North Am 2008;41:257–66.
4. Guerra S, Sherrill DL, Martinez FD, et al. Rhinitis as an independent risk factor for adult-onset asthma. J Allergy Clin Immunol 2002;109:419–25.
5. Corren J. Allergic rhinitis and asthma: how important is the link? J Allergy Clin Immunol 1997;99:S781–6.
6. Blomme K, Tomassen P, Lapeere H. Prevalence of allergic sensitization versus allergic rhinitis symptoms in an unselected population. Int Arch Allergy Immunol 2013;160(2):200–7.
7. Settipane RJ, Hagy GW, Settipane GA. Long-term risk factors for developing asthma and allergic rhinitis: a 23-year follow-up of college students. Allergy Proc 1994;15:21–5.
8. Leynaert B, Bousquet J, Neukirch C, et al. Perennial rhinitis: an independent risk factor for asthma in nonatopic subjects: results from the European Community Respiratory Health Survey. J Allergy Clin Immunol 1999;104(2):301–4.

9. Bousquet J, Van Cauwenberge P, Khaltaev N, ARIA Workshop Group, World Health Organization. Allergic rhinitis and its impact on asthma. J Allergy Clin Immunol 2001;108(5):147–336.
10. Meltzer EO, Hamilos DL, Hadley JA, et al. Rhinosinusitis: establishing definitions for clinical research and patient care. Otolaryngol Head Neck Surg 2004;131(6): S1–62.
11. Linneberg A, Henrick Nielsen N, Frolund L, et al. The link between allergic rhinitis and asthma: a prospective, population-based study, the Copenhagen Allergy Study. Allergy 2002;57:1048–52.
12. Möller C, Dreborg S, Ferdousi HA, et al. Pollen immunotherapy reduces the development of asthma in children with seasonal rhino-conjunctivitis (the PAT study). J Allergy Clin Immunol 2002;109(2):251–6.
13. Johnstone DE, Dutton A. The value of hyposensitization therapy for bronchial asthma in children–A 14 year study. Pediatrics 1968;42:793–802.
14. Jacobsen L, Nuchel Petersen B, Wihl HA, et al. Immunotherapy with partially purified and standardized tree pollen extracts. IV: results from long-term (6 year) follow-up. Allergy 1997;52:914–20.
15. Huse DM, Harte SC, Russel MW, et al. Allergic rhinitis may worsen asthma symptoms in children: the international Asthma Outcomes registry. Am J Respir Crit Care Med 1996;153:A860.
16. Stelmach R, do Patrocinio T Nunes M, Ribeiro M, et al. Effect of treating allergic rhinitis with corticosteroids in patients with mild-to-moderate persistent asthma. Chest 2005;128(5):3140–7.
17. Watson WT, Becker AB, Simons FE. Treatment of allergic rhinitis with intranasal corticosteroids in patients with mild asthma: effect on lower airway responsiveness. J Allergy Clin Immunol 1993;91:97–101.
18. Jani A, Hamilos DL. Current thinking on the relationship between rhinosinusitis and asthma. J Asthma 2005;42(1):1–7.
19. Lund V. The effect of sinonasal surgery on asthma. Allergy 1999;57: 141–5.
20. Aubier M, Neukirch C, Peiffer C, et al. Effect of cetirizine on bronchial hyperresponsiveness in patients with seasonal allergic rhinitis and asthma. Allergy 2001; 56:35–42.
21. Corey JP, Gungor A, Karnell M. Allergy for the laryngologist. Otolaryngol Clin North Am 1998;31(1):189–205.
22. National Heart, Lung, and Blood Institute: National Institute of Health; U.S. Department of Health and Human services: Expert panel report 3: guidelines for the diagnosis and management of asthma. NIH publication no. 07–4051, National Institutes of Health; National Heart, Lung, and Blood Institute; Bethesda (MD). 2007. Available at: http://www.nhlbi.nih.gov.libproxy.temple.edu/guidelines/asthma. Accessed March, 2013.
23. Expert panel report: guidelines for the diagnosis and management of asthma (EPR 1991). Bethesda (MD): US Department of Health and Human Services; National Institutes of Health; National Heart, Lung, and Blood Institute; National Asthma Education and Prevention Program; 1991.
24. Akinbami LJ. Asthma prevalence, health care use, and mortality: United States, 2005–2009. Natl Health Stat Report 2011;(32):1–16.
25. Schiller JS, Lucas JW, Peregoy JA. Summary health statistics for U.S. adults: National Health Interview Survey, 2011. National Center for Health Statistics. US Department of Health and Human Services Centers for Disease Control and Prevention. Vital Health Stat 2012;(252):1–207.

26. Bousquet J, Khaltaev N, Cruz AA, et al. Allergic Rhinitis and its Impact on Asthma (ARIA) 2008 update (in collaboration with the World Health Organization. GA(2)LEN and AllerGen). Allergy 2008;63(86):8–160.

27. Peat JK, Salome CM, Woolcock AJ. Longitudinal changes in atopy during a 4-year period: relation to bronchial hyperresponsiveness and respiratory symptoms in a population sample of Australian schoolchildren. J Allergy Clin Immunol 1990;85:65–74.

28. Jones C, Holt P. Immunopathology of allergy and asthma in childhood. Am J Respir Crit Care Med 2000;162:S36–9.

29. Prieto J, Gutierrez V, Berto JM, et al. Sensitivity and maximal response to methacholine in perennial and seasonal allergic rhinitis. Clin Exp Allergy 1996;26:61–7.

30. Lundback B. Epidemiology of rhinitis and asthma. Clin Exp Allergy 1998;2:3–10.

31. Dahl R, Andersen PS, Chivato T, et al. National prevalence of respiratory allergic disorders. Respir Med 2004;98(5):398–403.

32. Zemp E, Elsasser S, Schindler C, et al. Long term ambient air pollution and respiratory symptoms in adults (SAPALDIA Study). Am J Respir Crit Care Med 1999;159:1257–66.

33. Karvala K, Toskala E, Luukkonen R. New-onset adult asthma in relation to damp and moldy workplaces. Int Arch Occup Environ Health 2010;83(8):855–65.

34. Karjalainen A, Martikainen T, Klaukka T, et al. Risk of asthma among Finnish patients with occupational rhinitis. chest 2003;123:283–8.

35. Ameille J, Hamelin K, Andujar P, et al. Occupational asthma and occupational rhinitis: the united airways disease model revisited. Occup Environ Med 2013; 70:471–5.

36. Strachan DP, Cook DG. Health effects of passive smoking. 6. Parental smoking and childhood asthma: longitudinal and case control studies. Thorax 1998; 53(3):204–12.

37. Eisner MD, Yelin EH, Henke J, et al. Environmental tobacco smoke and adult asthma. The impact of changing exposure status on health outcomes. Am J Respir Crit Care Med 1998;158:170–5.

38. Ford ES. The epidemiology of obesity and asthma. J Allergy Clin Immunol 2005; 115(5):897–909.

39. Stein RT, Sherrill D, Morgan WJ, et al. Respiratory syncytial virus in early life and risk of wheeze and allergy by age 13 years. Lancet 1999;354(9178):541–5.

40. Johnston SL, Pattemore PK, Sanderson G, et al. Community study of role of viral infections in exacerbations of asthma in 9–11 year old children. BMJ 1995; 310(6989):1225–9.

41. Braunstahl GJ, Kleinjan A, Overbeek SE, et al. Segmental bronchial provocation induces nasal inflammation in allergic rhinitis patients. Am J Respir Crit Care Med 2000;161:2051–7.

42. Braunstahl GJ, Overbeek SE, Kleinjan A, et al. Nasal allergen provocation induces adhesion molecule expression and tissue eosinophila in upper and lower airways. J Allergy Clin Immunol 2001;107(3):469–76.

43. Braunstahl GJ, Overbeek SE, Fokkens WJ, et al. Segmental bronchoprovocation in allergic rhinitis patients affects mast cell and basophil numbers in nasal and bronchial mucosa. Am J Respir Crit Care Med 2001;164:858–65.

44. Fontanari P, Burnet H, Zatarra-Hartmann MC, et al. Changes in airway resistance induced by nasal inhalation of cold dry, dry, or moist air in normal individuals. J Appl Physiol 1996;81(4):1739–43.

45. Sarin S, Undem B, Sanico A, et al. The role of the nervous system in rhinitis. J Allergy Clin Immunol 2006;118(5):999–1014.

46. Lemanske RF, Busse WW. Asthma. J Allergy Clin Immunol 2003;111(2):502–19.
47. Erjavec F, Lembeck F, Florjanc-Irman T, et al. Release of histamine by substance P. Naunyn Schmiedebergs Arch Pharmacol 1981;317:67–70.
48. Piotrowski W, Foreman JC. Some effects of calcitonin gene-related peptide in human skin and on histamine release. Br J Dermatol 1986;114(1):37–46.
49. Mehta D, Malik AB. Signaling mechanisms regulating endothelial permeability. Physiol Rev 2006;86(1):279–367.
50. Canning BJ. Reflex regulation of airway smooth muscle tone. J Appl Phys 2006; 101(3):971–85.
51. Togias A. Rhinitis and asthma: evidence for respiratory system integration. J Allergy Clin Immunol 2003;111(6):1171–83.
52. Calderon M, Losewicz S, Prior A, et al. Lymphocyte infiltration and thickness of the nasal mucous membrane in perennial and seasonal allergic rhinitis. J Allergy Clin Immunol 1994;93:635–43.
53. Shturman-Ellstein R, Zeballos RJ, Buckley JM, et al. The beneficial effect of nasal breathing on exercise-induced bronchoconstriction. Am Rev Respir Dis 1978;118(1):65–73.
54. Hamilos D. Chronic sinusitis. J Allergy Clin Immunol 2000;106:213–27.
55. Bachert C, Vignola AM, Gevaert P, et al. Allergic rhinitis, rhinosinusitis, and asthma: one airway disease. Immunol Allergy Clin North Am 2004;24(1):19–43.
56. Alam R, Stafford RA, Forsythe P, et al. RANTES is a chemotactic and activating factor for human eosinophils. J Immunol 1993;150(8):3442–8.
57. Dunnill MS. The pathology of asthma with special reference to changes in the bronchial mucosa. J Clin Pathol 1960;13:27–33.
58. Dunnill MS, Massarella GR, Anderson JA. A comparison of the quantitative anatomy of the bronchi in normal subjects in status asthmaticus in chronic bronchitis, and in emphysema. Thorax 1969;24(2):176–9.
59. Kay AB. Asthma and inflammation. J Allergy Clin Immunol 1991;87(5):893–910.
60. Bousquet J, Jacquot W, Vignola M, et al. Allergic rhinitis: a disease remodeling the upper airways? J Allergy Clin Immunol 2004;113:43–9.
61. Romagnani S. Human TH1 and TH2 subsets: doubt no more. Immunol Today 1991;12(8):256–7.
62. Maddox L, Schwartz DA. The pathophysiology of asthma. Annu Rev Med 2002; 53:477–98.
63. Abbas AK, Murphy KM, Sher A. Functional diversity of helper T lymphocytes. Nature 1996;383:787–93.
64. Holt PG, Macaubas C. Development of long-term tolerance versus sensitisation to environmental allergens during the perinatal period. Curr Opin Immunol 1997; 9:782–7.
65. Ball TM, Castro-Rodriquez JA, Griffin KA, et al. Siblings, day-care attendance, and the risk of asthma and wheezing during childhood. N Engl J Med 2000; 343:538–43.
66. Fornadley JA, Corey JP, Osguthorpe JD, et al. Allergic rhinitis: clinical practice guideline. Committee on Practice Standards, American Academy of Otolaryngic Allergy. Otolaryngol Head Neck Surg 1996;115(1):115–22.
67. Greiner AN, Hellings PW, Rotiroti G. Allergic rhinitis. Lancet 2012;378(9809):2112–22.
68. Bush RK. The use of anti-IgE in the treatment of allergic asthma. Med Clin North Am 2002;86:1113–29.
69. Taramarcaz P, Gibson PG. Intranasal corticosteroids for asthma control in people with coexisting asthma and rhinitis. Cochrane Database Syst Rev 2003;(4):CD003570.

70. Dejima K, Hama T, Miyazaki M, et al. A clinical study of endoscopic sinus surgery for sinusitis in patients with bronchial asthma. Allerg Immunol 2005;
138(2):97–104.
71. Global initiative for asthma: global strategy for asthma management and prevention. 2013. Available at: www.ginasthma.org. Accessed April 9, 2013.
72. Dimov VV, Casale TB. Immunomodulators for asthma. Allergy Asthma Immunol
Res 2010;2(4):228–34.
73. Nelson HS, Weiss ST, Bleeker ER, et al. The Salmeterol Multicenter Asthma
Research Trial: a comparison of usual pharmacotherapy for asthma or usual
pharmacotherapy plus salmeterol. Chest 2006;129(5):15–26.

RADS and Its Variants
Asthma by Another Name

Annyce Mayer, MD, MSPH[a,b,*], Karin Pacheco, MD, MSPH[a,b]

KEYWORDS

- Reactive airways dysfunction syndrome • Work-exacerbated asthma
- Irritant exposures • Irritant asthma

KEY POINTS

- Acute high-level irritant exposures can cause asthma and exacerbate underlying asthma.
- Lower-level irritant exposures can at least exacerbate underlying asthma, although there is emerging consensus that recurrent lower-level exposures may also cause asthma.
- There is overlap between the exposures that have caused acute irritant-induced asthma and work-exacerbated asthma (WEA), many of which are also sensitizers.
- New-onset asthma in workers following lower-level irritant exposures, with no prior history of respiratory symptoms or asthma, may well be limited to a subset of "susceptible" hosts, such as those with asymptomatic airway hyperresponsiveness, atopy, and those who "outgrew" childhood asthma.
- The ATS statement on WEA has identified research needs to better define risk factors, biologic mechanisms, and outcomes in WEA, which should help facilitate necessary interventions in the medical system, as well as to formulate and apply strategies for prevention.

INTRODUCTION

Asthma is a chronic respiratory condition characterized by variable airflow obstruction, airways hyperresponsiveness, and airway inflammation. Approximately 7.7% of US adults of working age have asthma[1] and an estimated 16.3% of all cases of adult asthma have been attributed to asthma caused or exacerbated by workplace exposures.[2] Many other conditions and factors, such as rhinosinusitis, gastroesophageal reflux disease (GERD), vocal cord dysfunction, and cigarette smoking, may trigger symptoms that mimic asthma but are not, and these are covered elsewhere in this issue. Other, more serious conditions that mimic asthma include hypersensitivity

This article originally appeared in Immunology and Allergy Clinics of North America, Volume 33, Issue 1, February 2013.
[a] Division of Environmental and Occupational Health Sciences, Department of Medicine, National Jewish Health, 1400 Jackson Street, Denver, CO 80206, USA; [b] Department of Environmental/Occupational Health, Colorado School of Public Health - University of Colorado Denver, 13001 E. 17th Place, B119, Bldg. 500, 3rd Floor, Aurora, CO 80045, USA
* Corresponding author.
E-mail address: mayera@njhealth.org

pneumonitis, which can be caused by low molecular weight irritants that are also sensitizers,[3–6] bronchiolitis obliterans,[7,8] and irritant/odorant-triggered cough.[9–11] Whereas asthma caused by sensitization is well described and well accepted,[12–16] it is not the primary focus of this article. On the other hand, reactive airways dysfunction syndrome (RADS) and other variants of irritant-induced or irritant-exacerbated asthma may not always initially appear as asthma, but are, in fact, alternate presentations of asthma. Therefore, occupational and environmental exposures that can cause or exacerbate asthma should be considered as well. Although unique conditions exist in the workplace that more often lead to the type of exposures that can cause or exacerbate asthma, exposure to sensitizers and irritants that exacerbate or cause asthma can also occur in the home, during avocational activities, and following accidental industrial releases into the environment. Thus, although the terms occupational and workplace are used in this article, environmental sources of these exposures should also be considered.

The role of irritants in the causation of asthma is now well established. RADS was originally defined in 1981 by Brooks and Lockey[17] and detailed in case series of new-onset asthma syndrome within 24 hours following a single, high-level irritant exposure.[18] Since that time, modifications to the case definition have been proposed, and more recently the term "acute irritant asthma" has been used, with good consensus that this is not just an asthma syndrome but indeed occupational asthma.[14,16,19,20] Asthma has been reported after lower-level irritant exposures, with considerable controversy regarding whether or not the lower-level irritant exposure caused the asthma,[21,22] was a result of concurrent immunologic sensitization,[16,23] or caused an exacerbation of underlying asthma.[14–16,24,25] Work-exacerbated asthma (WEA) is defined as "preexisting or concurrent asthma that is worsened by workplace conditions,"[25] in which there is a temporal association between asthma exacerbations and work in a place where conditions exist that can exacerbate asthma, but that asthma caused by work (immunologic asthma and acute irritant asthma) is considered unlikely. WEA is often not compensable under workers' compensation.

This article covers the different clinical variants of irritant-induced asthma, specifically focusing on high level irritant-induced asthma and irritant-induced WEA reviews known causes, addresses the often adverse medical and socioeconomic outcomes of this complex condition, and considers issues of causation from an occupational and environmental medicine perspective.

CLINICAL VIGNETTE 1

John Adams is a 45-year-old city maintenance worker. He is a never-smoker and has no history of asthma or other medical problems. He performs maintenance inside city facilities, including the wastewater treatment plant. On one occasion, a regulator malfunction caused the sudden high-pressure release of 100% chlorine into the very small room where he was working. The sudden release caused him to take in a deep breath, and he experienced immediate cough, burning eyes and nose, chest burning and tightness, and shortness of breath. He was taken to the emergency department and placed on oxygen. He is not sure about what other treatment he received, but after a period of time he felt somewhat better and was discharged. Most of his symptoms continued to improve, but the dry cough persisted. He noted chest tightness and shortness of breath with exertion, such as walking in the mountains. His chest symptoms were also triggered by irritants, such as cigarette smoke, perfume, and dust, which had never bothered him before. He seeks medical attention for these symptoms 3 months later. Could this be asthma?

ACUTE IRRITANT ASTHMA

Yes, asthma should be considered as part of the differential diagnosis, and should be confirmed by methacholine challenge or bronchodilator responsiveness. The presentation is consistent with RADS, defined as asthma caused by a single, high level, irritant exposure hypothesized to cause acute bronchial mucosal damage leading to airways hyperresponsiveness. Whereas allergen exposures are well-documented causes of asthma, the role of irritants in the causation of asthma has been recognized only more recently. RADS was originally described as a "persistent asthma syndrome" after high-level irritant exposure.[17,18] Brooks noted that although the illness clinically simulated bronchial asthma and was associated with airways hyperreactivity, it differed from typical occupational asthma because of rapid onset (within 24 hours) after a single high-level environmental exposure, and this period of time is too short for the development of sensitization.[18] Although the validity of the syndrome as new-onset asthma was initially debated,[26,27] numerous case reports have followed,[9,28–32] and it is now widely accepted that acute high-level irritant exposures not only cause a syndrome that mimics asthma but can cause asthma itself.[14–16,19,20] Tarlo and Broder introduced the term "irritant-induced asthma" in 1989 to include workers in their case series who had high-level irritant exposure on more than one occasion,[33] which has been subsequently reported by others.[30] Other studies included those with onset of symptoms up to 7 days after a well-defined spill; they identified additional cases that otherwise met the case definition.[34] The term "acute irritant-induced asthma" was recently proposed,[16,20] and for workers without any prior history of asthma, the term is an accurate unifying descriptor. A list of some of the exposures reported to have caused acute irritant asthma, termed RADS and asthma after spills or accidental exposures, are shown in **Table 1**. The clinical criteria for RADS described by Brooks[18] and modifications that have been proposed are shown in **Box 1**.

In many cases, the symptoms resolve within months, but they can persist in some.[9,18,29–32,35,36] The long-term sequelae can be significant. One long-term follow-up study of workers (52% participation) with claims accepted by the workers' compensation agency in Quebec revealed significant ongoing respiratory impairment and psychosocial impact two years after initial symptoms. These patients presented with acute irritant-induced asthma due to a well-defined high-level accidental release (57% chlorine) and had symptoms that developed within 24 hours and persisted beyond 3 months. All subjects still had respiratory symptoms; 68% were on inhaled corticosteroids, there had been no significant improvement in forced expiratory volume in 1 second (FEV1) (mean FEV1 74.5% ± 19.5% predicted), and most still demonstrated airways hyperresponsiveness based on methacholine challenge or improvement after bronchodilator. There was a negative impact on quality of life, and about one-third had abnormal depression scores.[37] The long-term impact was similar to that reported in immunologic asthma.[38]

CLINICAL VIGNETTE 2

Michael Janvier is a 54-year-old insulator in a large plant. He has a 5-pack-year history and had stopped smoking at age 30. He has no prior history of respiratory symptoms. He has performed installation, repair, and routine maintenance on the pipes in a chrome-plating shop on and off over the past 10 years. Some of the pipes were located 4 to 5 feet above the acid baths. Depending on the job, he could spend several weeks or even months at a time in that shop. He sometimes felt burning in his eyes, nose, and throat, as well as some cough, although these symptoms were fairly mild and typically resolved later that evening or the next day. About a year ago, he began

Table 1
Reported high-level irritant exposures associated with development of acute irritant-induced asthma, along with pH, potential for thermal injury, and sensitizer potential

Author	Outcome	Reported Chemical	High or Low pH	Potential for Thermal Injury	Potential Sensitizer
Brooks et al,[18] 1985	RADS after single high-level exposure	Uranium hexafluoride			−
		Floor sealant			?
		Spray paint (3)			?
		35% hydrazine			
		Heated acid	+	+	
		Fumigating fog			?
		Metal coat remover	?		
		Fire/smoke		+	?
Tarlo and Broder,[33] 1989	RADS after 1 or more high-level exposures	Acids	+		
		Calcium oxide			
		Chlorine, sulfuric acid, sulfur dioxide	+		
		HCl, phosgene	+		
		Calcium oxide, welding fumes			?
		Burnt paint fumes		?	?
		Spray paint no isocyanate			
		Chlorine			
		Toluene diisocyanate			+
		Diphenyl methane diisocyanate			+
Chatkin et al,[45] 2007	Asthma after spills or accidental exposures	Isocyanates			+
		Paint			?
		Solvents			
		Chlorine			
		Ammonia	+		
		Calcium oxide	+		
		Acrylates			+
		Amines			+
		Epoxy resins			+
		Dyes			?
		Ozone			?
		Pesticides			
		Wood dust			?
		Methylmercaptan			

The "+" refers to the listed chemical exposures that have one or more of the other properties: high or low pH, potential for thermal injury and/or are potential sensitizers. The "?" refers to those chemical exposures that might have one of those properties, but there is insufficient information about the exposure to determine.

Abbreviation: RADS, reactive airways dysfunction syndrome.

to notice worsening shortness of breath while running and playing soccer. He also started awakening at night with chest tightness about once a week. A cardiac evaluation was negative, including a normal stress echocardiogram. His symptoms continue to worsen and he seeks further medical attention. Could this be this asthma?

ASTHMA FOLLOWING LOWER-LEVEL IRRITANT EXPOSURES

In 2005, Brooks[39] introduced the term "not-so-sudden onset" irritant-induced asthma to describe the exposures in a subgroup of subjects who had onset of asthma

---

Box 1
Clinical criteria for acute irritant-induced asthma[a]

1. A documented absence of preceding respiratory complaints.

2. The onset of symptoms occurred after 1 or more high-level exposures.[b]

3. The exposure was to a gas, smoke, fume, or vapor that was present in very high concentrations and had irritant qualities to its nature.

4. The onset of symptoms occurred within 24 hours[c] after the exposure and persisted for at least 3 months.

5. Symptoms simulated asthma with cough, wheezing, and dyspnea predominating.

6. Pulmonary function test may show airflow obstruction.

7. Methacholine challenge testing was positive.

8. Other types of pulmonary diseases were ruled out.

[a] Clinical criteria for RADS defined by Brooks[18] with minor modification as noted.

[b] Exposure to high-level irritant exposure on one or more occasions not confined to a single workplace event.[33]

[c] Others have used symptom onset up to 7 days after exposure.[34]

---

following longer and less intense irritant exposures. In a group of 71 subjects considered to be at moderate to high risk for RADS after repeated exposures to chlorine at a pulp and paper mill, 82% had persisting respiratory symptoms, 22% had evidence of reduced FEV1, and 41% had nonspecific airways hyperresponsiveness based on methacholine challenge that persisted 18 to 24 months after the end of exposure without clear host predisposition.[40] In contrast, long-term decline in lung function was seen in a longitudinal study of workers exposed to "puffs" of chlorine at a metal production plant; these exposures caused mild symptoms in those with a smoking history of 20-pack-years or more.[41] Kipen and colleagues[21] described a series of 10 cases of adult-onset asthma following "low-dose" irritant exposures, as shown in **Table 2**. Four of the cases were reported due to exposure to acid mist, whereas 4 or 5 of the other irritant exposures potentially also could have been sensitizers. In this series, another 5 cases had been excluded because of a history of asthma before the exposure, although 41% of the cases did meet the investigators' criteria for history of atopy (case history reviewed for seasonal allergy, rhinitis, atopic skin disease, or positive immediate hypersensitivity skin results). Host predisposition was also suggested as a mechanism in the subgroup with "not so sudden" irritant-asthma reported by Brooks and colleagues,[22] in which 88% were atopic (defined as allergen skin testing or radioallergosorbent tests positive, personal history of allergic disease, elevated total immunoglobulin E level, or family history of allergy) and 40% had a history of childhood asthma or asthma that had been quiescent at least 1 year.

It is important to recognize that a single, high-level exposure to a sensitizing chemical with irritant properties may also cause irritant asthma, although it may be difficult to exclude concurrent sensitization when that exposure is not confined to a single event.[18,33] Distinguishing between an immunologic and irritant mechanism can be difficult in the individual patient. This has been handled in a number of different ways: excluding those with exposure to irritants that were also sensitizers,[39,42] analyzing the chemical composition to exclude the presence of sensitizers to determine irritant mechanism,[43] using a specific inhalational challenge (SIC) in the laboratory or workplace to distinguish the two,[44] or including all high-level exposures regardless of SIC

Table 2
Reported low-dose irritant exposures, associated work-exacerbated asthma, and low-dose RADS, along with pH, potential for thermal injury, and sensitizer potential

Author	Outcome	Reported Chemical	High or Low pH	Potential for Thermal Injury	Potential Sensitizer
Chiry et al,[46] 2007	WEA with negative SIC	Flour			+
		Latex			+
		Isocyanates (3)			+
		Glutaraldehyde			+
		Triethanolamine			+
Lemiere et al,[47] 2012	WEA with negative SIC	Ammonia	+		
		Engine exhaust fumes			
		Pyrolysis fumes		?	?
		Metal fumes			?
		Silica			
		Mineral fibers			
		Metal compounds			?
		Animal-derived aerosol			?
		Wood			?
		Flour			+
		Acrylates			+
		Paints, including industrial and motor vehicle			+
		Adhesives			?
		Degreasing stripping agents			
		Hardeners			+
		Isocyanates			+
		Solvents			
Kipen et al,[21] 1994	Low-dose RADS	Bisulfite+SO2			
		Chemistry teaching laboratory	?		?
		Acid mist (4)	+		
		Cutting oil			?
		Cleaning agents			?
		Perfume agents			?
		New carpet installation			?

The "+" refers to the listed chemical exposures that have one or more of the other properties: high or low pH, potential for thermal injury and/or are potential sensitizers. The "?" refers to those chemical exposures that might have one of those properties, but there is insufficient information about the exposure to determine.

Abbreviations: RADS, reactive airways dysfunction syndrome; SIC, specific inhalation challenge; WEA, work-exacerbated asthma.

results.[45] The latter is not inconsistent with the original criteria proposed by Brooks and colleagues.[18] As shown in **Table 1**, many of the irritant exposures reported to cause acute irritant induced asthma are also potential sensitizers. Perhaps more important than establishing mechanism, establishing whether or not there is concurrent immunologic asthma has important implications for the degree of exposure control required for the worker to successfully remain in the workplace.

As described for high-level irritant exposures, lower-level exposures to sensitizing chemicals with irritant properties can also cause asthma either by an irritant or a sensitizing mechanism. Immunologic asthma has been differentiated from irritant-induced asthma in some studies by results from SIC.[46,47] As shown in **Table 2**, many of these irritant exposures in which sensitizers were not automatically excluded are very similar to the exposures reported with acute irritant asthma listed in **Table 1**. In a study by Kogevinas and colleagues,[48] occupations associated with excess risk of occupational asthma included farmers, painters, plastics workers, cleaners, spray painters, and agricultural workers; these are occupations in which there may be concurrent exposures to sensitizers. Overrepresentation of respiratory symptoms and asthma has been reported in workers repeatedly exposed to moderate to low-level irritant exposures that can also be sensitizers, such as cleaning workers[49–51] and hair dressers.[52]

CLINICAL VIGNETTE 3

Sandra Dalton is a 26-year-old woman with a prior history of childhood asthma and seasonal allergic rhinitis. Her asthma improved when she was an adolescent, and she used a bronchodilator only before exercise or for chest symptoms associated with an upper respiratory infection (URI). Six months ago she began a job with a company producing experimental semiconductors. She was responsible for loading panels of chips into a holder; this holder was then lowered into a nitric acid bath before the chips were removed and sent down the assembly line. Her job also involved refilling the nitric acid reservoir when levels were low. Although the bath was covered, it was opened to load and remove the computer chips. The room had an unpleasant acrid odor, and after about 3 months at work, she began to develop more frequent episodes of chest tightness that no longer completely resolved after using her bronchodilator. A recent URI triggered profound cough and wheezing, requiring a burst of oral steroids and the addition of a steroid inhaler to control symptoms. Is the patient's asthma exacerbation work related?

WORK-EXACERBATED ASTHMA

Yes, it is now widely accepted that low-level irritant exposures can exacerbate preexisting asthma.[14–16,24,25] WEA was recently defined by the American Thoracic Society as "preexisting or concurrent asthma that is worsened by workplace conditions," wherein the asthma either predates the exposure (preexisting) or is determined to have occurred independently, but concurrently with the workplace exposure (concurrent).[25] The diagnosis of WEA requires establishment of temporal association between asthma exacerbations and work in a workplace where conditions exist that can exacerbate asthma. WEA is common, reportedly occurring in 23% of adults within a health maintenance organization.[53]

Temporary Exacerbation Versus Permanent Aggravation of Preexisting or Concurrent Asthma

There is an assortment of irritant workplace exposures that may temporarily increase symptoms due to underlying asthma, or indeed any other chronic lung disease. Such increases in symptoms are often mild, temporary, and respond well to simple measures to decrease or avoid exposure, with the occasional additional use of short-acting bronchodilators. Patients with severe underlying asthma may not be tolerant of low level irritants that are present in many different environments. The problem occurs when there are specific exacerbating conditions that exist in the workplace, but the worker does not have control over mitigating them; such workers are often unable to remain in the workplace. A letter to the editor described the long-term impact of WEA in 10 cases 1 to 4 years after a diagnosis of WEA. None had been able to remain in the workplace because of their respiratory symptoms, and they also were unable to obtain any financial compensation from the Quebec Worker Compensation Board.[54] Although it is possible that medical treatment or enhanced ventilation or respiratory protection might have allowed these workers to remain in their jobs, outside of the workers' compensation system, such patients often do not have the authority to effect meaningful decreases in respiratory exposures in the workplace.

As a result, loss of employment, a need to change jobs, and other adverse socioeconomic effects,[55–58] as well as increased use of health care resources and decreased quality of life,[59] have been documented by a growing number of studies of workers after a diagnosis of WEA. If the worker does not return to baseline status despite optimized medical therapy, and reasonable exposure control measures have been implemented, such worsening would be considered a permanent aggravation, rather than a temporary exacerbation.

Although there are considerable data on disability and adverse socioeconomic outcomes in WEA, there are few clinical outcome studies.[25] There are also no clinical outcome data on workers who receive optimized medication therapy and reasonable workplace exposure controls, and their long-term ability to remain within the workplace (ie, the extent to which such cases of WEA could be limited to temporary exacerbations that are not associated with job loss and other socioeconomic disadvantages).

More concrete consideration of permanent aggravation can be made in the context of an acute irritant injury in a worker with preexisting asthma. The original clinical criteria proposed by Brooks and colleagues[18] excluded persons with preceding history of respiratory complaints. In most cases, it is impossible to verify a preexisting lack of airways hyperresponsiveness or airflow limitation. Multiple cases of high-level irritant exposures resulted in asthma that otherwise met the definition of RADS except for a prior history of mild asthma.[22,36,60,61] There is nothing about underlying asthma that would be expected to confer immunity from airways injury following such irritant exposures that cause RADS in a worker with normal airways. Indeed, one might postulate that those with preexisting asthma are even more susceptible to airways injury and persistent effects from irritant exposures, as is suggested by the 76% of subjects with a preexisting history of asthma who had accepted claims for asthma by the Ontario Workers' Compensation Board following high-level irritant exposures.[45] In many cases, with treatment, workers with preexisting asthma will be able to return to their baseline status in the same way as those with no prior history of asthma. In others, the condition does not return to baseline, and there is objective evidence of permanent worsening, such as a change in FEV1, methacholine PC-20, medication requirements, and/or the need for permanent removal from exposure even after optimized medical treatment and implementation of exposure controls. In this setting, the term "acute irritant-aggravated asthma" could be considered to describe the permanent change from the patient's baseline condition.

CHALLENGES IN THE DIAGNOSIS OF IRRITANT-INDUCED VERSUS IRRITANT-AGGRAVATED ASTHMA FROM AN OCCUPATIONAL AND ENVIRONMENTAL MEDICINE PERSPECTIVE DISTINGUISHING WORKERS WITH PREEXISTING OR CONCURRENT ASTHMA FROM NEW-ONSET ASTHMA

There can be difficulty distinguishing between new-onset occupational asthma caused by work, and WEA. For example, in a group of 53 workers with documented reversible airflow limitation or airways hyperresponsiveness and WEA, defined by worsening asthma symptoms at work and a negative SIC, only 20% reported a history of asthma before the exposure.[47] The investigators concluded that although it is often not possible to confirm by objective testing, a proportion of these subjects may suffer not from WEA, but from "low-dose irritant asthma" (ie, new-onset asthma). In another study, clinicians were not able to reliably differentiate the peak flow measurement pattern in workers with new-onset occupational asthma versus WEA on visual inspection or computer analysis.[46] In fact, the US National Institute for Occupational Safety and Health (NIOSH) Sentinel Event Notification Systems for Occupational Risks (SENSOR) program for surveillance of work-related asthma considered new-onset work-related asthma symptoms to be work-initiated asthma, even in the context of preexisting asthma that had been untreated or asymptomatic for at least 2 years before entering the workplace.[62]

Preexisting asymptomatic airways hyperresponsiveness (AHR) is well described as one of the factors that can predispose to asthma, and some investigators have argued that the existence of preexisting AHR precludes a diagnosis of RADS as new-onset asthma. The prevalence of asymptomatic airways hyperresponsiveness has ranged from 4% to 35% of the population depending on the definition used.[63] It is described with[64] and without[65] correlation with eosinophilia, which along with atopy can also predispose to asthma. A prior history of asthma, including childhood asthma, is also defined as preexisting asthma. The extent to which these are preexisting conditions, or simply markers of host risk factors for asthma, remains to be determined.[66]

In many of the US workers' compensation systems, work-related conditions are defined on a medically probable (greater than 50% likely) basis that the need for treatment in a case is the result of a work-related exposure when certain factors are present. These factors include: (1) the work exposure causes a new condition; or (2) the work exposure causes the activation of a previously asymptomatic or latent medical condition to become symptomatic and now require treatment; or (3) the work exposure aggravates a preexisting symptomatic condition that now requires treatment that was not needed before. A helpful approach to determining whether a condition is work-related is recommended by the Colorado Division of Workers' Compensation: would the patient need the recommended treatment if the work exposure had not taken place? If the answer is "no," then the condition is most likely work related.[67] To establish that the worker had preexisting or concurrent asthma, the physician would need to verify an asymptomatic or well-controlled stable asthma pattern that had clearly changed due to a well-defined workplace irritant exposure. It is also incumbent on the physician to rule out the contribution of nonoccupational causes to the asthma exacerbation, such as GERD, infection, or rhinosinusitis.

Defining High-Level Exposure

What constitutes a high-level exposure may or may not be obvious. In cases of very high-level accidental releases where no respiratory protection had been worn, the high-level exposure is obvious. A good example is the massive exposure to airborne alkaline particulates following the World Trade Center collapse in 2001; this led to the development of asthma in many of the first responders.[68–70] When explored, a dose-response has been noted,[28] but in most cases, no industrial hygiene monitoring data or dose reconstruction by an industrial hygienist are available. In less obvious cases, the physician can try to estimate the "dose" that was delivered to the lungs of the individual worker based on the intensity of the irritant exposure, the frequency, and the duration.

Intensity

Intensity is determined by the airborne concentration of the vapor, dust, gas, or fume, as well as the innate irritating properties of the chemical(s). Some chemicals are inherently more irritating than others.[9] For example, those with very low, or worse, very high pH, are extremely irritating. When heated chemicals are inhaled, thermal injury may compound the damage.

A release may or may not be large. A worker very close to the source of a release may have a high concentration in his or her breathing zone that is not shared by others a little farther away, as the concentration of irritants can be fairly quickly dissipated through dilution with ambient air currents. Airborne concentrations will be much higher within a confined space because there is no such potential for dilution. Chemicals with very low vapor pressure can quickly volatilize in considerable quantity, particularly when heated. The size of the chemical particle and its water solubility will determine deposition within the respiratory tract, with the smallest and most water-insoluble chemicals having the greatest potential to reach the lower airways.

However, there does not need to be a release or other recognized event to signal exposure to high-level irritants. Not all workplaces will have appropriate engineering controls in place, such as enclosures and local exhaust ventilation, which can greatly minimize exposure to vapors, dust, gas, and fumes. Such controls need to have been installed and used correctly to be effective. Unrecognized failures of these control measures may result in unrecognized excess exposures, although such exposures may be limited to only a few individuals who work directly in the area. Air monitoring by an industrial hygienist can determine actual airborne concentrations, although if interim control measures have been implemented, these may not reflect the actual concentration at the time of the release or engineering control failure.

The amount of the vapor, dust, gas, or fume that reaches the lungs of the worker will be considerably decreased if respiratory protection is used, but only if it was used and worn correctly, and the exposure did not exceed the respirator's protective limits. A filtering respirator needs to have the correct cartridges for the exposure. For example, particulate filtering cartridges are highly effective in trapping airborne particulates but do not filter out irritant gases. Combined particulate (P100) and organic vapor cartridges are highly effective protection against many gases and vapors, as well as fumes and particulates. Filtering facepiece respirators are considered protective at concentrations up to 10 times the Occupational Safety and Health Administration (OSHA) Permissible Exposure Limit (PEL) for half-face respirators and up to 50 times the PEL with full-face respirators. However, the respirator will only have been effective to that level if it was worn properly sealed to the skin without facial hair, and the adequacy of the seal was confirmed by fit testing.

Frequency

The frequency of the exposure is relevant in considering exposures not confined to a single event, and should be considered along with duration.

Duration

The duration of the exposure before moving to fresh air is another important factor in determining "dose" in both high-level and lower-level exposures. Moderate to heavy physical exertion will increase tidal volume and respiratory rate, thus effectively increasing the amount of the irritant delivered to the lungs per unit of time.

SUMMARY

Acute high-level irritant exposures can cause asthma and exacerbate underlying asthma. Lower-level irritant exposures can at least exacerbate underlying asthma, although there is emerging consensus that recurrent lower-level exposures may also cause asthma. There is overlap between the exposures that have caused acute irritant-induced asthma and WEA, many of which are also sensitizers. What constitutes an excessive level enough to cause asthma from acute high-level or recurrent lower-level accidental releases is not currently defined. New-onset asthma in workers following lower-level irritant exposures, with no prior history of respiratory symptoms or asthma, may well be limited to a subset of "susceptible" hosts, such as those with asymptomatic airways hyperresponsiveness, atopy, and those who "outgrew" childhood asthma. But it is reasonable to consider asthma to more likely than not have been caused by such irritant exposures when previously asymptomatic workers develop symptomatic asthma following clearly defined workplace irritant exposures, the asthma is confirmed by objective testing, and other lung diseases and nonoccupational causes of the asthma have been excluded. This attribution of work-relatedness should also apply to workers with prior well-controlled stable asthma who sustain objectively documented changes in the pattern of their asthma.

Workers with irritant-induced and WEA should receive optimized asthma therapy. Equally important is the reduction and control of their exacerbating workplace exposures. Without the ability to receive this combination treatment, it is likely these cases of WEA will not be limited to temporary exacerbations, but will continue to experience the long-term disability and socioeconomic disadvantage that has been repeatedly observed. The ATS statement on WEA has identified research needs to better define risk factors, biologic mechanisms, and outcomes in WEA,[25] which should help to facilitate necessary interventions in the medical system, as well as to formulate and apply strategies for prevention.

The informed clinician should be prepared to identify and treat both new-onset and work-exacerbated asthma, and to partner with occupational and environmental medicine clinicians to address the challenges inherent in the diagnosis and treatment of irritant-induced and irritant-aggravated asthma.

REFERENCES

1. National Center for Health Statistics. Asthma prevalence, health care use, and mortality: United States, 2003-05. Department of Health and Human Services; 2007.
2. Toren K, Blanc PD. Asthma caused by occupational exposures is common—a systematic analysis of estimates of the population-attributable fraction. BMC Pulm Med 2009;9:7.
3. Vandenplas O, Malo JL, Saetta M, et al. Occupational asthma and extrinsic alveolitis due to isocyanates: current status and perspectives. Br J Ind Med 1993; 50:213–28.
4. Baur X. Hypersensitivity pneumonitis (extrinsic allergic alveolitis) induced by isocyanates. J Allergy Clin Immunol 1995;95:1004–10.
5. Raulf-Heimsoth M, Baur X. Pathomechanisms and pathophysiology of isocyanate-induced diseases—summary of present knowledge. Am J Ind Med 1998;34:137–43.
6. Piirila P, Keskinen H, Anttila S, et al. Allergic alveolitis following exposure to epoxy polyester powder paint containing low amounts (<1%) of acid anhydrides. Eur Respir J 1997;10:948–51.

7. Konichezky S, Schattner A, Ezri T, et al. Thionyl-chloride-induced lung injury and bronchiolitis obliterans. Chest 1993;104:971–3.

8. Markopoulou KD, Cool CD, Elliot TL, et al. Obliterative bronchiolitis: varying presentations and clinicopathological correlation. Eur Respir J 2002;19:20–30.

9. Blanc P, Liu D, Juarez C, et al. Cough in hot pepper workers. Chest 1991;99: 27–32.

10. Ekstrand Y, Ternesten-Hasseus E, Arvidsson M, et al. Sensitivity to environmental irritants and capsaicin cough reaction in patients with a positive methacholine provocation test before and after treatment with inhaled corticosteroids. J Asthma 2011;48:482–9.

11. Schiffman SS, Williams CM. Science of odor as a potential health issue. J Environ Qual 2005;34:129–38.

12. Tarlo SM, Malo JL. An official ATS proceedings: asthma in the workplace: the Third Jack Pepys Workshop on Asthma in the Workplace: answered and unanswered questions. Proc Am Thorac Soc 2009;6:339–49.

13. Vandenplas O, Toren K, Blanc PD. Health and socioeconomic impact of work-related asthma. Eur Respir J 2003;22:689–97.

14. Bernstein IL, Bernstein DI, Chan-Yeung M, et al. Definition and classification of asthma in the workplace. In: Bernstein IL, Chan-Yeung M, Malo JL, et al, editors. Asthma in the workplace. 3rd edition. New York; 2006. p. 1–8.

15. Tarlo SM, Balmes J, Balkissoon R, et al. Diagnosis and management of work-related asthma: American College of Chest Physicians Consensus Statement. Chest 2008;134:1S–41S.

16. Malo JL, Vandenplas O. Definitions and classification of work-related asthma. Immunol Allergy Clin North Am 2011;31:645–62, v.

17. Brooks SM, Lockey J. Reactive airways disease syndrome (RADS): a newly defined occupational disease. Am Rev Respir Dis 1981;123(Suppl):133.

18. Brooks SM, Weiss MA, Bernstein IL. Reactive airways dysfunction syndrome (RADS). Persistent asthma syndrome after high-level irritant exposures. Chest 1985;88:376–84.

19. Alberts WM, do Pico GA. Reactive airways dysfunction syndrome. Chest 1996; 109:1618–26.

20. Francis HC, Prys-Picard CO, Fishwick D, et al. Defining and investigating occupational asthma: a consensus approach. Occup Environ Med 2007;64:361–5.

21. Kipen HM, Blume R, Hutt D. Asthma experience in an occupational and environmental medicine clinic. Low-dose reactive airways dysfunction syndrome. J Occup Med 1994;36:1133–7.

22. Brooks SM, Hammad Y, Richards I, et al. The spectrum of irritant-induced asthma: sudden and not-so-sudden onset and the role of allergy. Chest 1998;113:42–9.

23. Tarlo SM. Workplace irritant exposures: do they produce true occupational asthma? Ann Allergy Asthma Immunol 2003;90:19–23.

24. Goe SK, Henneberger PK, Reilly MJ, et al. A descriptive study of work aggravated asthma. Occup Environ Med 2004;61:512–7.

25. Henneberger PK, Redlich CA, Callahan DB, et al. An official American Thoracic Society statement: work-exacerbated asthma. Am J Respir Crit Care Med 2011; 184:368–78.

26. Kern DG, Sherman CB. What is this thing called RADS? Chest 1994;106:1643–4.

27. Kennedy SM. Acquired airway hyperresponsiveness from nonimmunogenic irritant exposure. Occup Med 1992;7:287–300.

28. Kern DG. Outbreak of the reactive airways dysfunction syndrome after a spill of glacial acetic acid. Am Rev Respir Dis 1991;144:1058–64.

29. Malo JL, Cartier A, Boulet LP, et al. Bronchial hyperresponsiveness can improve while spirometry plateaus two to three years after repeated exposure to chlorine causing respiratory symptoms. Am J Respir Crit Care Med 1994;150:1142–5.

30. Chan-Yeung M, Lam S, Kennedy SM, et al. Persistent asthma after repeated exposure to high concentrations of gases in pulpmills. Am J Respir Crit Care Med 1994;149:1676–80.

31. Harkonen H, Nordman H, Korhonen O, et al. Long-term effects of exposure to sulfur dioxide. Lung function four years after a pyrite dust explosion. Am Rev Respir Dis 1983;128:890–3.

32. Piirila PL, Nordman H, Korhonen OS, et al. A thirteen-year follow-up of respiratory effects of acute exposure to sulfur dioxide. Scand J Work Environ Health 1996;22:191–6.

33. Tarlo SM, Broder I. Irritant-induced occupational asthma. Chest 1989;96:297–300.

34. Cone JE, Wugofski L, Balmes JR, et al. Persistent respiratory health effects after a metam sodium pesticide spill. Chest 1994;106:500–8.

35. Takeda N, Maghni K, Daigle S, et al. Long-term pathologic consequences of acute irritant-induced asthma. J Allergy Clin Immunol 2009;124:975–81.e1.

36. Demeter SL, Cordasco EM, Guidotti TL. Permanent respiratory impairment and upper airway symptoms despite clinical improvement in patients with reactive airways dysfunction syndrome. Sci Total Environ 2001;270:49–55.

37. Malo J, L'Archeveque L, Gastellanos L, et al. Long-term outcomes of acute irritant-induced asthma. Am J Respir Crit Care Med 2009;179:923–8.

38. Maghni K, Lemiere C, Ghezzo H. Airway inflammation after cessation of exposure to agents causing occupational asthma. Am J Respir Crit Care Med 2004;169:367–72.

39. Brooks S, Hammad Y, Richards I, et al. The Spectrum of irritant-induced asthma. Chest 1998;113:42–9.

40. Bherer L, Cushman R, Courteau JP, et al. Survey of construction workers repeatedly exposed to chlorine over a three to six month period in a pulpmill: II. Follow up of affected workers by questionnaire, spirometry, and assessment of bronchial responsiveness 18 to 24 months after exposure ended. Occup Environ Med 1994;51:225–8.

41. Gautrin D, Leroyer C, Infante-Rivard C, et al. Longitudinal assessment of airway caliber and responsiveness in workers exposed to chlorine. Am J Respir Crit Care Med 1999;160:1232–7.

42. Wheeler S, Rosenstock L, Barnhart S. A case series of 71 patients referred to a hospital-based occupational and environmental medicine clinic for occupational asthma. West J Med 1998;168:98–104.

43. Burge PS, Moore VC, Robertson AS. Sensitization and irritant-induced occupational asthma with latency are clinically indistinguishable. Occup Med 2012;62: 129–33.

44. Leroyer C, Dewitte JD, Bassanets A, et al. Occupational asthma due to chromium. Respiration 1998;65:403–5.

45. Chatkin JM, Tarlo SM, Liss G, et al. The outcome of asthma related to workplace irritant exposures: a comparison of irritant-induced asthma and irritant aggravation of asthma. Chest 1999;116:1780–5.

46. Chiry S, Cartier A, Malo JL, et al. Comparison of peak expiratory flow variability between workers with work-exacerbated asthma and occupational asthma. Chest 2007;132:483–8.

47. Lemiere C, Begin D, Camus M, et al. Occupational risk factors associated with work-exacerbated asthma in Quebec. Occup Environ Med 2012;00:1–7.

48. Kogevinas M, Anto JM, Sunyer J, et al. Occupational asthma in Europe and other industrialised areas: a population-based study. European Community Respiratory Health Survey Study Group. Lancet 1999;353:1750–4.

49. Quirce S, Barranco P. Cleaning agents and asthma. J Investig Allergol Clin Immunol 2010;20:542–50 [quiz: 2p following 50].

50. Karjalainen A, Martikainen R, Karjalainen J, et al. Excess incidence of asthma among Finnish cleaners employed in different industries. Eur Respir J 2002; 19:90–5.

51. Rosenman KD, Reilly MJ, Schill DP, et al. Cleaning products and work-related asthma. J Occup Environ Med 2003;45:556–63.

52. Moscato G, Galdi E. Asthma and hairdressers. Curr Opin Allergy Clin Immunol 2006;6:91–5.

53. Henneberger PK, Derk SJ, Sama SR, et al. The frequency of workplace exacerbation among health maintenance organisation members with asthma. Occup Environ Med 2006;63:551–7.

54. Pelissier S, Chaboillez S, Teolis L, et al. Outcome of subjects diagnosed with occupational asthma and work-aggravated asthma after removal from exposure. J Occup Environ Med 2006;48:656–9.

55. Vandenplas O, Henneberger PK. Socioeconomic outcomes in work-exacerbated asthma. Curr Opin Allergy Clin Immunol 2007;7:236–41.

56. Larbanois A, Jamart J, Delwiche JP, et al. Socioeconomic outcome of subjects experiencing asthma symptoms at work. Eur Respir J 2002;19:1107–13.

57. Cannon J, Cullinan P, Newman TA. Consequences of occupational asthma. BMJ 1995;311:602–3.

58. Blanc PD, Ellbjar S, Janson C, et al. Asthma-related work disability in Sweden. The impact of workplace exposures. Am J Respir Crit Care Med 1999;160:2028–33.

59. Lemiere C. Occupational and work-exacerbated asthma: similarities and differences. Expert Rev Respir Med 2007;1:43–9.

60. Boulet LP. Increases in airway responsiveness following acute exposure to respiratory irritants. Reactive airway dysfunction syndrome or occupational asthma? Chest 1988;94:476–81.

61. Moore BB, Sherman M. Chronic reactive airway disease following acute chlorine gas exposure in an asymptomatic atopic patient. Chest 1991;100:855–6.

62. Jajosky RA, Harrison R, Reinisch F, et al. Surveillance of work-related asthma in selected U.S. states using surveillance guidelines for state health departments—California, Massachusetts, Michigan, and New Jersey, 1993–1995. MMWR CDC Surveill Summ 1999;48:1–20.

63. Boulet LP. Asymptomatic airway hyperresponsiveness: a curiosity or an opportunity to prevent asthma? Am J Respir Crit Care Med 2003;167:371–8.

64. Schwartz N, Grossman A, Levy Y, et al. Correlation between eosinophil count and methacholine challenge test in asymptomatic subjects. J Asthma 2012; 49:336–41.

65. Boulet LP, Prince P, Turcotte H, et al. Clinical features and airway inflammation in mild asthma versus asymptomatic airway hyperresponsiveness. Respir Med 2006;100:292–9.

66. Laprise C, Laviolette M, Boutet M, et al. Asymptomatic airway hyperresponsiveness: relationships with airway inflammation and remodelling. Eur Respir J 1999; 14:63–73.

67. State of Colorado Department of Labor and Employment Division of Workers' Compensation Level II Accreditation Course and Curriculum. Available at http://www.colorado.gov/cs/Satellite/CDLE-WorkComp/CDLE/1240336932511.

68. Prezant DJ, Levin S, Kelly KJ, et al. Upper and lower respiratory diseases after occupational and environmental disasters. Mt Sinai J Med 2008;75:89–100.
69. Prezant DJ, Weiden M, Banauch GI, et al. Cough and bronchial responsiveness in firefighters at the World Trade Center site. N Engl J Med 2002;347:806–15.
70. Banauch GI, Alleyne D, Sanchez R, et al. Persistent hyperreactivity and reactive airway dysfunction in firefighters at the World Trade Center. Am J Respir Crit Care Med 2003;168:54–62.

Asthma and Chronic Obstructive Pulmonary Disease
Similarities and Differences

Dirkje S. Postma, MD, PhD[a],*, Helen K. Reddel, MB, BS, PhD, FRACP[b],
Nick H.T. ten Hacken, MD, PhD[a], Maarten van den Berge, MD, PhD[a]

KEYWORDS

- Asthma • COPD • Inflammation • Remodeling • Overlap phenotype

KEY POINTS

- Asthma in childhood and chronic obstructive pulmonary disease (COPD) in smokers are easily distinguishable disease entities.
- There exist overlap phenotypes of asthma and COPD, such as asthma with neutrophilia and/or without bronchodilator response, and COPD with eosinophilia and/or some bronchodilator response.
- Differences in physiology, symptoms, inflammation, and remodeling between asthma and COPD are obscured by smoking. Hence asthma in a smoker and COPD appear similar (ie, they show phenotypic mimicry).
- A key component of overlap between asthma and COPD is the effect of aging.
- Some of the mechanisms driving airway obstruction and hyperresponsiveness are similar in asthma and COPD, and some are different.
- There is an unmet need to assess optimal treatment effects and safety in subphenotypes of asthma and COPD; phenotypes that have so far been excluded from pharmacologic studies.

INTRODUCTION

Asthma and chronic obstructive pulmonary disease (COPD) are both highly prevalent diseases worldwide. This issue of *Clinics in Chest Medicine* discusses different aspects of COPD, but in addition, the present article on overlap and differential signs and symptoms with asthma has been included. This is appropriate because it is often difficult to differentiate asthma from COPD, particularly at older ages. At that time in

This article originally appeared in Clinics in Chest Medicine, Volume 35, Issue 1, March 2014.
[a] University of Groningen, Department of Pulmonology, GRIAC research institute, University Medical Center Groningen, Hanzeplein 1, 9713 GZ Groningen, The Netherlands;
[b] Department of Medicine, Woolcock Institute of Medical Research, University of Sydney, 431 Gleve Point Road, Gleve NSW 2037, Australia
* Corresponding author.
E-mail address: d.s.postma@umcg.nl

life, patients with asthma may have developed persistent airway obstruction, a characteristic that is a prerequisite for diagnosis of COPD according to the GOLD (Global Initiative for Chronic Obstructive Lung Disease) criteria.[1] This feature would not be a problem if asthma and COPD had the same clinical prognosis and response to pharmacologic treatment, and required similar management of the disease in clinical practice. However, this is often not the case.[2]

Asthma and COPD have been defined over the years in many different ways, and the heterogeneity in definitions in the literature contributes to the difficulty of evaluating evidence about the extent to which they overlap. The problem is confounded by the necessary reliance in many epidemiologic studies on self-reported diagnosis of asthma and COPD, and because, in clinical practice, these diagnoses are often assigned without lung function testing having been performed.

Research on the clinical characterization, pathophysiology, prognosis, and management of asthma and COPD commenced with investigation of the extremes of the two conditions, namely:

1. Atopic individuals with asthma, never smokers or ex-smokers with less than 10 pack-year exposure, with significant bronchodilator reversibility at the time of study. These populations usually had an average age around 35 years.
2. Current or ex-smokers with fixed airway obstruction, generally with an age greater than 55 years.

This approach in research gave new insights into how best to treat the extreme phenotypes of asthma and COPD. However, many patients with asthma were excluded from these studies, particularly when they were smokers and showed no bronchodilator response at screening. Also excluded were many patients with COPD, especially when they showed an important reduction in airway obstruction after inhaling a bronchodilator.[3] As a result, such studies have not provided good insight into the management of asthma and COPD in daily practice, because it has been recognized that many patients do not fulfill the criteria of either asthma or COPD and show a mixture of both: the so-called overlap phenotype.[2] In the past, this concept was dismissed as representing the Dutch hypothesis,[4] but in more recent years the presence of overlap phenotypes has been widely accepted.[5–7]

When comparing asthma with COPD, it is important to realize that age has to be taken into account in every setting, because age induces changes in inflammation, immunologic responses, and mechanical properties of the lung.[8] Likewise, current smoking must be taken into account, because smoking induces inflammatory and remodeling changes in the lung and affects treatment response.[9,10] Hence it is not useful to compare young nonsmoking individuals with asthma and older smoking patients with COPD in their (dis)similarities in inflammatory cells and cytokines and in treatment response, because this is driven in both situations by differences in age and smoking status. Many studies in the past have overlooked the effects of both age and smoking and are therefore hampered in their interpretation as to whether asthma and COPD have comparable or distinct underlying mechanisms and treatment approaches.

This article discusses current knowledge on clinical features, inflammation and remodeling, genetics, and therapeutic response in asthma and COPD and discusses the overlap phenotypes.

DEFINITIONS

Asthma is currently defined as a chronic inflammatory disorder of the airways in which many cells and cellular elements play a role. The chronic inflammation is associated with airway hyperresponsiveness that leads to recurrent episodes of wheezing, breathlessness, chest tightness, and coughing, particularly at night or in the early morning. These episodes are usually associated with widespread, but variable, airflow obstruction within the lung that is often reversible either spontaneously or with treatment.[11,12] In contrast, COPD has for decades been defined as a preventable and treatable disease characterized by persistent airflow limitation that is usually progressive and associated with an enhanced chronic inflammatory response in the airways and the lung to noxious particles or gases. The following was added to this definition: "Exacerbations and comorbidities contribute to the overall severity in individual patients."[1] This definition of COPD is so vague that it fits many types of patients with distinct clinical characteristics, prognosis, and treatment response.[12] One of the important aspects here is that the airway obstruction in asthma, although often reversible, may be progressive in nature in a subset of patients with asthma,[13] leading to an overlap phenotype with COPD.

The definitions of asthma and COPD have been made to have a high sensitivity, but apparently their specificity is low. The problem is well acknowledged nowadays and recent studies suggest that 13% to 20% of patients with COPD have an overlap phenotype with asthma.[14] These patients have respiratory symptoms, have persistent airway obstruction, but some reversibility is still present after inhaling a bronchodilator and inflammatory markers are similar to those in asthma. Conversely, even 20% of patients with asthma at older ages have been given a diagnosis of COPD.[15]

CLINICAL FEATURES
Symptoms

It is difficult to differentiate asthma and COPD based on respiratory symptoms.[16] In the extremes with a sudden attack of wheeze and dyspnea after allergen exposure, it is clear that this is compatible with asthma. However, in the chronic forms, symptoms are many times more diffuse and patients with asthma may have symptoms of chronic cough and/or sputum production[17,18] formerly thought to imply COPD, especially when irreversible airway obstruction has developed.[19] In contrast, patients with COPD may have wheeze, a symptom formerly attributed solely to asthma.[20] Moreover, an increase in the number of cigarettes smoked is associated with development of wheeze in COPD.[20] Thus, symptoms alone cannot rule out one or the other condition. Chronic cough and sputum production are associated with worse outcome in COPD,[21] but how this affects asthma has not been evaluated yet. Interestingly, atopic patients with COPD more frequently develop symptoms of cough and sputum production over time than nonatopic patients.[22]

Airway Obstruction and Reversibility

Bronchodilator response has been assumed to be a key differential parameter between asthma and COPD. However, bronchodilator response is frequently observed in patients with COPD in clinical practice, as well as in more recently designed clinical trials and in observational studies in patients with COPD.[23] Up to 50% of patients with COPD in the Understanding Potential Long-term Impacts on Function with TIOTropium (UPLIFT) study showed some bronchodilator response.[24] In another study, patients with COPD without a history of asthma showed a prevalence of bronchodilator response of 44%, with bronchodilator response being more frequently present in more severe disease.[25] This pattern is compatible with findings in the Evaluation of COPD longitudinally to Identify Surrogate Endpoints (ECLIPSE) cohort investigating 1831 patients with COPD tested before and after salbutamol inhalation.[26] In this study, it was concluded that the magnitude of postsalbutamol forced expiratory volume in 1 second (FEV_1) change is comparable between patients with COPD and smoking controls, but is lower with more severe airway obstruction and in the presence of emphysema.[26] Bronchodilator response status varied temporally in the latter study, but patients with consistent bronchodilator response (n = 227) did not differ in mortality, hospitalization, or exacerbation frequency from those with a lack of bronchodilator response, after adjustment for differences in baseline FEV_1.[26] One study suggested that the bronchodilator response in COPD is associated with eosinophilia, whereas absence of this response is associated with neutrophilia, possibly also explaining why some studies suggest a better inhaled corticosteroid (ICS) response in patients with reversible COPD.[27] In addition, it is debatable whether significant airway obstruction needs to be a prerequisite to define COPD, because emphysema may exist even without the presence of airway obstruction.[28]

When investigating a group of 228 patients with asthma followed for 26 years, it was shown that asthmatic patients may develop irreversible airway obstruction.[19] Although all of this cohort had reversible airway obstruction at baseline, at follow-up, 16% had developed irreversible airway obstruction, 23% had reduced carbon monoxide transfer coefficient, and 5% had both. Persistent airway obstruction was predicted by lower lung function, lower bronchodilator response, and milder hyperresponsiveness at baseline and was accompanied by the development of symptoms of chronic cough and sputum production. Patients with asthma with low transfer factor at follow-up had a higher total lung capacity and residual volume at baseline, but in multiple regression analysis this was no longer significant when pack-years of smoking were entered; higher pack-years significantly contributed to a lower transfer factor, but smoking was not independently associated with persistent airway obstruction. These observations may suggest that subtle signs of future features of COPD may already be present in early asthma. Another important message of this study is that persistent airway obstruction and reduced transfer factor are both signs of COPD, but they are distinct entities in asthma in terms of symptoms and causes. This message may have consequences for treatment approaches in asthma and the overlap phenotypes.

Small airway obstruction has long been recognized as one of the underlying mechanisms of COPD. In the last decades, it has become evident that small airway obstruction also contributes to the clinical presentation of asthma, although it is not clear yet whether this is only present in severe asthma or in mild asthma as well.[29–31] This gap in knowledge is predominantly caused by the lack of accurate and reproducible measures of small airway function suitable for general use. Signs of small airway dysfunction can already be present even 1 month after birth and they constitute a predictor of subsequent development of asthma.[32] However, it remains to be seen whether small airway changes in asthma and COPD originate from similar underlying mechanisms. The difference between inspiratory and expiratory X5, a measure of small airway obstruction, is larger in patients with COPD than in patients with asthma despite similar degrees of large airway obstruction as assessed with FEV_1.[33] Moreover, patients with COPD have greater ventilation heterogeneity than patients with asthma, as measured with slope, acinar component of ventilation heterogeneity (S_{acin}), a measure of the smallest airways where gas exchange takes place. In contrast, people with asthma predominantly have abnormalities in S_{cond}, a measure of the more proximal small conducting airways that are located before the acinus.[34] An additional contrast is that treatment with a bronchodilator induces an improvement in S_{cond} in patients with asthma, whereas it improves S_{acin} in patients with COPD[35,36] Galban and colleagues[37] identified functional small airway disease from computed tomography (CT) imaging across the spectrum of COPD severity and provided suggestive evidence that small airway narrowing and obliteration precede the onset of emphysema in COPD. Together these findings may suggest that the most peripherally located small airway disease contributes to COPD, and that the more proximally located contributes to asthma.

Atopy

Most children with asthma, and a large proportion of adult patients with asthma, are atopic.[38] It has long been overlooked that patients with COPD can be atopic as well but it is unclear whether this has clinical implications. A European study on severe asthma identified features of severe asthma that were distinct from milder forms of asthma.[39] It showed that patients with severe asthma were less frequently atopic and more frequently lacked a bronchodilator response than patients with milder disease.[39] In addition, patients with asthma with atopy respond better to ICS treatment than those without atopy.[39] Therefore, recommendations for the treatment of allergy are also included in the treatment guidelines of asthma. Recent studies showed that atopy can be present in patients with COPD as well and that the presence of allergy is a risk factor for future development of COPD.[40,41] Around 18% of patients with COPD were shown to be atopic in the European Respiratory Society study on Chronic Obstructive Pulmonary Disease (EUROSCOP) study,[22] and logistic regression provided evidence that atopic patients were more likely male, younger, and with a higher body mass index. Of importance, the presence of atopy was not associated with more severe airway obstruction.[22] Atopic patients with COPD more frequently develop symptoms of cough and sputum production when not using ICS treatment.[22] These symptoms were more likely to improve after ICS treatment of 2 years in atopic than in nonatopic patients with COPD. This finding is compatible with data from 1978 showing that atopic patients with COPD are the ones who benefit most from corticosteroid treatment.[42]

Airway Hyperresponsiveness

Airway hyperresponsiveness is a risk factor for development both of asthma and of COPD, as well as for a more rapid decline in lung function.[43] In general, most patients with asthma express hyperresponsiveness, in contrast with about 60% of patients with COPD, even with mild disease in which the level of FEV_1 does not impinge on the severity of hyperresponsiveness.[44] However, the drivers of hyperresponsiveness in asthma and COPD, and whether different mechanisms are responsible for this phenomenon, have not been elucidated. There are many physiologic changes that may contribute to hyperresponsiveness: airway luminal diameter, airway wall thickness, smooth muscle mass, vascular engorgement, elastic recoil, airway inflammation, epithelial injury, and neural activity. Short-term treatment with ICS improves hyperresponsiveness in asthma, in conjunction with improvement of eosinophilic inflammation. After long-term ICS treatment, hyperresponsiveness may even disappear in a subset of patients with asthma.[45,46] In contrast, hyperresponsiveness improves to a smaller extent in COPD, in which it almost never disappears. One study investigating patients with asthma and COPD showed that a higher level of total serum immunoglobulin E predicted improvement in hyperresponsiveness with ICS.[47] This finding has not been investigated in other studies, but remains an interesting observation because this was present both in asthma and in COPD.[47] Although a common characteristic, this may be caused by different underlying mechanisms, which have only been studied to a limited extent in COPD. Chanez and colleagues[48] found that patients with COPD with asthmalike features (ie, eosinophilia and airway hyperresponsiveness) had thicker basement membranes than those without these features. Finkelstein and colleagues[49] investigated hyperresponsiveness in patients with COPD and showed that the airway wall internal to the smooth muscle layer of the small airways was thickened. A thicker airway wall was associated with more severe hyperresponsiveness. However, smooth muscle mass contributed more to hyperresponsiveness than adventitial or submucosal thickening.[50,51] This finding is similar with asthma, in which an increase in smooth muscle mass has also been shown to contribute to the presence and severity of hyperresponsiveness.[52,53] Even within asthma, different mechanisms contribute to severity of hyperresponsiveness. In older patients, this is predicted by air trapping and ventilation heterogeneity in the most distal small airways (S_{acin}), whereas ventilation heterogeneity in the more proximal small airways (S_{cond}) and inflammation predicts the severity of hyperresponsiveness in younger individuals with asthma.[54] Of interest, exhaled bronchial nitric oxide (NO), a parameter of large airway inflammation (usually related to eosinophilia) improved by ICS treatment in younger patients with asthma in conjunction with S_{cond}. However, the severity of hyperresponsiveness remaining after 3-month ICS treatment was best predicted by S_{cond} levels only.[55] It has yet to be established how small airway obstruction affects the severity of hyperresponsiveness in COPD. A recent cross-sectional and longitudinal study in COPD did not assess small airway function directly, but showed that a more severe hyperresponsiveness was associated with higher residual volume, a measure of air trapping related to small airway function, and with airway inflammation reflected by a higher number of neutrophils, macrophages, and lymphocytes in sputum and bronchial biopsies.[56] Severity of hyperresponsiveness was not associated with eosinophilic inflammation as suggested by Chanez and colleagues,[48] again suggesting that the mechanisms underlying hyperresponsiveness in asthma and COPD are at least partially different.

The Overlap Phenotype

There is no extensive literature available comparing the overlap phenotype with asthma on one hand and COPD on the other hand.[6,7,14,57,58] Some reviews have tried to give an overview[2,59,60] or to develop consensus on how best to define the overlap phenotype.[61] In epidemiologic studies in the United States and United Kingdom, 17% to 19% of patients with obstructive airway disease reported having both asthma and COPD, and these patients accounted for as many as 50% of patients with obstructive airway disease more than 50 years of age.[7] Thus, patients reporting to have been diagnosed with both asthma and COPD are generally older. However, as indicated earlier, diagnoses in population studies are often not based on lung function testing. When analyzing 175 individuals from a random population sample with objective measures, Weatherall and colleagues[58] performed a cluster analysis and showed 5 clusters: (1) severe and markedly variable airway obstruction with features of atopic asthma, chronic bronchitis, and emphysema; (2) features of emphysema alone; (3) atopic asthma with eosinophilic airway inflammation; (4) mild airway obstruction without other dominant phenotypic features; and (5) chronic bronchitis in nonsmokers. These findings make the situation even more complex. These investigators identified clusters 2 and 3 as clear emphysema and clear asthma respectively, whereas clusters 1, 4, and 5 represented various other overlapping phenotypes in asthma and COPD. However, Weatherall and colleagues[58] did not examine the extent to which patients in these clusters differed with respect to other clinical or physiologic characteristics. In addition, these 5 clusters remain to be confirmed in other studies. Kauppi and colleagues[62] based an asthma and COPD diagnosis on UK guidelines and American Thoracic Society/European Respiratory Society criteria respectively. In this large group of patients with clinical disease, 1084 had asthma only, 237 COPD only, and 225 the overlap phenotype.[62] As expected, patients with asthma were younger, more frequently female, and less frequently had a history of smoking.[62] In addition, 26% of patients with asthma had been smoking for more than 10 years, compared with 72% and 76% of patients with COPD and the overlap phenotype respectively. The overlap group was between the asthma and COPD groups in other characteristics like gender, disease duration, pack-years smoking, lung function parameters, and comorbidities. These findings are compatible with those reported by Gibson and Simpson[2] in their review (ie, it was present in 64% of patients with the overlap syndrome, intermediate between a prevalence of 100% of patients with asthma and 25% of patients with COPD). Hypertension was highly prevalent as comorbidity with 32% in asthma, 41% in the overlap group, and 45% in patients with COPD, ages being on average 53, 61, and 64 years. However, it is also clear that the prevalence of comorbidities is higher in COPD than in asthma (**Table 1**), either as a result of long-standing smoking in COPD or because of the systemic inflammation present in COPD. In addition, patients with the overlap syndrome are more likely frequent exacerbators (ie, >2 exacerbations per year), have more gas trapping on CT, worse quality of life, more respiratory symptoms, more hospitalizations, and consume much more health care resources than pure asthmatics.[6,7,14,57–62] Moreover, patients with the overlap phenotype are reported to have higher mortalities,[63] especially when peripheral blood eosinophilia is present.[64] Hardin and colleagues[14] additionally found that subjects with both COPD and asthma combined frequently have rhinitis, although it still remains to be established whether or not this reflects underlying atopy. Overall, data show that the overlap syndrome has characteristics between those of asthma and COPD, and is frequently present, irrespective of whether reported by patients or doctors, or objectively characterized.

GENETICS AND ENVIRONMENT

Genetic factors contribute to the development of both asthma and COPD, in conjunction with environmental factors. Many environmental factors contribute to both asthma and COPD and some only to either asthma or COPD alone. **Table 2** shows an overview of these factors as published in a recent review.[65] More severe airway hyperresponsiveness, lower lung function, maternal smoking during pregnancy, air pollution, and personal cigarette smoking are risk factors for development of both asthma and COPD. One of the features that drive several of these risk factors may be abnormal lung development in utero. It may be that this abnormal lung development, for instance caused by maternal smoking, drives one of the underlying mechanisms of the abnormal lung response that patients with asthma and COPD express after inhalation of noxious stimuli that all individuals encounter, which then results in abnormal

Table 1
Proportion of patients with comorbidities

	Asthma (n = 1084)	Overlap (n = 225)	COPD (n = 237)
Hypertension	32.3	41.3	44.7
Coronary disease	7.7	19.1	25.3
Diabetes	6.8	12.9	19.8
Cerebrovascular disease	3.2	7.1	10.1
Peripheral vascular disease	0.6	3.6	7.2

Data from Kauppi P, Kupiainen H, Lindqvist A, et al. Overlap syndrome of asthma and COPD predicts low quality of life. J Asthma 2011;48(3):279–85.

Table 2
Risk factors for asthma and COPD

Host factors	Male sex in childhood, female sex in adulthood	Family history of COPD
	(Family) history of asthma	Family history asthma/atopy
	Genetic constitution	Genetic constitution
	Airway hyperresponsiveness	Airway hyperresponsiveness
	Atopy	—
	Low lung function	Low lung function
	Overweight	—
Perinatal factors	Maternal smoking	Maternal smoking
	Maternal diet	—
	Mode of delivery	—
Childhood exposures	Viral respiratory infections	Respiratory tract infections
	No breastfeeding	—
	Microbial deprivation	Maternal smoking
	Environmental tobacco smoke exposure	Indoor air pollution
	Air pollution	—
Adult exposures	Occupational exposures	Occupational exposures
	Cigarette smoking	Cigarette smoking
	Outdoor air pollution	Outdoor air pollution
	—	Indoor air pollution

From Postma DS, Kerkhof M, Boezen HM, et al. Asthma and chronic obstructive pulmonary disease: common genes, common environments? Am J Respir Crit Care Med 2011;183(12):1588–94; with permission.

lung function measures, caused by airway inflammation and remodeling superimposed on this abnormal lung development. This mechanism would also explain, at least partially, the overlap syndrome if abnormal lung development in utero is the underlying mechanism of asthma and COPD.

There are additional differences in asthma and COPD caused by differences in the underlying genetic makeup of these two diseases. Genome-wide association studies (GWAS) have shown differential genes to be associated with COPD and asthma.[65,66] Recent GWAS have identified loci that harbor susceptibility genes for asthma and other pulmonary conditions. Many of the genes at these loci have unknown functions and have not previously been considered biologically plausible candidates for disease pathogenesis. Genes found by GWAS in asthma are *ORMDL3, GSMDB, IL18R1, IL1RL1, IL33, SMAD3, IL2RB, DENND1B, HLA-Dr/DQ* region, *PDE4D2, RAD50-IL13, WDR36, TLE4,* and *MYB*.[67] Studies have recently started to investigate the genome for subphenotypes of asthma. Thus, Himes and colleagues[68] found that the presence of a bronchodilator response is associated with *SPATS2*. However, this has not been tested in COPD so far. In addition, the level of lung function and its accelerated decline were investigated specifically in asthma.[69] Unfortunately, the numbers of individuals investigated were too small to find significant genome-wide associations. Nevertheless, this is the way forward to assess whether similar genes are associated with development of a fixed airflow obstruction in asthma and a more severe disease with a higher level of lung function decline in COPD. This research may determine whether similar and/or differential mechanisms are underlying the fixed airflow obstruction in asthma and COPD.

Several genes have been associated with COPD (defined usually by low FEV_1 and FEV_1/forced vital capacity <70%) in GWAS (ie, *CHRNA3, CHRNB3/4, HHIP,* and *FAM13A*). Furthermore, several genes have been associated with a lower lung function in the general population, like *AGER, GPR126, GSTCD, HTR4, THSD4*, and *TSN1*. However, a low lung function, in the general population without further testing, may reflect asthma, COPD, or both, especially at older age, which hampers the interpretation of genetics of COPD to a large extent. Therefore, the genes published so far might not be specific to asthma or COPD, but it could be hypothesized that they reflect abnormal lung development in utero, which by itself has not been tested so far. Moreover, because COPD encompasses several phenotypes such as chronic bronchitis, airway obstruction, and emphysema, and asthma may encompass individuals with persistent airway obstruction, it is not possible to tell which genes are associated with which phenotype of COPD if not tested formally.

Overlap of Asthma and COPD

Many candidate genes and genes found by GWAS have been associated on multiple occasions with asthma, and sometimes with COPD as well.[65] Bosse[66] recently published an overview of COPD genes found by GWAS and frequently replicated candidate genes. **Table 3** combines the data on the number of publications with association of genes with asthma and with COPD as reviewed in these two articles.[65,66] The common genes identified for both asthma and COPD are *ADRB2, GSTM1, GSTP1, IL13, TGFB1*, and *TNF*.[65] We reported that this, so far limited, list of candidate genes underlying both asthma and COPD might be extended in the near future, because some genes identified in COPD have not been studied yet in asthma or too few studies have been performed that have tried to replicate genes associated with asthma in COPD. In addition, it is likely that genes that affect lung development in utero and lung growth in early childhood in interaction with environmental detrimental stimuli, such as smoking and air pollution, are contributing to asthma in childhood, progression of asthma to a phenotype with persistent airway obstruction, as well as development of COPD (**Fig. 1**).[65] Additional genes and environmental factors drive specific immunologic mechanisms that underlie asthma (like the Th2/Th1 (Thelper2/Thelper1) balance) and these may also contribute to the overlap phenotype of asthma and COPD (**Fig. 2**).

One approach to studying shared genes may be to compare the top hits of GWAS in distinct asthma and COPD populations. However, to unravel whether there exists an overlap phenotype that is genetically driven, a more fruitful method might be to search for shared genetics of asthma and COPD by performing a GWAS in one cohort including patients across the spectrum of chronic airways disease, and then examining whether the overlap phenotype has shared or distinct genes with asthma and with COPD. Such a study would require a large number of well-characterized patients, but it seems the way forward.

INFLAMMATION AND REMODELING

Inflammation and remodeling are present in COPD throughout the bronchial tree and lung tissue. There are 3 distinct processes present, and in different combinations in COPD: (1) chronic sputum production and cough, so called chronic bronchitis; (2) small airway disease; and (3) emphysema, which is the loss of elastic tissue in the peripheral lung.[70] Respiratory bronchioles of young smokers are already inflamed,[70] likely reflecting early signs of COPD. This inflammation has been shown to predominantly comprise mononuclear cells in the airway wall and macrophages in the small airway lumen. In the peripheral airways of patients with established COPD, there is also an inflammatory infiltrate, in which neutrophils and predominantly CD8-positive lymphocytes as well as mast cells predominate (mast cells particularly in patients

Table 3
Number of reports showing genes that are replicated in asthma more than 10 times, and their positive reports in COPD, and the converse number of reports with more than 10 times replication of association with COPD and their reports in asthma

	Number of Reports in Asthma	Number of Reports in COPD
Genes >10 Times in Asthma and also Reported in COPD		
ADAM33	23	6
ADRB2	46	12
CCL5	12	1
CD14	34	2
GSTM1	6	16
GSTP1	17	16
HLA	15	2
IL4	23	3
IL10	18	7
IL13	38	9
IL1B	12	6
IL4R	43	2
LTA4	12	5
STAT6	15	1
TGFB1	12	13
TNF	28	20
Genes >10 Times in Asthma but not in COPD		
HLADRB1	32	Not reported
FCERB1	22	Not reported
FLG	18	Not reported
NPSR1	12	Not reported
ORMDL3	12	0
Genes >10 Times in COPD, but not in Asthma		
EPHX	Not tested	25
SERPINA1	0	19

From Postma DS, Kerkhof M, Boezen HM, et al. Asthma and chronic obstructive pulmonary disease: common genes, common environments? Am J Respir Crit Care Med 2011;183(12):1588–94, with permission; and Bosse Y. Updates on the COPD gene list. Int J Chron Obstruct Pulmon Dis 2012;7:607–31, with permission.

with centrilobular emphysema).[71,72] In addition, squamous cell metaplasia, fibrosis, and increased smooth muscle mass, associated with hypertrophy and hyperplasia of smooth muscle cells, are present.[73] Each of these components may contribute to airway narrowing, with consequences for severity of the disease and of respiratory symptoms. Moreover, goblet cell hyperplasia is frequently present and may contribute to chronic cough and phlegm in COPD, next to the contribution of increased mucus tenacity resulting from changes in soluble factors in the mucus, components that are different in asthma and COPD.[5] These types of inflammation and remodeling processes are also present in asthma (ie, increased numbers of eosinophils, CD4-positive lymphocytes and mast cells have been shown in both diseases).[5] Fabbri and colleagues[74] showed that patients with a history of asthma or a history of COPD with a similar level of airway obstruction and hyperresponsiveness have

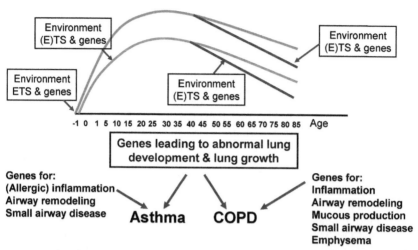

Fig. 1. Lung development, growth, and decline in interaction with genetic and environmental factors. Green line represents normal lung development, growth, and decline. Orange line represents abnormal prenatal lung development and growth. Red line represents abnormal lung decline caused by exposure to tobacco smoke. (E)TS, (environmental) tobacco smoke. (*From* Postma DS, Kerkhof M, Boezen HM, et al. Asthma and chronic obstructive pulmonary disease: common genes, common environments? Am J Respir Crit Care Med 2011;183(12):1588–94, copyright © 2011, American Thoracic Society; with permission.)

different inflammatory patterns (eosinophils in asthma and neutrophils in COPD), suggesting that there is no overlap in inflammatory pattern between asthma and COPD. However, in this case patients with COPD were all ex-smokers and current smokers and, as mentioned earlier, this may have skewed findings in the inflammatory pattern toward neutrophils, particularly because inflammation persists after smoking cessation in COPD.[75,76] Furthermore, although there was a significant difference in airway inflammation at a group level, there was also considerable overlap between asthma and COPD. Thus, these findings do not exclude an overlap phenotype of asthma and COPD.

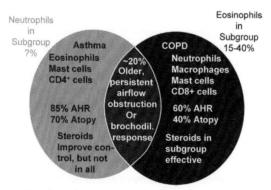

Fig. 2. The characteristics of patients with asthma, COPD, and the overlap phenotype. AHR, airway hyperresponsiveness.

Smoking induces inflammation in the lung with increased numbers of CD8 cells, neutrophils, mast cells, and macrophages in COPD.[77] It is not surprising that smoking in asthma induces comparable changes in inflammation (ie, more mast cells and fewer eosinophils in airway wall biopsies).[9] In addition, there is more remodeling in smokers with asthma, as reflected by more goblet cells and mucus-positive epithelium, increased epithelial thickness, and a higher proliferation rate of intact and basal epithelium in smokers with asthma.[9,22] Although asthma outside the context of smoking does not generally lead to neutrophilia, severe asthma is accompanied by a more neutrophilic inflammation compared with milder forms of asthma,[5,78] and some investigators have reported neutrophilic inflammation in patients with milder disease.[79] In contrast, severe asthma has a distinctive inflammatory phenotype as well: Benayoun and colleagues[80] showed that particularly high numbers of fibroblasts and airway smooth muscle hypertrophy in the proximal airways differentiates severe persistent asthma from milder asthma and COPD. Whether this is also the case in the smaller airways remains to be established. Next to neutrophilic asthma, there also exists a subset of patients with COPD with eosinophilia. The prevalence of eosinophilic COPD has been reported to range between 12% and 25% or even higher (up to 50% of stable patients with COPD).[81] This type of inflammatory cell in particular increases during exacerbations of COPD.[82] Bafadhel and colleagues[83] showed that the presence of blood eosinophilia (>2%) during an exacerbation of COPD may be a useful biomarker to direct corticosteroid therapy. In addition, it has been shown that stable patients with COPD and sputum eosinophilia can be effectively treated with inhaled steroids.[84]

Next to inflammation, remodeling plays a role in the clinical expression of asthma and COPD. It has been postulated that airway remodeling underlies the phenotypic overlap in asthma and COPD.[22] Airways are thickened in both asthma and COPD. However, Kuwano and colleagues[85] showed that the small airways in asthma are thicker than in COPD and healthy controls. Moreover, despite thickening of the airway wall in asthma, the airway lumen is larger[86] than in COPD, suggesting differential effects of airway wall thickening in asthma and COPD, possibly reflecting different underlying remodeling processes. This finding is underscored by the observation that patients with asthma generally do not develop emphysema. Parenchymal changes occur in asthma, in the sense of abnormal alveolar attachments and reduced numbers and changed geometry of elastic fibers.[87,88] These changes occur in the peribronchial region, whereas in emphysema there are widespread changes in lung tissue, not only in the peribronchiolar region, which differentiates people with asthma from patients with COPD with emphysema. However, there are also similarities with respect to remodeling in asthma and COPD, as recently pointed out in a review by Mauad and colleagues,[5] namely that structural changes occur in both diseases because of chronic inflammatory tissue injury, especially in the most severe cases. Because there are limited patterns of repair in the lungs, similar structural abnormalities may exist in some patients, possibly contributing to the clinical overlap. The latter review by Mauad and colleagues[5] and the studies discussed earlier show that some changes are characteristic of each disease (emphysema in COPD, epithelial desquamation and prominent increases in airway smooth muscle mass in the central airways in asthma), but in the overlap phenotype changes of both asthma and COPD may be present.

PHARMACOLOGIC RESPONSES

One of the difficulties in discussing treatment response in asthma and COPD is that patients with overlap phenotypes of asthma and COPD have been systematically excluded from drug trials, which are designed to include patients with pure COPD and pure asthma. This exclusion represents a problem for evidence-based guidelines on obstructive airway disease. Travers and colleagues[89] showed that only 5 of 100 individuals identified with COPD in a general population survey would fulfill inclusion criteria for major randomized controlled trials and reported comparable findings for asthma.[90] Thus, it is difficult to predict in an evidence-based way what the response to antiinflammatory and/or bronchodilator treatment would be in the full spectrum of COPD and the full spectrum of asthma.

Treatment of asthma and COPD is based on targeting inflammation and remodeling as well as counteracting contraction of the smooth muscles around the airways. Treatment is driven by the manifestations of disease both in asthma and COPD and aims to reduce symptoms, exacerbation frequency, and to improve health status, and, with severe disease, to improve exercise tolerance.[11] A proportion of patients with asthma or COPD does not achieve an acceptable level of control despite combination treatment with ICSs and long-acting bronchodilators, and has a more rapid loss of FEV_1 over time. This finding has been attributed to unresponsiveness of the underlying inflammatory and remodeling processes in the airways in the case of COPD. However, as mentioned earlier, it may also represent an overlap syndrome with neutrophilia in severe or persistent asthma, or clinicians may be treating patients with large-particle drugs, so the small airways are not being reached and inflammation and remodeling are not being adequately treated in either asthma or COPD.[30]

In general, lung function does not improve to a large extent in COPD and randomized studies have shown that the accelerated lung function decline, a major clinical characteristic of COPD, is not affected to a large extent by pharmacotherapy. However, 2 recent studies suggested that the decline in lung function can be significantly attenuated with ICS treatment, at least in a subset of patients with COPD, irrespective whether long acting beta agonists (LABAs) were added.[91,92] A recent meta-analysis showed that ICSs have immune-modulating effects in COPD,[93] hence this may be plausible. However, most studies do not show effects on lung function decline and the parameters that can predict a favorable ICS response in COPD remain to be determined.[94] Siva and colleagues[94] recently showed that patients with COPD with sputum eosinophilia (>3%) may respond better to ICS with respect to reduction in exacerbations, whereas the Groningen Leiden Universities Corticosteroids in Obstructive Lung Disease (GLUCOLD) study suggested that the presence of hyperinflation (a sign of small airway involvement) may predict a better response to ICS with respect to lung function decline, whereas disturbed diffusion capacity, a marker of emphysema, predicts a worse response.[95] Here, eosinophilia in sputum did not predict a better or worse response, suggesting that some markers associate with exacerbation frequency and others with lung function loss. The observation that signs of emphysema predict worse ICS response is plausible because regeneration of destroyed alveoli has never been shown in COPD, or in any other lung disease.

In eosinophilic asthma, ICS doses can be downtitrated based on sputum eosinophilia. Whether this is also the case in COPD, in which ICS doses have typically been much higher than in asthma, needs to be firmly established in future studies, but a pilot study suggested that this may be a good approach,[84] particularly given the concern about pneumonia with ICS in COPD (although not in asthma). However, in clinical practice it is difficult to perform sputum induction on regular basis, and, at least in asthma, the inflammatory profile can vary from visit to visit[96]; thus new inflammatory markers have to be found for optimal initiation and downtitration of ICS.

If a diagnosis of asthma or COPD is not reached, it could be worth establishing in all patients with airway obstruction, either asthma or COPD or overlap phenotypes, whether sputum eosinophilia is present, and, if so, initiating ICS treatment.[61] In addition, it could be worth starting long-acting bronchodilators if symptoms persist, because this improves clinical stability further. Welte and colleagues[97] showed that triple therapy (ICS with LABA and long-acting muscarinic anticholinergic) has great benefit in COPD, with many patients showing considerable bronchodilator responses (up to 50%). From this, it could be inferred that the overlap phenotype, in more severe disease, could benefit from triple therapy as well, which is also consistent with the observations of Magnussen and colleagues[98] showing that patients with COPD and concomitant asthma improve considerably with tiotropium bromide with respect to lung function and need for rescue medication.

SUMMARY

It is easy to differentiate pure asthma from pure COPD, because they reflect the extremes of a spectrum. However, in many, especially older, patients, features of both asthma and COPD can be present, leading to an overlap phenotype. There is no extensive literature available on the overlap phenotype, and interpretation of studies thus far has been hampered by differential age and smoking status in asthma and COPD. The balance of evidence so far suggests that the severity of airway obstruction and hyperresponsiveness in asthma, COPD, and the overlap phenotypes is driven by some similar and some different mechanisms. In addition, there is an unmet need to assess treatment effects in individuals with the overlap phenotype of asthma and COPD, because they have been consistently excluded from pharmacologic studies.

REFERENCES

1. Global initiative for chronic obstructive lung disease (GOLD). 2013. Available at: www.goldcopd.org.
2. Gibson PG, Simpson JL. The overlap syndrome of asthma and COPD: what are its features and how important is it? Thorax 2009;64(8):728–35.
3. Hanania NA, Celli BR, Donohue JF, et al. Bronchodilator reversibility in COPD. Chest 2011;140(4):1055–63.
4. Postma DS, Boezen HM. Rationale for the Dutch hypothesis. Allergy and airway hyperresponsiveness as genetic factors and their interaction with environment in the development of asthma and COPD. Chest 2004;126(Suppl 2):96S–104S.
5. Mauad T, Dolhnikoff M. Pathologic similarities and differences between asthma and chronic obstructive pulmonary disease. Curr Opin Pulm Med 2008;14(1): 31–8.
6. Contoli M, Baraldo S, Marku B, et al. Fixed airflow obstruction due to asthma or chronic obstructive pulmonary disease: 5-year follow-up. J Allergy Clin Immunol 2010;125(4):830–7.
7. Soriano JB, Davis KJ, Coleman B, et al. The proportional Venn diagram of obstructive lung disease: two approximations from the United States and the United Kingdom. Chest 2003;124(2):474–81.
8. Knudson RJ, Clark DF, Kennedy TC, et al. Effect of aging alone on mechanical properties of the normal adult human lung. J Appl Physiol 1977;43(6):1054–62.
9. Broekema M, ten Hacken NH, Volbeda F, et al. Airway epithelial changes in smokers but not in ex-smokers with asthma. Am J Respir Crit Care Med 2009; 180(12):1170–8.
10. Tomlinson JE, McMahon AD, Chaudhuri R, et al. Efficacy of low and high dose inhaled corticosteroid in smokers versus non-smokers with mild asthma. Thorax 2005;60(4):282–7.

11. Global INitiative for Asthma (GINA) guidelines. 2012. Available at: www. ginasthma.org.

12. Postma DS, Brusselle G, Bush A, et al. I have taken my umbrella, so of course it does not rain. Thorax 2012;67(1):88–9.

13. Broekema M, Volbeda F, Timens W, et al. Airway eosinophilia in remission and progression of asthma: accumulation with a fast decline of FEV(1). Respir Med 2010;104(9):1254–62.

14. Hardin M, Silverman EK, Barr RG, et al. The clinical features of the overlap between COPD and asthma. Respir Res 2011;12:127.

15. Akgun KM, Crothers K, Pisani M. Epidemiology and management of common pulmonary diseases in older persons. J Gerontol A Biol Sci Med Sci 2012; 67(3):276–91.

16. Levy ML, Fletcher M, Price DB, et al. International Primary Care Respiratory Group (IPCRG) Guidelines: diagnosis of respiratory diseases in primary care. Prim Care Respir J 2006;15(1):20–34.

17. Rogers DF. Airway mucus hypersecretion in asthma: an undervalued pathology? Curr Opin Pharmacol 2004;4(3):241–50.

18. Thiadens HA, de Bock GH, Dekker FW, et al. Identifying asthma and chronic obstructive pulmonary disease in patients with persistent cough presenting to general practitioners: descriptive study. BMJ 1998;316(7140):1286–90.

19. Vonk JM, Jongepier H, Panhuysen CI, et al. Risk factors associated with the presence of irreversible airflow limitation and reduced transfer coefficient in patients with asthma after 26 years of follow up. Thorax 2003;58(4):322–7.

20. Watson L, Schouten JP, Lofdahl CG, et al. Predictors of COPD symptoms: does the sex of the patient matter? Eur Respir J 2006;28(2):311–8.

21. Prescott E, Lange P, Vestbo J. Chronic mucus hypersecretion in COPD and death from pulmonary infection. Eur Respir J 1995;8(8):1333–8.

22. Fattahi F, ten Hacken NH, Lofdahl CG, et al. Atopy is a risk factor for respiratory symptoms in COPD patients: results from the EUROSCOP study. Respir Res 2013;14(1):10.

23. Tashkin DP, Celli B, Decramer M, et al. Bronchodilator responsiveness in patients with COPD. Eur Respir J 2008;31(4):742–50.

24. Tashkin DP, Celli B, Senn S, et al. A 4-year trial of tiotropium in chronic obstructive pulmonary disease. N Engl J Med 2008;359(15):1543–54.

25. Bleecker ER, Emmett A, Crater G, et al. Lung function and symptom improvement with fluticasone propionate/salmeterol and ipratropium bromide/albuterol in COPD: response by beta-agonist reversibility. Pulm Pharmacol Ther 2008; 21(4):682–8.

26. Albert P, Agusti A, Edwards L, et al. Bronchodilator responsiveness as a phenotypic characteristic of established chronic obstructive pulmonary disease. Thorax 2012;67(8):701–8.

27. Papi A, Romagnoli M, Baraldo S, et al. Partial reversibility of airflow limitation and increased exhaled NO and sputum eosinophilia in chronic obstructive pulmonary disease. Am J Respir Crit Care Med 2000;162(5):1773–7.

28. Mohamed Hoesein FA, de HB, Zanen P, et al. CT-quantified emphysema in male heavy smokers: association with lung function decline. Thorax 2011;66(9):782–7.

29. Van den Berge M, ten Hacken NH, Cohen J, et al. Small airway disease in asthma and COPD: clinical implications. Chest 2011;139(2):412–23.

30. Van den Berge M, ten Hacken NH, Van der Wiel E, et al. Treatment of the bronchial tree from beginning to end: targeting small airway inflammation in asthma. Allergy 2013;68(1):16–26.

31. Van der Wiel E, ten Hacken NH, Postma DS, et al. Small-airways dysfunction associates with respiratory symptoms and clinical features of asthma: a systematic review. J Allergy Clin Immunol 2013;131(3):646–57.

32. Turner SW, Palmer LJ, Rye PJ, et al. Infants with flow limitation at 4 weeks: outcome at 6 and 11 years. Am J Respir Crit Care Med 2002;165(9): 1294–8.

33. Paredi P, Goldman M, Alamen A, et al. Comparison of inspiratory and expiratory resistance and reactance in patients with asthma and chronic obstructive pulmonary disease. Thorax 2010;65(3):263–7.

34. Verbanck S, Schuermans D, Paiva M, et al. Nonreversible conductive airway ventilation heterogeneity in mild asthma. J Appl Physiol 2003;94(4):1380–6.

35. Verbanck S, Schuermans D, Noppen M, et al. Evidence of acinar airway involvement in asthma. Am J Respir Crit Care Med 1999;159(5 Pt 1):1545–50.

36. Verbanck S, Schuermans D, Van MA, et al. Conductive and acinar lung-zone contributions to ventilation inhomogeneity in COPD. Am J Respir Crit Care Med 1998;157(5 Pt 1):1573–7.

37. Galban CJ, Han MK, Boes JL, et al. Computed tomography-based biomarker provides unique signature for diagnosis of COPD phenotypes and disease progression. Nat Med 2012;18(11):1711–5.

38. Kay AB. Overview of 'allergy and allergic diseases: with a view to the future. Br Med Bull 2000;56(4):843–64.

39. The ENFUMOSA cross-sectional European multicentre study of the clinical phenotype of chronic severe asthma. European Network for Understanding Mechanisms of Severe Asthma. Eur Respir J 2003;22(3):470–7.

40. Sparrow D, O'Connor G, Weiss ST. The relation of airways responsiveness and atopy to the development of chronic obstructive lung disease. Epidemiol Rev 1988;10:29–47.

41. Weiss ST. Atopy as a risk factor for chronic obstructive pulmonary disease: epidemiological evidence. Am J Respir Crit Care Med 2000;162(3 Pt 2):S134–6.

42. Sahn SA. Corticosteroids in chronic bronchitis and pulmonary emphysema. Chest 1978;73(3):389–96.

43. Postma DS, Kerstjens HA. Characteristics of airway hyperresponsiveness in asthma and chronic obstructive pulmonary disease. Am J Respir Crit Care Med 1998;158(5 Pt 3):S187–92.

44. Tashkin DP, Altose MD, Bleecker ER, et al. The lung health study: airway responsiveness to inhaled methacholine in smokers with mild to moderate airflow limitation. The Lung Health Study Research Group. Am Rev Respir Dis 1992; 145(2 Pt 1):301–10.

45. Kerstjens HA, Brand PL, Hughes MD, et al. A comparison of bronchodilator therapy with or without inhaled corticosteroid therapy for obstructive airways disease. Dutch Chronic Non-Specific Lung Disease Study Group. N Engl J Med 1992;327(20):1413–9.

46. Reddel HK, Jenkins CR, Marks GB, et al. Optimal asthma control, starting with high doses of inhaled budesonide. Eur Respir J 2000;16(2):226–35.

47. Kerstjens HA, Schouten JP, Brand PL, et al. Importance of total serum IgE for improvement in airways hyperresponsiveness with inhaled corticosteroids in asthma and chronic obstructive pulmonary disease. The Dutch CNSLD Study Group. Am J Respir Crit Care Med 1995;151(2 Pt 1):360–8.

48. Chanez P, Vignola AM, O'Shaugnessy T, et al. Corticosteroid reversibility in COPD is related to features of asthma. Am J Respir Crit Care Med 1997; 155(5):1529–34.

49. Finkelstein R, Ma HD, Ghezzo H, et al. Morphometry of small airways in smokers and its relationship to emphysema type and hyperresponsiveness. Am J Respir Crit Care Med 1995;152(1):267–76.
50. Wiggs BR, Bosken C, Pare PD, et al. A model of airway narrowing in asthma and in chronic obstructive pulmonary disease. Am Rev Respir Dis 1992;145(6):1251–8.
51. Rutgers SR, Timens W, Kauffman HF, et al. Markers of active airway inflammation and remodelling in chronic obstructive pulmonary disease. Clin Exp Allergy 2001;31(2):193–205.
52. Blacquiere MJ, Timens W, Melgert BN, et al. Maternal smoking during pregnancy induces airway remodelling in mice offspring. Eur Respir J 2009;33(5):1133–40.
53. Black JL, Panettieri RA Jr, Banerjee A, et al. Airway smooth muscle in asthma: just a target for bronchodilation? Clin Chest Med 2012;33(3):543–58.
54. Hardaker KM, Downie SR, Kermode JA, et al. Predictors of airway hyperresponsiveness differ between old and young patients with asthma. Chest 2011;139(6):1395–401.
55. Downie SR, Salome CM, Verbanck S, et al. Ventilation heterogeneity is a major determinant of airway hyperresponsiveness in asthma, independent of airway inflammation. Thorax 2007;62(8):684–9.
56. Van den Berge M, Vonk JM, Gosman M, et al. Clinical and inflammatory determinants of bronchial hyperresponsiveness in COPD. Eur Respir J 2012;40(5):1098–105.
57. Shaya FT, Dongyi D, Akazawa MO, et al. Burden of concomitant asthma and COPD in a Medicaid population. Chest 2008;134(1):14–9.
58. Weatherall M, Travers J, Shirtcliffe PM, et al. Distinct clinical phenotypes of airways disease defined by cluster analysis. Eur Respir J 2009;34(4):812–8.
59. Guerra S. Overlap of asthma and chronic obstructive pulmonary disease. Curr Opin Pulm Med 2005;11(1):7–13.
60. Buist AS. Similarities and differences between asthma and chronic obstructive pulmonary disease: treatment and early outcomes. Eur Respir J Suppl 2003;39:30s–5s.
61. Soler-Cataluna JJ, Cosio B, Izquierdo JL, et al. Consensus document on the overlap phenotype COPD-asthma in COPD. Arch Bronconeumol 2012;48(9):331–7.
62. Kauppi P, Kupiainen H, Lindqvist A, et al. Overlap syndrome of asthma and COPD predicts low quality of life. J Asthma 2011;48(3):279–85.
63. Meyer PA, Mannino DM, Redd SC, et al. Characteristics of adults dying with COPD. Chest 2002;122(6):2003–8.
64. Hospers JJ, Schouten JP, Weiss ST, et al. Asthma attacks with eosinophilia predict mortality from chronic obstructive pulmonary disease in a general population sample. Am J Respir Crit Care Med 1999;160(6):1869–74.
65. Postma DS, Kerkhof M, Boezen HM, et al. Asthma and chronic obstructive pulmonary disease: common genes, common environments? Am J Respir Crit Care Med 2011;183(12):1588–94.
66. Bosse Y. Updates on the COPD gene list. Int J Chron Obstruct Pulmon Dis 2012;7:607–31.
67. Hao K, Bosse Y, Nickle DC, et al. Lung eQTLs to help reveal the molecular underpinnings of asthma. PLoS Genet 2012;8(11):e1003029.
68. Himes BE, Jiang X, Hu R, et al. Genome-wide association analysis in asthma subjects identifies SPATS2L as a novel bronchodilator response gene. PLoS Genet 2012;8(7):e1002824.

69. Imboden M, Bouzigon E, Curjuric I, et al. Genome-wide association study of lung function decline in adults with and without asthma. J Allergy Clin Immunol 2012;129(5):1218–28.

70. Niewoehner DE, Kleinerman J, Rice DB. Pathologic changes in the peripheral airways of young cigarette smokers. N Engl J Med 1974;291(15):755–8.

71. Battaglia S, Mauad T, van Schadewijk AM, et al. Differential distribution of inflammatory cells in large and small airways in smokers. J Clin Pathol 2007;60(8): 907–11.

72. Ballarin A, Bazzan E, Zenteno RH, et al. Mast cell infiltration discriminates between histopathological phenotypes of chronic obstructive pulmonary disease. Am J Respir Crit Care Med 2012;186(3):233–9.

73. Baraldo S, Turato G, Saetta M. Pathophysiology of the small airways in chronic obstructive pulmonary disease. Respiration 2012;84(2):89–97.

74. Fabbri LM, Romagnoli M, Corbetta L, et al. Differences in airway inflammation in patients with fixed airflow obstruction due to asthma or chronic obstructive pulmonary disease. Am J Respir Crit Care Med 2003;167(3):418–24.

75. Rutgers SR, Postma DS, ten Hacken NH, et al. Ongoing airway inflammation in patients with COPD who do not currently smoke. Thorax 2000;55(1):12–8.

76. Willemse BW, ten Hacken NH, Rutgers B, et al. Effect of 1-year smoking cessation on airway inflammation in COPD and asymptomatic smokers. Eur Respir J 2005;26(5):835–45.

77. Hogg JC, Chu F, Utokaparch S, et al. The nature of small-airway obstruction in chronic obstructive pulmonary disease. N Engl J Med 2004;350(26):2645–53.

78. Shaw DE, Berry MA, Hargadon B, et al. Association between neutrophilic airway inflammation and airflow limitation in adults with asthma. Chest 2007;132(6): 1871–5.

79. McGrath KW, Icitovic N, Boushey HA, et al. A large subgroup of mild-to-moderate asthma is persistently noneosinophilic. Am J Respir Crit Care Med 2012;185(6):612–9.

80. Benayoun L, Druilhe A, Dombret MC, et al. Airway structural alterations selectively associated with severe asthma. Am J Respir Crit Care Med 2003; 167(10):1360–8.

81. Saha S, Brightling CE. Eosinophilic airway inflammation in COPD. Int J Chron Obstruct Pulmon Dis 2006;1(1):39–47.

82. Bathoorn E, Liesker JJ, Postma DS, et al. Change in inflammation in out-patient COPD patients from stable phase to a subsequent exacerbation. Int J Chron Obstruct Pulmon Dis 2009;4:101–9.

83. Bafadhel M, McKenna S, Terry S, et al. Blood eosinophils to direct corticosteroid treatment of exacerbations of chronic obstructive pulmonary disease: a randomized placebo-controlled trial. Am J Respir Crit Care Med 2012;186(1):48–55.

84. Brightling CE, McKenna S, Hargadon B, et al. Sputum eosinophilia and the short term response to inhaled mometasone in chronic obstructive pulmonary disease. Thorax 2005;60(3):193–8.

85. Kuwano K, Bosken CH, Pare PD, et al. Small airways dimensions in asthma and in chronic obstructive pulmonary disease. Am Rev Respir Dis 1993;148(5): 1220–5.

86. Carroll N, Elliot J, Morton A, et al. The structure of large and small airways in nonfatal and fatal asthma. Am Rev Respir Dis 1993;147(2):405–10.

87. Carroll NG, Perry S, Karkhanis A, et al. The airway longitudinal elastic fiber network and mucosal folding in patients with asthma. Am J Respir Crit Care Med 2000;161(1):244–8.

88. Mauad T, Silva LF, Santos MA, et al. Abnormal alveolar attachments with decreased elastic fiber content in distal lung in fatal asthma. Am J Respir Crit Care Med 2004;170(8):857–62.

89. Travers J, Marsh S, Caldwell B, et al. External validity of randomized controlled trials in COPD. Respir Med 2007;101(6):1313–20.

90. Travers J, Marsh S, Williams M, et al. External validity of randomised controlled trials in asthma: to whom do the results of the trials apply? Thorax 2007;62(3): 219–23.

91. Lapperre TS, Snoeck-Stroband JB, Gosman MM, et al. Effect of fluticasone with and without salmeterol on pulmonary outcomes in chronic obstructive pulmonary disease: a randomized trial. Ann Intern Med 2009;151(8):517–27.

92. Celli BR, Thomas NE, Anderson JA, et al. Effect of pharmacotherapy on rate of decline of lung function in chronic obstructive pulmonary disease: results from the TORCH study. Am J Respir Crit Care Med 2008;178(4):332–8.

93. Jen R, Rennard SI, Sin DD. Effects of inhaled corticosteroids on airway inflammation in chronic obstructive pulmonary disease: a systematic review and meta-analysis. Int J Chron Obstruct Pulmon Dis 2012;7:587–95.

94. Siva R, Green RH, Brightling CE, et al. Eosinophilic airway inflammation and exacerbations of COPD: a randomised controlled trial. Eur Respir J 2007;29(5): 906–13.

95. Snoeck-Stroband JB, Lapperre TS, Sterk PJ, et al. Fewer packyears smoking and less signs of emphysema predict long-term inhaled corticosteroid response in moderate to severe COPD: analysis of a randomized trial cohort. Abstract ATS. 2012.

96. Hancox RJ, Cowan DC, Aldridge RE, et al. Asthma phenotypes: consistency of classification using induced sputum. Respirology 2012;17(3):461–6.

97. Welte T, Miravitlles M, Hernandez P, et al. Efficacy and tolerability of budesonide/formoterol added to tiotropium in patients with chronic obstructive pulmonary disease. Am J Respir Crit Care Med 2009;180(8):741–50.

98. Magnussen H, Bugnas B, van NJ, et al. Improvements with tiotropium in COPD patients with concomitant asthma. Respir Med 2008;102(1):50–6.

The Overlap of Bronchiectasis and Immunodeficiency with Asthma

Tho Truong, MD

KEYWORDS

- Bronchiectasis • Asthma • Immunodeficiency • Atopy • B lymphocyte
- T lymphocyte

KEY POINTS

- Bronchiectasis should be considered as both a differential diagnosis for, as well as a co-morbidity in, patients with asthma, especially severe or long-standing asthma.
- Chronic airway inflammation is thought to be the primary cause of bronchiectasis, as seen in chronic or recurrent pulmonary infections and autoimmune conditions that involve the airways.
- Consequently, immunodeficiencies with associated increased susceptibility to respiratory tract infections or chronic inflammatory airways also increase the risk of developing bronchiectasis.
- Chronic bronchiectasis is associated with impaired mucociliary clearance and increased bronchial secretions, leading to airway obstruction and airflow limitation, which can lead to the exacerbation of underlying asthma or an increase in asthma symptoms.

INTRODUCTION

Bronchiectasis should be considered as both a differential diagnosis for, as well as a comorbidity in, patients with asthma, especially severe or long-standing asthma. Chronic airway inflammation is thought to be the primary cause of bronchiectasis, as demonstrated in chronic or recurrent pulmonary infections and autoimmune conditions that involve the airways. Consequently, immunodeficiencies with associated increased susceptibility to respiratory tract infections or chronic inflammatory airways also increase the risk of developing bronchiectasis. Chronic bronchiectasis is associated with impaired mucociliary clearance and increased bronchial secretions, leading to airway obstruction and airflow limitation, which can lead to the exacerbation of underlying asthma or an increase in asthma symptoms.

The Definition of Bronchiectasis

Chronic and abnormal dilation of the airways characterizes bronchiectasis. This persistent enlargement of the bronchi results in decreased clearance of respiratory

This article originally appeared in Immunology and Allergy Clinics of North America, Volume 33, Issue 1, February 2013.
Allergy and Clinical Immunology, National Jewish Health, Denver, CO, USA
E-mail address: truongt@njhealth.org

secretions, which then may lead to symptoms of airflow obstruction and increased mucus production and retention. Airflow limitation in bronchiectasis may be reversible as well as fixed. These postobstructive changes further increase the risk of respiratory infection and inflammatory damage in the airways, which in turn can worsen the bronchiectasis. These conditions also produce an airway environment that predisposes to persistent abnormal colonization of microflora, further driving the bronchiectasis. In addition to infection and autoimmune disease, significant chronic aspiration of oropharyngeal or gastric contents as well as chronic exposure to toxic inhalants may also contribute to or result in bronchiectasis.

The Diagnosis of Bronchiectasis

The current defining test for bronchiectasis is radiographic, using high-resolution computed tomography (HRCT) of the chest. The patient's clinical history is also taken into account. A luminal airway diameter that is more than 1.5 times the adjacent blood vessel supports the presence of cylindrical bronchiectasis; a normal luminal airway diameter is usually 1.0 to 1.5 times the size of an adjacent vessel. Other features are also considered besides airways dilation, such as a lack of tapering of the airways when dilation is present, bronchial wall thickening in the dilated airways, the presence of cysts adjacent to the luminal wall of the dilated bronchiole, and mucopurulent plugs. When there is involvement of the smaller airways, there can be irregular, more peripherally located linear branch markings (2–4 mm), a so-called tree-in-bud pattern. Bronchial wall thickening has been suggested as the best predictor of functional decline, and the presence of cysts off of the bronchial wall may signal more destructive bronchiectasis. Although also described with emphysema, blebs can also appear more distally but are generally thinner in wall thickness and are not accompanied by proximal airway changes as seen in emphysema. Evidence for chronic infection, such as consolidation, lymphadenopathy, and vascular disruption, may also be seen.[1]

Bronchiectasis and Asthma

There have been many studies that demonstrate considerable overlap between asthma and bronchiectasis. For instance, investigators[2–4] studied 245 patients characterized as having severe asthma. Of these patients, 24.8% had radiographic evidence of bronchiectasis on CT of the chest. In another study of 1680 patients with a diagnosis of asthma, about 3% had radiographic bronchiectasis. In contrast to age- and gender-matched patients with asthma without bronchiectasis who generally had only mild intermittent or mild persistent asthma (69.4%), most of those patients with asthma with bronchiectasis had severe persistent asthma (49.0%). Not surprisingly, these patients had a much higher rate of pulmonary complications and hospitalizations for respiratory failure.[5]

Bronchiectasis and Immunodeficiency States

Because the presence of bronchiectasis may significantly alter the prognosis of patients with asthma, it is important to optimize the management of its known causes and contributors. There is some evidence to suggest that the diagnosis and treatment of underlying immunodeficiency can prevent or slow the deterioration of pulmonary outcomes in patients with bronchiectasis and certain immunodeficiency states. A longitudinal study of children with primary immunodeficiency showed that children diagnosed with bronchiectasis at a median age of 3 years and subsequently diagnosed with and treated for primary humoral immunodeficiency did not have deterioration of pulmonary function at 9 years of age, based on pulmonary function studies and HRCT scores.[6] Another study on the efficacy of intravenous immunoglobulin treatment in children with common variable immunodeficiency (CVID) found that treatment with a sufficient replacement dose of intravenous gamma globulin (IVIG) significantly reduced the mean number of respiratory infections per patient per year, from 10.2 to 2.5. The annual number and length of hospital stays per patient also decreased significantly from 1.36 to 0.21 admissions and 16.35 to 6.33 days, respectively. Additionally, the mean annual number of antibiotics used per patient decreased significantly from 8.27 to 2.50. These investigators suggested that age at diagnosis, diagnostic delay, number of respiratory tract infections, and number of antibiotics were found to be significantly higher in patients with bronchiectasis. Thus, an evaluation for immunodeficiency states should be considered in all patients with bronchiectasis to optimize its management and minimize adverse sequelae.

Immunodeficiency, Atopy, and Asthma

In addition to sinopulmonary infections playing a role in poorly controlled asthma, patients with certain primary and secondary immunodeficiency diagnoses also have an increased risk for atopic disease. For instance, up to 50% of children with selective immunoglobulin A (IgA) deficiency have been observed to have allergic disease.[7] In a prospective study of children with selective IgA or IgG4 subclass deficiency, the occurrence of allergic disease and asthma increased with decreased levels of IgA and/or IgG4 in serum and salivary IgA. Another study showed that not only was the prevalence of atopy higher in a group of children with selective IgA deficiency compared with the control population, but also that the children with selective IgA deficiency had more frequent concomitant airways hyperresponsivity to the dust mite *Dermatophagoides pteronyssinus*.[8–10] It is thought that deficient mucosal immunity in IgA deficiency plays a role in the dysregulation of tolerance to allergens.

Perhaps counter to intuition, even patients with profound defects in antibody production, including IgE, have demonstrated a relatively high incidence of asthma and atopic disease. In 2008, Shabestari and Rezaei[11] reported a case in which a patient with Bruton agammaglobulinemia, with essentially absent serum concentrations of all immunoglobulin isotypes and virtually absent CD19+ lymphocytes, had a positive skin prick test to multiple airborne allergens. He also had bronchial hyperresponsivity by allergen challenge and spirometry. It is speculated that a bias toward T-helper cell type 2 (Th2)-mediated immune response accounts for this.

This Th2-bias has also been suggested in patients with CVID through the demonstration of increased interleukin 4 (IL-4) and IL-10 production. A high incidence of asthma, usually diagnosed after the initial presentation, was seen in 83% of pediatric patients with CVID.[12] Similarly, in another study, 9 out of 18 patients who had a diagnosis of CVID and a clinical history suggestive of allergic asthma tested positive to bronchoprovocation with histamine or specific allergen challenge; 6 of those patients had positive placebo-controlled bronchoprovocation to a specific allergen despite negative allergen-specific IgE and skin testing.[13,14]

Patients with secondary immunodeficiency, such as human immunodeficiency virus (HIV) infection, have also demonstrated clinical atopy, and in some studies, increased IgE-mediated atopy. Some data support that patients who are HIV positive present with a higher incidence of atopy in the earlier stages of HIV infection compared with the general population. Multivariate analysis of 74 hospitalized patients with HIV demonstrated that a personal history suggestive of allergic disease and serum IgE level >150 ku/L were predictors of atopy; gender, HIV risk group, CD4+ T cells, CD23 expression on B cells, and AIDS were not associated.[15] This study speculated that because allergic reactions could accelerate HIV infection by increasing the type 2 cytokines, identifying the atopic state in patients with HIV, especially those with IgE greater than 150 ku/L or a personal history that suggests allergy, was important to optimizing control of the HIV infection.

Immunodeficiency

Both primary and secondary immunodeficiencies should be considered in patients with bronchiectasis. Both primary and secondary immunodeficiency can increase the risk for sinopulmonary infections, leading to bronchiectasis. The evaluation for immunodeficiency is guided by the clinical presentation, such as patient age and gender, past medical history, present health, nutritional status, as well as history of infections (including severity, infectious organisms, and involved organ systems).

Secondary Immunodeficiency

Systemic illnesses, such as diabetes, hematologic malignancies, and chronic infections; immunosuppressive treatments, such as chemotherapy and radiation; and protein-losing syndromes may cause secondary immunodeficiency. Secondary immunodeficiency may also occur in critically ill and older hospitalized patients because prolonged serious illness and poor or diminished nutrition can lead to impaired immune responses. Frequently, secondary immunodeficiency can be corrected if the underlying problem resolves.

Protein loss

Serum protein loss through the kidneys, gastrointestinal (GI) tract, or skin, as with severe burns or dermatitis, can lead to immunodeficiency, particularly because of the loss of IgG and albumin. Enteropathy can also result in lymphopenia with the loss of both T and B lymphocytes. In intestinal lymphangiectasia, there is abnormal dilatation of intestinal mucosal lymphatic channels, which leads to the loss of immunoglobulins and lymphocytes into the gut lumen. The disorder may be congenital or result from processes that obstruct lymph drainage of the gut or cause an increased central venous pressure. These disorders can mimic B- and T-cell deficiencies, but treatment with a diet high in medium-chain triglycerides may decrease the loss of immunoglobulins and markedly improve lymphocyte counts.

Nutrition

Undernutrition also impairs immune responses. It should be considered as a cause for immunodeficiency states, particularly in elderly, chronically ill, institutionalized, or homebound patients. Calcium, vitamin E, and zinc play essential roles in immunity. The risk for calcium deficiency is increased in the elderly because of decreased calcium absorption from the GI tract as well as decreased ingestion of calcium from the diet. Institutionalized or homebound elderly patients are also more likely to have zinc deficiency than the general population.

Immune function and aging

Normal decreases in immune function have been described in healthy aging patient populations. For instance, cellular immunity may be reduced because the thymus generally produces fewer naïve T cells. The total number of T lymphocytes does not decrease, but naïve T cells potentiate the response to new antigens. The preexisting T-cell repertoire can only recognize a limited number of antigens. In addition, impaired cellular signal transduction has been demonstrated, and this could lead to decreased signaling to B cells to make antibodies and decrease the T-cell response to antigen. Neutrophils are also less effective in phagocytosis and have decreased microbicidal activity.

Hematological malignancies

Although hematologic malignancy has been reported in up to 30% of patients with primary immunodeficiencies, secondary immunodeficiency can be seen in patients with primary lymphoproliferative disorders. Cellular and humoral immune deficiencies have been described in acute and chronic leukemias, myeloma, and lymphomas. Because these conditions can result in B and T lymphocyte dysfunction, patients are more susceptible to recurrent lung infections and the development of bronchiectasis.[16–19] Additionally, chemotherapeutic agents used to treat these conditions often result in profound immunodeficiency (See "Medication that may cause immunodeficiency" slide).

Some medications which may cause immunodeficiency	
Anti convulsants	**Chemotherapeutic drugs**
Carbamazepine	Busulfan
Phenytoin	Cyclophosphamide
Valproate	Docetaxel
Anti hypertensives	Epirubicin
Amlodipine	Imatinib
Captopril	Melphalan
Enalapril	**NSAIDs**
Hydralazine	Diclofenac
Hydrochlorothiazide	Fenclofenac
Anti microbials	Meloxicam
Amphotericin B	Naproxen
Anti-virals (ie acyclovir, cidovir, foscarnet)	**Steroid-sparing Immunosuppressives**
Antimalarial agents (ie chloroquine)	Azathioprine
	Cyclopsorine
Cephalosporins/Penicillins	Gold salts
Ethambutol	Mycophenolate mofetil
Tetracycline/Doxycycline	Penicillamine
Biologics/Immunologicals	Sirolimus
Abatacept	Sulfasalazine
Alemtuzumab	Tacrolimus
Belatacept	**Other**
Certolizumab	Glipizide
Muromonab	Gabapentin
Rituximab	Penicillamine
Corticosteroids	Proton pump inhibitors (esomeprazole, lansoprazole, omperazole)
	Metoclopramide

HIV infection

The progression of disease in individuals infected with HIV varies greatly, but in most untreated patients, there is a progressive T-cell defect that results in a declining trend in CD4+ T-helper cell number. This declining trend may lead to decreased cellular immunity as well as T-cell–independent immunity, such as with local macrophage- and monocyte-dependent pulmonary immunity. Additionally, although most adult patients may have hypergammaglobulinemia with HIV infection, infants who are HIV positive can demonstrate severe hypogammaglobulinemia, suggesting that the development of humoral immunity is also affected.[20] Consequently, patients who are HIV positive are more prone to recurrent infections, both with usual and opportunistic pulmonary pathogens, including mycobacterium and *S pneumonia*.

Secondary Immunodeficiencies and Bronchiectasis

Reliable data regarding the relationship between secondary immune deficiencies and bronchiectasis are limited. Most of this data come from studies of patients with infectious complications caused by hematologic malignancy or the treatment of hematologic malignancy and patients who are HIV positive. It is generally regarded that other secondary causes of immunodeficiency do not result in a significant increased risk for recurrent pulmonary infection and bronchiectasis.

Hematological malignancies and bronchiectasis

A handful of case reports and series have described bronchiectasis complicating chemotherapy in acute myelogenous leukemia, CLL, multiple myeloma, and lymphomas. Multiple myeloma and CLL seem to be more commonly associated with bronchiectasis than the other hematologic malignancies, but there are no well-established incidence rates of bronchiectasis in patients with hematological malignancies. This lack may be caused by the combination of prolonged survival in patients with these malignancies and the higher frequency of secondary hypogammaglobulinemia in CLL and myeloma than in other hematologic disorders. It is suggested that patients with radiographic-proven bronchiectasis be assessed for hypogammaglobulinemia and considered for IVIG therapy. Bronchiectasis has also been reported, though less frequently, in acute hematological malignancies, perhaps as a consequence of severe lung infections or in the setting of profound immunodeficiency after chemotherapeutic intervention.[16,18,21]

Posttransplantation bronchiectasis

Hematopoietic stem cell transplantation (HSCT) is associated with an increased incidence of respiratory infections and prolonged defects in both cellular and humoral immunity in survivors.[22–26] These factors could predispose to bronchiectasis; in fact, serial CT scans after allograft HSCT can demonstrate rapidly developing bronchiectasis over a period of weeks to months. In addition, up to 10% of HSCT allograft recipients will develop bronchiolitis obliterans, which is the main pulmonary manifestation of graft-versus-host disease. This precedes the appearance of diffuse bronchiectasis in approximately 40% of cases.[27] Likewise, patients who develop bronchiolitis obliterans after lung transplantation may also have CT evidence of bronchiectasis, and there are cases of bronchiectasis developing after the transplantation of other solid organs, presumably because of impaired pulmonary immunity secondary to immunosuppressive therapy.[28]

HIV and bronchiectasis

The cause of HIV-related bronchiectasis is not well understood because of multiple confounding factors, such as concurrent pneumonia or tuberculosis; some studies also suggest an association of HIV in adults with an increase in chronic obstructive pulmonary disease. More reliable data may be from longitudinal pediatric studies. Up to 16% of children infected with HIV develop bronchiectasis.[20] Because of much better recent survival rates, the incidence of bronchiectasis in adults infected with HIV may also be significant. Bronchiectasis in children who are HIV positive is more likely in patients with CD4 counts less than 100 mm^3 or who have had recurrent pneumonia. Interestingly, there is also a specific association with lymphocytic interstitial pneumonitis (LIP), with up to 40% of HIV-infected children with LIP developing bronchiectasis.[29–31] There are no comparative data on the pattern and progression of bronchiectasis in patients who are HIV positive versus patients with bronchiectasis from other causes. More prevalence data and stratification of risk groups in HIV-positive patients are needed to direct recommendations for the management of bronchiectasis to prevent or slow the progression of lung disease.

Primary Immunodeficiencies

Primary immunodeficiencies are genetically predetermined disorders of the immune system, which result in decreased immunity and subsequent increase in susceptibility to infection. There are other diseases that result in recurrent or persistent infections, such as cystic fibrosis (CF) and ciliary dyskinesia, that also have a molecular genetic basis; these are discussed briefly but have generally not been thought to be predominantly driven by a functional defect within the immune system, although newer data suggest mucosal immunity is significantly diminished in these diseases. The molecular basis for about 70% to 80% of the more than 200 primary functional immune deficiencies that have been clinically described is known. For many of these diagnoses, the severity and spectrum of disease can vary widely. These conditions generally present during childhood, with about 70% of patients aged less than 20 years at the onset, with unusually frequent/recurrent infection or infection with uncommon organisms. Overall, about 60% of patients are male because many of the described disorders are X-linked. It is estimated that the incidence of symptomatic disease is about 1 out of 280 people.[32]

Primary immunodeficiencies are currently classified by the deficient immune system components involved, such as the B lymphocytes and immunoglobulins, T lymphocytes and natural killer (NK) cells, phagocytic cells, complement proteins, and receptor proteins, although there can be considerable overlap in immune function for these components, and combinations of deficiencies have been described in several clinical immunodeficiency diseases or syndromes.[32]

B lymphocyte disorders and hypogammaglobulinemia

It has been generally presumed that antibody deficiencies, which account for more than 50% of the described primary immunodeficiencies, result mostly from B-cell defects. Selective IgA deficiency is the most common B-cell disorder, and others are CVID and X-linked agammaglobulinemia (XLA). Patients with these diseases may have low or absent quantitative immunoglobulin isotypes and, in the case of CVID and XLA, low or absent specific antibody titers that can predispose them to infections with encapsulated gram-positive bacteria.

T lymphocyte disorders

Approximately 5% to 10% of primary immunodeficiencies are T-cell disorders. These diseases predispose patients to infection by viruses and opportunistic organisms, such as *Pneumocystis jiroveci* and fungi, as well as many common respiratory tract pathogens. Some T-cell disorders also cause immunoglobulin deficiencies because

B lymphocyte and T lymphocyte crosstalk is essential to generate specific antibodies. The more common T-cell disorders are DiGeorge syndrome, ZAP-70 deficiency, X-linked lymphoproliferative syndrome, and chronic mucocutaneous candidiasis.[33]

Disorders with combined B- and T-cell defects

Severe combined immunodeficiency (SCID) describes a set of disorders based on molecular defects affecting both B-cell and T-cell function. Several forms have been described and linked to specific genetic mutations, such as purine nucleoside phosphorylase deficiency. Immunoglobulin levels are normal or elevated with this deficiency, but because of inadequate T-cell function, antibody formation is impaired. Other genetic mutations identified in SCID include adenosine deaminase deficiency as well as mutations in the common gamma chain (encoded by the gene IL-2 receptor gamma), Janus kinase-3, and Artemis/DCLRE1C (which is essential to DNA repair).[34]

Disorders of innate immunity

Clinically significant primary NK cell defects are very rare and predispose patients to viral infections and tumors. Defects in the phagocytic and direct pathogen killing function of cells, such as macrophages, neutrophils, and monocytes, may account for 10% to 15% of described primary immunodeficiencies. Patients may have recurrent cutaneous staphylococcal and gram-negative infections. The most common phagocytic cell defects are chronic granulomatous disease (CGD), leukocyte adhesion deficiency, and Chédiak-Higashi syndrome.[32]

Complement deficiencies and more newly described toll-like receptor protein deficiencies are rare ($\leq$2% of described primary immunodeficiencies). Complement deficiencies can result in defective opsonization, phagocytosis, and lysis of pathogens, causing susceptibility to several bacteria. They can also cause defective clearance of antigen-antibody complexes, resulting in autoimmune inflammatory damage to an end-organ system (such as in lupus glomerulonephritis). Complement deficiency can also include the deficiency of C1 inhibitor, which underlies hereditary angioedema but is not associated with abnormal frequency or type of infections. C1 inhibitor deficiency is autosomal dominant, whereas the other complement deficiencies are autosomal recessive; the exception is properdin, which is X linked.[32]

The Relationship Between Immunodeficiency and Bronchiectasis

Infections as a cause for bronchiectasis in immunodeficiency

Almost all of the described immunodeficiencies and immunodeficiency syndromes can theoretically lead or contribute to bronchiectasis by increasing the risk of chronic or abnormally frequent and serious sinopulmonary infections. Overall, immunodeficiency is considered to be a rare cause of bronchiectasis in adults (0.5% to 2.4% versus 2% to 10% in the pediatric population).[5,35] However, some other reviewers have noted that of those presenting with bronchiectasis, as many as 7% of the adult population or one-third of the pediatric population have a primary immunodeficiency.[36] There are relatively few studies in the current literature that evaluate the incidence of immunodeficiency in patients with bronchiectasis, and most of these studies have been done at hospitals or academic centers specializing in respiratory diseases. Thus, the true incidence of immunodeficiency, especially particular immunodeficiencies, in patients with bronchiectasis is really unknown.

The pathophysiologic process leading to bronchiectasis is characterized by airway injury and dilation, which is then thought to promote the persistent colonization of pathogens in the affected bronchi as well as denude the airways of mucociliary structures that provide clearance of secretions. Common nasopharyngeal pathogens, such as *Streptococcus pneumoniae* and *Haemophilus influenzae*, infect both adults and children to cause acute bronchitis and pneumonia. It is speculated that impaired host immunity to these pathogens initiates the development of bronchiectasis, which then further compromises mucosal structures and immune defenses to permit infection and/or chronic colonization with environmental bacteria, such as with *Pseudomonas aeruginosa.*[36]

Because antibody-mediated immunity underlies the recognition of polysaccharide encapsulated respiratory pathogens, such as *S pneumoniae* and *H influenzae,* primary humoral immunodeficiency or antibody deficiency secondary to lymphoproliferative malignancies have been the most identified and studied in bronchiectasis patients. In one London hospital study, 122 out of 165 patients with radiographic evidence of bronchiectasis had an identifiable cause. Of those 122 patients, 11 had immunodeficiency compared with 17 with primary ciliary dyskinesia, 2 with cystic fibrosis, and 13 with allergic bronchopulmonary aspergillosis; the remaining majority of patients had a postinfectious cause or idiopathic bronchiectasis. Immunodeficiency in those 11 patients was diagnosed by low quantitative IgG levels as well as low postvaccination pneumococcal antibody titers, which characterize humoral immunodeficiency. Seven of these patients had common variable immunodeficiency with panhypogammaglobulinemia, and 4 patients had humoral immunodeficiency secondary to lymphoma or leukemia.[37]

Autoimmune or autoinflammatory disease as a cause for bronchiectasis in immunodeficiency

It is well accepted that certain systemic autoimmune diseases, such as rheumatoid arthritis (RA) and primary Sjögren disease, can lead to bronchiectasis. In an older study of 52 patients with a diagnosis of idiopathic bronchiectasis, there was a very high prevalence of rheumatoid factor (52%) and an increased prevalence of antinuclear factor (10%) in the patients with bronchiectasis compared with the control groups. The presence of these autoantibodies did not correlate closely with the severity of disease. Ten patients with bronchiectasis (19%) had one or more previously diagnosed autoimmune disorders; similarly, bronchiectasis was present in 2 out of 12 patients with recent-onset inflammatory RA.[38,39] In a more recent prospective series, HRCT demonstrated bronchiectasis in 6 out of 42 patients with autoantibody positivity for RA (positive anticyclic citrullinated peptide and/or 2 rheumatoid factor isotypes) but no inflammatory arthritis, and 2 of those patients then presented with frank RA within 13 months.[40–43] Reciprocally, it is well established that a significant number of patients with primary immunodeficiency, especially CVID, develop manifestations of autoimmunity. It is not clear whether the patients with RA and bronchiectasis have had significant infections or immunosuppression that contributed to their bronchiectasis,[44,45] or if there is an inflammatory phenomena independent from infection that underlies the mechanism for bronchiectasis in patients with immune dysregulation.

Humoral Immunodeficiencies Associated with Bronchiectasis

The development of humoral immunodeficiencies

There are multiple steps in B-cell differentiation and signal transmission that, if compromised, may lead to clinically significant antibody deficiency. Variable defects leading to a compromised antibody response to antigens result in CVID, which is actually a heterogeneous group of disorders with only a partially characterized molecular cause. A blockade in the maturation process from pre–B cell to immature B cell has been well characterized by a mutation in Bruton tyrosine kinase, which results in XLA. There have also been genetic mutations affecting the early pre–B-cell repertoire, such as with recombination-activating gene; this mutation also affects T-cell development and results in SCID. Defects in class switching and somatic hypermutation result in hyper IgM syndromes.

CVID

CVID is the second most common adult primary immunodeficiency (after selective IgA deficiency) and is characterized by low serum concentrations of IgG in combination with other isotypes, poor responses to immunizations, and recurrent sinopulmonary infections. The serum IgG level must be 2 standard deviations lower than normal. The underlying genetics of this heterogeneous group of disorders have only been partially described. About 10% to 20% of cases are familial; the first associated genes described have been inherited in an autosomal-dominant fashion, often with variable penetrance. Some of the more recently identified genetic defects associated with CVID have an autosomal recessive inheritance pattern. Of the 10% to 15% of patients with CVID who have had an underlying genetic abnormality described, most patients have defects in the transmembrane regulator, calcium modulator, and cyclophilin ligand interactor. Much smaller populations of people with CVID have had B- or T-cell anomalies related to surface receptors involved in crosstalk between the two sets of lymphocytes, such as with mutations of the inducible T-cell surface expressed CD28 costimulatory molecule and the B-cell activating factor receptor, which is the CD19 component of the coreceptor for the B-cell antigen receptor.[32]

This variety of mutations affecting the different components involved in the process of antibody production may also explain the diversity of clinical presentations and outcomes in patients with CVID. For example, as mentioned earlier, up to 25% to 30% of patients with CVID also develop autoimmune and/or lymphoproliferative sequelae, including inflammatory arthritis, colitis, lymphocytic lung disease, or granulomatous disease. These proinflammatory complications of immunodeficiency, thought to be caused by dysregulated immune cell signaling, may arguably contribute to the development of bronchiectasis independent of the problem of higher susceptibility to infection caused by the immunodeficiency.

The treatment of CVID with IVIG has been shown to both reduce the incidence of respiratory tract infections[46,47] and decrease inflammation associated with bronchiectasis.[48,49] Thus, early identification and treatment of CVID with IVIG may arguably improve prognostic outcomes associated with bronchiectasis. Traditionally, the dose of replacement IVIG given is based on keeping the IgG trough level, which often resulted in dosing that kept the trough at the lower end of the normal range. However, more recent studies have advocated that individualized dosing, based on infection end points in patients, may be needed to minimize the risk of bronchiectasis and chronic, progressive lung disease.[50]

XLA

Despite the absence of all antibody isotypes in agammaglobulinemia, the relative risk for patients with agammaglobulinemia of developing structural lung damage is reportedly less than patients with CVID.[51] XLA has been associated with up to 3% of cases of childhood bronchiectasis[39,52] but is only a rare cause in adults. No specific pattern of bronchiectasis in patients with XLA has clearly been described. The long-term prognosis has improved with aggressive treatment with IVIG and antibiotic therapy, although there are few data on the rate of progression of bronchiectasis, and chronic lung disease remains a significant cause of death.[53]

Selective IgA, IgM, and IgG subclass deficiencies

There are no clear data to support that isolated IgA, IgM, or IgG subclass deficiency is clinically relevant or if any specific chronic management or treatment is indicated. IgA deficiency is relatively common, with a prevalence of about 1 in 600. However, it is unlikely that, in the absence of concurrent IgG subclass deficiency or specific antibody deficiency, isolated IgA or IgM deficiency would lead to bronchiectasis and progressive lung disease.[54–56] However, IgG subclass deficiency, especially IgG2, has been associated with bronchiectasis in children.[57] However, because the incidence of IgG subclass deficiency in patients with bronchiectasis varies so greatly (anywhere from 4% to nearly 50%), the clinical significance of this correlative data is called into question. IgG subclass deficiency is a relatively common finding in the general population and may reflect transient, normal fluctuations in the immune system.[58] Nonetheless, it should be noted that IgG2 deficiency has been associated with low specific antibody responses to *S pneumoniae* or *H influenzae* bacteria that are associated with bronchiectasis.[59]

Specific antibody deficiency

In one small population study without matched controls, up to 58% of patients with idiopathic bronchiectasis were identified with specific antibody deficiency to polysaccharide antigens. This and other similar studies used the measurement of antibody titers to *S pneumoniae* and *H influenzae* after vaccination in comparison with the antibody response to protein antigen vaccination, such as tetanus or diphtheria, to identify patients with specific antibody deficiency to these polysaccharide-encapsulated organisms; the lower-limit threshold to define the criteria for this immunodeficiency has been frequently debated, and there is still no clear concensus.[59] Antibody responses to vaccination with polysaccharide antigens are variable and affected by age, and up to 10% of the normal population may be nonresponders.[60–62] A larger series of adult patients with bronchiectasis suggest specific antibody deficiency has an incidence varying from 4% to 11%.[60,63–65] An impaired specific antibody response was associated with selected IgG subclass deficiencies in some patients.[57] It is clear that higher-powered, control-matched studies are needed to evaluate any relationship between specific antibody deficiency and bronchiectasis.

Other Primary Immunodeficiencies and Bronchiectasis

Transporter antigen peptide deficiency syndrome

Transporter antigen peptide (TAP) proteins are required for the transfer of peptide antigens from the cytosol into the endoplasmic reticulum, where they associate with human leukocyte antigen (HLA)-1 for presentation on cell surfaces. Autosomal recessive mutations in the TAP1 or TAP2 genes result in reduced HLA-1 expression and CD8 lymphocyte numbers but increased NK and γδ T cells.[36,66,67] Most patients with TAP deficiency have recurrent sinopulmonary infections with common respiratory tract bacterial pathogens and develop bronchiectasis.[66,67] Only a handful of families with TAP deficiency have been described, and this genetic defect will be responsible for a vanishingly small proportion of cases of bronchiectasis. However, the association of TAP deficiency and other very rare familial T-cell disorders with bronchiectasis[68–70] demonstrates that there are previously unsuspected mechanisms of immunity to extracellular bacterial pathogens involving CD8 lymphocytes that require further investigation. In addition, it has been suggested that an excess of NK and γδ T cells might promote bronchiectasis because of a dysregulated inflammatory response to infection with bacterial pathogens.

Macrophage or neutrophil functional deficiencies

There have been many inherited disorders affecting neutrophil function described, such as CGD, leukocyte adhesion deficiency, and Chédiak-Higashi syndrome. Although these disorders are extremely rare, making it difficult to accurately evaluate their clinical associations, neutrophil disorders classically lead to recurrent pneumonia. In a relatively large series of adult patients with bronchiectasis, tests of neutrophil function, such as flow cytometry for DHR, could only occasionally identify patients with abnormal responses. Even in these patients, the relationship of the defect to bronchiectasis is not clear. CGD has been associated with cases of bronchiectasis in some pediatric case reports, but these reports have significant selection bias. There is only a weak association of neutrophil defects with bronchiectasis and this may be attributable to the fact that the range of pathogens these patients are most susceptible to includes *Staphylococcus aureus*, *Nocardia*, *Aspergillus*, and *Candida* species but excludes *S pneumoniae* and *H influenzae*, which are the pathogens most closely associated with development of bronchiectasis.[52,71,72]

Primary defects of macrophage function generally affect intracellular killing and lead to increased incidences of infection with intracellular pathogens (such as mycobacteria, *Histoplasma*, *Listeria*, and *Salmonella* species) and have not been associated with the development of bronchiectasis. The extent to which functional polymorphisms of phagocytic receptors, such as Fc gamma RIIA H/R 131, or pattern recognition receptors, such as toll-like receptors, may predispose to bronchiectasis is unclear.[71,72]

Hyper IgE syndrome

Hyper IgE syndrome (Job syndrome) is a rare autosomal-dominant inherited syndrome that causes susceptibility to a range of infections and presents with a characteristic set of bone, dental, vascular, and joint abnormalities. Most patients have the classic clinical triad of extremely high elevations in serum IgE levels, recurrent pneumonias, and soft tissue abscesses.[32,36] Patients have impaired T-helper cell type 17 (Th17) CD4 response, which has a role in mucosal immunity to some respiratory pathogens, such as *Klebsiella pneumoniae* and *S pneumoniae*, as well as *S aureus* and *Candida*. Th17 CD4 immune responses aid in neutrophil recruitment to sites of infection and to the local mucosal communities. Pneumonias in patients with hyper IgE syndrome can be complicated by pneumatoceles but can also lead to bronchiectasis in a significant proportion of patients.[73–79]

Inherited disorders of DNA repair

Ataxia telangiectasia, an inherited disorder of DNA repair, and Wiskott-Aldrich syndrome, an X-linked immunodeficiency caused by mutations in the WASP gene, increase the risk of infections by affecting the development of adaptive immunity. Many of these patients are antibody deficient and have bronchiectasis.[80] Mutations in the WASP gene can result in low levels of T and B lymphocytes, NK cells, and serum IgM. Patients subsequently tend to develop infections with encapsulated organisms and therefore are at risk of bronchiectasis.[81] Both of these disorders are rare causes of bronchiectasis in pediatric case series.[52,72]

Complement deficiency found in patients with bronchiectasis

Immunity to extracellular bacterial pathogens relies on the complement system; thus, it is not surprising that inherited complement deficiencies, such as C2 or mannose-binding lectin (MBL) deficiency, have been associated with recurrent respiratory infections. As a consequence, there are reports of MBL deficiency isolated in patients with bronchiectasis; however, it should be noted that MBL deficiency figures to be a relatively common condition, affecting up to 25% of the population, and the reports of bronchiectasis with this condition are quite rare. It is speculated that concurrent MBL deficiency in patients with CVID and CF may increase the incidence and severity of bronchiectasis. Lower levels of L-ficolin, another MBL pathway opsonin, has also been found in patients with bronchiectasis compared with controls, but those data have not been replicated. Other complement deficiencies are very rare, and there are no data on these deficiencies and bronchiectasis.[36]

Cystic fibrosis and ciliary dyskinesia

Patients with CF and ciliary dyskinesia will likely develop bronchiectasis caused by persistently poor mucociliary clearance. Neither had been thought to be true genetic defects of the immune system. However, more recent data suggest mutations of the CF transmembrane conductance regulator in CF also cause a variety of defects in immune cell function involved in mucosal innate immunity. Studies have demonstrated impaired phagocyte function, reduced efficacy of antibacterial peptides, failure of bacterial internalization by epithelial cells, and an exaggerated inflammatory response to infection. Aside from a problem with mucociliary clearance, multiple defects in innate immunity could play a significant role in the development of bronchiectasis in patients with CF, but further research is required.[82]

Causes of hypogammaglobulinemia	
Non Malignant Systemic Conditions	**Infectious Diseases**
	HIV
Immunodeficiency caused by hypercatabolism of immunoglobulin	Congenital Rubella
	Congenital infection with CMV
Immunodeficiency caused by excessive loss of immunoglobulins (nephrosis, severe burns, lymphangiectasia, severe diarrhea)	Congenital infection with Toxoplasma gondii
	Epstein-Barr Virus
	Malignancy
Genetic Disorders (Other than CVID)	Chronic Lymphocytic Leukemia
	Immunodeficiency with Thymoma
Ataxia Telangiectasia	Non Hodgkin's lymphoma
Autosomal forms of SCID	B cell malignancy
Hyper IgM Immunodeficiency	Myelofibrosis
Transcobalamin II deficiency	Metastatic solid cancers (brain, lung, intestinal)
X-linked agammaglobulinemia	
X-linked lymphoproliferative disorder (EBV associated)	**Medications**
	Antimalarial agents
X-linked SCID	Captopril
Some metabolic disorders	Carbamazepine
Chromosomal Anomalies	Glucocorticoids
Chromosome 18q- Syndrome	Fenclofenac
Monosomy 22	Gold salts
Trisomy 8	Penicillamine
Trisomy 21	Phenytoin
	Sulfasalazine
	Rituximab

Suggested Immunologic Evaluation of Patients with Bronchiectasis

The identity of the infecting organisms are of most value to direct laboratory investigations; encapsulated bacteria suggest B-cell immunodeficiencies; fungi, viruses, and mycobacteria usually present in T-cell immunodeficiencies; and catalase-positive organisms (eg, *Staphylococcus*, *Aspergillus*) suggest a neutrophil dysfunction. Generally, a sequential approach to investigating immune function in patients with bronchiectasis or recurrent infections is recommended. Initial measurements of total serum Ig, IgG subclasses, specific antibody levels before and after vaccination (See Secondary Causes of Hypogammabulinemia slide) should be performed, secondary causes of hypogammaglobulinemia should be considered, as well as HIV testing if there is clinical indication. Further testing and referral to an immunologist may then be considered; additional evaluation may include tests to evaluate cellular function (such as T- and B-cell immunophenotyping) and innate immunity (such as neutrophil superoxide measurements (CGD) and complement). Lastly, gene sequencing and functional assays may be considered.[32,36]

Relationship Between Immunodeficiency, Bronchiectasis, and Asthma

In summary, the concomitant presence of immunodeficiency in patients with existing asthma and chronic airway obstruction increases susceptibility to recurrent or persistent infections and/or airway inflammation. This susceptibility may drive the process of bronchiectasis and result in increased airway secretions, thereby further increasing the risk for pulmonary infection. This promotes a cycle of airway inflammation, bronchial obstruction, and poorly controlled asthma. There is a high incidence of bronchiectasis in patients with severe asthma, although the precise frequency of bronchiectasis causing asthma is unclear, as both asthma and irreversible airway obstruction can also be complications of chronic bronchiectasis due to persistent bronchial wall inflammation. In patients with bronchiectasis, if humoral immunodeficiency such as CVID is identified and treated with IVIG, there is a reduction in frequency and severity of pulmonary infections. Better control of infection risk in patients with immunodeficiency and bronchiectasis will lead to better control of asthma and potentially prevent or mitigate chronic lung disease sequelae caused by both uncontrolled asthma and progressive bronchiectasis.

REFERENCES

1. Barker AF. Clinical manifestations and diagnosis of bronchiectasis in adults. UpToDate; 2012.
2. Bisaccioni C, Aun MV, Cajuela E, et al. Comorbidities in severe asthma: frequency of rhinitis, nasal polyposis, gastroesophageal reflux disease, vocal cord dysfunction and bronchiectasis. Clinics (Sao Paulo) 2009;64(8):769–73.
3. Boyton RJ, Smith J, Ward R, et al. HLA-C and killer cell immunoglobulin-like receptor genes in idiopathic bronchiectasis. Am J Respir Crit Care Med 2006;173:327–33.
4. Boyton RJ, Smith J, Jones M, et al. Human leucocyte antigen class II association in idiopathic bronchiectasis, a disease of chronic lung infection, implicates a role for adaptive immunity. Clin Exp Immunol 2008;152:95–101.
5. Oguzulgen IK, Kervan F, Ozis T, et al. The impact of bronchiectasis in clinical presentation of asthma. South Med J 2007;100(5):468–71.
6. Haidopoulou K, Calder A, Jones A, et al. Bronchiectasis secondary to primary immunodeficiency in children: longitudinal changes in structure and function. Pediatr Pulmonol 2009;44(7):669–75.

7. Klemola T. Deficiency of immunoglobulin A. Ann Clin Res 1987;19:248–57.
8. Szczawinska-Poplonyk A. An overlapping syndrome of allergy and immune deficiency in children. J Allergy (Cairo) 2012;2012:658279 [E-Review article].
9. Taylor AE, Finney-Hayward TK, Quint JK, et al. Defective macrophage phagocytosis of bacteria in COPD. Eur Respir J 2010;35:1039–47.
10. Tanawuttiwat T, Harindhanavudhi T. Bronchiectasis: pulmonary manifestation in chronic graft versus host disease after bone marrow transplantation. Am J Med Sci 2009;337:292.
11. Shabestari MS, Rezaei N. Asthma and allergic rhinitis in a patient with BTK deficiency. J Investig Allergol Clin Immunol 2008;18(4):300–4.
12. Ogershok PR, Hogan MB, Welch JE, et al. Spectrum of illness in pediatric common variable immunodeficiency. Ann Allergy Asthma Immunol 2006;97(5): 653–6.
13. Agondi RC, Barros MT, Rizzo LV, et al. Allergic asthma in patients with common variable immunodeficiency. Allergy 2010;65(4):510–5.
14. Amorosa JK, Miller RW, Laraya-Cuasay L, et al. Bronchiectasis in children with lymphocytic interstitial pneumonia and acquired immune deficiency syndrome. Plain film and CT observations. Pediatr Radiol 1992;22:603–6.
15. Corominas M, Garcia JF, Mestre M, et al. Predictors of atopy in HIV-infected patients. Ann Allergy Asthma Immunol 2000;84(6):607–11.
16. Kearney PJ, Kershaw CR, Stevenson PA. Bronchiectasis in acute leukaemia. Br Med J 1977;2:857–9.
17. Kilpatrick DC, Chalmers JD, MacDonald SL, et al. Stable bronchiectasis is associated with low serum L-ficolin concentrations. Clin Respir J 2009;3:29–33.
18. Knowles GK, Stanhope R, Green M. Bronchiectasis complicating chronic lymphatic leukaemia with hypogammaglobulinaemia. Thorax 1980;35:217–8.
19. Lambrecht BN, Neyt K, GeurtsvanKessel CH. Pulmonary defense mechanisms and inflammatory pathways in bronchiectasis. Eur Respir Mon 2011;52:11–21.
20. Love JT Jr, Shearer WT. Hypogammaglobulinemia in HIV-infected infants. N Engl J Med 1995;333(5):321–2.
21. Okada F, Ando Y, Kondo Y, et al. Thoracic CT findings of adult T-cell leukemia or lymphoma. AJR Am J Roentgenol 2004;182:761–7.
22. Morehead RS. Bronchiectasis in bone marrow transplantation. Thorax 1997;52: 392–3.
23. Parkman R. Antigen-specific immunity following hematopoietic stem cell transplantation. Blood Cells Mol Dis 2008;40:91–3.
24. Paganin F, Seneterre E, Chanez P, et al. Computed tomography of the lungs in asthma: influence of disease severity and etiology. Am J Respir Crit Care Med 1996;153:110–4.
25. Patel IS, Vlahos I, Wilkinson TM, et al. Bronchiectasis, exacerbation indices, and inflammation in chronic obstructive pulmonary disease. Am J Respir Crit Care Med 2004;170:400–7.
26. Pasteur MC, Helliwell SM, Houghton SJ, et al. An investigation into causative factors in patients with bronchiectasis. Am J Respir Crit Care Med 2000;162: 1277–84.
27. Gunn ML, Godwin JD, Kanne JP, et al. High-resolution CT findings of bronchiolitis obliterans syndrome after hematopoietic stem cell transplantation. J Thorac Imaging 2008;23:244–50.
28. de Jong PA, Dodd JD, Coxson HO, et al. Bronchiolitis obliterans following lung transplantation: early detection using computed tomographic scanning. Thorax 2006;61:799–804.

29. Baris S, Ercan H, Cagan HH, et al. Efficacy of intravenous immunoglobulin treatment in children with common variable immunodeficiency. J Investig Allergol Clin Immunol 2011;21(7):514–21.
30. Berman DM, Mafut D, Djokic B, et al. Risk factors for the development of bronchiectasis in HIV-infected children. Pediatr Pulmonol 2007;42:871–5.
31. Sheikh S, Madiraju K, Steiner P, et al. Bronchiectasis in pediatric AIDS. Chest 1997;112:1202–7.
32. Buckley RH. Overview of immunodeficiency disorder. Merck manual. 2008.
33. Buckley RH. Primary immunodeficiency diseases due to defects in lymphocytes. N Engl J Med 2000;343:1313–24.
34. Yee A, De Ravin SS, Elliott E, et al. Severe combined immunodeficiency: a national surveillance study. Pediatr Allergy Immunol 2008;19(4):298–302.
35. Bilton D, Jones AL. Bronchiectasis: epidemiology and causes. Eur Respir Mon 2011;52:1–10.
36. Brown JS, Baxendale H, Floto RA. Immunodeficiencies associated with bronchiectasis. Eur Respir Mon 2011;52:178–91.
37. Shoemark A, Ozerovitch L, Wilson R. Aetiology in adult patients with bronchiectasis. Respir Med 2007;101:1161–70.
38. Hilton AM, Doyle L. Immunological abnormalities in bronchiectasis with chronic bronchial suppuration. Br J Dis Chest 1978;72(3):207–16.
39. Lieberman-Maran L, Orzano IM, Passero MA, et al. Bronchiectasis in rheumatoid arthritis: report of four cases and a review of the literature–implications for management with biologic response modifiers. Semin Arthritis Rheum 2006; 35:379–87.
40. Demoruelle MK, Weisman MH, Simonian PL, et al. Brief report: airways abnormalities and rheumatoid arthritis-related autoantibodies in subjects without arthritis: early injury or initiating site of autoimmunity? Arthritis Rheum 2012; 64(6):1756–61.
41. Dhasmana DJ, Wilson R. Bronchiectasis and autoimmune disease. Eur Respir Mon 2011;52:192–210.
42. Dogru D, Ozbas Gerceker F, Yalcin E, et al. The role of TAP1 and TAP2 gene polymorphism in idiopathic bronchiectasis in children. Pediatr Pulmonol 2007; 42:237–41.
43. Doring G, Gulbins E. Cystic fibrosis and innate immunity: how chloride channel mutations provoke lung disease. Cell Microbiol 2009;11:208–16.
44. Cooper N, Arnold DM. The effect of rituximab on humoral and cell mediated immunity and infection in the treatment of autoimmune disease. Br J Haematol 2010;149:3–13.
45. Cooper N, Davies EG, Thrasher AJ. Repeated courses of rituximab for autoimmune cytopenias may precipitate profound hypogammaglobulinaemia requiring replacement intravenous immunoglobulin. Br J Haematol 2009;146:120–2.
46. Busse PJ, Razvi S, Cunningham-Rundles C. Efficacy of intravenous immunoglobulin in the prevention of pneumonia in patients with common variable immunodeficiency. J Allergy Clin Immunol 2002;109:1001–4.
47. Casanova JL, Abel L. Human genetics of infectious diseases: a unified theory. EMBO J 2007;26:915–22.
48. Eijkhout HW, van Der Meer JW, Kallenberg CG, et al. The effect of two different dosages of intravenous immunoglobulin on the incidence of recurrent infections in patients with primary hypogammaglobulinemia. A randomized, double-blind, multicenter crossover trial. Ann Intern Med 2001;135:165–74.

49. Eisen DP. Mannose-binding lectin deficiency and respiratory tract infection. J Innate Immun 2010;2:114–22.

50. Lucas M, Lee M, Lortan J, et al. Infection outcomes in patients with common variable immunodeficiency disorders: relationship to immunoglobulin therapy over 22 years. J Allergy Clin Immunol 2010;125:1354–60.

51. Aghamohammadi A, Allahverdi A, Abolhassani H, et al. Comparison of pulmonary diseases in common variable immunodeficiency and X-linked agammaglobulinaemia. Respirology 2010;15:289–95.

52. Li AM, Sonnappa S, Lex C, et al. Non-CF bronchiectasis: does knowing the aetiology lead to changes in management? Eur Respir J 2005;26:8–14.

53. Howard V, Greene JM, Pahwa S, et al. The health status and quality of life of adults with X-linked agammaglobulinemia. Clin Immunol 2006;118:201–8.

54. Jeurissen A, Bossuyt X, Snapper CM. T cell-dependent and -independent responses. J Immunol 2004;172:2728.

55. Jonsson G, Truedsson L, Sturfelt G, et al. Hereditary C2 deficiency in Sweden: frequent occurrence of invasive infection, atherosclerosis, and rheumatic disease. Medicine (Baltimore) 2005;84:23–34.

56. Stead A, Douglas JG, Broadfoot CJ, et al. Humoral immunity and bronchiectasis. Clin Exp Immunol 2002;130:325–30.

57. Umetsu DT, Ambrosino DM, Quinti I, et al. Recurrent sinopulmonary infection and impaired antibody response to bacterial capsular polysaccharide antigen in children with selective IgG-subclass deficiency. N Engl J Med 1985;313:1247–51.

58. Nahm MH, Macke K, Kwon OH, et al. Immunologic and clinical status of blood donors with subnormal levels of IgG2. J Allergy Clin Immunol 1990;85:769–77.

59. van Kessel DA, van Velzen-Blad H, van den Bosch JMM, et al. Impaired pneumococcal antibody response in bronchiectasis of unknown aetiology. Eur Respir J 2005;25:482–9.

60. Go ES, Ballas ZK. Anti-pneumococcal antibody response in normal subjects: a meta-analysis. J Allergy Clin Immunol 1996;98:205–15.

61. Gregersen S, Aalokken TM, Mynarek G, et al. Development of pulmonary abnormalities in patients with common variable immunodeficiency: associations with clinical and immunologic factors. Ann Allergy Asthma Immunol 2010;104:503–10.

62. Rodrigo MJ, Miravitlles M, Cruz MJ, et al. Characterization of specific immunoglobulin G (IgG) and its subclasses (IgG1 and IgG2) against the 23-valent pneumococcal vaccine in a healthy adult population: proposal for response criteria. Clin Diagn Lab Immunol 1997;4:168–72.

63. Lipsitch M, Whitney CG, Zell E, et al. Are anticapsular antibodies the primary mechanism of protection against invasive pneumococcal disease? PLoS Med 2005;2:e15.

64. Litzman J, Freiberger T, Grimbacher B, et al. Mannose-binding lectin gene polymorphic variants predispose to the development of bronchopulmonary complications but have no influence on other clinical and laboratory symptoms or signs of common variable immunodeficiency. Clin Exp Immunol 2008;153:324–30.

65. Miravitlles M, Vendrell M, de Gracia J. Antibody deficiency in bronchiectasis. Eur Respir J 2005;26:178–80.

66. Gadola SD, Moins-Teisserenc HT, Trowsdale J, et al. TAP deficiency syndrome. Clin Exp Immunol 2000;121:173–8.

67. Zimmer J, Andres E, Donato L, et al. Clinical and immunological aspects of HLA class I deficiency. QJM 2005;98:719–27.

68. Chatila T, Wong R, Young M, et al. An immunodeficiency characterized by defective signal transduction in T lymphocytes. N Engl J Med 1989;320: 696–702.
69. Contoli M, Message SD, Laza-Stanca V, et al. Role of deficient type III interferon-lambda production in asthma exacerbations. Nat Med 2006;12:1023–6.
70. Crothers K, Butt AA, Gibert CL, et al. Increased COPD among HIV-positive compared to HIV-negative veterans. Chest 2006;130:1326–33.
71. Andrews T, Sullivan KE. Infections in patients with inherited defects in phagocytic function. Clin Microbiol Rev 2003;16:597–621.
72. Nikolaizik WH, Warner JO. Aetiology of chronic suppurative lung disease. Arch Dis Child 1994;70:141–2.
73. Aujla SJ, Dubin PJ, Kolls JK. Th17 cells and mucosal host defense. Semin Immunol 2007;19:377–82.
74. Holland SM, DeLeo FR, Elloumi HZ, et al. STAT3 mutations in the hyper-IgE syndrome. N Engl J Med 2007;357:1608–19.
75. Holmes AH, Pelton S, Steinbach S, et al. HIV related bronchiectasis. Thorax 1995;50:1227.
76. Holmes AH, Trotman-Dickenson B, Edwards A, et al. Bronchiectasis in HIV disease. Q J Med 1992;85:875–82.
77. Paulson ML, Freeman AF, Holland SM. Hyper IgE syndrome: an update on clinical aspects and the role of signal transducer and activator of transcription 3. Curr Opin Allergy Clin Immunol 2008;8:527–33.
78. Pijnenburg MW, Cransberg K, Wolff E, et al. Bronchiectasis in children after renal or liver transplantation: a report of five cases. Pediatr Transplant 2004;8: 71–4.
79. Zhang Z, Clarke TB, Weiser JN. Cellular effectors mediating Th17-dependent clearance of pneumococcal colonization in mice. J Clin Invest 2009;119: 1899–909.
80. Bott. 2007.
81. Ochs HD, Filipovich AH, Veys P, et al. Wiskott-Aldrich syndrome: diagnosis, clinical and laboratory manifestations, and treatment. Biol Blood Marrow Transplant 2009;15:84–90.
82. Moskwa P, Lorentzen D, Excoffon KJ, et al. A novel host defense system of airways is defective in cystic fibrosis. Am J Respir Crit Care Med 2007;175:174–83.